CONCEPTUAL FOUNDATIONS

THE BRIDGE TO PROFESSIONAL NURSING PRACTICE

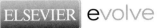

YOU'VE JUST PURCHASED
MORE THAN
A TEXTBOOK!

Evolve Student Resources for *Friberg: Conceptual Foundations: The Bridge to Professional Nursing Practice, Sixth Edition,* include the following:

- **Case Studies** designed to apply knowledge and stimulate critical thinking
- **100 NCLEX-RN style questions** for review, reflection, and further study of chapter content

Activate the complete learning experience that comes with each textbook purchase by registering at

http://evolve.elsevier.com/Friberg/bridge/

REGISTER TODAY!

CONCEPTUAL FOUNDATIONS

THE BRIDGE TO PROFESSIONAL NURSING PRACTICE

SIXTH EDITION

ELIZABETH E. FRIBERG, DNP, RN
Associate Professor
University of Virginia School of Nursing
Charlottesville, Virginia

JOAN L. CREASIA, PhD, RN
Dean and Professor Emerita
College of Nursing
University of Tennessee
Knoxville, Tennessee

ELSEVIER

ELSEVIER

3251 Riverport Lane
St. Louis, Missouri 63043

CONCEPTUAL FOUNDATIONS: THE BRIDGE TO PROFESSIONAL
NURSING PRACTICE, SIXTH EDITION

ISBN: 978-0-323-29993-0

Previous editions copyrighted 2011, 2007, 2001, 1996, and 1991.

Library of Congress Cataloging-in-Publication Data

Conceptual foundations : the bridge to professional nursing practice /
[edited by] Elizabeth E. Friberg, Joan L. Creasia. -- Sixth edition.
    p. ; cm.
Includes bibliographical references and index.
ISBN 978-0-323-29993-0 (pbk. : alk. paper)
I. Friberg, Elizabeth E., editor. II. Creasia, Joan L., editor.
[DNLM: 1. Nursing--United States. 2. Nursing Care--United States. WY 16 AA1]
RT86.7
610.73--dc23

2014042671

Senior Content Strategist: Sandra Clark
Content Development Specialist: Jennifer Wade
Publishing Services Manager: Jeff Patterson
Senior Project Manager: Tracey Schriefer
Design Direction: Amy Buxton

Printed in the United States of America

Last digit is the print number: 9 8 7 6 5 4 3 2 1

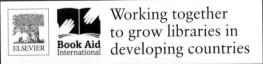

Marianne Baernholdt, PhD, MPH, RN, FAAN
Director, Langston Center for Quality, Safety, and Innovation
Professor, School of Nursing
Virginia Commonwealth University
Richmond, Virginia

Camille Burnett, PhD, MPA, APHN-BC, DSW
Assistant Professor and Roberts Scholar
Department of Family, Community and Mental Health Systems
University of Virginia School of Nursing
Charlottesville, Virginia

Cathy L. Campbell, PhD, RN, ANP-BC
Associate Professor
Department of Acute and Specialty Care
University of Virginia School of Nursing
Charlottesville, Virginia;
Visiting Research Fellow in Nursing
Department of Nursing
University of Birmingham, School of Health and Population Sciences, College of Medical and Dental Sciences
Birmingham, West Midlands
United Kingdom

Kimberly R. Cash, RN, MSN, CNML
Patient Safety Officer
CoxHealth
Springfield, Missouri

Katharine C. Cook, PhD, RN
Dean and Professor
School of Nursing
Notre Dame of Maryland University
Baltimore, Maryland

Regina M. DeGennaro, DNP, RN, AOCN, CNL
Assistant Professor
Acute and Specialty Care
University of Virginia School of Nursing
Charlottesville, Virginia

Elizabeth G. Epstein, PhD, RN
Associate Professor
University of Virginia School of Nursing
Charlottesville, Virginia

Elizabeth E. Friberg, DNP, RN
Associate Professor
University of Virginia School of Nursing
Charlottesville, Virginia

Vicki S. Good, MSN, RN, CENP, CPPS
Administrative Director of Patient Safety
CoxHealth
Springfield, Missouri

Mary Gunther, PhD, RN
Associate Professor; Executive Associate Dean for Academic Affairs
University of Tennessee College of Nursing
Knoxville, Tennessee

L. Louise Ivanov, PhD, RN, FAAN
Professor
School of Nursing
University of North Carolina–Greensboro
Greensboro, North Carolina

Arlene Wynbeek Keeling, PhD, RN, FAAN
Centennial Distinguished Professor of Nursing; Director, The Eleanor Crowder Bjoring Center for Nursing Historical Inquiry; Chair, Department of Acute and Specialty Care
University of Virginia School of Nursing
Charlottesville, Virginia

Kathryn Laughon, PhD, RN, FAAN
Associate Professor
University of Virginia School of Nursing
Charlottesville, Virginia

Dale Halsey Lea, MPH, RN, CGC
Cumberland Foreside, Maine

Patricia C. McMullen, PhD, JD, CRNP, FAANP
Dean and Ordinary Professor
School of Nursing
The Catholic University of America
Washington, DC

Brenda C. Morris, EdD, MS, RN, CNE
Associate Dean for Academic Affairs and Clinical Associate Professor
College of Nursing and Health Innovation
Arizona State University
Phoenix, Arizona

Kelly K. Near, MLS, MSN, RN, WHNP-BC
Hospital and Community Services Librarian
Claude Moore Health Sciences Library
University of Virginia
Charlottesville, Virginia

Nayna C. Philipsen, JD, PhD, RN, CFE, FACCE
Professor
College of Health Professions
Coppin State University
Baltimore, Maryland

Kathryn B. Reid, PhD, RN, FNP-BC, CNL
Associate Professor
University of Virginia School of
    Nursing
Charlottesville, Virginia

Richard A. Ridge, MBA, PhD, RN, NEA-BC, CENP
Director of Nursing Innovation and
    Outcomes
Texas Children's Hospital
Houston, Texas

Karen J. Saewert, PhD, RN, CPHQ, CNE, ANEF
Clinical Professor
College of Nursing & Health
    Innovation
Senior Director of Educational
    Support Services and Director of
    E³: Evaluation and Educational
    Excellence
College of Nursing & Health
    Innovation and College of Health
    Solutions
Arizona State University
Phoenix, Arizona

Julie Schexnayder, DNP, MPH, ACNP-BC
Nurse Practitioner
Department of Medicine
University of Virginia
Charlottesville, Virginia

Audrey E. Snyder, PhD, RN, ACNP-BC, CEN, CCRN, FAANP, FAEN
Assistant Professor
School of Nursing
University of Northern Colorado
Greeley, Colorado

Teresa Maggard Stephens, PhD, MSN, RN
Clinical Assistant Professor, RN-BSN
    Coordinator
College of Nursing
University of Tennessee
Research Coordinator
The University of Tennessee Medical
    Center
Knoxville, Tennessee

Jennifer Casavant Telford, PhD, ACNP-BC
Assistant Professor
School of Nursing and Department of
    History
University of Connecticut
Storrs, Connecticut

Sandra P. Thomas, PhD, RN, FAAN
Professor and Chair, PhD Program in
    Nursing
University of Tennessee Knoxville
Knoxville, Tennessee

Debra C. Wallace, PhD, RN, FAAN
Daphine Doster Mastroianni
    Distinguished Professor of Nursing
Family and Community Nursing
University of North Carolina at
    Greensboro
Greensboro, North Carolina

Frances Rieth Ward, PhD, RN, MBE
Associate Professor
School of Nursing
Rutgers University
Newark, New Jersey

Ishan C. Williams, PhD
Assistant Professor
School of Nursing
University of Virginia
Charlottesville, Virginia

Mary Catherine T. Winston, DNP, RN, ANP-BC
Nurse Practitioner
Family Medicine
Maury River Family Practice
Glasgow, Virginia

Marylee Bressie, DNP, RN, CCRN, CCNS, CEN
Core Faculty/Nurse Planner
The School of Nursing and Health
 Sciences
Capella University
Minneapolis, Minnesota

Michele Bunning, RN, MSN
Associate Professor
Good Samaritan College of Nursing
 and Health Science
Cincinnati, Ohio

Kelly A. Crum, MSN, RN
Dean, School of Nursing; Associate
 Professor of Nursing
Maranatha Baptist University
Watertown, Wisconsin

Nancy Diede, EdD, MS, RN, CNE
Department Head and Associate
 Professor of Nursing
Health Sciences
Rogers State University
Claremore, Oklahoma

Maurice Espinoza, MSN, RN, CNS, CCRN
Clinical Nurse Specialist
University of California Irvine Health
Orange, California

Carol A. Fanutti, EdD, MS, RN, CNE
Trocaire College
Buffalo, New York

Christine Finn, PhD, FNP, MBA, MA, MS, BSN, SANE, FNE, CPHQ, CEN
Associate Professor
Regis University
Denver, Colorado

Sylvie Grignon, RN, pedagogical advisor nursing program
Services aux Entreprises et
 Collectivités
CEC Chibougamau, Québec
Chibougamau, Québec
Canada

Kathleen S. Jordan, DNP, MS, RN, FNP-BC, ENP-BC, SANE-P
Nurse Practitioner
Mid-Atlantic Emergency Medicine
 Associates
Clinical Associate Professor
The University of North Carolina at
 Charlotte
Charlotte, North Carolina

Eileen M. Kaslatas, MSN RN CNE
Professor
Health and Human Services
Macomb Community College
Clinton Township, Michigan

Patsy Love, DNP, RN, CNOR
Assistant Professor
Bethune-Cookman University
Daytona Beach, Florida

Lauro Manalo Jr., RN, MSN
Professor
Health Sciences
Allan Hancock College
Santa Maria, California

Deborah K. Peetz, MSN, RN
Assistant Professor
BSN-Completion Program
Viterbo University
La Crosse, Wisconsin

Michele J. Upvall, PhD, RN, CRNP
Professor
School of Nursing
Carlow University
Pittsburg, Pennsylvania

The sixth edition of *Conceptual Foundations: The Bridge to Professional Nursing Practice* brings a change in editorial leadership and engagement, several changes in chapter contributing authors and chapter approach, and the addition of three new chapters. After more than 20 years of dedication to this text, Joan Creasia, PhD, RN, FAAN, has passed all editorial tasks to her colleague, Elizabeth E. Friberg, DNP, RN. Previous contributors of chapters or professional profiles in practice are acknowledged altogether at the end of this preface. Their work provided a foundation on which new chapters were based, expanded, and revised. Our new contributing authors eagerly took on the task of updating and verifying existing work while presenting the material in a creative or fresh format to encourage student engagement. We have added three new chapters, on information management, global rural nursing practice, and telehealth, all areas in which nursing provides significant leadership. As we go to press, we have made every effort to integrate the most current information on the *health care reform initiatives* and *Healthy People 2020.* It is a period of dynamic change.

Since 2011 and the release of the fifth edition of this text, the profession and practice of nursing has faced many challenges, launched new initiatives, and taken leadership roles in various aspects of health care and health care service delivery. With the influence of the 1965 American Nurses Association (ANA) recommendation that the minimum educational preparation for professional nurses be at a baccalaureate level; the Institute of Medicine's *The Future of Nursing: Leading Change, Advancing Health* (2010); and the Carnegie Foundation for the Advancement of Teaching's *Educating Nurses: A Call for Radical Transformation* (2010), educational pathways to increase the number of professional nurses and advanced practice nurses have created multiple models for professional entry and advancement. Nursing workforce challenges and other national agendas, such as patient safety and health care reform, have created a demand for professional nurses in a variety of health care delivery settings and academia. The demands of practice complexity, professional career advancement, and nurse/faculty shortages provide the stimulus for many associate degree and diploma program graduates to consider educational advancement.

The first edition of *Conceptual Foundations* targeted the RN-BSN student by focusing on the context, dimensions, and themes of professional nursing practice. The *context* of professional nursing practice sheds meaning on the nursing profession and the conditions that must be present for societal recognition of nursing as a profession from historical aspects to the future *NOW* within the reality of current policy climates. The *dimensions* of professional practice are the spatial influences on professional nursing practice that may evolve over time, such as the economic issues, communication, clinical reasoning, ethical comportment, legal aspects, information management, and teaching and learning principles. *Themes* in professional nursing practice reflect a sampling of nursing leadership areas of interest as the profession assumes its societal role as a recognized profession in a changing health care delivery infrastructure. Since the first edition, nursing programs other than completion programs have used this text in foundational courses at the baccalaureate and graduate levels. We believe that the content of this sixth edition remains relevant for use in these programs, but we have retained language targeted at a postlicensure audience seeking to advance professional careers.

APPROACH

The rapid changes in the health care delivery system continue to influence nursing education and practice. With the passage of a landmark health care reform initiative and the explosion of health care technology and informatics, professional nursing has provided extensive leadership and received public role recognition for its contributions. From planning and delivery to patient safety, consumer/patient-centric services, quality improvement, cost containment, community-based services, health promotion, and disease prevention, nursing has emerged as the pivotal coordinator to ensure high-quality care at reasonable cost. Now more than ever, nurses need strong foundations in the political, legal, economic, population, systems, and ethical aspects of health care in general and nursing care specifically. This text provides that foundation and relates those general concepts to the professional practice of nursing.

Nursing education programs have diverse student populations that span multiple ages and cultural and life experience parameters that bring a richness and depth to their educational advancement. Many are adult learners with increased capacity for critical thinking and self-directed learning. Others are advancing their education while working or raising a family. Some are pursuing their advanced education using distance-learning pedagogies. *Conceptual Foundations* provides a meaningful and diverse conceptual approach to nursing practice that encourages exploration of original theorists, critical analysis of issues and concepts, and applicability to diverse client populations and clinical settings. The text frames the professional practice of nursing by using a variety of subject matter experts and reflective profiles of practicing professional nurses.

The editor recognizes that multiple educational pathways exist toward professional nursing education and practice, including a variety of entry-level and seamless academic progression models. The American Association of Colleges of Nursing (AACN) and the National League for Nursing (NLN) are key stakeholders in the nursing education arena and provide programmatic guidance frameworks for determining the essentials of nursing education programs and ultimate competencies of graduates from those programs. However, this text has not organized its content to map to any specific nursing education guidance framework. Instead we have approached the text content from the previously discussed framework of *context*, *dimensions* and *themes*. This provides flexibility for nursing educators to utilize the text in a variety of educational pathways to fit their institution's adopted educational framework and philosophy. Chapter titles provide sufficient information to crosswalk to both guidance frameworks.

The reader will find both *client* and *patient* terminology used, at times interchangeably, to reflect changes in nursing practice and delivery settings. Although philosophically we believe a distinction exists, to maintain the flow of the content we allowed authors the liberty to use these terms interchangeably.

ORGANIZATION

The text is divided into three parts: **Part I, Context of Professional Nursing Practice,** explores a brief history of professional nursing in the United States, pathways of nursing education, development of professional

identity (beyond socialization), professional nursing roles, theories and frameworks for professional nursing practice, and health policy and planning within the nursing practice environment. The historical chapter provides a brief history of professional nursing in the United States and its relevance to current practice by engaging students in a flow of issues, instead of using the typical timeline approach, and framing a future professional nursing vision. The nursing education chapter includes current enrollment statistics and discussion of the most recent pathway changes. *Beyond Professional Socialization* takes an expanded approach, moving students into discussions of professional identity formation consistent with the IOM report on the *Future of Nursing (2010)* and the Carnegie report on *Educating Nurses (2010)*. The chapter on roles addresses various professional roles as well as the dynamics of role stress in the work environment. Theories and frameworks provide links to the classic works of original theorists using their own words while updating these concepts with current research applications in nursing. The chapter on health policy provides a framework for understanding policy and politics, the legislative process, implementation and regulation, and the stakeholders and leadership involved. Additionally, the chapter summarizes major historical policy eras and their impact on nursing practice, especially the recent health care reform initiatives passed under the Patient Protection and Affordable Care Act of 2010.

Part II, Dimensions of Professional Nursing Practice, explores economic issues; effective communication; "thinking-like-a-nurse" (critical thinking, clinical reasoning, and the nursing process); 21st Century teaching and learning principles; legal aspects of nursing practice; ethical dimensions of nursing and health care (day-to-day ethics); information management; and diversity in health and illness. Economic issues that currently drive health care delivery and practice reform, including current and future nursing practice, are presented in a manner that engages students in the complexities of the current economic climates. The chapter on effective communications covers intrapersonal/interpersonal communication, context, self-awareness, active listening, therapeutic communication, organizational communication, and group dynamics of a high-reliability organization (HRO). Using a fresh approach, *Think-Like-a-Nurse* explores the relationship among critical thinking disposition, clinical reasoning, and the nursing decision-making process including the outcomes of clinical judgment. Using a fresh approach, the teaching and learning chapter discusses 21st Century theories and strategies including the role of technology and health literacy in designing effective teaching-learning experiences for individuals and groups. The chapter on legal aspects provides a basic understanding of statutory, public, and private law and covers topics such as licensure, delegation, and practice acts in a format that makes these legal aspects easily accessible to the student. The chapter on ethics takes a new approach and identifies resources and strategies to address everyday practice problems, defines key terms in ethics language, and provides an ethical framework for use in day-to-day practice at four professional levels: patient, unit, organization, and national/global. The chapter on information management is a new chapter that distinguishes between informatics, information management, and information literacy, and provides a rationale for standardized languages and the need for controlled vocabulary searching for evidence-based practice using answerable clinical questions. The chapter on diversity in health and illness explores cultural competency and culturally relevant care including the CLAS Act standards.

Part III, Themes in Professional Nursing Practice, explores subjects and topics in which professional nursing is demonstrating leadership, such as health and health promotion, genetics and genomics, global rural health, violence against women, telehealth, and patient safety. The chapter on health and health promotion emphasizes preventive services; the concepts of behavioral and lifestyle change, self-efficacy, and environmental influences and the *Healthy People 2020* agenda. The chapter on genetics and genomics provides a foundation for the rapid developments in this area and nursing's role, especially in the family history pedigree and referral for genetic testing and counseling. The discussion on global rural health is a new chapter that explores the new local and international rural context of nursing practice and the impact of social determinants of health (SDH). Violence is a very broad topic, therefore we have taken a fresh approach to focusing on a specific aspect of violence at an epidemic level. The chapter on violence against women explores a specific type of violence as a global and national health issue, and the associated assessment and intervention aspects of effective nursing

care. The chapter on telehealth is a new chapter that focuses on nurses' role in emerging interventions using telehealth technology to address access and improve outcomes for patient-care, including policy implications and evaluations of local capability. The chapter on patient safety explores the critical role that nursing performs in providing a safe health care environment for the delivery of health care services in a variety of settings consistent with current national quality and safety initiatives.

PEDAGOGY

Each chapter is organized to direct the attention of the student or faculty reader and developed in a similar format. Chapters begin with learning **Objectives** followed by a reflective **Profile in Practice** related to the chapter topic. The text includes an opening **Introduction** to explain the approach of the chapter and closes with a **Summary** of the chapter content. The editor follows the Summary with two newly labeled sections, Salient Points (formerly Key Points) and Critical Reflection Exercises (formerly Critical Thinking Exercises) to capture the nursing profession's transformations in nursing education. **Salient Points** emphasize the major take-away concepts from each chapter to help students develop a sense of discernment and prioritization about the content. This models a way of thinking about implications for practice. Chapter content flows from the general concept to application in nursing practice. **Key terms** are presented in italics, and **definitions** are embedded in the text for reading ease. The structure of text chapters allows for significant flexibility in sequencing of topics and is not intended to be read in sequential order. The nature of the content creates the need for **cross-references** of topics that are addressed by multiple chapters. The editor provides those cross-references where she feels they are most useful to the reader. **Boxes, Tables,** and **Figures** are used throughout for emphasis and provide a visual reinforcement for important content. **Internet links** are embedded within the text or provided in **Website Resources** when websites other than those referenced in the chapter may be useful for both the student and faculty. **Critical Reflection Exercises** are provided at the end of each chapter to expand the student's exploration of key concepts, reflect on practice implications, and stimulate further group discussions. Critical reflection is necessary for accountable professional practice now and in the future in an ever-changing practice environment.

References, either classic or current (within the past 5 years), are provided for all citations. The authors have chosen to reference classic works where appropriate to instill in students a sense of the richness of nursing's body of knowledge that supports current professional practice. Evidence- and research-based references are largely current except where a classic reference is better suited. We have retained our practice of providing classic references for major theorists and use of the actual theorist's language/words in describing their theories. This practice provides the opportunity for students and faculty to experience their work first-hand and refer to their original writings. Current research and evidence-based application are integrated throughout the content.

This format challenges the reader to discover new knowledge or reframe prior learning on a more conceptual and universally applicable level in professional practice. The contextual, dimensional, and theme-based approach provides a comprehensive source text for exploring foundational concepts of professional nursing practice targeted to transition or completion programs but applicable in a variety of educational programs. Nursing practice as it is today and will be in the future is supported by these foundational concepts and the ever-expanding nursing knowledge base that flows from them.

SPECIAL FEATURES

A website, http://evolve.elsevier.com/Friberg/bridge/, provides student resources as well as these instructor resources: TEACH for Nurses (a faculty instruction manual), test bank, image collection, and PowerPoint presentation for each chapter.

CONTRIBUTORS TO PREVIOUS EDITION

The editor wishes to thank the following individuals who contributed chapters or profiles in practice to the prior edition of this text:

Chapter 1
Laura J. Robinson (Profile in Practice)
Chapter 2
Joan L. Creasia, PhD, RN

Chapter 3
Cynthia A. Holcomb, BSN, MS, RN, BC (Profile in Practice)
Chapter 4
Sarah A. Delgado, RN, MSN, ACNP
Elke Jones Zschaebitz, MSN, FNP-BC
Elizabeth E. Friberg, DNP, RN
Chapter 6
Maureen Nalle, PhD, RN (Profile in Practice)
Chapter 7
Mattia J. Gilmartin, RN, MBA, PhD
Chapter 8
Barbara Moran, PhD, CNM (Profile in Practice)
Chapter 10
Tami H. Wyatt, PhD, RN, CNE
Patricia Biller Krauskopf, PhD, RN, FNP-BC (Profile in Practice)
Chapter 12
Heather Vallent, RN, MS
Pamela J. Grace, PhD, APRN
Chapter 13
Teresa L. Panniers, PhD, RN
Susan Kaplan Jacobs, MLS, MA, RN, AHIP
Elizabeth A. Drew, MSN, RN (Profile in Practice)
Chapter 14
Anne Harrington, BSN, RN (Profile in Practice)
Lindsey Wilson, BSN, RN (Profile in Practice)
Audrey Snyder, PhD, RN, ACNP-BC, CEN, FAANP (Profile in Practice)
Chapter 17
Vickie H. Southall, MSN, RN
Melissa A. Sutherland, PhD, FNP-C (Profile in Practice)
Chapter 19
Marilyn Grace O'Rourke, DNP, APHN-BC
Carol Wardlaw, MSN, APRN (Profile in Practice)
Elizabeth Herzan-Taylor, MS, APRN (Profile in Practice)

Elizabeth E. Friberg, DNP, RN

Dedicated to

Joan L. Creasia, PhD, RN,

for her dedication to this text for more than 20 years

CONTENTS

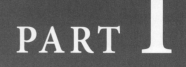

PART I

Context of Professional Nursing Practice

A Brief History of Professional Nursing in the United States

Jennifer Casavant Telford, PhD, ACNP-BC and Arlene Wynbeek Keeling, PhD, RN, FAAN

http://evolve.elsevier.com/Friberg/bridge/

OBJECTIVES

At the completion of this chapter, the reader will be able to:

- Describe the relevance of the study of history to clinical practice and health policy in the 21st century.
- Discuss the impact of Florence Nightingale's model and the American Civil War on mid to late–19th-century American nursing education.
- Describe the transition of nursing education from the hospital to collegiate programs.
- Discuss the role of nursing licensure in safeguarding the public and developing educational and clinical nursing standards.
- Discuss the development of advanced clinical practice nursing and doctoral education for nurses from the 1960s to the present and the context in which these developments occurred.

PROFILE IN PRACTICE

Sharon Casavant

Honors Bachelor's Student, University of Connecticut, School of Nursing

As an undergraduate nursing student in my junior year, I focused on developing knowledge and skills in the care of patients. The importance of studying nursing history evaded me. The pivotal moment in which history became less distant and more relevant was during my interaction with Connecticut Commissioner of Veteran's Affairs, Dr. Linda Schwartz. As a lover of history, she escorted me and our school's historian, Dr. Jennifer Telford, down to the bellows of the Veteran's Home, in search of historical nursing artifacts. We were to preserve these items as part of the Josephine A. Dolan's Collection of Nursing Artifacts at the University of Connecticut, School of Nursing.

On our walk, the Commissioner graciously indulged my curiosity about her own history as a military veteran. She was injured during a helicopter crash while she was serving in Vietnam. Her willingness to share her experiences helped me realize that personal experiences and the study of nursing history are closely related. With each step down the hall, she greeted every veteran whom she addressed by name, stopped to inquire how his or her new medication was working or whether the location of the new apartment was closer to the bus stop. Each veteran lit up when they saw her. I began to think about their service to our country and how these experiences shaped their lives. Had they been physically or mentally injured during their service? How had war changed them? It is clear that as a nurse and the Commissioner of Veterans Affairs this woman had profound impact in their lives. Watching the Commissioner's interactions with the veterans from my novice lens led me to conclude how military veterans possess unique perspectives on life and that their military experiences are likely to shape health care practices.

For veterans, telling their stories is imperative. For nursing students, listening to them is educational. Nursing history came alive for me through their stories. I took it upon myself to search and access recorded oral histories of military nurse veterans housed in the School of

Nursing *(http://archives.lib.uconn.edu/islandora/object/ 20002%3A20100100)*. Veterans' stories of self-sacrifice were rich with humor, compassion, and some sadness. I am in awe of their ingenuity and fortitude in the face of tragedy and terrible conditions. Their stories helped me realize the importance of the history of nursing. The challenges, faced by both the wartime nurses and the veterans they cared for, serve as good models for current and future nursing care. I finally understand what Dr. Telford meant when she said, "Nursing's past is prologue."

INTRODUCTION

On September 21, 2001, the Board of Directors of the American Association for the History of Nursing adopted a position paper in which the authors make a substantial argument for the integration of the study of the history of nursing in all levels of nursing education. In this paper, the authors argue that studying nursing history provides nursing students with a "sense of professional identity, a useful methodological research skill, and a context for evaluating information" (Keeling & Ramos, 1995). Other research has shown that the conduct of historical inquiry contributes to the overall knowledge base of health care practitioners and goes beyond rounding out university education with some humanities content. In spite of these strong and evidence-based recommendations, the study of nursing history has all but been eliminated from most nursing curricula. To argue effectively for the reintroduction or continued inclusion of history in the heavily science-based nursing curricula (Toman & Thifault, 2012), Toman examined the ways in which students who use primary source historical data during their nursing education begin to use more complex, critical analyses of health care issues—skills that will serve them well as practicing nurses. Toman's study supports the relevance of the history of nursing to contemporary nursing practice, as discussed in Borsay's 2009 publication, "Nursing History: An Irrelevance for Nursing Practice?"

Because of the breadth and depth of the history of nursing in the United States, this chapter provides only select highlights, supporting student learning with historical information based on primary source documents. It can stand alone to provide the reader with information about the history of modern nursing in the United States from the middle of the 19th century to today. Topics include Florence Nightingale's influential nursing practice and the spread of her ideas about nursing education from Britain to the United States; issues surrounding the development of professional and educational standards for nurses; the influence of science and technology on the development of nursing; and the rise of nurse practitioner (NP) programs and doctoral education for nurses. These events and topics did not happen in isolation from the history of medicine and the health care system. Therefore that context is considered, as well as how nursing has shaped—and has been shaped by—a confluence of factors.

Nursing has indeed evolved over the course of more than 150 years since the inception of the first Nightingale schools in the United States, but it has not done so without facing significant challenges. Many of these challenges persist today, including issues surrounding gender, race, socioeconomic status, educational requirements for entry into practice, professional licensure, nursing shortages, pandemic disease, and wars.

Historically women have been charged with providing physical care to those who are sick or injured. Women's role in society as mothers and caregivers coincided with their domestic duties and was accepted as a natural extension of the homemaker role. To assist mid-19th-century women with their caretaker role, Florence Nightingale published *Notes on Nursing: What It Is and What It Is Not*. In the preface of this book, first published in 1859, Nightingale explained that her notes on nursing were "meant simply to give hints for thought to women who have personal charge of the health of others. Every woman … or at least almost every woman has, at one time or another of her life, charge of the personal health of somebody, whether child or invalid—in other words, every woman is a nurse" (Nightingale, 1859, p. 8). Although more than 150 years have passed since Nightingale wrote her book, and today's nurses are professionals, many of her notes on nursing continue to be relevant to contemporary nursing practice.

British Origins of Nursing Training Programs

Florence Nightingale is well known for her work during the Crimean War in which she revolutionized the care provided to British soldiers (1853 to 1856). Her wartime experiences not only improved military medicine and nursing, but also shaped her ideas about the value of the trained nurse. Indeed her commitment to improving nursing in England was later the impetus for the creation of the Nightingale Training School for Nurses at St. Thomas's Hospital in London in 1860.

Just as Nightingale's work in the Crimea was an impetus for instituting a training school for nurses in England, the provision of nursing care by American women during the United States Civil War (1861 to 1865) was the impetus for the establishment of nurse training programs in the United States. During the war, volunteer women demonstrated the effectiveness of skilled nursing on improving outcomes for sick and injured soldiers. After the firing on Fort Sumter, thousands of women from both Northern and Southern states lent their services to care for the injured, sick, and dying soldiers in homes, hospitals, infirmaries, and on battlefields. Their success in reducing morbidity and mortality in the military provided evidence that trained nurses could be of benefit. Thus in the years following the war, philanthropic women in the United States devoted their energies to establishing nurse training schools that were based on the Nightingale apprenticeship model (Dock, 1907; Woolsey, 1950).

The Nightingale model had "pupil" nurses training on hospital wards under the direction of a nursing superintendent. It not only provided hospitals with an inexpensive and skilled workforce, but also gave working-class women an opportunity for employment outside the home that was an alternative to factory work. In 1873, the first three U.S. training schools were established: Bellevue Hospital in New York City, Connecticut Hospital in New Haven, and Massachusetts General Hospital in Boston. In exchange for 2 to 3 years of intense work, pupil nurses acquired the necessary knowledge and skills to find employment as graduate private duty nurses following graduation. In addition, working-class women who graduated from these programs quickly acquired an elevated social status as "trained nurses."

In 1873 fewer than 200 hospitals existed in the entire United States. In a relatively short time hospitals proliferated and training schools gained in popularity. By 1900 the United States had 432 hospital-based nursing schools (Roberts, 1954), and by 1910 there were more than 4000 hospitals in existence (Melosh, 1982).

The training in these hospital-based schools was arduous, requiring long days of patient service on the wards after which students attended classes. In addition to providing direct patient care, students performed housekeeping tasks, prepared meals, cleaned the wards and operating rooms, sterilized instruments, and assisted physicians. A 1902 textbook of nursing described the relationship between physicians and nurses during this era: "To the doctor, the first duty [of the nurse] is that of obedience—absolute fidelity to his orders, even if the necessity of the prescribed measures is not apparent to you. You have no responsibility beyond that of faithfully carrying out the directions received" (Weeks-Shaw, 1902, p. 4).

Professionalism Through Organization

Obedience to the physician and long days on the wards did not create an environment conducive to learning, nor did it promote nursing as a profession. Superintendents of nursing, responsible for student learning within nurse training schools, expressed their concern about the demands on students to staff hospital wards (Figure 1-1). To address their concerns, Isabel Hampton, Superintendent of the Johns Hopkins Hospital School of Nursing, assembled superintendents of America's largest schools at the 1893 Chicago World's Fair. Discussions among these women resulted in a movement to raise and standardize requirements for the training of nurses (Draper, 1893/1949).

In January 1894 the superintendents created the Society of Superintendents of Training Schools for Nurses of the United States and Canada (later renamed the National League for Nursing Education [NLNE] in 1912). The goals of the Society of Superintendents were "to promote fellowship of members, to establish and maintain a universal standard of training, and to further the best interests of the nursing profession" (American Society of Superintendents of Training Schools for Nurses, 1897, p. 4). Shortly thereafter the national government released data revealing that there were almost 109,000 "untrained nurses and midwives competing with 12,000 graduate nurses" for nursing positions (U.S. Bureau of Census, 1900, p. xxiii). Although the NLNE was concerned with the educational standards for nurses, the Nurses' Associated Alumnae of the United States and Canada (renamed the American Nurses Association [ANA] in 1912) focused on achieving legal recognition for trained nurses.

To protect the public from nurses who lacked formal training, the Nurses' Associated Alumnae began to pursue legal registration for trained nurses. Superintendent Isabel Hampton argued in support of this measure, because at that time a trained nurse meant "… anything, everything, or next to nothing" (Hampton, 1893/1949, p. 5). Securing legal recognition was seen as a way to

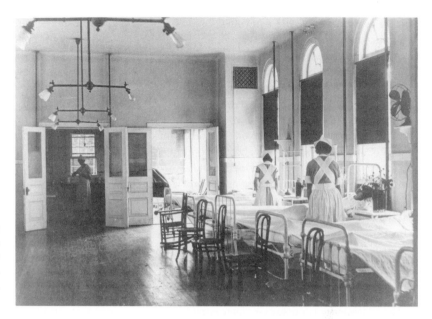

FIGURE 1-1 Student nurses on wards, circa 1900. (Courtesy Eleanor Crowder Bjoring Center for Nursing Historical Inquiry, The University of Virginia, School of Nursing, Charlottesville, VA.)

counter the prevailing belief in society that "an ignorant woman, who was not fit for anything else, is good enough for a nurse" (Draper, 1893/1949, p. 151). The Nurses' Associated Alumnae, composed of alumnae associations from schools of nursing, quickly moved to establish associated state organizations so that nurses could undertake the necessary political lobbying for the enactment of state registration laws. Their mission was to "strengthen the union of nursing organizations, to elevate nursing education, [and] to promote ethical standards" for the profession (Nurses' Associated Alumnae of the United States, 1902/2007, p. 766). The two substantive issues that concerned this group were the establishment and maintenance of a journal, the *American Journal of Nursing*, and securing state registration for nurses. The latter was of particular importance because it "would achieve legal recognition of nursing as a profession and provide a means for distinguishing trained nurses from those who purported to be but whose preparation for the practice of nursing fell short of standards" (Daisy, 1996, p. 35).

The efforts of the Nurses' Associated Alumnae resulted in nursing registration legislation in March 1903 in North Carolina, followed by New Jersey, New York, and Virginia later that same year. These acts defined for the public that a "registered nurse" had attended an acceptable nursing program and passed a board evaluation examination. Still lacking, however, were national educational standards and an agreed-upon definition of professional nursing

practice. Following the enactment of nurse licensure, leaders of the profession created state nursing boards and empowered them to use their legal authority to protect the public from unfit nurses. Ironically women who lacked the legal right to vote in 1910 aided 27 states in enacting nurse registration laws. By 1923 all the states in the nation, along with Hawaii and the District of Columbia, had enacted nurse registration laws (Bullough, 1975). Although many nursing leaders praised the accomplishment of the enactment of registration laws for nurses, one did not. Annie Goodrich, Inspector of Nurses Training Schools for the New York State Education Department (and later dean of the Yale School of Nursing), noted that the boards were "conspicuously weak and inefficient in every state" (Goodrich, 1912, p. 1001).

Nursing Practice in Early 20th-Century America

Employment opportunities for graduate nurses in the early 20th century were, for the most part, limited to caring for ill persons in their own homes; hospitals were seen as places to care for those who had no one else to care for them. Nursing students staffed the hospital, under the direction of the head nurse who was usually a training school graduate. Head nurses and nurse anesthetists were the few who worked as graduates inside hospitals. Most nursing school graduates eagerly donned their white uniforms, caps, and nursing pins and joined a "registry," allowing them to practice as private duty nurses in patients' homes. Nurse registries, operated by hospitals, professional organizations, or private businesses, provided sites where the public could acquire the services of these private duty nurses. Families could contract for the services of a nurse for a day or a few hours to care for their loved ones either at home or in the hospital (Whelan, 2005). Although physicians' orders were required, private duty in the home provided graduate nurses with the venue and the opportunity to break away from the rigid hospital routine and allowed for a more autonomous practice. These nurses provided care to patients with contagious diseases such as pneumonia and typhoid fever, aided women after childbirth, and supported patients with fractures, infected wounds, strokes, and mental diseases. Private duty nurses lived with and worked for their patients, providing 24-hour care, often for weeks at a time (Stoney, 1919).

For the most part, middle- and upper-class households employed private duty nurses. Graduate nurses were generally pleased with their role as private duty nurses, but their employment was seasonal and sporadic. Because of the onslaught of contagious diseases in the cold months of the year, winters were busy and summers slow. Average annual income of a private duty nurse in the late 1910s was approximately $950, a sum that sustained her but left little savings for future needs (Reverby, 1987). Nonetheless, the trend toward private duty prevailed. By the 1920s 70% to 80% of graduates worked as private duty nurses.

During the early 20th century, however, new medical discoveries led the public to hospitals for the latest in scientific care. To deal with the increasing hospital census in the 1920s, nursing superintendents were pressured to admit more students into school programs. In turn the increase of nursing students resulted in an increase of graduate nurses, thus creating a surplus. In 1926 the ANA and NLNE grew concerned about the economic plight of graduate nurses and authorized a comprehensive study of the working conditions of graduate nurses. The study, later known as the *Burgess Report*, documented that registered nurses faced widespread underemployment and harsh working conditions (Burgess, 1928). Another survey, conducted by Janet Geister, underscored the private duty nurses' economic plight. According to Geister, 80% of nurses' patient cases lasted only 1 day. This level of employment earned them approximately $31.26 a week, or 49 cents an hour—less than the income of scrubwomen, who earned 50 cents an hour (Geister, 1926). A few years later, with the collapse of the stock market

and the subsequent economic depression that enveloped the country, even the lowest-paying jobs for private duty nurses disappeared. Private duty nursing became a "luxury" few could afford. This reality combined with the fact that patients would soon prefer the scientific medical care offered in hospitals, created a gloomy occupation outlook for private duty nurses.

Despite the increasing complexity of hospital work, administrators and physicians simply could not justify hiring large numbers of graduate nurses when they had an inexpensive nursing student workforce readily available. Employing registered nurses would increase overhead costs immensely; moreover, physicians were afraid that graduate nurses would get involved with decision making in the hospital. As noted by one physician-hospital administrator, nursing was "only a differentiation of domestic duty" and the graduate nurse a "half-baked social product thrust into the fulfillment of an uncertain social need" (Howard, 1912). Although private duty nurses outnumbered other professional nurses, and many were members of the ANA Private Duty Nurses Section, they lacked leaders at both the national and state levels. Without leaders, private duty nurses failed to unite or develop effective strategies to upgrade their clinical standards or improve their economic conditions. However, many private duty nurses, who diligently upgraded their medical knowledge and skills, did achieve individual distinction and respect in their communities. These nurses fared much better economically than other graduates because physicians and families requested their services. For most graduates, however, job opportunities would not improve until the late 1930s when hospitals began to add registered nurses to their staffs (Roberts, 1954).

Progressivism and Public Health Nursing

During the same time period in which nursing was establishing, the United States was undergoing social changes that would also affect the profession. Urbanization, industrialization, and the influx of European immigrants, especially into the northeastern section of the country, soon resulted in overcrowded tenement slums, filthy streets, and poor working conditions. Communicable diseases ran rampant. One young nurse, Lillian Wald, saw the conditions in New York City as her opportunity to care for the poor and to establish a role for nursing in the community. According to Wald, the needs of these New York City residents were limitless.

"There were nursing infants, many of them with the summer bowel complaint that sent infant mortality soaring during the hot months; there were children with measles, not quarantined; there were children with ophthalmia, a contagious eye disease; there were children scarred with vermin bites; there were adults with typhoid; there was a case of puerperal septicemia, lying on a vermin-infested bed without sheets or pillow cases; a family consisting of a pregnant mother, a crippled child and two others living on dry bread …; a young girl dying of tuberculosis amid the very conditions that had produced the disease" (Wald, quoted in Duffus, 1938, p. 43).

In response to these conditions, in 1895 Wald and her colleague Mary Brewster founded the Henry Street Settlement House and Henry Street Visiting Nurse Services (Keeling, 2007; Wald, 1938). Wald's work promoting health and preventing disease improved condition for the poverty-stricken immigrants on New York City's Lower East Side. The visiting nurses' work quickly expanded to include new services, most notably school nursing, industrial nursing, tuberculosis nursing, and infant welfare nursing. Later Wald joined forces with the Metropolitan Life Insurance Company to send nurses into the homes of the company's customers when they became ill (Hamilton, 1989; Struthers, 1917).

In 1912 Wald founded the National Organization for Public Health Nursing (NOPHN)—nursing's first specialty organization. That year there were approximately 3000 public health nurses working throughout the United States (Gardner, 1936). The major goals of the NOPHN were to develop adequate numbers of public health nurses to meet the needs of the public and to link the emerging field of public health nursing to preventive medicine (Brainard, 1922).

The creation of the federally based Children's Bureau, also in 1912, as well as the passage of the Maternal and Infant Act (Sheppard-Towner) in 1921, reflected the federal government's growing concern for the health of women and children during the Progressive era. Public health nurses served as the backbone of new initiatives under the Sheppard-Towner Act, traveling to remote areas in their states to bring clinics and health services to those most in need. Although the federal programs experienced opposition, especially from physicians, in the 8 years of their existence, the programs demonstrated the effectiveness of nurses in the screening of patients and referring them to physicians. The

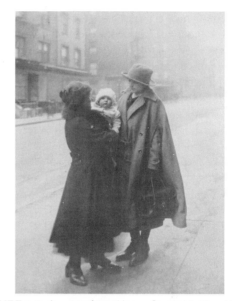

FIGURE 1-2 A nurse from Henry Street Visiting Nurses Services stops to inquire about the health of a baby she had known through visiting the family, 1925. (Courtesy Josephine A. Dolan Collection at the University of Connecticut, School of Nursing.)

programs also brought health education to thousands of American families (Meckel, 1990) (Figure 1-2).

The development of community health nursing was important to the nation and to the nursing profession because it brought essential health services to the public. It also provided nurses with unique opportunities to integrate epidemiological knowledge and sanitation practices—as well as medical science—into the care and education of the public. Community nurses, using their hospital training, expanded the domain of nursing practice to include individuals, families, and communities. Their pioneering activities in health promotion and disease prevention, along with their stand on health and welfare issues, have proved essential in shaping America's health system and the discipline of nursing (Bullough & Bullough, 1978).

Nurses in War

As noted, during the American Civil War (1861 to 1865), both Union and Confederate leaders sought women's help in the care of sick and wounded soldiers. Providing support through Ladies' Aid Societies and the U.S. Sanitary Commission, numerous white middle-class women volunteered to practice nursing. In the South, many elite women brought along their black female slaves to help, and throughout the Confederacy hundreds of black men (both slave and free) served as nurses. In addition, Catholic nuns and Lutheran deaconesses provided care to the soldiers. However, there were no trained nurses and no military nurses at this time.

It would not be until 1898, during the Spanish-American War, that trained nurses volunteered to serve in the army to care for soldiers suffering from yellow fever. This experience helped to convince military physicians and Congress that trained female nurses should become permanent members of the nation's defense forces. It set the stage for the creation of the Army Nurse Corps in 1901 and the Navy Nurse Corps in 1908 (Sarnecky, 1999).

Both the Army Nurse Corps and the Navy Nurse Corps would serve in World War I during the next decade. Although the United States' formal involvement in World War I (1917 to 1919) was short, it was important in documenting the ability of trained nurses to work effectively in war. Nursing leaders cooperated with the federal government in a major recruitment and mobilization campaign to remedy the profound shortage of nursing personnel that existed in the spring of 1917. As part of that effort, the American Red Cross, led by Jane Delano, conducted an ambitious campaign to draw women into the war effort. Meanwhile nursing leaders debated the issue of who was qualified to serve in the war. In the existing environment of patriotic fervor, many women of higher society, as well as thousands of minimally trained nurses' aides, wished to serve as nurses; however, leaders of the nursing profession insisted on the use of properly trained nurses. A dual solution was reached: the creation of an innovative program at Vassar College and the establishment of an Army School of Nursing, both designed to increase the supply of trained nurses for the military (Clappison, 1964). During the war even those who were properly trained faced challenges. Tested by harsh conditions on the European front, severe nursing shortages, and the occurrence of a devastating influenza pandemic, white female nurses demonstrated their effectiveness (Telford, 2007). Because of the segregated nature of American society at the time, black nurses, both male and female, were denied the opportunity to participate (Figure 1-3).

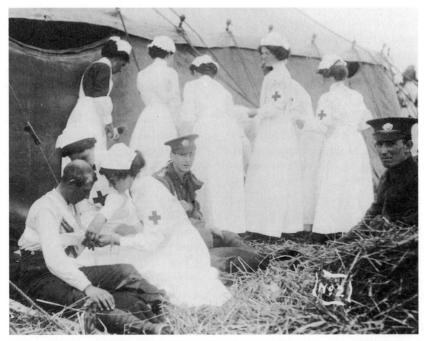

FIGURE 1-3 Nursing in World War I, circa 1918. (Courtesy Camilla Louise Wills Collection at the Eleanor Crowder Bjoring Center for Nursing Historical Inquiry, The University of Virginia, School of Nursing, Charlottesville, VA.)

Hospitals Become Businesses

After World War I hospitals continued to grow in both number and size. Between 1925 and 1929 $890 million was spent on their construction. The use of x-rays, the introduction of new drugs such as sulfa and insulin, and the reliance on laboratory tests such as urinalysis and the complete blood count revolutionized modern medicine, just as the introduction of aseptic techniques and developments in anesthesia had revolutionized surgery at the turn of the century (Howell, 1996). Modern obstetrics, with its promise of "twilight sleep" to reduce the pain of childbirth, brought women who previously had their babies at home into hospitals. Over the course of the next few decades, the addition of pediatric, psychiatric, and physical therapy services, as well as the introduction of private patient rooms, enhanced the hospital's image and attracted thousands of new patients into hospitals (Roren, 1930). Indeed, the 20th century saw America's appreciation of the benefits of scientific medicine (Howell, 1996). With the growth of hospitals, the social and economic status of staff physicians and hospital directors also increased. The status of nurses did not increase, however, and nursing administrators continued their struggle to convince hospitals that graduate nurses, rather than nursing students, should be responsible for patient care. Meanwhile nurse educators urged that students spend more time in formal classroom instruction. This struggle continued even after the Goldmark Report revealed shocking deficiencies in the education of nursing students (Goldmark, 1923).

It would take the stock market crash of 1929 and the subsequent national economic depression of the 1930s to change the hospital staffing situation. Indeed the economic depression that gripped the country caused serious financial, social, and health problems for the nation. Business failures and unemployment spread; by 1932, 25% of working Americans had lost their jobs (Blum, 1981). As fewer and fewer patients were able to pay for private duty nurses, physicians, or medical and surgical procedures, hospital administrators were forced to examine the costs of providing care. Maintaining a nursing school was expensive, and many small hospitals had to close their schools. In fact, 570 training programs were closed during the 1930s (Roberts, 1954). To keep the remaining nursing schools intact, their budgets were seriously curtailed and students' education was further compromised.

At the same time, large hospitals, especially municipal hospitals, experienced a large influx of patients seeking charitable care. The Social Security Act of 1935, with its financial aid for the elderly and its Title V health care benefits for disabled children, had provided some relief, but it was not until the development of Blue Cross, a revolutionary prepaid health insurance plan (Numbers, 1978), that hospitals found a solution. Selling health plans to workers able to pay for future hospitalizations proved to be an engaging idea because it helped to ensure the financial stability of hospitals that became Blue Cross associates. The public was demanding hospital care, and Blue Cross could pay for it.

Members of the American Medical Association (AMA), however, rejected the new Blue Cross health plan, characterizing it as "economically unsound, unethical and inimical to the public interests" (Kimball, 1934, p. 45). In spite of the AMA's opposition, Blue Cross proved to be attractive to patients and hospitals. Moreover, because it filled hospital beds with paying patients, it was formally endorsed by the American Hospital Association in 1937. As a hospital official noted, "Blue Cross was sired by the Depression and mothered by hospitals out of desperate economic necessity" (Sommers & Sommers, 1961). More than 1 million people participated as members of Blue Cross in 1937, providing hospitals with adequate incomes to remain open and plan for their futures.

As the economy slowly improved in the late 1930s, training school costs continued to be viewed as a burden to hospital budgets. Hospitals that closed their schools substituted untrained attendants for student workers, but it soon became evident, especially to physicians, that additional graduate nurses were needed to provide patients with safe and effective nursing care. This realization, coupled with new sources of income from health insurance and government relief programs and the availability of unemployed private duty nurses willing to work for minimum wages, encouraged administrators to add graduate nurses to their staffs (Fitzpatrick, 1975). The increase of registered nurses on hospital staffs—from 4000 positions in 1929 to 28,000 in 1937 and to more than 100,000 by 1941—helped improve the quality of patient services.

Paradoxically, graduate nursing staffs also introduced a new professional tension within the hospital system (Cannings & Lazonick, 1975). Hospital administrators, accustomed to a docile and inexpensive student workforce, considered graduate nursing services costly and only partially necessary. In addition, administrators and physicians saw registered nurses as potential threats because they were less compliant than students. The nurses used their own judgment in providing patient care, basing their decisions on their professional knowledge and experiences rather than simply following orders.

Tensions resulted. As independent practitioners working in private homes, the nurses had worked autonomously to give the quality of care they believed patients needed. Now, as staff nurses working in the hospital setting, they were part of a bureaucracy that demanded loyalty to physicians and the hospital itself rather than to patients. In addition, the hospitals' employment of subsidiary nursing and housekeeping staff added managerial tasks to their responsibilities. Moreover, the strict institutional control of their clinical practice reminded them of the exploitation, harsh discipline, and regimentation they had experienced in their training schools (Flood, 1981).

Given the economic realities of the Depression, however, graduate nurses and hospitals began an uneasy working alliance. Learning how to interact successfully with professional graduates rather than a student workforce challenged hospital administrators and nursing superintendents, who struggled to establish personnel policies that professional nurses would accept. Nonetheless, for the most part, hospitals offered registered nurses "low pay, long hours, split shifts, authoritarian supervision, and rigid rules" (Reverby, 1987, p. 192).

By the 1950s hospitals had become the major employers of nurses. As such, they gained the power to set nursing wages and working conditions and often thwarted nurses in their quest for adequate compensation and the right to participate in hospital decisions regarding patient care (Reverby, 1987). Likely fueled by their lack of autonomy and their plight as subservient members of a hierarchical hospital system, nurses identified education as a potential pathway to leadership.

Collegiate Nursing Education: The Early Years

Throughout the early years of the 20th century, some nurse educators believed that the profession's superintendents, faculty, and public health nurses should have postgraduate education in institutions of higher learning. As early as 1899, Teachers College at Columbia University offered a post-diploma hospital economics program. Mary Adelaide Nutting and Isabel Stewart directed this program and offered innovative programs in administration, education, and public health nursing to thousands of nurses from the United States and abroad (Christy, 1969).

In 1909 the University of Minnesota established the first permanent undergraduate nursing educational program in the United States. For most students, however, admission to college was prohibited by cost and the time required to complete the program. Thus enrollment in these institutions remained low compared with diploma programs. By 1923 only 17 collegiate schools nationwide offered 5-year degree programs. Although the profession had made some progress toward collegiate status, it still lacked the social endorsement and financial support that had paved the way for medical education to move into universities.

Medical education experienced a very different trajectory from nursing. Large financial endowments, primarily from the Rockefeller, Carnegie, and Commonwealth foundations, had propelled medical education into the mainstream of university education. Data from the famous 1910 Abraham Flexner Report had demonstrated inadequacies in medical education, acting as a catalyst for reform. The Rockefeller General Education Board alone funneled more than $91 million into medical schools (Starr, 1982). Although nursing leaders sought similar assistance for nursing education, only the Rockefeller Foundation was persuaded to endow the establishment of two university-based nursing schools—Yale in 1924 and Vanderbilt in 1930 (Abram, 1993). Annie Goodrich, a noted nursing educator, directed the first independent nursing collegiate school at Yale University. This baccalaureate program was based on the premise that nursing concepts pertinent to acute illness, the psychosocial dimensions of illness, and public health principles were essential components of educational programs for professional nurses (Sheahan, 1979).

By 1935 sufficient numbers of collegiate programs provided the catalyst for the organization of the Association of Collegiate Schools of Nursing, an organization whose mission was to establish collegiate nursing programs in American universities. Its early members strongly maintained that nursing could not develop into a profession until it could generate scientifically sound nursing knowledge that could sustain the practice of nursing (Stewart, 1943). Although this group later disbanded, in 1969 a small group of deans of collegiate and university programs established the Conference of Deans of Colleges and University Schools of Nursing, known today as the American Association of Colleges of Nursing (AACN; Keeling, Kirchgessner, & Brodie, 2009). The AACN continues to play an essential role in nursing education, research, and health policy. Ironically, however, the nursing profession continues to allow many pathways into practice and has yet to reach a consensus about the educational qualifications needed by entry-level practicing nurses.

World War II

The United States' entry into World War II in 1941, after the bombing of Pearl Harbor, immediately increased the demand for skilled nurses to care for sick and injured soldiers as well as patients on the home front. To meet the increased demands, the federal government created two new programs: the American Red Cross volunteer nurse's aides program in 1941 and the Cadet Nurse Corps in 1943 (Johnston, 1966).

The loss of professional and nonprofessional staff to the military and defense industry left hospitals and public health agencies in need of auxiliary help to care for citizens at home. Through a joint venture with the Office of Civilian Defense and the American Red Cross, more than 200,000 women volunteered to become certified nurse's aides and work under nursing supervision to provide nursing services. This venture proved to be an important step in the stratification of nursing into registered, practical, and aide levels. Its success encouraged hospitals to continue to use auxiliary nursing personnel after the war to ease the nation's postwar shortage of nurses (Bullough & Bullough, 1978).

In 1943 Frances Payne Bolton, a congresswoman from Ohio, sponsored a bill that authorized the U.S. Public Health Service to establish the Cadet Nurse Corps. This was the most significant federally sponsored program to increase the supply of professional nurses in the 1940s. The bill subsidized the education of students who agreed, upon graduation, to serve in military or civilian health agencies for the duration of the war. Students were provided tuition, fees, and books, plus a monthly stipend throughout their training. Participating schools also received funds for instructional facilities and postgraduate education for their nursing faculty (Figure 1-4).

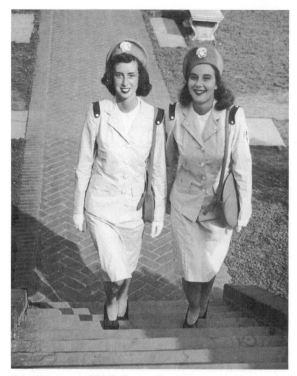

FIGURE 1-4 USPHS Cadet Corp Nurses—Bishop Sisters, 1944. (Courtesy Eleanor Crowder Bjoring Center for Nursing Historical Inquiry, The University of Virginia, School of Nursing, Charlottesville, VA.)

Although the cadet corps accepted students for only 2 years (July 1943 to October 1945), almost 170,000 cadets entered 1125 participating schools, and two thirds of them graduated. The program recruited a large number of graduates to the profession and led to major changes in nursing education. The government's requirements of a modified program, including policies of nondiscrimination on the basis of race and marital status, allowed an opportunity to redesign nursing education. In addition, because nursing school directors rather than hospital administrators were required to administer the federal funds, the actual costs of the nursing program and the services provided to hospitals by students became known. Armed with this information, nursing directors were better equipped to negotiate with administrators for funds to upgrade their programs after the war (Brueggemann, 1992).

African-American Nurses

Unlike their predecessors, nursing leaders during World War II attempted to remedy the shortage of nursing personnel by employing people belonging to two groups that had been previously excluded from mainstream nursing: men and African-American women. Since their inception in the late 19th century, most nursing schools had excluded men and African-American women from admission, based on discriminatory and restrictive policies. To ensure that African-American patients received medical care and that African-American physicians and nurses had opportunities to become professionals, separate African-American hospitals and schools were created in the late 1800s (Gamble, 1989). African-American graduates of these programs faced further discrimination as registered nurses because many hospitals and community health agencies refused to employ them, citing objections from white patients to being cared for by African-American nurses. African-American nurses faced additional discrimination when they attempted to join most of the state associations of the ANA. To overcome such overt and covert forms of discrimination, the National Association of Colored Graduate Nurses (NACGN) was formed in 1908. The NACGN fought for almost 50 years to end the social, economic, and professional injuries inflicted on African-American graduate nurses (Staupers, 1951). It would not be until 1945 that discriminatory policies would change.

Stirred by patriotism, many young African-American women had entered the Cadet Nurse Corps because that program prohibited discrimination based on race. However, throughout World War II the Army Nurse Corps maintained restrictive racial quotas, whereas the Navy Nurse Corps excluded all African Americans. By 1944 public opinion had turned against the armed services' discriminatory policies, and in January 1945 both corps lifted their racial restrictions and accepted African-American female nurses into their ranks.

When World War II came to an end, the presence of many more African-American registered nurses, many of whom were graduates of the Cadet Nurse Corps, caused state nurses associations to remove racial barriers to membership. General integration into the ANA was hastened in 1948, when its House of Delegates granted individual membership to African-American nurses barred from their state associations and called for the establishment of biracial integration at district and state levels. In 1950 only two state associations retained racial restrictions, allowing the NACGN to announce its dissolution. By 1952, all state nurses associations had removed racial discriminatory policies for ANA membership.

Unfortunately, the end of overt racial discrimination against African-American nurses did not eradicate the more subtle and entrenched forms of prejudice. For black nurses the struggle to be fully accepted as professionals by patients, hospitals, and fellow heath care colleagues continued. This deep-seated discrimination led to the emergence of the National Black Nurses Association in 1971. As was its predecessor (the NACGN), the National Black Nurses Association was (and continues to be) committed to acting as an advocate for improvement of the health care for blacks and to ensuring that African-American nurses participate fully in the nursing profession and the larger health care system (Carnegie, 1995).

Male Nurses

The longstanding bias against male nurses that was present in the opening decades of the 20th century was based on society's belief that nursing was a feminine skill and therefore men should not be nurses (Nurses' Associated Alumnae of the United States, 1902/2007). In the late 19th and early 20th centuries, most men who wanted to be nurses attended all-male programs sponsored by religious groups or affiliated with psychiatric hospitals. Some hospital administrators hired male graduate nurses but often treated them as orderlies rather than as nursing professionals (Craig, 1940).

Within the military, male nurses faced a more entrenched form of discrimination than did their African-American female nurse counterparts. Tradition and sentiment had long dictated that nursing was a woman's field, and when Congress established the nurse corps, it had mandated that *only women* could be appointed as military nurses. Male nursing students and graduates were subject to the Selective Service Act draft, but most volunteered for service rather than waiting to be drafted. Once in, male nurses were denied professional nursing status; most served as enlisted personnel in health-related positions (Rose, 1947). It would not be until 1955, after the Korean conflict, that Congress passed legislation allowing the appointment of male nurses as reserve officers in the Army, Navy, and Air Force Nurse Corps (Sarnecky, 1999).

Post–World War II Era

America emerged from World War II profoundly changed as a people, society, and country. After years of war, with the rationing of resources and lack of individual choices, Americans wanted better lives for themselves and their families. In particular, they wanted quality health care and educational opportunities. In response to citizens' needs, the federal government formulated new health priorities and policies and funded health initiatives. One of the first of these was the Hospital Survey and Reconstruction Act (the Hill-Burton Act) of 1946, which began to provide federal funds for hospital construction and new health centers. Over the next decade these funds significantly expanded and updated the nation's hospitals, increased bed capacity, and transformed hospitals into scientific and technical medical centers (Risse, 1999).

At mid-century, the public's growing belief in the power of modern medicine was sustained by impressive advances in pharmacology, medicine, and surgery. Penicillin, one of the earliest "miracle drugs," successfully treated serious infections and, in preventing postoperative infections, opened the door to radically new surgical procedures. The dramatic advances in pharmacology, medical sciences, and technology enticed health professionals and patients alike to believe in the possibility that humans might conquer all diseases. The public encouraged the federal government to continue its large appropriations for medical research, education, and services (Stevens, 1989).

The Nursing Shortage

With a rise in the number and size of hospitals, an explosive rise in U.S. population, and an increase in the incidence of chronic disease, the nation's demand for nurses increased dramatically after World War II. Seventy-eight million children were born between 1946 and 1964 (later known as the *baby boom generation*). This phenomenon was coupled with a rise in chronic disease among a growing elderly population. Demand for hospital beds was at an all-time high. The problem was that there were not enough nurses.

Faced with this problem, hospital administrators were forced to restrict admissions. They also had to seek solutions, initially focusing on acquiring more nurses rather than on creating ways to improve the education of nurses (Lynaugh & Brush, 1996). Other strategies to address the shortage followed. These included the employment of ward clerks, the use of volunteers, practical nurses, and aides to help nurses provide patient care, the initiation of team nursing, the importation of foreign nurses, and improvement in nurses' salaries and working conditions.

Federal funding for nursing education remained modest until 1964, when Congress passed the *Nurse Training Act* in response to pressure from the American Medical Association and the American Hospital Association about the need for nurses. This landmark legislation awarded $242.6 million for nursing student scholarships, loans, recruitment, school construction and maintenance, and special educational projects (Kalisch & Kalisch, 1995). The success of these initiatives helped diminish the nation's shortages of nurses. Between 1950 and 1967 the number of registered nurses rose by 67%, the number of practical nurses rose by 134%, and the number of nursing aides/assistants rose by 244% (U.S. Public Health Service, 1976).

NURSING IN INSTITUTIONS OF HIGHER EDUCATION

Baccalaureate Programs

In addition to other legislation after the war, in 1946 Congress passed the GI Bill of Rights, enabling veterans to acquire vocational training or a college education (Kiester, 1994). Nurse veterans took advantage of the opportunity to enroll in college programs and earned degrees in nursing education and administration. The increased enrollment provided a new direction for collegiate nursing programs. Beginning in the 1950s, entry-level baccalaureate nursing programs were opened to high school graduates throughout the nation. In 1962 178 colleges offered undergraduate degrees in nursing, and the pool of baccalaureate-educated nurses, essential to the creation of advanced nursing educational programs, dramatically expanded (Brown, 1978).

Community College Programs

The severity of the nursing shortage in the postwar years encouraged faculty to develop new entry-level nursing programs. In 1951 nurse educator Mildred Montag proposed an innovative program to prepare nurse technicians in 2-year associate degree (AD) community colleges. A 5-year study of AD programs found that their graduates were able to pass state nursing licensure examinations. They demonstrated an adequate level of clinical nursing competency and were employed as graduate nurses (Haase, 1990).

The results of this study launched the AD educational movement. Securing funding from the Nurse

Training Act of 1964, community colleges opened AD programs at a phenomenal rate. From 1952 to 1974, the number of AD programs in the country doubled every 4 years. During one period, new programs opened at the rate of one per week (Rines, 1977).

Several important goals were attained by the AD programs' success. A new pool of students, including men, married women with children, and older-than-typical undergraduates, were now able to choose nursing careers. The AD graduates helped minimize the nursing shortages of the 1970s and 1980s; this encouraged hospital directors to close their expensive 3-year diploma programs and let colleges and universities educate nurses. Soon diploma education disappeared in most states (Lynaugh & Brush, 1996). Today AD programs are the major point of entry into nursing; as reflected in a 2003 survey of nursing programs and graduates, AD programs prepared more graduates than did the combined baccalaureate and diploma programs (National League for Nursing, 2003).

Although AD education opened nursing education to a broader student population, the existence of three entry-level educational programs—diploma, associate, and baccalaureate degree, all leading to registered nurse licensure and beginning positions—has led to confusion among the public and the profession as to the exact requirements for a credential as a professional nurse. What is becoming clearer with recent research, however, is that BSN-prepared graduates give care that is evidence-based and improves patient outcomes. Today there is a focus on hospitals hiring more nurses prepared at the BSN level.

Graduate Programs

In the mid-1950s the need for nurses prepared at the graduate level to direct nursing service departments and teach in baccalaureate programs encouraged faculty to develop more master's-level programs. These earlier programs focused on preparing educators and administrators rather than clinicians. However, in the 1960s, as the pace of medical innovation increased and new clinical subspecialties such as cardiology, nephrology, and oncology came into existence, master's programs shifted their focus to preparing clinical nurse specialists and NPs.

Although nurses have earned doctoral degrees since the mid-1920s, most of them acquired their education in related disciplines such as education and sociology. In the late 1960s aided by funds from the federal government, doctoral nursing programs began to appear (Grace, 1978). Nursing doctoral programs provided

the profession with the rigorous academic credentials it needed to develop its unique disciplinary knowledge and prepare its future researchers and scholars. Questions about the nature of nursing, its mission and goals, and the scope of nurses' roles drove nurse educators to consider the answers to these questions and present them in a more coherent whole. These questions grew out of an interest in changes in the educational preparation of nurses from diploma to baccalaureate programs, as well as concerns about what to include or exclude in curricula and what nurses needed to learn to function as nurses (Meleis, 2004).

To begin to answer questions about the discipline of nursing, schools and colleges of nursing were incorporated into institutions of higher education devoted to scholarly inquiry and research. One of these was Columbia University Teachers College. Many of the prominent nursing leaders of the 1950s took courses in education and administration at Teachers College. Some of these nursing leaders received a doctoral degree in education (EdD).

Teachers College can also be credited with the birth of nursing theory (Omery, Kasper, & Page, 1995). The earliest nursing theories were similar to system and physiological models. These models reflected the paradigm that was strongly supported by the field of education at the time: the received view of science. Other disciplines considered these tenets to be *one* way of gaining knowledge in the sciences; however, education—and therefore nursing—held that these tenets were the *only* way. Nurses then adopted this paradigm as truth. This view was not without its problems; as nurses restricted themselves to objective data based on quantitative methods of inquiry, they simultaneously restricted knowledge development in the discipline (Telford, 2004). Only later did the profession's leaders incorporate other ways of knowing, including clinical expertise, qualitative methods, and historical research.

RISE OF ADVANCED PRACTICE NURSING IN CLINICAL SETTINGS

Acute Care Nurse Specialist

Advances in medical science and technology through the latter half of the 20th century radically changed the practice of medicine and the treatment of hospitalized patients. However, the newly constructed hospitals, with their private rooms and long hallways caused new problems for an already short-handed nursing staff, as patients could no longer be seen from a central nurses' station. Moreover, many nurses were unskilled and unfamiliar with the new treatments and new technologies. As a result, nurse and physician teams initiated the concept of the intensive care unit (ICU), a large room in which the hospital's most experienced and competent nurses could work with critically ill patients. Within these new units, the care of the critically ill changed, as did the nurses' role. Their success paved the way for the creation of acute care nurse specialist roles (Fairman & Lynaugh, 1998; Lynaugh & Brush, 1996).

An example of one of these units was the coronary care unit (CCU). Influenced by research on the success of cardiopulmonary resuscitation and cardiac defibrillation, and interested in using electronic monitoring technology for improving the care of cardiac patients, physicians, and nurses opened CCUs to manage patients with acute myocardial infarction. Supported by federal appropriations for medical research, CCUs proliferated. Central to the coronary care specialist movement was the nurses' drive toward independent practice, nurse-derived standards of care, and a collegial relationship with the units' physicians. Working together, nurses and physicians shared the emerging clinical knowledge for managing critically ill patients. They mastered new medical technology and wrote standard "order sets," educating nurses to identify changes in cardiac rhythms and to treat patients without waiting for physicians' orders. Gaining acceptance as essential members of the CCU team, nurses stretched the boundaries of nursing practice and laid the foundation for a more autonomous practice for other master's-prepared nurses (Keeling, 2004).

As these highly specialized nurses realized their need for continuing education, ICU nurses formed national specialty organizations, including the American Association of Cardiovascular Nurses (AACN) in 1969, renamed the American Association of Critical Care Nurses in 1972. These organizations established practice standards and developed continuing education programs and certification for their respective emerging clinical specialties. The success of ICU nurses paved the way for the creation of many subspecialty units (including units for neonatology, burns, renal dialysis, and oncology) and marked a significant advance in the scope of practice for nurses and opportunities for professional growth (Fairman & Lynaugh, 1998; Keeling, 2004) (Figure 1-5).

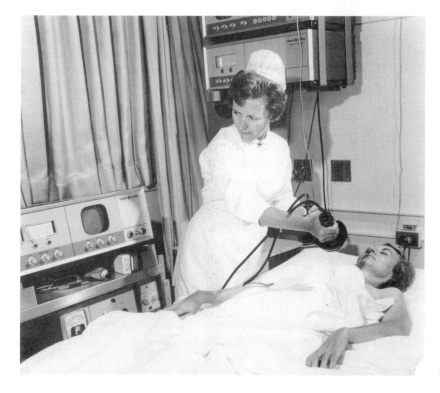

FIGURE 1-5 Rose Pinneo, RN—Cardiac defibrillation, circa 1963. (Courtesy Eleanor Crowder Bjoring Center for Nursing Historical Inquiry, The University of Virginia, School of Nursing, Charlottesville, VA.)

Primary Care Nurse Practitioners

At the same time that acute care specialist roles were emerging in hospitals, the primary care NP movement crystallized (Keeling, 2007) (Figure 1-6). The idea of an advanced practice role for pediatric nurses, the rise of medical specialization, the concurrent shortage of primary care physicians (especially in rural areas), and the public's demand for improved access to health care all helped foster the movement.

In 1965 Loretta Ford and Henry Silver opened the first pediatric NP program at the University of Colorado. This collaborative project, designed by a nurse and a pediatrician, prepared professional nurses to provide well child care and manage the care of children with common childhood illnesses. Its success

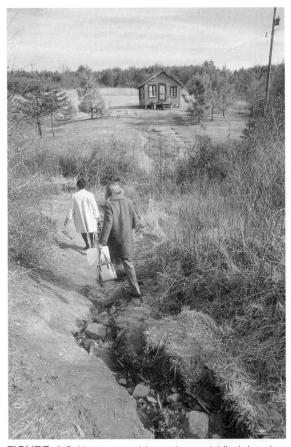

FIGURE 1-6 Nurse practitioner in rural Virginia, circa 1970s. (Courtesy Eleanor Crowder Bjoring Center for Nursing Historical Inquiry, The University of Virginia, School of Nursing, Charlottesville, VA.)

would lead to federal funding for the education of NPs in other clinical areas.

Similar to acute care specialists, primary care NPs developed organizations that created certification requirements and clinical standards. However, because NPs assumed diagnostic and treatment responsibilities outside the confines of the hospital, they also set in place legal certification at the state level and began to seek prescriptive authority (Fairman, 1999, 2008; Keeling, 2007).

By the 1970s NPs were employed in a variety of primary care settings, including physicians' offices, clinics, and schools. In addition, some practiced in hospitals in subspecialty areas such as nephrology, oncology, and neonatology. In the early 1990s, in response to the growing shortage of medical residents in subspecialty areas and the need to manage patients with increasingly complex medical needs (e.g., heart and lung transplants), acute care nurse practitioner (ACNP) programs began to develop across the nation. Today numerous ACNPs work in acute care hospitals in various subspecialties—some as "nurse hospitalists." In addition, states are beginning to require that NPs have the proper educational requirements (e.g., ACNP versus primary care NP) related to their specific job requirements and scope of practice.

Clinical Nurse Leader and Doctor of Nursing Practice

At the turn of the 21st century, the development of a new role for nurses came about as a response to growing patient care needs and to the changing health care delivery environment. In February 2004, the American Association of Colleges of Nursing Board approved a new model of nursing practice and nursing education at the master's level—the clinical nurse leader (CNL) (AACN, 2004). The CNL, a generalist master's-prepared clinician, was to provide care in all health care settings at the point of care. He or she was to be accountable for client care outcomes by coordinating, delegating, and supervising the care provided by the health care team. The CNL was not considered to be an advanced practice nurse. According to AACN, if the education of the *generalist* nurse was elevated to the master's degree level, it was reasonable to assume that *specialty* education, and the education of those individuals prepared for the highest level of nursing practice, would occur at the doctoral level. Thus the Doctor of Nursing Practice (DNP) degree was proposed. It would be a terminal doctorate, equivalent to a PhD, but with a focus on practice rather than research. It would be a degree, not a new "role."

The *practice-focused* doctoral degree was not a new idea. The first such program, offering the Nursing Doctorate (ND), was established at Case Western Reserve University in 1979 and offered an entry-level nursing degree. Since then, numerous practice-focused doctoral programs were begun throughout the country (AACN, 2004). There are now 241 DNP programs currently enrolling students at schools of nursing nationwide, and an additional 59 DNP programs are in the planning stages and DNP programs are now available in 40 states plus the District of Columbia. From 2012 to 2013, the number of students enrolled in DNP programs increased from 11,575 to 14,699. During that same period, the number of DNP graduates increased from 1858 to 2443 (AACN, 2014). If AACN leadership holds sway, the DNP will be the requisite preparation for all advanced practice nursing roles, including the NP, CNS, certified nurse midwife, and certified registered nurse anesthetist (CRNA) in the near future.

SUMMARY

This chapter provides a brief overview of the history of American nursing from the middle of the 19th century to the present day. Highlights include the impact of Florence Nightingale's ideas about nursing and nurse training, issues surrounding the development of professional and educational standards for nurses, the role of nurses in war, and the development of NP programs and doctoral education for nurses. These events and topics did not happen in isolation; rather they occurred in the context of the development of the practice of medicine and the rise of science and the health care system. Therefore the chapter discusses how nursing was influenced by these events, as well as how nursing has also shaped its own progress.

The chapter also discusses the challenges the profession has faced in the last 150 years. Many of the issues that nurses faced in the past persist today. Among these are the issue of equal opportunity for all races, genders, and classes, and the issue of professional consensus about the educational requirements for entry into practice.

The context in which the nursing profession exists is also still a consideration as the world faces the implications of a global society and the challenges of potential pandemic diseases, persistent wars, and continuing nursing shortages. The future of nursing will likely continue to demand nursing care that is innovative, efficient, cost effective, and responsive to human needs in all settings. As in the past, the decisions made by nursing leaders today in response to these forces are already shaping the profession's future. Those decisions can be better made with an understanding of the profession's past.

SALIENT POINTS

- The first hospital-based nurse training schools, built on the apprenticeship model of learning, had the dual task of providing care to patients and educating students to become professional nurses.
- Nursing state licensure, begun in 1903, is important because it protects the public and defines the role and scope of nursing practice.
- Nurses have played a major role in providing essential health services to the community for more than a century, especially for the poor and chronically ill.
- During World War II, the U.S. Public Health Service Cadet Nurse Corps attracted thousands of students to the profession and provided essential nursing services in civilian hospitals.

- Nursing, still a predominately Caucasian and female-oriented profession, needs to continue to recruit outside of this domain.
- Associate degree programs, begun in 1952, opened the nursing profession to a more diverse population than had existed with diploma and baccalaureate education.
- Advanced clinical practice nurses, as acute care nurses and NPs, expanded the boundaries of the profession.
- Graduate programs prepared nursing educators, directors, clinical specialists, researchers, and administrative leaders needed by the health care system and society. The CNL role and the DNP degrees continue to evolve.

CRITICAL REFLECTION EXERCISES

1. Reflect and discuss how the past informs the present in relation to two of the following current issues:
   - Nurses practicing to the full extent of their education and experiences
   - Nurses practicing as full partners in redesigning health care in the United States
   - Diversity in gender, race, and class in the nursing profession
   - Disaster preparedness and response
   - Health care for all
   - Health promotion and disease prevention
   - Health service delivery value (Triple Aim)
   - Aging of the population
   - Increase in chronic diseases
   - Emerging technologies
   - Expanding knowledge and information in the sciences and nursing profession
   - Nursing education mobility/progression models

REFERENCES

Abram, S. (1993). Brilliance and bureaucracy: Nursing and changes in the Rockefeller Foundation. 1915–1930. *Nursing History Review, 1,* 119–138.

American Association of Colleges of Nursing (AACN). (2004). *AACN position statement on the practice doctorate in nursing.* Retrieved from http://www.aacn.nche.edu/DNP/DNPPositionStatement.htm

American Association of Colleges of Nursing (AACN). (2014). *DNP fact sheet.* Retrieved from http://www.aacn.nche.edu/media-relations/fact-sheets/dnp

American Society of Superintendents of Training Schools for Nurses. (1897). *First and second annual reports.* Harrisburg, PA: Harrisburg Publishing.

Blum, J. (1981). The end of an era. In J. Blum (Ed.), *The national experience* (pp. 652–669). New York: Harcourt Brace Jovanovich.

Borsay, A. (2009). Monica Baly lecture: Nursing history: An irrelevance for nursing practice? *Nursing History Review, 17,* 14–27.

Brainard, A. (1922). *The evolution of public health nursing.* Philadelphia: Saunders.

Brown, J. (1978). Master's education in nursing, 1945–1969. In M. L. Fitzpatrick (Ed.), *Historical studies in nursing* (pp. 104–130). New York: Teachers College.

Brueggemann, D. (1992). *The United States Cadet Nurse Corps 1943–1948: The Nebraska experience.* Omaha, NE: University of Nebraska. Unpublished master's thesis.

Bullough, B. (1975). The first two phases in nursing licensure. In B. Bullough (Ed.), *The law and the expanding nurse's role* (pp. 7–21). New York: Appleton-Century-Crofts.

Bullough, V., & Bullough, B. (1978). *The care of the sick: The emergence of modern nursing.* New York: Prodist.

Burgess, M. (1928). *Nurses, patients and pocketbooks.* New York: National League for Nursing Education, Committee on the Grading of Nursing Schools.

Cannings, K., & Lazonick, W. (1975). The development of the nursing labor force in the United States: A brief analysis. *International Journal of Health Services, 5,* 185–217.

Carnegie, M. (1995). *The path we tread: Blacks in nursing 1854–1984.* Philadelphia: Jones & Bartlett.

Christy, T. (1969). *Cornerstone for nursing education.* New York: Teachers College.

Clappison, G. B. (1964). *Vassar's rainbow division 1918.* Lake Mills, IA: Graphic Publishing.

Craig, L. (1940). Opportunities for men nurses. *American Journal of Nursing, 40,* 667–670.

Daisy, C. (1996). *Keeping the flame: The influence of Agnes Ohlson on licensure and registration for nurses: 1936–1963* (Unpublished doctoral dissertation).

Dock, L. (1907). *A history of nursing* (Vol. 2). New York: G.P. Putnam's Sons.

Draper, E. A. (1893/1949). Necessity of an American Nurses' Association. In J. S. Billings, & H. M. Hurd (Eds.), *Nursing of the sick* (pp. 149–153). New York: McGraw-Hill.

Duffus, R. L. (1938). *Lillian Wald, neighbor and crusader.* New York: Macmillan.

Fairman, J. (1999). Delegated by default or negotiated by need? Physicians, nurse practitioners, and the process of clinical thinking. *Medical Humanities Review, 13*(1), 38–58.

Fairman, J. (2008). *Making room in the clinic: Nurse practitioners and the evolution of modern health care.* New Brunswick, NJ: Rutgers University Press.

Fairman, J., & Lynaugh, J. (1998). *Critical care nursing: A history.* Philadelphia: University of Pennsylvania.

Fitzpatrick, M. L. (1975). Nurses in American history: Nursing and the great depression. *American Journal of Nursing, 75,* 2188–2190.

Flood, M. (1981). *The troubling expedient: General staff nursing in United States hospitals in the 1930s: A means to institutional, educational, and personal ends.* Berkeley, CA: University of California (Unpublished doctoral dissertation).

Gamble, V. (1989). *Making a place for ourselves.* New York: Oxford University.

Gardner, M. (1936). *Public health nursing* (3rd ed.). New York: Macmillan.

Geister, J. (1926). Hearsay and fact in private duty. *American Journal of Nursing, 26,* 515–528.

Goldmark, J. (1923). *Nursing and nursing education in the United States: Report of the committee for the study of nursing education.* New York: Macmillan.

Goodrich, A. W. (1912). A general presentation of the statutory requirements of the different states. *American Journal of Nursing, 12,* 1001–1008.

Grace, H. C. (1978). The development of doctoral education in nursing: A historical education perspective. *Journal of Nursing Education, 17,* 17–27.

Haase, P. (1990). *The origins and rise of associate degree nursing education.* Durham, NC: Duke University Press.

Hamilton, D. (1989). The cost of caring: The Metropolitan Life Insurance Company's visiting nurse service, 1909–1953. *Bulletin of the History of Medicine, 63,* 414–434.

Hampton, I. A. (1893/1949), Educational standards for nurses. In *Nursing of the sick* (pp. 1–12). New York: McGraw-Hill. Reprinted from J. S. Billings, & H. M. Hurd (Eds.). (1894). *Hospitals, dispensaries and nursing: Papers and discussions in the International Congress of Charities, Correction, and Philanthropy, Section III, Chicago, June 12th to 17th, 1893. Part III, Nursing of the sick.* Baltimore: Johns Hopkins University Press.

Howard, H. B. (1912). The medical superintendent (section on hospitals). *American Medical Association Transactions, 76.*

Howell, J. (1996). *Technology in the hospital: Transforming patient care in the early twentieth century.* Baltimore: Johns Hopkins University Press.

Johnston, D. F. (1966). *History and trends of practical nursing.* St Louis: Mosby.

Kalisch, P., & Kalisch, B. (1995). *The advance of American nursing* (3rd ed.). Philadelphia: Lippincott.

Keeling, A. (2004). Blurring the boundaries between medicine and nursing: Coronary Care nursing, 1960s. *Nursing History Review, 12,* 139–164.

Keeling, A. (2007). *Nursing and the privilege of prescription, 1893–2000.* Columbus, OH: Ohio State University Press.

Keeling, A., Kirchgessner, J., & Brodie, B. (2009). *A history of the American Association of Colleges of Nursing.* Washington, DC: AACN.

Keeling, A., & Ramos, M. C. (1995). The role of nursing history in preparing nursing for the future. *Nursing and Health Care, 16*(1), 30–34.

Kiester, E. (1994). The GI Bill may be the best deal ever made by Uncle Sam. *Smithsonian, 25*(8), 128–139.

Kimball, J. F. (1934). Prepayment plan of hospital care. *American Hospital Association Bulletin, 8,* 45.

Lynaugh, J., & Brush, B. (1996). *American nursing: From hospitals to health systems.* Cambridge, MA: Blackwell.

Meckel, R. (1990). *Save the babies.* Baltimore: Johns Hopkins University Press.

Meleis, A. I. (2004). *Theoretical nursing development & progress.* Philadelphia: Lippincott Williams & Wilkins.

Melosh, B. (1982). *The physician's hand.* Philadelphia: Temple University.

National League for Nursing. (2003). Annual Report, 2003. *Nursing data review, academic year, 27.*

Nightingale, F. (1859). *Notes on nursing: What it is and what it is not.* New York: D Appleton and Company, 1860.

Numbers, R. (1978). The third party: Health insurance in America. In J. Leavitt, & R. Numbers (Eds.), *Sickness and health in America* (pp. 142–145). Madison, WI: University of Wisconsin.

Nurses' Associated Alumnae of the United States. (1902/2007). Proceedings of the fifth annual convention. In C. O'Lynn, & R. E. Tranbarger (Eds.), *Men in nursing: History, challenges, and opportunities* (pp. 743–809). New York: Springer.

Omery, A., Kasper, C. E., & Page, G. G. (1995). *In search of nursing science.* Thousand Oaks, CA: Sage.

Reverby, S. (1987). *Ordered to care.* New York: Cambridge University.

Rines, A. (1977). Associate degree nursing education: History, development and rationale. *Nursing Outlook, 25,* 496–501.

Risse, G. B. (1999). *Mending bodies, saving souls: History of hospitals.* New York: Oxford University.

Roberts, M. (1954). *American nursing: History and interpretation.* New York: Macmillan.

Roren, R. (1930). *The public's investment in hospitals* (Committee on the Costs of Medical Care, Publication No. 7). Chicago, IL: The University of Chicago Press.

Rose, J. (1947). Men nurses in military service. *American Journal of Nursing, 47,* 147–148.

Sarnecky, M. (1999). *History of the Army Nurse Corps.* Philadelphia: University of Pennsylvania.

Sheahan, D. (1979). *The social origins of American nursing and its movement into the university. (Unpublished doctoral dissertation).* New York: New York University.

Sommers, H., & Sommers, A. (1961). *Patients and health insurance.* Washington, DC: Brookings Institution.

Starr, P. (1982). *The social transformation of American Medicine.* New York: Basic Books.

Staupers, M. (1951). Story of the NACGN. *American Journal of Nursing, 51,* 221–222.

Stevens, R. (1989). *In sickness and in wealth.* New York: Basic Books.

Stewart, I. (1943). *The education of nurses.* New York: Macmillan.

Stoney, E. (1919). *Practical points in nursing.* Philadelphia: Saunders.

Struthers, L. (1917). *The school nurse.* New York: G.P. Putnam's Sons.

Telford, J. (2004). *The liberation of the minds and practices of nurses: The evolution and adoption of the Received View to enlightenment in nursing science, circa 1873-present* (Unpublished).

Telford, J. (2007). *American Red Cross nursing during World War I: Opportunities and obstacles* (Unpublished doctoral dissertation).

Toman, C., & Thifault, M. C. (2012). Historical thinking and the shaping of nursing identity. *Nursing History Review, 20,* 184–204.

U.S. Bureau of Census. (1900). *Special reports: Occupation roles, and gender.* Washington, DC: U.S. Government Printing Office.

U.S. Public Health Service. (1976). *The consumer and health planners.* Washington, DC: U.S. Government Printing Office.

Wald, L. (1938). *The house on Henry Street.* New York: Henry Holt.

Weeks-Shaw, C. (1902). *A text-book of nursing, for the use of training schools, families, and private students.* New York: Appleton.

Whelan, J. (2005). A necessity in the nursing world: Chicago Nurses Professional Registry 1918–1950. *Nursing History Review, 13,* 49–76.

Woolsey, A. H. (1950). *A century of nursing, with hints toward the organization of a training school (originally published 1876), and Florence Nightingale's historic letter on the Bellevue School, September 18, 1872.* New York: Hospitals and training schools; report to the Standing Committee on Hospitals of the State Charities Aid Association. May 24, 1876. To which is added: "Founding of the Bellevue Training School for Nurses," Chapter 6 of Recollections of a Happy Life, by E. Christophers Hobson (originally published 1916). New York: Putnam.

Pathways of Nursing Education

Kathryn B. Reid, PhD, RN, FNP-BC, CNL and Elizabeth E. Friberg, DNP, RN

ℯ http://evolve.elsevier.com/Friberg/bridge/

OBJECTIVES

At the completion of this chapter, the reader will be able to:

- Trace the history of nursing education from its inception to the present.
- Compare nursing education programs for similarities and differences.
- Classify nursing education programs according to role preparation, scope of practice, eligibility for licensure, and eligibility for specialty certification.

- Identify and analyze trends in nursing program development, including eligibility for admission, career mobility and advancement opportunities, and program accessibility.
- Evaluate the effectiveness of mechanisms to ensure program quality.
- Analyze the merits and shortcomings of the current nursing education system.

👤 PROFILE IN PRACTICE

Mary Gunther, PhD, RN

Associate Professor, Executive Associate Dean for Academic Affairs, University of Tennessee College of Nursing, Knoxville, Tennessee

I was never one of those little girls who wanted to be a nurse. In fact, if early favorite toys and after-school activities had been a predictor, I now would be a truck driver or a librarian. Typical of times, the high school I attended did not provide academic counseling to educate families about tuition assistance or scholarships. My grandmother, who was raising me, made it clear that a college education was beyond our financial means. It was her fervent wish that I always be able to take care of myself (i.e., be able to get a well-paying job) without relying on anyone else. She gave me two choices: become a nun or study nursing. I chose the latter.

I completed a 2-year nursing diploma program at a community hospital in Chicago. It was the type of program common at the time: Students staffed the hospital around the clock 5 days a week and worked weekends for pay. The opportunity for hands-on clinical experience was unsurpassed. When it came time to look for a job, I chose to specialize in pediatrics, because children were less intimidating to me than adults. Furthermore, they were easier

to physically move! Over the first 10 years of my career I became "a good nurse," developing both my intuitive and technical skills. I could recognize what needed to be done and when. What I did not know was why. I decided to take advantage of working at a university hospital and returned to school. It took me 15 years of on-again, off-again study to get my BSN. (Obviously, I was not exactly driven; it's more like I meandered through the undergraduate program.) By that time, I was a head nurse and had a whole new set of management and administrative skills to learn.

Flushed with the success of being the first one in my family ever to graduate from college, I went back for a master's degree in nursing administration. What a difference! Almost everyone in my class had worked as a nurse for several years. Everyone had a story to tell about where they had been and where they wanted to go. The classes were not necessarily harder than those in the undergraduate program—just more interesting because they were directly applicable to our various jobs. I fell in love with nursing all over again. I finished my MSN degree in 18 months, just in time to become the direc-tor of a large pediatric nursing department. Within a few years, I was the budget director for the entire division of nursing. Suddenly I was explaining to administrators just what it is that nurses do that makes them irreplaceable and invaluable. It was a very challenging and stressful (although not necessarily intellectually stimulating) job. I was homesick for the College of Nursing. There were so many more things I wanted to know. So back I went.

My days as a doctoral student were among the hap-piest in my life. It was both the hardest and the most rewarding program I had undertaken. I also found out that I enjoy teaching, mainly because I like to talk about nursing and its place and the value it contributes in the real world. Over the past several years, I have become in-creasingly interested in nursing conceptual models and theories and their role in guiding nursing research, prac-tice, and education. Studying the various models has given me an appreciation of the values and philosophies of nursing, while enabling me to answer clearly the ques-tion, "What is it that nurses do, and why do they do it?" I hope the fascination never wanes.

INTRODUCTION

For individuals seeking a career in nursing, deciphering the various types of educational programs and the rela-tionship of each program type to future nursing practice can be daunting. Many types of programs at all levels pro-vide multiple pathways to one or more nursing credential. Chapter 1 describes the social, political, and economic forces that influenced the evolution of nursing as a pro-fession and the system of nursing education. This chap-ter analyzes the various educational opportunities with some considerations for selecting among the options. A brief historical overview of each type of program helps build greater understanding of the factors influencing nursing education. More important, this chapter high-lights the contributions each type of program provides for contemporary health care systems, advancement of the nursing profession, and promotion of a professional workforce dedicated to lifelong learning.

In 1965 the American Nurses Association (ANA) designated the baccalaureate degree as the educational entry point into professional nursing practice (ANA, 1965). Now, almost 50 years later, three educational pathways for registered nurse (RN) licensure still exist: baccalaureate, associate degree, and diploma programs (Figure 2-1). The existence of multiple pathways con-tributes to a confusing landscape of nursing education and creates challenges for aspiring nurses as they try to choose the most appropriate program in which to enter the profession. No matter which type of entry into practice program one chooses, "the demands placed on nursing in the emerging health care system are likely to require a greater proportion of RNs who are prepared beyond the associate degree or diploma level" (Pew Health Professions Commission, 1998, p. 64). With evidence supporting improved patient safety and out-comes related to the educational level of the nursing

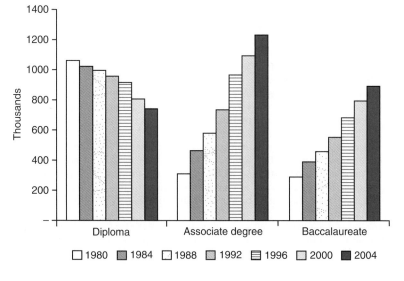

FIGURE 2-1 Initial nursing prepara-tion of the registered nurse population, 1980 to 2004. (From U.S. Department of Health and Human Services, Health Resources and Services Administra-tion. [2006]. Preliminary findings: 2004 national sample survey of registered nurses. [Online]. Retrieved from http://bhpr.hrsa.gov/healthworkforce/reports/rnpopulation/preliminaryfindings.htm.)

staff, serious attention is now focused on shifting the educational level of the professional nursing workforce to the baccalaureate level in earnest (Benner et al., 2009; Institute of Medicine [IOM], 2010). Employers are preferentially hiring nurses prepared at the baccalaureate level, particularly in hospital settings (AACN, 2013). In many cases employment of nurses prepared at the diploma or associates degree level includes a condition of continuing education so as to sustain employment. In short, nurses are asked to develop and implement a plan for obtaining the baccalaureate degree within a certain time frame, usually between 3 and 5 years. The landmark report issued by the Institute of Medicine in 2010, *The Future of Nursing*, calls for raising the number of baccalaureate-prepared nurses in the workforce to 80%, as well as doubling the number of nurses with doctoral degrees (IOM, 2010). The nursing education system is challenged to balance the goal of providing adequate numbers of new baccalaureate-prepared nurses while advancing the educational level of nurses who were initially prepared at the associate degree or diploma level.

HISTORY OF NURSING EDUCATION IN THE UNITED STATES

Diploma Programs

The first formal nursing education program in the United States was a 4-month hospital-based diploma program at the Boston Training School for Nurses at Massachusetts General Hospital. That program, established in 1873, was originally intended to emulate the apprenticeship model put forward by Florence Nightingale when she established collegiate nursing in London in 1860. Anti-collegiate forces prevailed, however, and the hospital-based diploma program became the predominant model for nursing education in the United States. The model, in fact, flourished for nearly a century and still exists today. At their peak in 1958, diploma programs numbered 944. At that time and during the decade that followed, diploma graduates constituted nearly the entire RN workforce. In 1963 the Surgeon General's Report indicated that 86% of working nurses were diploma graduates. The decline in the number of programs began in earnest in the 1960s and 1970s and continues even today. By 1993, 126 diploma programs existed in 26 states, with more than half of the programs in three states: Ohio, New Jersey, and Pennsylvania. In 2013, 47 accredited diploma programs remained in

16 states, and more than half of them were located in two states: Pennsylvania with 19 programs and New Jersey with 8 programs (Accreditation Commission for Education in Nursing [ACEN], 2014). Diploma programs are typically 2 to 3 years in length, and graduates are eligible to take the RN licensure examination (NCLEX-RN®), but do not earn a college degree at either the associates or baccalaureate level. As the length of diploma programs increased over the years from four months to three years, nursing students were increasingly used to meet hospital staffing needs rather than function in the student role. This exploitation of nursing students was addressed in several landmark studies of nursing and nursing education, and student life eventually became more compatible with sound educational practices. Many of these same studies also encouraged the profession to move its programs into collegiate settings (Brown, 1948; Goldmark & the Committee for the Study of Nursing Education, 1923) and to abandon the apprenticeship model. Ultimately, the high cost of these programs to students and to the hospitals that offered them, coupled with an increasing number of collegiate options, brought about the closure of many diploma programs.

Some diploma programs, rather than closing outright, began to align themselves with academic institutions. Others actually joined forces with academic institutions and began to offer joint degrees. Some became freestanding degree-granting institutions in their own right and now grant associate or baccalaureate degrees in nursing. These programs have been accredited by the regional accrediting body and have also achieved professional nursing accreditation from one of the specialized accrediting agencies.

Baccalaureate Degree Education

The first baccalaureate nursing program was established in the United States at the University of Minnesota in 1909. The baccalaureate phenomenon caught on slowly and did not gain much momentum until after World War II. Until the mid-1950s many baccalaureate programs were 5 years in length and consisted of 2 years of general education followed by 3 years of nursing academics and clinical practice. The main difference between the 3 years of nursing in baccalaureate and diploma programs was the inclusion of public health nursing as part of the baccalaureate curriculum. Eventually the nursing content in baccalaureate programs was strengthened and expanded.

The proliferation of baccalaureate programs was slowed by the paucity of faculty members qualified to teach in these programs. Although this was understandable given the relative youth of nursing in academic centers, it created reluctance on the part of college and university administrators to establish baccalaureate nursing programs. The programs that were established were often forced to hire nursing faculty who would not otherwise qualify for university faculty appointments. This deficit has taken several decades to correct itself, but nursing faculty teaching in baccalaureate programs today are for the most part bona fide members of their respective academic communities.

Most baccalaureate programs are now 4 academic years in length, and the nursing major is typically concentrated at the upper division level, although many programs provide core-nursing coursework throughout all 4 years. Graduates are prepared as generalists to practice nursing in beginning leadership positions in a variety of settings, and they are eligible to take the NCLEX-RN. To prepare nurses for this multifaceted role, several components are essential for all baccalaureate programs. These components are liberal education, quality and patient safety, evidence based practice, information management, health care policy and finance, communication/collaboration, clinical prevention/population health, and professional values (American Association of Colleges of Nursing [AACN], 2008). The number of BSN programs has continued to increase over the past several years. In 2013 the number was 846 (AACN, 2014a, p. 9).

Accelerated BSN Programs. As the nursing shortage gained national recognition during the 1980s and 1990s, accelerated BSN programs emerged to hasten the time to graduation for select groups of students. Some programs accept non-nurse college graduates, and the curriculum is designed for completion in less time than the traditional BSN program through a combination of "bridge" and transition courses. These programs are especially attractive for individuals desiring a career change. In 2013, 256 colleges and universities offered accelerated BSN prdograms for non-nurse college graduates (AACN, 2014a, p. 9). Accelerated BSN programs also serve as an important point of entry into professional nursing for those whose backgrounds are underrepresented in nursing, including men and individuals from racial and ethnic minorities. The Robert Wood Johnson Foundation established the New

Careers in Nursing scholarship program in 2008. This program was specifically designed to recruit individuals from under-represented groups (men and those from racial and ethnic minorities) into nursing through these accelerated programs. (http://www.newcareers-innursing.org/)

RN-BSN Track. The majority of baccalaureate programs admit both pre-licensure students and RNs who are graduates of diploma and associate degree nursing programs, but some programs admit only RNs. The general education requirements are the same for all students. Although some content in the RN track may be configured differently, both RN and pre-licensure students meet the same program objectives. Licensed practical nurses (LPNs) may also be given credit for prior learning when they enroll in baccalaureate programs. The baccalaureate in nursing degree is the most common requirement for admission to graduate nursing programs, but it is not the only route to graduate nursing education.

The RN-BSN track or option in the baccalaureate program is designed to recognize and reward prior learning and to capitalize on the characteristics of the adult learner. Several models of awarding academic credit to RNs for prior education and experience exist to facilitate educational mobility. These include direct transfer of credits, credits awarded by examination, variable credits awarded after portfolio review of educational and professional experiences, the holding of lower division nursing credits in "escrow" until completion of the program, and a number of other innovative models. This reflects the AACN's assertion that "educational mobility options should respect previous learning that students bring to the educational environment … and build on knowledge and skills attained by learners prior to their matriculation" (AACN, 1998, p. 1). In 2013 there were 668 RN-BSN programs offered nationwide (AACN, 2014a, p. 9).

Vocational Education

Practical/vocational nurse programs started in 1942 in response to the acute shortage of licensed nurses in the United States created by World War II. Because of the dramatic influx of RNs into the various military branches, U.S. hospitals were largely staffed by nurse's aides, volunteers, and other unlicensed personnel. Practical/vocational nurse programs were established to provide some formal training for those who were entering the nursing workforce with little or no knowl-edge about nursing care and few, if any, nursing skills. The programs eventually led to a new kind of licensure for nurses, namely, licensed practical nurse/licensed vocational nurse (LPN/LVN). The license is awarded by the state board of nursing after the graduate has passed the NCLEX-PN® examination.

LPN/LVN programs are typically located in techni-cal or vocational education settings. Programs are 9 to 15 months long, require proof of high school gradua-tion or its equivalent for admission, and are designed to prepare graduates to work with RNs and be supervised by them. Programs lead to a certificate of completion and eligibility to take the NCLEX-PN. More than 2000 state-approved practical/vocational nursing programs currently exist in the United States (NCSBN, 2014). Because many courses taken by practical nurse students do not carry academic credit, these programs do not always articulate well with collegiate nursing programs. Associate degree programs, however, often have proce-dures for accommodation of practical nurses into their programs by way of advanced placement.

Associate Degree Education

In 1952 the associate degree in nursing (ADN) became another program option for those desiring to become RNs. Designed by Mildred Montag, these programs were intended to be a collegiate alternative for the prep-aration of technical nurses and a response to the nurs-ing shortage (Haase, 1990). In 1958 the W. K. Kellogg Foundation funded a pilot project at seven sites in four states. The success of the pilot project led to a phe-nomenal growth of associate degree programs in the United States. These programs multiplied in commu-nity colleges and also began to appear at 4-year colleges and universities. By 1973 approximately 600 associate degree programs existed in the United States. Today almost 1400 state-approved associate degree nursing programs exist (NCSBN, 2014).

Associate degree nursing programs are designed to be 2 years in length and consist of basic general edu-cation requirements necessary for entry into clinical nursing courses, all of which carry academic credit. Associate degree nursing programs prepare technical bedside nurses for secondary care settings, such as com-munity hospitals and long-term health care facilities. Montag's intent was for nurses with associate degrees to work under the direction of registered professional

nurses who were prepared at the baccalaureate level. Some confusion arose about roles and relationships, and by the time the first groups of students had gradu-ated from ADN programs, they were declared eligible for the RN licensure examination, as were their BSN-prepared counterparts, an eligibility that graduates of these programs retain today. The degree most often awarded on completion of the associate degree pro-gram is the ADN. A few institutions award the associate of arts in nursing (AAN) degree.

Master's Degree Education

While the establishment of associate and baccalaure-ate degree nursing programs was proceeding, master's programs were beginning to emerge on university campuses. The need for nursing faculty to teach in all the new and developing nursing education programs was apparent. Interest in master's-prepared nurses also surged in the service sector as the roles of clinical nurse specialists, nurse practitioners, nurse anesthe-tists, nurse midwives, and nurse administrators became more clearly defined.

Master's education in nursing traces its origins to 1899, when Teachers College in New York began to offer graduate courses in nursing management and nursing education. However, master's programs did not begin to escalate and become nationally visible until the late 1950s and early 1960s. The first programs were strong on role preparation for administration and teaching but light on advanced nursing content. This was not sur-prising because the nurses teaching in these programs did not themselves hold graduate degrees in nursing. As advanced nursing content became more clearly defined, and as increasing numbers of nursing faculty became proficient at teaching, strong advanced nursing content became the prevailing characteristic of master's pro-grams in nursing. Role preparation received less atten-tion as clinical emphasis increased, and by the 1990s advanced practice became the predominant focus for most master's degree programs. The expanding author-ity of advanced practice nurses (APNs) to serve as autonomous providers of care requires the education of the clinicians be sound and consumers of APN care be able to have confidence in the quality of the educational experience (Booth & Bednash, 1994).

Master's programs in nursing are typically 1 to 2 years of full-time study and are built on the baccalaure-ate nursing major. The program content includes a set of graduate-level foundational (core) courses, including a research component and clinical specialty courses. Other recommended core content areas include clinical prevention and population health for improving health; interprofessional collaboration for improving patient and population health outcomes; health policy and advocacy; informatics and health care technologies; translating and integrating scholarship into practice; quality improvement and safety; organizational and systems leadership; and finally a background in science from the sciences and humanities. For specialty tracks that prepare APNs, an additional clinical core consists of advanced pathophysiology, pharmacology, and advanced health/physical assessment; and clinical specific courses (AACN, 2011).

Master's degree programs in nursing have experienced phenomenal growth over the past several decades. In 1973 only 86 such programs existed. In 2014 there are 483 master of science in nursing (MSN)-accredited programs, a notable fact in light of the recent dramatic growth in new Doctor of Nursing Practice programs (ACEN, 2014; Commission on Collegiate Nursing Education [CCNE], 2014). Master's degree programs currently are offered in all states and territories of the United States.

RN-MSN and Non-Nurse Master's Entry Options.
The bachelor of science in nursing (BSN) degree or its equivalent is usually a requirement for admission to a master's program in nursing, but several interesting models that accommodate other types of students have emerged. Some master's programs admit RNs without a baccalaureate degree or with a baccalaureate degree in another field into a streamlined track that includes both baccalaureate and master's level courses. Other programs admit students who are not nurses at all. Approximately 155 RN-MSN programs are in existence nationwide (AACN, 2014a, p.13).

The impetus for opening admissions to other types of students was the recognition of the kinds of students who were applying in significant numbers to associate degree and baccalaureate nursing programs. Frequently non-nurses with baccalaureate or graduate degrees in other fields were seeking admission to basic nursing programs. RNs from associate degree and diploma programs who had completed baccalaureate degrees in fields other than nursing were applying for admission to baccalaureate nursing programs to present the appropriate credential for admission to

a master's program in nursing. These students brought a rich and diversified background to their educational programs and were highly motivated, self-directed adult learners with a strong and clearly defined career orientation. Some of these students were well served by an accelerated second baccalaureate degree offered by several institutions, but master's programs could clearly accommodate them and take them to the master's level in educationally sound and cost-effective ways.

Master's programs in nursing that admit non-nurse college graduates and RNs without a baccalaureate degree in nursing take the necessary steps to ensure that both groups complete whatever undergraduate or graduate prerequisite courses are needed to acquire the equivalent of a baccalaureate nursing major. They then pursue the same graduate-level foundational, specialty, and cognate courses required of master's students; thus they exit the program having met the same program objectives that all graduates of both programs must meet. Non-nurses are eligible to take the NCLEX-RN examination on completion of the generalist or baccalaureate equivalent portion of the program or at program completion. In 2013, 155 MSN for nurses with non-nursing college degrees and 145 MSN for non-nursing college graduates (2nd degree programs) existed (AACN, 2014a, p.13).

Dual Degree Programs.
Another option regarding master's programs in nursing is the joint program leading to two master's degrees awarded simultaneously. This type of program is especially relevant for nurses seeking administrative positions that require both advanced nursing knowledge and business management skills. Several joint program models now exist across the country, reflecting nursing's responsiveness to documented student need and interest, as well as demonstrating nursing's ability to collaborate with other academic disciplines. Among the available programs in conjunction with the master's degree in nursing are the master's degree in business administration (MSN/MBA), master's degree in public administration (MSN/MPA), master's degree in public health (MSN/MPH), master's degree in divinity (MSN/MDiv), master's degree in juris doctor (MSN/JD), and master's degree in hospital administration (MSN/MHA). Degree candidates must be admitted to both programs and must fulfill requirements for both programs. However, requirements common to both programs may be consolidated. In 2013, 104 such programs were in

existence, with several more in development (AACN, 2014a, p.13).

Clinical Nurse Leader Program. In 2004 a new nursing role emerged, the clinical nurse leader (CNL), a master's-prepared nurse who "oversees the care coordination of a distinct group of patients and actively provides direct patient care in complex situations" (AACN, 2005b, p. 1). The concept was developed in collaboration with leaders from education and practice settings. The AACN (2003) further describes the CNL role: "Along with the authority, autonomy, and initiative to design and implement care, the CNL is accountable for improving individual care outcomes and care processes in a quality cost-effective manner" (p. 7). The CNL role differs from advanced practice nursing roles in that the CNL is a generalist and not a specialist, as are nurse practitioners and clinical specialists. A more in-depth presentation of the role and expectations of the CNL can be found in the White Paper on the Role of the CNL (AACN, 2007). Approximately 100 schools of nursing partnering with almost 200 health care delivery organizations in 35 states and Puerto Rico were involved in a pilot project to develop the CNL role, integrate it into the health care system, and evaluate the outcomes. In 2013 there were 94 schools admitting students into CNL programs, and more than 3000 nurses who had achieved CNL certification (AACN, 2014a, p.14).

A number of master's programs in nursing across the United States have multiple entry options such as those described in this chapter, and more are being developed as adult learners from diverse backgrounds migrate toward nursing. The degree most often awarded on completion of a master's degree program is the master of science in nursing degree (MSN). At least 90% of nursing master's degrees are MSN degrees. Other degree designations include the master's degree in nursing (MN), master of science degree with a major in nursing (MS), and master of arts degree with a major in nursing (MA). The degree designation is more a matter of institutional policy than a reflection of program type or content. In fact no substantive distinction can be made among these various degree designations for master's-level nursing programs.

Doctoral Education

As might be expected, given nursing's relative youth in academe, the profession has only recently carved out a major doctoral presence in the academic community.

Until 1970 less than a dozen doctoral programs with a major in nursing existed across the United States. Most nurses who earned doctoral degrees did so in related disciplines such as sociology, anthropology, education, psychology, or physiology. In 1983, 27 doctoral programs in nursing existed. By 1990, only 7 years later, their number had nearly doubled. As the movement toward the practice doctorate gained momentum, the number of doctoral programs in nursing increased rapidly. In 2010 the landmark Institute of Medicine report on the Future of Nursing recommended that the number of nurses with a doctorate be doubled by 2020 (IOM, 2010). In 2013 the number of doctoral programs more than doubled to 374, primarily because of the advent of doctor of nursing practice (DNP) programs, with 133 programs delivering the PhD, and 241 delivering the DNP (AACN, 2014b). At present two pathways to the doctoral degree in nursing can be taken: research-focused programs (doctor of philosophy or PhD) and practice-focused programs (doctor of nursing practice or DNP). As is evident from their titles, these programs have different emphases.

Research-Focused Programs. The degree most commonly awarded for the research-focused doctorate in nursing is the doctor of philosophy (PhD) with a major in nursing. Other degrees awarded include the doctor of nursing science (DNS or DNSc) and the doctor of science in nursing (DSN), although with the advent of the doctor of nursing practice (DNP) (see the following section), these are slowly being phased out. The varying degree designations do not necessarily distinguish one program from another in terms of content, rigor, or research emphasis, but some programs may have a heavier clinical emphasis than others. In most instances the degree designation is specified for the discipline by the institution that awards the degree. Although some are still questioning nursing's readiness to join the doctoral community of scholars, the profession is quietly preparing an array of scholars and researchers whose contributions to the health and nursing literature are qualitatively and quantitatively impressive.

Most research-focused doctoral programs admit students with an MS degree, but a few admit students with a BSN. These programs range in length from three to five years of full-time study or that equivalent in part-time work. The curriculum includes advanced content in concept and theoretical formulations and testing, theoretical analyses, advanced nursing, supporting cognates, and in-depth research. The culminating requirement for the degree is the completion and defense of the doctoral dissertation. In 2013, 133 research-focused doctoral programs maintained an enrollment of more than 5000 students, and graduated more than 600 students, a trend that has remained stable and shows steady growth over time (AACN, 2014a, p. 9, 13, 25 and 47).

Practice-Focused Programs. The clinical practice doctorate in nursing is the DNP. Conceptualized as the highest degree for nursing practice, the DNP program prepares graduates to identify emerging clinical patterns and problems within a practice setting; synthesize data, information, and knowledge for developing evidence based practice care regimens; demonstrate advanced levels of clinical judgment, cultural sensitivity, and systems thinking; and work collaboratively with other health professionals, consumers, and policy makers (AACN, 2005b). As noted by Edwardson (2004), "the graduates of these programs will not represent a point on a continuum between researchers and practitioners but rather will be highly specialized practitioners of the profession engaged in either direct or indirect clinical activities" (p. 44).

Rather than focusing on the generation of new knowledge, practice-focused doctoral programs emphasize the translation and application of new knowledge to practice. Thus students in these doctoral programs are encouraged to develop projects grounded in clinical practice as opposed to creating new knowledge or science. In 2005 only 10 DNP programs existed. In 2014 the number of accredited DNP programs remains steady at 162 (AACN, 2014a; ACEN, 2014), with many more programs in various stages of development and implementation. In 2013, 240 DNP programs exist nationally, with many of these pursuing initial accreditation (AACN, 2014a, p. 13). The rapid increase in the number of DNP programs is a response to the AACN position that by 2015 the education of APNs should be moved from the master's to the doctoral level (AACN, 2014b).

An earlier model of practice-focused doctoral education was the nursing doctorate (ND). First conceptualized by Rozella Schlotfeldt as analogous to medical, dental, and legal models of education, the ND program was designed to prepare graduates for licensure and professional practice in their field (Schlotfeldt, 1978).

According to Jones and Lutz (1999), "an ND is a clinically focused degree that emphasizes research utilization (not generation) in patient care and health care policy. The goal for ND programs is to produce highly specialized practitioners for practice, teaching, consultation, and management" (p. 246).

The first ND program was established in 1979 at the Frances Payne Bolton School of Nursing, Case Western Reserve University. This 4-year program admitted students with a baccalaureate degree in another field; on completion of the generalist component of the program they were eligible to take the NCLEX-RN. As part of the academic program, students also acquired an advanced practice specialty. This program model did not enjoy much growth. With the emergence of the DNP described in the preceding paragraphs, ND programs made the transition to the DNP model.

To put the various educational programs in perspective, a comparison of their characteristics is presented in Table 2-1. The changes in the highest educational preparation of the nursing workforce from 1977 to 2004 are presented in Figure 2-2.

CONSIDERATIONS IN SELECTING A NURSING EDUCATION PROGRAM

A number of considerations influence an individual's choice in selecting either a basic or a graduate-level nursing program. Perhaps among the most important are cost to the student, quality of the program, and accessibility. Refer to student-consumer portals where selective schools pay to advertise, such as www.allnursingschools.com and www.aacn.nche.edu, or membership associations for colleges of nursing for additional information.

Cost

Colleges, national summary documents, and public libraries provide relevant cost information on public and private institutions that offer nursing education programs. From this information some generalizations can be made. First, state-supported community or junior colleges tend to be less expensive than state-supported 4-year colleges and universities. Second, state-supported institutions of higher education usually give a substantial tuition reduction to in-state students. Third, state- or government-supported higher

TABLE 2-1   Comparison of Nursing Education Programs by Year Established

	DIPLOMA PROGRAMS	BACCALAUREATE PROGRAMS	PRACTICAL/VOCATIONAL NURSE PROGRAMS	ASSOCIATE DEGREE PROGRAMS	MASTER'S PROGRAMS	RESEARCH-FOCUSED DOCTORAL PROGRAMS	PRACTICE-FOCUSED DOCTORAL PROGRAMS
Year established	1873	1909	1942	1952	Late 1950s	1960s	1979 (ND) 2004 (DNP)
Location	Hospitals	4-Year colleges and universities; a few in community colleges	Vocational/technical schools	Community, junior, or 4-year colleges and universities	Universities and colleges	Universities and colleges	Universities and colleges
Accessibility	Limited; phasing out by converting to degree programs (AD and BS)	Universal; all states, most cities; some are RN-BSN only	Universal; all states, most cities;	Universal; all states, almost all cities;	Very good; 475 programs with at least 1 in every state	Somewhat limited; 133	Somewhat limited but increasing rapidly as APRN programs convert to DNP
Length	2–3 years	4 years	9–15 months	2 years	1–2 years for full-time post-baccalaureate BSN-prepared nurses; additional work for other types of students	3–5 years post-master's; 4–5 years post-baccalaureate	3–4 years post-baccalaureate; 2–3 years post-master's
Cost	A few hundred dollars per term	Highly variable; a few thousand to several thousand dollars per year	Minimal; mostly books and cost of living	Reasonable in state or other public colleges; a few hundred to a few thousand dollars per year	Variable; several hundred to several thousand dollars per term	Several thousand dollars per term	Several thousand dollars per term
Purpose	Prepare clinically competent bedside nurses	Prepare professional nurse generalists for acute care settings, community-based practice, and beginning leadership/management positions	Prepare assistive licensed nurse workers	Prepare competent technical bedside nurses for secondary care settings	Prepare nurse generalists (CNLs) or APNs in a clinical specialty	Prepare leaders for education, administration, clinical practice, and research	Prepare clinically adept APNs for leadership positions in clinical settings
Advanced placement or acceleration opportunities	For LPNs or LVNs	For LPNs/LVNs or RNs from diploma and associate degree nursing programs	None	For LPNs or LVNs	For non-nurse college graduates, RNs with degrees in other fields, some RNs without degrees	For BSNs (limited number of programs)	Varies by program
Degree/certificate	Diploma	BSN	Certificate of completion	ADN (usually) or AAN	MSN (most common) or MN, MS, MA	PhD (most common) or DSN, DNS, DNSc, EdD	DNP
License eligibility	RN	RN (if not already licensed)	LPN/LVN	RN	RN if unlicensed at entry	Not applicable	Not applicable
Certification eligibility	None	Limited	None	None	Multiple	None	Multiple

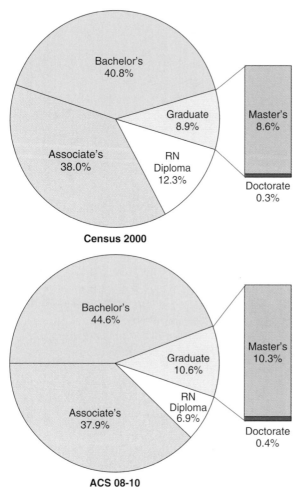

Census 2000

Bachelor's 40.8%

Graduate 8.9%

Master's 8.6%

Associate's 38.0%

RN Diploma 12.3%

Doctorate 0.3%

ACS 08-10

Bachelor's 44.6%

Graduate 10.6%

Master's 10.3%

Associate's 37.9%

RN Diploma 6.9%

Doctorate 0.4%

FIGURE 2-2 RN Workforce Education: Highest degree held by RNs, Census 2000 and American Community Survey (ACS) 2008 to 2010. (From Health Resources and Services Administration, Bureau of Health Professions National Center for Health Workforce Analysis. [2013]. The U.S. Nursing Workforce: Trends in supply and education. [Online]. Retrieved from http://bhpr.hrsa.gov/healthworkforce/reports/nursingworkforce/nursingworkforcefullreport.pdf.)

education is almost always significantly less expensive than private education, but this fact should not deter investigation of private institutions because of the availability of financial aid.

Financial Assistance. Financial aid packages at most institutions are somewhat commensurate with actual costs. Assistance can take the form of scholarships, loans, work-study appointments, employment opportunities within the institution, assistantships, tutoring assignments, or some combination of these or other options. Many of these options are no longer limited to full-time students. Financial assistance awards may be based on scholarship, need, competitive performance, or a combination of two or more of these factors. Financial support may be, and in most cases should be, sought from more than one source. Although most financial assistance awards are administered and awarded by the institution, a variety of packages are available from community- or government-based agencies and organizations. Examples of such agencies include state and local governments, the military, chambers of commerce, minority organizations, churches, community clubs, and local or state chapters of health-related organizations (e.g., March of Dimes, American Red Cross, and American Heart Association). Financial institutions may have attractive student loan packages. Local hospitals and other health care agencies often sponsor or support nursing students in exchange for a commitment from the student to work for the sponsoring agency for a specified period of time after graduation.

To determine how entry-level nursing students financed their education, a study was conducted with a national sample of 496 students (Norman et al., 2005). Financial aid was the major source of funding for 32% of the students, followed by parental support (18%), personal savings (16%), government loans (15%), institutional scholarships (8%), and bank loans (5%). Many students also held part-time jobs. The researchers postulated that nursing students may not be aware of or have a full understanding of the benefits of federal student loan programs, which may forgive a portion of the balance each year in exchange for working in an underserved area or teaching in a school of nursing. Significant financial resources are available to support students in their nursing education, and additional information is readily available on major websites, including the ANA, AACN, and NLN. Nursing program administrators also assist students in identifying sources of financial aid beyond what is available from the institution.

Quality

Issues of program quality relate to the quality of the educational program itself, as well as the eligibility of its graduates to become licensed or certified. Regarding program quality, how are prospective students protected from program mediocrity? And how is the public protected from low-quality nursing practice, which can frequently be traced to low-quality programs?

The public is protected by licensure and certification procedures that ensure a standardized level of competence. The student is protected from marginal programs by institutional accreditation through regional accrediting bodies, specialized accreditation of the nursing program(s) by the Commission on Collegiate Nursing Education (CCNE) or the Accreditation Commission for Education in Nursing (ACEN), and approval from the legal regulatory body for programs preparing for licensure, specifically the respective state boards of nursing. Appropriate questions to ask about the quality of nursing programs include the following:

- Is the parent institution accredited by the appropriate regional accrediting body?
- Is the nursing program unconditionally approved by the state board of nursing and fully accredited by a professional accrediting agency (if eligible)?
- What is the usual pass rate for first-time writers of the licensure examination from the school or program of interest?
- Is the faculty appropriately credentialed for the area of responsibility?
- Is each faculty member certified in his or her clinical specialty, if appropriate?
- Are graduates of the program eligible for the appropriate certification examination for the program being pursued?
- Does the program have a troubled history regarding licensure examination performance, accreditation, or state approval?

Specialized Accreditation. Major changes in the accreditation of nursing education programs have occurred in the past 15 years. Until 1999 the National League for Nursing (and subsequently, the NLNAC) was the specialized accrediting body for all nursing programs, LPN/LVN through master's degree. In 2000 the CCNE was approved by the Department of Education as an official accrediting agency for baccalaureate and graduate nursing education programs, thus offering a choice of accrediting agencies for those programs. In 2013 ongoing dispute between the NLN and the NLNAC led to severing ties between the two organizations and the creation of the ACEN (ACEN, 2014). Because accreditation is a voluntary process, programs

are not required to seek professional accreditation to continue to operate (although all programs must be approved by their respective state boards of nursing). Virtually all baccalaureate and master's programs are accredited by either the CCNE or ACEN. Students should recognize that attending a non-accredited program may limit access to federal loans and scholarships. In addition, most graduate schools will accept only students who have earned degrees from accredited schools.

In the past, when a master's program received accreditation by a specialized accrediting body, the accreditation covered all specialties that were offered within the master's program. However, when a nurse-midwifery program was one of the options in the master's program, even though it was covered by master's program accreditation, separate specialized accreditation for the nurse-midwifery program was sought from the American College of Nurse Midwives so that graduates of that program could take the midwifery license/certification examination and therefore practice as nurse-midwives. Now nurse anesthesia programs have been upgraded from diploma or certificate programs to master's-level programs. Although many nurse anesthesia programs are accredited as one of the offerings within the master's program, these programs also seek and receive specialized accreditation from their specialty organization, the American Association of Nurse Anesthetists. This practice will continue so that nurse anesthetists are eligible for the credentials that enable them to practice their specialty. Other nursing specialties may possibly seek programmatic accreditation that goes beyond the broader accreditation that the ACEN or CCNE makes available. This movement is closely tied to the increasing emphasis on specialty certification and the organizations in the best position to provide it. Persons pursuing advanced specialty preparation need to monitor this issue with vigilance.

Certification. The certification of individual nurses is a growing quality-control activity being implemented by a variety of nursing and nursing-related organizations. Certification is directed toward attesting to or endorsing the demonstrated knowledge base and clinical practice behaviors associated with high-quality performance in an area of specialization.

Certification protects the public by enabling anyone to identify competent people more readily. Simultaneously it aids the profession by encouraging and recognizing professional achievement. Certification also recognizes specialization, enhances professionalism and, in some cases, serves as a criterion for financial reimbursement (American Nurses Credentialing Center [ANCC], 2009). This movement is a very important one for the profession. Initiatives are in place to make eligibility and certification requirements more uniform, reduce duplicate or similar certification requirements among organizations, and match certification programs with the specialties being practiced.

Currently the American Nurses Credentialing Center (ANCC) (an arm of the American Nurses Association) offers nearly 40 certification examinations, 24 of which are for advanced practice in a variety of specialties. Fifteen baccalaureate and/or associate degree/diploma level certification examinations in selected clinical specialties are also available. In addition, examinations for nursing case management, ambulatory care nursing, and pain management are offered (ANCC, 2014). The Commission on Nurse Certification, an autonomous arm of the AACN, offers the certification exam for the CNL.

Other certification examinations are offered by a variety of nursing specialty organizations. Some certifications are highly specialized in such areas as addiction, diabetes, neuroscience, nephrology, ophthalmology, perioperative nursing, oncology, critical care, and occupational health. Many nursing specialty organizations that offer certification examinations are members of the American Board of Nursing Specialties. This board has a national peer-review program that sets standards for certification and approves certification programs. All certification efforts are designed to recognize the competence of nurses in specific areas and to protect the public from unsafe or uninformed nursing practice.

Accessibility: Distance Education

To improve accessibility in terms of geographic location and scheduling of classes, some nursing programs offer all or part of their curriculum through distance education technologies. Distance or distributive education is a method of teaching and learning that takes place outside the traditional classroom setting. Often students are in locations that are remote from the site where the course is taught. A variety of technologies are used to deliver education at a distance, including interactive television, e-mail and facsimile transmissions, and Internet-based courses with real-time interactive chat

rooms. Students learn in either a synchronous format (at the same time as their peers) or in an asynchronous format (independent of their peers). Less-sophisticated and readily available technologies include audiocassettes, videotapes, and CD-ROM media. The potential benefits of distance education were recognized by the AACN (1999): "Careful use of technology in education may well enhance the profession's ability to educate nurses for practice, prepare future nurse educators, and advance nursing science in an era when the number of professional nurses, qualified nurse faculty, and nurse researchers is well below national need" (p. 3).

As this movement gains momentum in nursing education, a number of issues need to be addressed, including the following:

- What is the effect of distance education on the cost and quality of the program?
- What equipment is needed by both the teacher and learner to maximize distance learning?
- What impact does distance education have on the process of professional socialization/formation?
- How can teaching strategies best match learner needs?
- What policies exist to clarify intellectual property rights and the use of copyrighted material in distance education courses?
- What effect, if any, does distance education have on student financial aid support?

The answers to these questions will likely challenge traditional assumptions about the effectiveness of various teaching-learning strategies and their relationship to program quality. A further discussion of distance learning occurs in Chapter 10.

OBSERVATIONS AND ANALYSIS

Many have argued that regardless of the reasons, the system of nursing education to both gain entry into the profession as well as advance within the profession is chaotic, confusing, and redundant. Some hold out for the day when there will be only one way to become a nurse, only one degree to be obtained, only one license to be acquired, and only one way to be approved and recognized as a specialist. That, after all, is the way medicine, dentistry, pharmacy, and law do it. Can nursing look to any more likely professions for modeling and emulation? Probably not.

But consider for a moment how different the evolution of medicine has been. Consider the venerable age of the profession. Consider how readily and completely the European model for medical education was transplanted unchanged to the United States. Consider the unquestioned dominance of the medical profession in the United States from the time the health care system was first defined until it began to crumble. And now that it is crumbling, consider the serious criticism being leveled at the medical profession—criticism about education, practice, costs, and societal insensitivities. Medical reform is being demanded by the federal and state governments, consumers, and the profession itself. And this reform must be conducted and completed by those who entered that profession in good faith and with a set of information-based expectations they thought would last a lifetime. This state of affairs is by no means an indictment of the medical profession or the majority of its members. It is, instead, an example of what can happen when the status quo is unquestioned, when a service profession loses touch with its constituencies, and when hard questions are not answered because they are not asked.

Wherever the nursing education system is right now, it is clearly in a better place than many of its other health profession counterparts. Nursing does not necessarily need to look to other health professions to take the right cues or develop the right models. Rather, it needs to look within itself to examine what has been created; to retain, build on, and reconfigure as needed that which is good; to abandon or revamp that which is no longer germane; to clarify ambiguities; to underline uniqueness; to stay in touch with its consumers; and to continue the trend of the profession to embrace and participate fully in the higher-education academic community, enjoying, and benefiting from all the collegial and professional relationships that accrue from participation. Those, after all, are relationships that can only get better.

With those observations as a backdrop, an analysis of strengths, weaknesses, and areas needing attention is presented. The information is organized around program types and educational level.

Practical/Vocational Nurse Programs

Strengths. Programs are short, economical, and accessible. Programs prepare assistive nurse workers who are eligible to take the NCLEX-PN.

Weaknesses. Programs are not collegiate based. Graduates are not prepared to do what they are often called on to do in the workplace. Practical nurses are exploited and are frequently called on to perform functions beyond their legally defined scope of practice.

Recommendations. Elevate these programs to the community college level and award the associate's degree. Adjust enrollments downward to reflect market demands.

Diploma Programs

Strength. Programs prepare competent bedside nurses who are eligible to take the NCLEX-RN.

Weaknesses. Programs, for the most part, are not collegiate based, and nursing courses may not be readily transferable for educational advancement. In addition, they are expensive to operate.

Recommendation. Continue admirable and effective efforts to align with degree-granting institutions or become degree-granting as newly established academic institutions.

Associate Degree Programs

Strengths. Programs are offered in academic/collegiate settings and are affordable and accessible. Programs prepare competent technical bedside nurses who are eligible to take the NCLEX-RN.

Weaknesses. Some programs may require as many as 75 course credits and take three years or longer to complete (Nelson, 2002). Programs and their graduates go beyond the purposes and scope of the practice envisioned by the program founder. When combined with practical nurses, the total number of technical nurse types being produced is excessive given current and future market demands (Benner et al., 2009).

Recommendations. Collaborate with the LPN/LVN leadership to develop one program type that prepares the technical nurse, using what is most effective from both programs to bring about this outcome. Once the two programs have become one, assess the marketplace and consumer needs for this type of nurse and adjust the program output accordingly. Some states are exploring transitioning associate degree programs to the baccalaureate level. Community colleges are encouraged to partner with baccalaureate programs whenever possible to achieve this goal (AACN, 2005b).

Baccalaureate Programs

Strengths. Programs provide a solid liberal education and a substantive upper-division nursing major.

Both components are combined in ways that prepare a nurse generalist who is able to provide professional nursing services in beginning leadership positions in a variety of settings and who is eligible to take the NCLEX-RN. Programs are accessible and many accommodate RNs who are graduates of associate degree and diploma programs. Baccalaureate programs in nursing have been designated by the ANA as the entry point for professional practice (ANA, 1965) and this was reaffirmed by the Institute of Medicine (2010).

Weaknesses. The legal scope of practice for associate degree–prepared and baccalaureate-prepared nurses is undifferentiated because both groups are awarded the same license. This limits differentiated roles in work settings and hinders the reward system for leadership responsibilities.

Recommendations. Consider a different license for baccalaureate-prepared nurses. Give additional emphasis to health care costs, evidence based practice, management/delegation, health promotion/wellness care, and informatics in the curriculum (Speziale & Jacobson, 2005). Strive to reach the goal recommended by the National Advisory Council for Nursing Education that at least two thirds of the nursing workforce hold a baccalaureate or higher degree (Division of Nursing, 1996; IOM, 2010).

Master's Programs

Strengths. Programs are accessible and prepare graduates for advanced practice in a clinical specialty. Some of the programs admit non-nurse college graduates, RNs with baccalaureate degrees in other fields, and some RNs without baccalaureate degrees. Graduates of these programs are prepared to function as CNLs or engage in advanced practice nursing as nurse practitioners, clinical nurse specialists, nurse anesthetists, or nurse-midwives, as well as in other specialty practices.

Weaknesses. Non-nurses take the same licensure examination (NCLEX-RN) as associate degree and baccalaureate graduates. Certificate programs for master's-prepared nurses are not uniformly consistent in terms of eligibility requirements and examination rigor.

Recommendations. Collaborate with baccalaureate nurse educators and other interested professionals in bringing to fruition a different examination for professional nurses. Bring greater uniformity and meaning to certification programs. Monitor the status of transitioning advanced practice nursing education to the DNP.

Doctoral Programs in Nursing

Strengths. Programs prepare leaders and clinicians for responsible advanced positions in nursing education, nursing administration, nursing research, nursing practice, or some combination of these roles. Programs are fairly accessible compared with doctoral programs in other disciplines.

Weakness. Proliferation of research-focused programs may result in the use of some unqualified faculty members for program delivery.

Recommendations. Stabilize growth of research-focused programs at the current level so faculty can fine-tune their qualifications and participate more fully in the life of scholarship. Market the practice-focused doctorate as the preferred route to preparation for advanced practice nursing in the clinical setting.

IMPACT OF STUDIES OF THE PROFESSION

Throughout this chapter the history of nursing education has been traced from professional, organizational, regulatory, and institutional perspectives. The system has been described, analyzed, compared within itself, and presented for what it is and what it is becoming. One frame of reference not formally considered from the standpoint of impact or programmatic direction is that provided by the multiple studies published regarding nursing and nurses. Many such studies have been conducted by nurses, the federal government, and human behavior experts from other disciplines (e.g., sociology, anthropology). Results from all of these efforts by nurses and on behalf of nursing have been used to bring about improvements and needed change.

To analyze these studies and their impact on the evolution of nursing education would constitute a book in its own right. The analysis of nursing education that completes this chapter is presented without direct reference to these studies, while recognizing fully that these studies are quite directly related to what is and what will be in nursing education. The following studies are recommended to the reader for serious review:

- The Goldmark Report: Nursing and Nursing Education in the United States (1923)
- The Brown Report: Nursing for the Future (1948)
- The Lysaught Report: An Abstract for Action (1970)
- The Institute of Medicine reports: Nursing and Nursing Education: Public Policy and Private Ac-

tions (1983); Crossing the Quality Chasm: A New Health System for the 21st Century (2001); Health Professions Education: A Bridge to Quality (2003); The Future of Nursing: Leading Change, Advancing Health (2010)

- The Pew Health Professions Commission reports: Healthy America: Practitioners for 2005 (Sugars, O'Neil, & Bader, 1991) and Recreating Health Professional Practice for a New Century (Pew, 1998)
- Educating Nurses: A Call for Radical Transformation (Benner et al., 2009).

LOOKING TOWARD THE FUTURE

However nursing education programs are configured for the future, facets of the system must be retained that ensure continued and growing representation of the gender and cultural diversity that exists in American society. Efforts to attract ethnic and racial minorities and men to nursing must be intensified. Ethnic and racial minority enrollment in baccalaureate and graduate programs is showing a slight increase, and in 2013, accounts for 26.9% to 41.7% of student enrollments across BSN, MSN, and doctoral programs (AACN, 2014a). African-Americans represent the largest minority group (11%) in all levels of nursing education (AACN, 2014a, p. 21). Male nurses are still a minority, but their ranks are also increasing. In 2013 approximately 11.4% of baccalaureate students, 10.3% of master's students, and 8.7-11.3% of all doctoral students (research-focused, DNP, and post-doctoral) were male (AACN, 2014a).

Historically, transformations in nursing and nursing education have been driven by major socioeconomic factors, developments in health care, and professional issues unique to nursing. Trends to watch in terms of their potential impact on nursing education for the future are the following (Heller, Oros, & Durney-Crowley, 2000):

- The changing demographics and increasing diversity of society
- The technological explosion
- The globalization of the world's economy and society
- The era of the educated consumer, alternative therapies, genomics, and palliative care
- The shift to population-based care and the increasing complexity of client care
- The cost of health care and the challenge of managing and coordinating care
- The impact of health policy and regulation, including health care reform
- The growing need for interdisciplinary education for collaborative practice
- The current nursing shortage and opportunities for lifelong learning and workforce development
- Advances in nursing science and research

A system of nursing education that is responsive to society and maximizes career development of nurses and advancement of the profession must be maintained. Greater clarity and meaning must be brought to licensure and certification programs. And the kinds and numbers of nurses we educate to meet societal and professional needs must be monitored and controlled (Bellack & O'Neil, 2000). If this chapter conveys a message of endorsement and enthusiasm for the nursing profession and most components of its educational enterprise, a major outcome has been realized. Every reason exists to believe our successes will continue and our problems can be solved. Nursing is a profession in which exciting things are happening and the best is yet to come.

SUMMARY

This chapter has analyzed the various pathways to several types of nursing credentials and has offered considerations for choosing among those educational opportunities. The various pathways are linked to the historical social, political, and economic forces that influenced the development of nursing as a profession. The contributions of each pathway to our contemporary health system, the profession of nursing, and the professional workforce are highlighted. The existence of multiple educational pathways contributes to the confusion of aspiring nurses and the public. The health care system of the future will require a greater proportion of RNs prepared beyond the diploma or associate-degree level. This creates a challenge for the nursing education system to meet the demand for adequate numbers of baccalaureate-prepared nurses while advancing the educational level of nurses prepared at the diploma or associate-degree level. Additionally, nursing education programs must address the shifting demographics and diversity of our society; advances in science, technology, and care practices (e.g., genomics, palliative care, alternative therapies, collaborative practice, population based practice); globalization; health policy impacts; educated consumers; workforce shortages and lifelong learning needs; as well as advances in nursing science and research.

SALIENT POINTS

- Health care needs in society, along with certain historical events, influenced the development of multiple tracks of nursing education.
- Hospital-based diploma programs were the predominant model of nursing education in the United States for nearly 100 years.
- Although the first baccalaureate program in nursing was established in 1909, the development of significant numbers of these programs progressed slowly.
- Practical/vocational nursing programs were established to provide formal training for unlicensed personnel who, in large numbers, staffed U.S. hospitals during World War II.
- As a reaction to the vocational model of practical nursing, associate degree programs were established to educate technical nurses in collegiate programs.
- Master's programs prepare APNs, other nurse specialists, and CNLs to assume significant roles in a variety of health care settings.

- Practice-focused doctoral programs are designed to prepare graduates for the highest level of clinical nursing practice.
- Research-focused doctoral programs in nursing are designed to prepare scholars and researchers to expand the body of nursing knowledge.
- Cost and quality are two major considerations in selecting educational programs in nursing.
- Indicators of academic program quality include the status of program accreditation and approval, pass rates on licensure examinations, and pass rates on certification examinations.
- Although each nursing education program has unique strengths, each also has weaknesses to which attention must be given.
- The tapestry of nursing education has the potential to be affected by societal and professional trends and issues.

CRITICAL REFLECTION EXERCISES

1. Consider your current position in the "tapestry" of nursing education, then reflect and discuss potential opportunities for (a) your academic progression pathway, and (b) your personal lifelong learning strategy for advancement or maintenance of competency.

2. Given current trends in socioeconomic factors and developments in health care technology, the nursing profession's transformation, and nursing education, envision and discuss the potential impact these trends may have on your own nursing practice and career trajectory in the future.

REFERENCES

American Association of Colleges of Nursing. (1998). *Position statement on educational mobility*. Washington, DC: Author.

American Association of Colleges of Nursing. (1999). *Distance technology in nursing education*. Washington, DC: Author.

American Association of Colleges of Nursing. (2003). *Working paper on the role of the clinical nurse leader*. Retrieved from http://www.aacn.nche.edu/Publications/WhitePapers/ClinicalNurseLeader.htm

American Association of Colleges of Nursing. (2005a). *The essentials of doctoral education for advanced nursing practice*. Retrieved from http://www.aacn.nche.edu/DNP/pdf/Essentials5-06.pdf

American Association of Colleges of Nursing. (2005b). *Position statement on baccalaureate programs offered by community colleges*. Retrieved from http://www.aacn.nche.edu/Publications/positions/ccbsn.htm

American Association of Colleges of Nursing. (2007). *White paper on the education and role of the clinical nurse leader*. Retrieved from http://www.aacn.nche.edu/Publications/WhitePapers/ClinicalNurseLeader07.pdf

American Association of Colleges of Nursing. (2008). *Essentials of baccalaureate education for professional nursing practice*. Washington, DC: Author.

American Association of Colleges of Nursing. (2011). *Essentials of masters education for advanced practice nursing.* Washington, DC: Author.

American Association of Colleges of Nursing. November 25, 2013 [Press Release]. New AACN data confirms that Baccalaureate prepared nurses are more likely to secure jobs. Retrieved from http://www.aacn.nche.edu.

American Association of Colleges of Nursing. (2014a). *2013-2014 Enrollments and graduations in baccalaureate and graduate programs in nursing.* Washington, DC: Author.

American Association of Colleges of Nursing. (2014b). *Doctor of nursing practice.* Retrieved from http://www.aacn.nche.edu/Media/FactSheets/dnp.htm

Accreditation Commission for Education in Nursing. (2014). 2013-2014 ACEN Annual Report. Retrieved from http://www.acenursing.org

American Nurses Association. (1965). *Educational preparation for nurse practitioners and assistants to nurses: A position paper.* New York: ANA.

American Nurses Credentialing Center. (2009). *Frequently asked questions about ANCC certification.* Retrieved from http://www.nursecredentialing.org/FunctionalCategory/FAQ/CertiticationFAQs.aspx

American Nurses Credentialing Center. (2014). *ANCC nurse certification.* Retrieved from http://www.nursecredentialing.org/certification.aspx

Bellack, J., & O'Neil, E. H. (2000). Recreating nursing practice for a new century: Recommendations and implications of the Pew Health Professions Commissions final report. *Nursing and Health Care Perspectives,* *21*(1), 14–21.

Benner, P., Sutphen, M., Leonard, V., & Day, L. (2009). *Educating nurses: A call for radical transformation.* San Francisco: Jossey-Bass.

Booth, R. Z., & Bednash, G. (1994). *Syllabus: The newsletter of the American Association of Colleges of Nursing,* *20*(5), 2.

Brown, E. L. (1948). *Nursing for the future.* New York: Russell Sage Foundation.

Commission on Collegiate Nursing Education (CCNE). (2014). *Find accredited programs.* Retrieved from http://www.aacn.nche.edu/ccne-accreditation

Division of Nursing. (1996). *National Advisory Council on Nurse Education: Report to the Secretary of the Department of Health and Human Services.* Washington, DC: U.S. Government Printing Office.

Edwardson, S. R. (2004). Matching standards and needs in doctoral education in nursing. *Journal of Professional Nursing,* *20*(1), 40–46.

Goldmark, J., & The Committee for the Study of Nursing Education (1923). *Nursing and nursing education in the United States.* New York: Macmillan.

Haase, P. (1990). *The origins and rise of associate degree nursing education.* Chapel Hill, NC: Duke University Press.

Heller, B. R., Oros, M. T., & Durney-Crowley, J. (2000). The future of nursing education: 10 trends to watch. *Nursing and Health Care Perspectives,* *21*(1), 9–13.

Institute of Medicine. (1983). *Public policies and private actions.* Washington, DC: National Academy Press. [p.35]

Institute of Medicine. (2001). *Crossing the quality chasm: A new health system for the 21st century.* Washington, DC: National Academy Press. [p.35]

Institute of Medicine. (2003). *Health professions education: A bridge to quality.* Washington, DC: National Academy Press. [p.35]

Institute of Medicine. (2010). *The future of nursing: Leading change, advancing health.* Washington, DC: National Academies Press.

Jones, K. D., & Lutz, K. F. (1999). Selecting doctoral programs in nursing: Resources for students and faculty. *Journal of Professional Nursing, 15,* 245–252.

Lysaught, J. (1970). *An abstract for action.* New York: McGraw-Hill. [p.35]

National Council for State Boards of Nursing (NCSBN). (2014). *NCLEX Educational Program Codes.* Retrieved from https://www.ncsbn.org/NCLEX_Educational_Program_Codes.pdf

Nelson, M. A. (2002). *Education for professional nursing practice: Looking backward into the future.* Retrieved from http://www.nursingworld.org/ojin/topic18/tpc18_3.htm

Norman, L., Buerhaus, P. I., Donelan, K., McCloskey, B., & Dittus, R. (2005). Nursing students assess nursing education. *Journal of Professional Nursing, 21*(3), 150–158.

Pew Health Professions Commission. (1998). *Recreating health professional practice for a new century.* San Francisco: Author.

Schlotfeldt, R. M. (1978). The professional doctorate: Rationale and characteristics. *Nursing Outlook, 26,* 302–311.

Speziale, H. J. S., & Jacobson, L. (2005). Trends in registered nurse education programs 1998–2008. *Nursing Education Perspectives, 26*(4), 230–235.

Sugars, D. A., O'Neil, E. H., & Bader, J. D. (1991). *Healthy America: Practitioners for 2005. An agenda for action for U.S. health professional schools.* Durham, NC: The Pew Health Professions Commission.

U.S. Department of Health and Human Services, Health Resources and Services Administration. (2006). Preliminary findings: 2004 national sample survey of registered nurses. Retrieved from http://bhpr.hrsa.gov/healthworkforce/reports/rnpopulation/preliminaryfindings.htm

Beyond Professional Socialization

Karen J. Saewert, PhD, RN, CPHQ, CNE, ANEF

OBJECTIVES

At the completion of this chapter, the reader will be able to:

- Contrast professional socialization with professional identity formation.
- Discuss the key messages of the Institute of Medicine's report: *The Future of Nursing: Leading Change, Advancing Health* as it relates to professional identity formation.
- Engage in identifying personal commitments to advance professional identity formation.
- Reflect on a recent academic and/or professional learning experience and its impact on beliefs about self-development and professional engagement.

PROFILE IN PRACTICE

Gloria Adriana Perez, PhD, ANP-BC, FAAN

Assistant Professor and Southwest Borderlands Scholar; Co-Director, Hartford Center of Gerontological Nursing Excellence; John A. Hartford Foundation Claire M. Fagin Fellow.

The first professional nurse I ever met was my grandmother in Mexico. My sister, brother, and I spent every summer in Mexico from elementary school through high school. In the evenings I loved going with my aunt to pick up my grandmother at the hospital after her shift, and I fondly remember how she would interact with her co-workers—demonstrating respect, compassion, and wisdom. She wore her white uniform, her long hair was always pulled back, and her shoes were always clean. My grandmother would tell me that if I became a nurse, God would always have mercy on me. Indeed my grandmother was right.

I have been truly fortunate to have mentors at every stage of my professional development, starting with my grandmother. During my senior year of high school my English teacher gave us an assignment to examine our career choice. I researched nursing to better understand the demand for the profession, the work environment, the challenges of practicing nurses, and opportunities for advancement. I knew before I became a nurse that the work of nursing was demanding and that I could prepare to become a Registered Nurse through a community college or university educational pathway. I chose to stay in my hometown, Yuma, Arizona and attend the local community college to be close to family and save money so that I could work when I transferred to the university. I had a summer job before I started college, answering phones at the Arizona Department of Economic Security. I learned valuable skills about how to work with the public and communicate professionally. My mentor was an older gentleman with whom I shared my nursing research paper. He told me he thought I would make an excellent nurse because his wife and daughter were both nurses and I was intelligent and compassionate like they were. I was afraid to start college but he made me feel like I could do it.

I had several mentors in my associate degree program at Arizona Western College. I admired the faculty so much and was inspired by their professionalism. Both in the classroom and clinical setting, they were always prepared; serious, yet approachable. Their expectations were shared on the first day of our program—that this would only be a first step into our nursing career and we would all continue on to earn a Bachelor of Science degree in nursing. I developed close, supportive relationships with other students, forming strong beliefs in the power of peer-mentorship. Never one to have good study habits, my nursing peers invited me to study groups, and together we were successful. After my first year and summer semester I was licensed as a practical nurse and worked in a nursing home. My passion for the care of older adults began as a result of this experience. I knew that if I wanted to improve their care, I would need to reach my highest potential in nursing.

This realization motivated me to make an appointment to meet with a student advisor at Arizona State University (ASU)—my dream school. The college of nursing had a "minority recruiter" who spent time with me reviewing the necessary steps, courses, and resources available to me to complete by bachelor's degree at ASU. She confirmed what I had already experienced in my clinical rotations—there was a shortage of ethnic minority nurses! She told me that less than 3% of nurses were Hispanic and even less had advanced degrees or doctoral education. I was compelled to make a difference.

I transferred to ASU immediately upon graduation. Although I missed my family, I enjoyed my independence. As a new graduate the RN-BSN program introduced me to other nurses, most of us from small towns, although many had been practicing nurses for years. I knew that I eventually wanted to be a nurse practitioner, but financially I needed to work, save money, and apply for scholarships. While in the RN-BSN program I worked in a telemetry unit at St. Joseph's Hospital & Medical Center in Phoenix, Arizona. I chose a Catholic hospital because it reminded me of my grandmother. To this day I feel that some of the most valuable lessons I learned about professional nursing and leadership grew out of experiences at this hospital. I was promoted to supervisor after 3 years, a position that included formal leadership training and socialization with our executive nursing team. As a young nurse I worked with nurses who were mostly older than me. This practice extended into my own personal life. For the first time I joined a professional nursing organization—the National Association of Hispanic Nurses (NAHN)—and while nurses my age would get together for social events, I was having 1:1 "cafecitos" with the founders of the organization.

I still read the email I received while in the adult nurse practitioner program from one of my professors inviting me to work as a Graduate Research Assistant (GRA). She wanted me to be part of her research team on a study promoting physical activity among older adults with arthritis. Although there were tough days on the clinical unit, working as a GRA helped me to develop into a global thinker. I learned how to ask research questions based on what I experienced in the clinical setting. I wanted to know more about the lives of older Hispanic women because I saw them experience cardiovascular disease differently than other patients. I grew interested in keeping them healthy and figuring out the best way to approach the clinical problem from their perspective. As

a graduate student I had the opportunity to evolve my own thinking as I worked on my thesis, "The Cultural Meaning of Heart Health among Hispanic Women." During a research team meeting my faculty mentors began talking about my next step as a PhD student. Until that point I had not thought about life beyond my nurse practitioner program, but the way doctoral education was discussed seemed so attainable.

The best academic experience I had was in a new PhD in Nursing and Healthcare Innovation program at ASU—with only three of us in this first cohort, we received individualized attention. For the first time, I felt I could fully take advantage of the many socialization opportunities, interact with other doctoral students and faculty both within and outside of ASU, and attend research conferences. I made the time to immerse myself in the PhD student life, applying for research grants, writing, and strengthening my communication skills while actively conducting and presenting my research. I achieved some of my proudest accomplishments during this time. I was the first PhD student at the ASU College of Nursing and Health Innovation to be awarded both a National Institutes of Health/National Institute of Nursing Research Award and a National Hartford Center of Gerontological Nursing Excellence (NHCGNE) Patricia G. Archbold predoctoral scholarship. Although the financial support was significant, the training and mentorship I received annually during the NHCGNE Leadership Conference was key to my overall success. I had the honor of meeting and developing both personal and professional relationships with both senior mentors and more than 200 other alumni sponsored by the John A. Hartford Foundation. Although NAHN has always been my anchor professional organization, the Hartford Gerontological Nursing Leaders alumni group has been like a second family. I have access to top gerontological nursing scientists, leaders, and clinicians at some of the most prestigious universities in the country. My confidence, knowledge, and professionalism have grown leaps and bounds as a result. Although in many ways I feel like the impact I can have as a nurse—in education, practice, and research—is just beginning, I am excited to mentor the next generation of nurses. As President of the National Association of Hispanic Nurses in Phoenix, I am using my knowledge and skills to grow and strengthen a network of nurses who can advance the health of our diverse and growing community. My work in this area has propelled me forward, and provided opportunities to work with other prestigious teams and learn new skills in health policy while working with other disciplines, consumers, and policy makers. I am extending my professional growth and development in the direction of making meaningful contributions as a member of the national *Campaign for the Future of Nursing* at the *Center to Champion Nursing in America* and as an appointed board member of the *American Organization of Nurse Executives*. I remain excited and passionate about my future as a nurse!

INTRODUCTION

Knowledge, values, skills, behaviors, and norms relevant and appropriate to professional nursing practice are acquired over time through interactive and repetitive processes. Like any life experience, professional identity formation is a process, not an event, nested within everyday experience (Crigger & Godfrey, 2011). The processes of learning and incorporating aspects of a profession into one's professional identity are collectively termed *socialization.*

Nursing education is strong in ways of teaching that effectively assist students to develop a deep sense of professional identity, commit to the values of the profession, and act with ethical comportment (Benner, Sutphen, Leonard, & Day, 2010). As such, socialization begins in the basic nursing program educational setting and continues throughout one's professional nursing career. This process is reactivated at a number of junctures: (1) when a new graduate leaves the educational setting and begins professional nursing practice; (2) when an experienced nurse changes work settings, either within the same organization or in a new organization; and (3) when a nurse undertakes new roles, such as returning to school or assuming a leadership role. Whichever the juncture, socialization involves personal change, as a new professional self-identity is re-formed or re-defined. Consequently, nurses are either in the process of developing a growing sense of professional identity and flourishing or failing to expand their notion of professional identity (Crigger & Godfrey, 2011).

LOOKING BACK

Although historical continuity gives shape, context, and perspective to nursing's values and responsibilities as the largest group of health care providers in the health care arena (Fairman, 2012), new technologies and evolving roles demand continuous adaptation (Lai & Lim, 2012) and more autonomous practitioners (Eckhardt, 2002). However, it is important not to fail to *build* on the past in the rush toward innovation while at the same time let go of past difficulties (Lee & Fawcett, 2013) to help craft the message of what professional identity means in our field, and to clearly communicate what nurses do and how nurses contribute (Shekleton, 2012). Embracing new ideas will mean having the courage to let go of

familiar processes, which in turn may mean letting go of familiar tasks and roles so that patients receive the benefit of each nurse's professional role (Battié, 2013).

A robust understanding of the professional identity of nursing—both at the individual and disciplinary level—empowers nurses to (1) assume a professional identity that reflects a more responsible and equitable role, (2) challenge the traditional way nurses perceive themselves and are perceived by others, and (3) develop a more relevant notion of professional identity (Crigger & Godfrey, 2011). Nurses share a responsibility for understanding and communicating the direction that nursing and health care are taking, critical to nursing's visibility, credibility, clout, and momentum to lead (not follow) into the future (Cardillo, 2011). It is also crucial to the continuous development of the professional discipline of nursing that its members embrace not only their role as members of the professional discipline, but also embrace continuous changes in self, others, and the knowledge and practice of the discipline (Lee & Fawcett, 2013).

MOVING FORWARD

The Future of Nursing: Leading Change, Advancing Health is the second-largest comprehensive study of the nursing profession published by the Institute of Medicine (IOM) since 1983. It has had and will continue to have a profound effect on nursing education, practice, and research (Chard, 2013). Its key messages and related recommendations affirm and encourage professional nurses to practice fully, achieve higher levels of education, become full partners in providing and reforming health care, and develop an infrastructure for workforce data collection (IOM, 2010). This influential report provides the discipline of nursing with an exciting and historic opportunity to transform health care systems using the expertise and power of nurses and nursing (Shekleton, 2012) in calling for broad changes in the nursing profession for the benefit of society and patients, the ultimate recipients of these transformations (Thibault, 2011).

THE *NOW* FUTURE

As the information about *The Future of Nursing* report has been disseminated, it describes the future of nursing as *now*—situated in a health care world where nurses are not only significant, but essential in providing high-quality, safe, and patient-centered care (Fights, 2012). *Now* is the time to develop a more relevant notion of professional identity and bring forward words that better explain the contemporary view of nursing and collectively move us forward in responding to the recommendations (Crigger & Godfrey, 2011)

The IOM has identified nurses as key leaders in driving the reform and work to be done to reshape health care delivery in the United States. It is important that all nurses become educated and knowledgeable about this report, understand its implications for the future of the discipline, identify ways that individual nurses can get involved in implementing the recommendations, and educate others on what needs to be done (Battié, 2013; Shekleton, 2012).

STATE OF BEING TRANSFORMATION

Being a nurse professional is a dynamic process—one with many possibilities for action, influence, and transformation (Godfrey & Crigger, 2012). Although not exhaustive or exclusive, these possibilities include nurse as: *innovation catalyst, interprofessional collaborator, engaged stakeholder, expert learner, knowledge worker, agent of inquiry, voice for action, assimilator,* and/or *reflective practitioner.*

NURSE AS INNOVATION CATALYST

Nurses, with the capacity for lifelong and expert learning, are preparing for new challenges and opportunities by moving beyond the *process* of professional socialization to *learning* that promotes new capabilities to *see, do,* and *be* anchored in the fundamental purposes of nursing. For true innovation to occur within the context of complexity and rapid change, old ways of thinking and acting must also radically change (Shekleton, 2012).

NURSE AS INTERPROFESSIONAL COLLABORATOR

Interprofessional education is one strategy to strengthen nursing education and enhance the role of nurses as collaborative leaders in the health care system. For nurses to practice at the highest level for which they are educated, for there to be uniformly high standards

for nursing education, and for nurses to successfully partner with physicians and other health professionals in redesigning our health care system, then rigorous, structured interprofessional education experiences can be one of the tools used in accomplishing these goals (Thibault, 2011).

Improved systems are frequently the result of collaboration among health care professionals who are first committed to improving their own practice; accordingly, insights into improved systems begin in a nurse's own practice (Armstrong & Sherwood, 2012). The increased complexity of providing patient care demands an educational process that includes how to "be" a nurse in an interprofessional environment, develops the nurse's ability to make clinical judgments, uses and coordinates interdisciplinary approaches to care, yet focuses on the specific needs of the patient (Fights, 2012). It is in the "being" that nurses have the voice and strength of advocacy and systems-level change and the capacity to serve as champions for patient-, family-, and community-based perspectives in an interprofessional environment (Bleich, 2013).

NURSE AS EXPERT LEARNER, KNOWLEDGE WORKER, AND AGENT OF INQUIRY

Many students entering RN-BSN programs already have a strong sense of clinical competence and a variety of diverse practice-based experiences but may enroll without a clear understanding of nursing as a professional discipline and what it means to be a member of a professional discipline (Lee & Fawcett, 2013). Increasing the competency and education of the nursing workforce is a new necessity in keeping with the shifting standards of all health care professions that may require changing individual beliefs about self-development and professional engagement on the never-ending road to professionalism in nursing (Bleich, 2013; Morris & Faulk, 2012). *The Future of Nursing* report calls for every nurse to engage in lifelong learning (Fights, 2012). This process and adaptation of learning is one by which nurses continually seek new information, receive clarity on the information, synthesize the new information into practice, and prepare to learn new information again (Candela, 2012).

Patient care is but one part of the overall system through which nurses can direct their energy and articulate their position as full partners in redesigning health care (Chard, 2013). Engagement in the exploration and investigation of care activities and the research and documentation of nursing practice (Fights, 2012) is needed to further knowledge and skill. This knowledge can come from many sources that can enhance evidence based practice in nursing care delivery; nurses do gather such knowledge every day but often do not appreciate or acknowledge its occurrence and their role as knowledge workers in health care delivery (Foster, 2012).

NURSE AS ASSIMILATOR AND REFLECTIVE PRACTITIONER

Without forward movement in both practice and education it will be difficult to accept and institute change (Godfrey & Crigger, 2012). Sullivan (2005) as cited by Day (2011) identified three high-level professional apprenticeships that form the background to all the Carnegie Foundation studies of professional education: the cognitive apprenticeship (knowledge base required for practice), the skills-based apprenticeship (judgment and know-how), and the apprenticeship of ethical comportment (professional behavior), with assimilation of these apprenticeships essential to integrated professional performance and practice.

Reflection becomes essential to systematic thinking about our actions and responses in a manner that allows transformed perspective and reframing for determination of future actions and response (Sherwood & Horton-Deutsch, 2012). Integrating reflective practices into nursing education and professional development has a significant impact on the quality of work processes and their outcomes by considering what we know, believe, and value (Horton-Deutsch & Sherwood, 2008; Sherwood & Horton-Deutsch, 2012).

NURSE AS ENGAGED STAKEHOLDER AND VOICE FOR ACTION

Agreeing with the IOM message is not enough. Nurses have remained too silent in a system that favors other health professionals—so much so that among some people, there is a public image that we exist in service to these other health care disciplines, patients, and their family members, and in care delivery models and processes that favor labor-intensive efforts (Bleich, 2013). The need for a full partnership and the large responsibility it carries will require individual nurses to enhance their leadership skills and competencies and position themselves as advocates for patient care, professional nursing, and effective health care policy to realize the goal of the IOM message (Chard, 2013).

▌ SUMMARY

Benner, Sutphen, Leonard, and Day (2010) hold that rather than being taught knowledge and skills to perform nursing care, students must learn to *be* nurses through powerful and integrative learning experiences. Nursing is not something that is simply done, but is rather an embodied state of being. Within this identity the professional nurse integrates scientific knowledge (cognitive apprenticeship), judgment and know how (skill apprenticeship), and ethics (ethical comportment apprenticeship) daily in unique and changing situations. Fluid use of these three apprenticeships is essential for practice excellence (Handwerker, 2012). Incorporating the key messages of the IOM report and using the report as an evidence-based blueprint for change will require a commitment from all stakeholders in a shared vision for a better health care system (Chard, 2013).

Whether the IOM's key messages and recommendations become the reality of nursing's future is up to each of us; every nurse—from bedside to the boardroom—has a role in transforming nursing (Fights, 2012; Thibault, 2011). Nurses and supportive stakeholders have a blueprint for meeting the public's need to promote health, mitigate illness, and enhance quality-of-life care (Bleich, 2013). Although the IOM report reinforces the need for all nurses to make a personal commitment to lifelong learning and education so that they are increasingly well prepared for their roles in a reformed health care system, each nurse must consider personal and professional goals and find a part of this process that means something to him or her and become involved (Battié, 2013).

If nursing doesn't answer the call of policymakers to share the future of health care, others will (Fights, 2012). How will you lead from where you stand?

SALIENT POINTS

- Socialization to professional nursing is an interactive, dynamic, lifelong process that includes internalization of its attitudes, behaviors, skills, and values.
- Professional identify formation transcends the socialization process; nursing is not something that is simply done, but is rather an embodied state of being.
- The IOM messages and recommendations focus on advancing the profession of nursing to enhance the preparation of nurses to function to the full extent of their education in an envisioned and transformed health care system.
- Interprofessional education can be a strategy to improve nursing education and enhance the role of nurses as collaborative leaders in the health care system.
- Every nurse has a professional role and responsibility to participate in realizing the vision and reality of the *Future of Nursing* report and its recommendations.

CRITICAL REFLECTION EXERCISES

1. Specify five commitments you are willing to make to advance your professional identity formation. What resources will you need to fulfill the identified commitments and overcome any obstacles you may encounter?
2. Consider an action you can take and/or have taken as a member of the professional nursing community to advance a key message of the IOM report. What is/was the catalyst for selection of this action?
3. Share a recent academic and/or professional learning experience and its impact on your beliefs about self-development and professional engagement. What insights do you have about the impact of this experience?
4. What personal and professional transformations can you envision making to enhance the integration of *innovation catalyst, interprofessional collaborator, engaged stakeholder, expert learner, knowledge worker, agent of inquiry, voice for action, assimilator,* and/or *reflective practitioner* in your way of being a nurse? Share the rationale for your choice(s).

REFERENCES

Armstrong, G., & Sherwood, G. D. (2012). Reflection and mindful practice: A means to quality and safety. In G. D. Sherwood, & S. Horton-Deutsch (Eds.), *Reflective practice: Transforming education and improving outcomes* (pp. 21–39). Indianapolis, IN: Sigma Theta Tau International.

Battié, R. N. (2013). The IOM Report on the Future of Nursing: What perioperative nurses need to know. *AORN, 98*(3), 227–234.

Benner, P. A., Sutphen, M., Leonard, V., & Day, L. (2010). *Educating nurses: A call for radical transformation.* Stanford, CA: Jossey-Bass.

Bleich, M. R. (2013). The Institute of Medicine Report on the Future of Nursing: A transformational blueprint. *AORN, 98*(3), 214–217.

Candela, L. (2012). From teaching to learning: Theoretical foundations. In D. M. Billings, & J. A. Halstead (Eds.), *Teaching in nursing: A guide for faculty* (4th ed.) (pp. 202–243). St Louis: Saunders.

Cardillo, D. (2011). Nursing: The future is yours! *NSNA Imprint, 58*(5), 36–38.

Chard, R. (2013). The personal and professional impact of the Future of Nursing report. *AORN, 98*(3), 273–280.

Crigger, N., & Godfrey, N. (2011). *The making of nurse professionals: A transformational, ethical approach.* Sudbury, MA: Jones & Bartlett.

Day, L. (2011). Using unfolding case studies in a subject-centered classroom. *Journal of Nursing Education, 50*(8), 447–452.

Eckhardt, J. A. (2002). Effects of program design on the professional socialization of RN-BSN students. *Journal of Professional Nursing, 18*(3), 157–164.

Fairman, J. (2012). History for the future (of nursing). *Nursing History Review, 20*(1), 10–13.

Fights, S. D. (2012). Nurses lead from where we stand: How can you impact the future of nursing? *MEDSURG Nursing, 21*(2), 57–58.

Foster, C. W. (2012). Institute of Medicine The Future of Nursing report, lifelong learning, and certification. *MEDSURG Nursing, 21*(2), 115–116.

Godfrey, N., & Crigger, N. (2012). Forming a professional identity: an important key to nursing's future. *Missouri Nurse,* 12–13.

Handwerker, S. (2012). Transforming nursing education: A review of current curricular practice in relation to Benner's latest work. *International Journal of Nursing Education Scholarship*, *9*(1), 1–16.

Horton-Deutsch, S., & Sherwood, G. D. (2008). Reflection: An educational strategy to develop emotionally competent nurse leaders. *Journal of Nursing Management*, *16*(8), 946–954.

Institute of Medicine. (2010). The future of nursing: Leading change, advancing health. Retrieved from http://www.iom.edu/Reports/2010/The-Future-of-Nursing-Leading-Change-Advancing-Health.aspx.

Lee, R. C., & Fawcett, J. (2013). The influence of the metaparadigm of nursing on professional identity development among RN-BSN students. *Nursing Science Quarterly*, *26*(1), 96–98.

Lai, P. K., & Lim, P. H. (2012). Concept of professional socialization in nursing. *International e-Journal of Science, Medicine & Education*, *6*(1), 31–35.

Morris, A. H., & Faulk, D. R. (Eds.). (2012). The road to professionalism: Transformative learning for professional role development. In *Transformative learning in nursing: A guide for nurse educators* (pp. 91–103). New York, NY: Springer.

Sullivan, W. (2005). *Work and integrity: The crisis and promise of professionalism in America* (2nd ed.). San Francisco, CA: Jossey-Bass.

Shekleton, M. E. (2012). The Institute of Medicine Report on the Future of Nursing: New horizons for nursing and healthcare. *CHART Journal of Illinois Nursing*, *110*(4), 14–17.

Sherwood, G. D., & Horton-Deutsch, S. (2012). Turning vision into action. In G. D. Sherwood, & S. Horton-Deutsch (Eds.), *Reflective practice: Transforming education and improving outcomes* (pp. 3–19). Indianapolis, IN: Sigma Theta Tau International.

Thibault, G. E. (2011). Interprofessional education: An essential strategy to accomplish the Future of Nursing goals. *Journal of Nursing Education*, *50*(6), 313–317.

Professional Nursing Roles

Regina M. DeGennaro, DNP, RN, AOCN, CNL

ⓔ http://evolve.elsevier.com/Friberg/bridge/

OBJECTIVES

At the completion of this chapter, the reader will be able to:

- Articulate the impact of culture on perceptions of the professional nursing role.
- Discuss the role and identity dyads in the framework of the nursing profession.
- Describe the roles commonly assumed by professional nurses and the associated identity characteristics.
- Discuss the impact of the multiple roles experienced by the professional nurse.
- Differentiate the common sources of role stress and resultant role strain.
- Identify the strategies for managing role stress and strain.

PROFILE IN PRACTICE

Kristi D. Wilkins, MSN, RN, CCRN, CCNS
University of Virginia Health System, Charlottesville, Virginia

Each step in my health care profession has shaped my ability to better serve as the clinical nurse specialist (CNS) for the Surgical Trauma Burn Intensive Care Unit at the University of Virginia Health System. My student job in the Laboratory for Clinical Learning in nursing school gave me first-hand experience in developing and implementing effective processes to educate others. Working as a patient care assistant allowed me the opportunity to learn to communicate and collaborate effectively with patients, families, and the interdisciplinary team. My first position as a new nurse sparked my interest in the care of the burn patient and subsequently my specialty in graduate school. Specialty practice is defined population focus, care setting, or disease process. For me this is the critical care setting because I care for patients with a diverse spectrum of conditions and needs: trauma, traumatic brain injury, burn, solid organ transplant, complex wounds and reconstructive surgery, and an array of other surgical diagnoses. An additional complexity is the care of patients across the care continuum from critically ill to acute care because the unit may care for patients at both ends of the care dichotomy. Tackling specialty knowledge in all of these patient populations is daunting; therefore my practice relies on effective utilization of resources and navigation of the health system.

A single day of practice provides a multitude of pivotal intersects to influence the care of a patient. This may be as simple as collaboration with physician colleagues during patient rounds or empowering a patient and/or family member to be an active partner in establishing care goals. Or it may be as complex as ensuring effective glycemic control across the critical care division. It may include formally educating professional colleagues at surrounding hospitals in the care of the burn patient. Evaluating outcomes and implementing evidence based strategies to prevent complications, shorten length of stay, and lower health care costs are some of the results that validate the role of the CNS.

The population within my care domain is patients and their families but also nursing and interdisciplinary colleagues—as well as the health care system as a whole. My day-to-day practice includes educating and mentoring clinical staff in care standards, health care technology, preventative care, and patient advocacy. The professional development of others is one of the most rewarding aspects of my role. I am expected to promote certification, to assist clinicians in furthering their careers by challenging the clinical ladder, and to enable clinicians to contribute to nursing knowledge by creating clinical research. I often find myself explaining this aspect of my role to colleagues this way: *Simply put, I enable and empower you to better care for our patients.*

I believe the CNS or advanced practice nurse has the responsibility to influence nursing and medicine beyond one's immediate reach. This can be accomplished through a variety of mechanisms: active participation in one's professional organization, contributing to professional publications or presentations, or educating the next generation of nursing colleagues. Health care and health care systems are dynamic. The CNS, at any one moment of time, may focus on just one aspect of his or her arsenal of competencies, but it is the synthesis of all of these elements that allow the role to be effective and vital in health care excellence.

INTRODUCTION

In today's rapidly changing health care environment, the professional nursing role is becoming less traditional and increasingly diverse and expanded in response to the growing complexity in health care. As the professional disciplines are called upon to lead expanded and more diverse health care services in a wide variety of settings, the traditional structure of provider roles is challenged. Nursing is responding to this challenge by examining the nature of the professional role, exploring its underlying values and identity, and adapting it to better meet the needs of a dynamic health care system. In recent years, rapid advances in science and treatments, improved disease management with integration of new technologies, and shifts in care delivery have contributed to the need for contemporary nurses to be well educated and experienced. Demographics continue to change with the aging and increasingly diverse public. This chapter focuses on role taking in nursing by examining stereotypes of nursing in the common culture, reviewing the historical development of nursing roles, identifying the types of roles nurses commonly assume and the associated identity characteristics, exploring the relevance of education and work environment to practice roles, and finally, addressing aspects of role dynamics, sources of role stress, and strategies for resolving role stress.

NURSING ROLES, FUNCTIONS, AND CHARACTERISTICS

Nursing Role Stereotypes

To examine the professional nursing role, first consider the kaleidoscope of media and culture and their impact in shaping the way society sees nurses. This is vital during a time in which there is a shortage of nurses and an emerging dissonance between nursing education and the experiences of nurses in health care. Research illustrates representations of professional roles and gender in media and the arts can shape a society's view of that profession's work. Dr. Stanley, a lecturer in the School of Nursing and Midwifery at Curtin University of Technology in Perth, remarked, "Public perceptions of different professions are strongly influenced by the media, and in the past the way that nurses have been represented in featured films has often been at odds with the way nurses perceive their profession" (Stanley, 2008, para 3).

Images of interprofessional critical thinking and decision making that occur in health care settings between nurses and colleagues seem to be absent from the current media. The 2010 Institute of Medicine report on the future of nursing reveals the need for nurses to be transformational in the delivery of health care. Perhaps illustrating the rigorous preparation that comprises nursing education might allow for a change in the image and perception of nursing. Working within complex systems demands leadership skills that guide solutions to improve the quality and safety of patients and families.

Nurses have often been portrayed in film and television as comedic sex kittens—from B-movie productions in the 1970s such as *Private Duty Nurses* (Armitage, 1971) to Hot Lips Houlihan in the acclaimed television series *M∗A∗S∗H∗* (Hornberger, 1972) to contemporary productions such as the television series *ER* (Burns, 1994), *Scrubs* (Lawrence, 2001), *Nightingales* (Cramer, 1988), and *Grey's Anatomy* (Corn, 2005). In these portrayals, the nurse as caregiver is often twisted into an individual with uncontrolled libidinal impulse. Stanley (2008) noted, "Just over a quarter of the films I reviewed featured an overtly sexual representation of nurses … an image that has negative implications for nursing professionals" (para 9).

In addition to sexualized roles, nurses have also been portrayed as harsh disciplinarians with an unyielding, even sadistic, worldview. Examples of these menacing roles include the ghoulish nurse in *The Lost Weekend* (Brackett & Wilder, 1945), the murderous caregiver in Stephen King's *Misery* (Reiner, Scheinman, Stott, & Nicolaides, 1990), and most notably, the sinister and terrifying Nurse Ratched, who provoked emotional breakdowns in her emasculated, unstable, male patients in the Oscar-winning movie, *One Flew Over the Cuckoo's Nest* (Douglas & Zaentz, 1975).

Because nursing is often seen as a female profession, these portrayals reflect society's view of women, which shifted with the advent of the feminist movement, when women challenged sexist limitations on professional roles. Stanley believes, for instance, that the portrayal of nurses as sadistic coincided with the liberation of a repressed inner-self in line with the development of women's power (Stanley, 2008).

As women become more socially, professionally, and politically active, opportunities for women in the nursing field have also expanded. For example, military nurses are portrayed as heroes and heroines. The television show *China Beach* (Wells, 1988) was critiqued as "focusing on the women at the base, an emphasis fundamentally intended to undermine vainglorious heroism and to portray war instead, through women's eyes, as a vast and elaborate conceit. Contemporary critics divided between those applauding the program's feminine deflation of war, and those who regarded the characters and their orientations toward war as wholly stereotypical invocations of femininity" (Saenz, 1988, para 3).

Recent films such as *Pearl Harbor* (Bruckheimer & Bay, 2001) and Ian McEwan's 2007 film from the honored book *Atonement* (McEwan, 2001) portray war nurses as heroines and self-sacrificing women. In the Academy Award–winning film *The English Patient* (Zaentz & Minghella, 1996), the nurse Hanna's selfless dedication to her craft and patient leads her to stay with him under desperate wartime conditions, her skilled compassion guiding her to assist him as he is dying.

Recent films and television illustrate improvements in the portrayal of nurses, such as Hanna in *The English Patient* (Zaentz & Minghella, 1996) or actress Julianna Margulies' nursing role in *ER* (Spielberg, 1994). Nurse-focused television roles include examples of gender and ethnic diversity of the professional nurse, for example, *HawthoRNe* with Jada Pinkett Smith in the role of Christina (Masius, 2009), and *Mercy* with Jamie Lee Kirchner as Sonia Jimenez (Heldens, 2009). *Nurse Jackie* (Brixius, Dunskey, & Wallem, 2009) depicts

diverse nurse characters with critical thinking skills and acknowledges a real problem that exists in the nursing profession, and one that she experiences and manages with an addiction to pain medications. However, substantial obstacles and stereotypes still exist, driven by the gender-bound thinking attached to the nursing role. One barrier includes the limited preparation in media training and opportunities for nurses to engage in communicating with the media.

In 2012 the UCLA School of Nursing hosted a symposium entitled: "Nurses and the Media: A Call to Action," sharing the message that nurses need to teach the world about their profession (Wood, 2012). Nurses' perspectives differ from other health professionals' knowledge, experience, and perspectives. Their expertise can be shared with the public. Nurses can improve the professional image through investing in presenting nursing and increasing local involvement. *The Truth about Nursing* is a nonprofit organization focused on improving the image of nursing in the media, founded by Sandy Summers, RN, MSN, MPH in 2001 after recognizing the lack of understanding about the profession (Summers, 2001).

A major obstacle is demonstrated in the wildly successful film *Meet the Parents* (Tenenbaum, 2000), which reinforces how nursing struggles with its identity as gender-specific to women. Actor Ben Stiller's character, Greg Focker, is a nurse who comically raises our consciousness of the negative perceptions of men in nursing. In one critical scene Greg is staying at his new girlfriend's house in order to meet her father, Jack Byrnes, along with several other relatives, including two male physicians. When Greg arrives at the breakfast table—the only person in the house clad in pajamas—Jack introduces the bedraggled Greg to the group:

Jack Byrnes: Greg's a male nurse.

Greg Focker: Yes, thank you, Jack.

Kevin Rowley (surgeon): Wow, that's great. I'd love to find time to do some volunteer work. Just the other day I saw a golden retriever, he had like a gimp, and you know I wish I could have done something.

Greg Focker: Yeah, well I get paid too so it's sort of an "everyone wins" thing.

The stereotype that the male nurses are "less than male" and "do women's work" is still an image reflected in contemporary U.S. culture despite a long history of men in nursing. In fact, as early as the 4th and 5th centuries, men worked as nurses (Evans,

2004). Today one of the little-known facts of military nursing is the high percentage of men performing nursing roles in all three service branches. In the Army 35.5% of its 3381 nurses are men; in the Air Force, 30% of 3790 nurses are men; and in the Navy, 36% of the 3125 nurses are men. By contrast, in 2009 men made up only 6% of the nursing workforce in the United States (Lucas, 2009). As of 2011, 9.6% of all registered nurses in the United States were male, up from 2.7% in 1970 (U.S. Census Bureau, 2012). Peter Buerhaus, a professor of nursing at Vanderbilt University, noted that social stigmas associated with men in nursing seem to be disappearing based on the growth of the number of work opportunities in nursing in recent years (USA Today, 2013).

Actual Nursing Roles

Distinct from the stereotypes portrayed in the media, including film and television, the actual roles nurses play are uniquely multifaceted. The scope of these roles is a provocative one that incites many opinions within and external to the profession since Florence Nightingale first examined the role of nursing in her publication *Notes on Nursing: What It Is and What It Is Not* (1860). The wisdom and vision of Nightingale were clear as she refrained from pigeonholing the profession in the context of time and space: "I do not pretend to teach her how, I ask her to teach herself, and for this purpose I venture to give her some hints" (Nightingale, 1860, p. 8). Educators often find themselves getting out of the way of nursing students, allowing their wisdom to shine.

Nightingale saw nursing as an art and, as such, the various roles in nursing as multilayered and fluid defined by the context and demands of the environment in which that nurse works. Professional nurses today function as researchers, administrators, community organizers, policy makers, clinicians, and educators, in a multitude of settings, with each context helping to set roles, expectations, and limitations. Furthermore, many nurses do not stop being a nurse when they leave the hospital, clinic, school, tent, office, lab, or mobile unit where they happen to work; many carry the identity of being a nurse into their personal lives.

Kathy Douglas, RN, MHA, is chief nursing officer for API Healthcare and the president of the nonprofit organization On Nursing Excellence. She directed the 2012 documentary *NURSES: If Florence Could See Us Now*, in an effort to provide a real picture of nurses today. Nurses in various roles were interviewed with no script, and spoke from the heart. They shared stories with the goal of educating the public and inspiring nurses. Douglas offers some insight into the complexities of being a nurse and explores the many roles that nurses play as over 100 nurses offer a snapshot of nursing in this film by First Run Features (Douglas, 2012).

Being a nurse is about executing a number of roles in service to health and health care that are intertwined with the identity, talents, and values of each individual. That is, nurses are defined by the roles they play and their personal identity, which provides the substance and motivation for their work. When this complex tangle of role and identity is bifurcated and nursing practice is industrialized, the meaning of being a nurse is diminished. Critically, this professional alignment of role and identity leads to personal and professional happiness; hence understanding the nature of role and identity and their interconnection is essential in evaluating the roles played by professional nurses.

The *Merriam-Webster Online Dictionary* defines *role* as "a socially expected behavior pattern usually determined by an individual's status in a particular society" (2013). The word *role* may be interpreted as a set of behaviors and expectations, rights and obligations, as conceptualized by actors in a situation guided by individuals with social position who set these behaviors. Roles are associated with social positions (status, power) and are shaped by the expectations of others in an individual's workplace or social network (Biddle, 1979). Although structure and function are essential to an understanding of role, to define nursing in the context of expected behaviors would then interpret actions as solely prescribed by rules outlined in policy and procedure or a job description. From this functional perspective, the meaning of *role* is shallow and lacking the underpinnings of the individual's professional identity, which underscores the motivation for selecting the profession.

The *Merriam-Webster Online Dictionary* defines *identity* as "the distinguishing character or personality of an individual," and the word *identification* is defined as "a psychological orientation of the self in regard to something (as person or group) with resulting feeling of close emotional association" (2013). There is no set identity in nursing, because the profession consists of individuals with unique values and experiences. Nursing roles are guided by a derived identity and sense of self gathered from the professional organizations or work groups to which nurses belong (Hogg & Terry, 2000). From this perspective identity can be understood as how a person sees himself or herself in a particular role; what a person believes about the world, moral choices, and social justice; and a person's sense of profession and being in relationship to a work role.

According to one paradigm model, an individual's sense of identity is determined mostly by the explorations and commitments that she or he makes regarding certain personal and social traits (Marcia, 1966). In this framework the identity of a nurse is determined by how that individual views, imagines, and experiences nursing.

Praxis and the Nursing Meta-Dyad

The fusion of role and identity set in an understanding of the cultural context of nursing represents praxis, the integration of action and reflection, which is essential to any transformative helping profession. To better understand this complex interplay of role and identity and the harmony and disunity it can create, it is helpful to use the theoretical construct of a dyad. The word *dyad* comes from the Greek *dyas*, which stands for the number two and represents the principle of "two-ness" or otherness. The *Merriam-Webster Online Dictionary* defines *dyad* as "a pair maintaining a sociologically or physically significant relationship" (2013). This can serve as a model for holding together, through exploration, the critical functions of nursing with personal identity that make up the individual nurse's professional role identity.

Bringing together role and identity integrates nursing into the surrounding culture and opens up a broader understanding of the profession. For example, whereas role is about health and the interaction of person and disease, identity is about individual values and approaches concerning illness and wellness. When these concepts are combined, the result represents the fullness of nursing praxis. In terms of the individual nurse, this integration of

role and identity allows balance. The nursing identity embraces wellness; the nursing role manages health and disease.

What infuses the art and practice of nursing is a single overarching dyad, a meta-dyad of the professional nurse role, driven by an intrinsic personal identity of being other-centered (other-centeredness). For the professional nursing role, the core identity is that of caring for others or other-centeredness—the conscious movement of care directed to and with another human being or a community of human beings.

When one explores the meaning of the professional nursing role, most definitions lead to dyads that partner expressions of highly educated, highly skilled professionals with definitions of individuals who care for others with great empathy and compassion. Nurses combine scientific clinical reasoning with people skills. A frequent expression is that nursing is both high tech and high touch.

These definitions invariably go on to indicate that professional nurses are educators as well as managers, colleagues, mentors, researchers, and advocates for health. An understanding of these roles and their parallel identity characteristics is essential for a nurse to be successful. The nurse must be grounded in the concept of other-centeredness as opposed to being egocentric. An exceptional demonstration of this other-centeredness is nursing's central ethical doctrine, which holds that a nurse's first obligation is to the patient (Siefert, 2009).

Moral theorist and feminist thinker Carol Gilligan's work speaks to the morality of care defining the preservation of relationships as the highest level of moral reasoning. From her perspective of the nature of moral development, nursing based on other-centeredness represents the final stage in moral development. What underlies the skill and knowledge of professional nursing is caregiving, empathy, and compassion (McFadden, 2006).

Essential Role Functions and Characteristics

Embedded within this overarching construct of the role of the nurse with an identity of other-centeredness are seven key dyads that are essential to any exploration of nursing. These roles and the corresponding identity characteristics that infuse these roles (Figure 4-1) constitute an overlapping mosaic

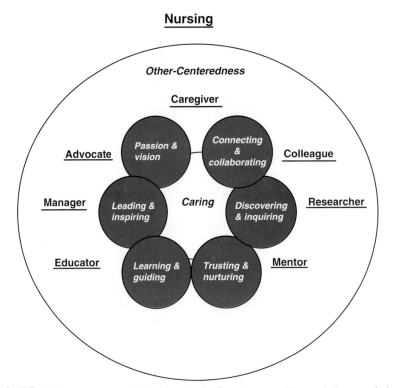

FIGURE 4-1 The nursing role identity dyads. Functions and internal characteristics.

that is not exclusive but is foundational to the professional role of nurse. This mosaic of nursing role and identity dyads can be viewed as role progression as professional experience ensues.

Caregiver—Caring, Compassion, and Empathy.

Compassion is that which makes the heart of the good move at the pain of others. It crushes and destroys the pain of others.

Buddha

If the act of caregiving drives the health care delivery role, compassion is an essential identity characteristic that guides the actions of assessment, planning, intervention, and evaluation. When asked about the most important role of a nurse, most nurses respond with one word: caregiving. The nursing profession is grounded in the phenomenon of caring (Leininger, 1988). Leininger discovered that patients from diverse cultures valued care differently than nurses did. Gradually, Leininger became convinced of the need for a theoretical framework

to discover, explain, and predict dimensions of care and developed culture care theory, the only nursing theory that focuses on culture (Leininger & McFarland, 1997). This theory defines caring behaviors on the part of a caregiver as those that are congruent with the beliefs, values, and expressions of the care recipient. Similarly, Jean Watson's theory of caring describes the scientific basis of nursing as extending beyond human interaction, to a moral concern for preserving human dignity and respect for the wholeness of the care recipient (Childs, 2006). Both of these theories demonstrate the link between the caregiver role and the identity characteristics of compassion and empathy.

Caring is an essential feature of the profession, one that is central to a nurse's identity and that serves to facilitate health and healing. Because of this fundamental maxim, preparing the nurse for the caregiving role is an established practice in nursing education. It is more difficult, however, to describe and teach fostering caring through compassion. Although "teaching" identity is a complex process, nurses need to be taught a deepening awareness of the emotions prompted by the pain and suffering of others. This begins with teaching self-assessment, self-care, and reflective practices of inquiry, self-evaluation and stress management techniques. Grounded in the development of empathy, caring is the vigorous attempt not only to feel another's pain but to take steps to alleviate suffering and to seek the wellness within that person. Covington (2005) states, "Caring presence is mutual trust and sharing, transcending connectedness, and experience. This special way of being a caring presence involves devotion to a client's well-being while bringing scientific knowledge and expertise to the relationship" (p. 169). Kathy Robinson (2003), former president of the Emergency Nurses Association, writes, "No technology in health care replaces the critical thinking of a human mind, the caring of a human soul, the proficiency and skill of a human hand, and the warmth of a human heart in healing the sick and injured. That is nursing, esteemed colleagues; that is you" (p. 200).

Colleague—Collaborating and Connecting. The role of nurse as colleague is not only essential to collaborative clinical and research practices, but integral to the team process in dynamic health care. Working together toward common purposes, improving health, respecting shared strengths, offering effective peer review, caring and compassion—these are fundamental to the profession. For example, in 2009, 90% of American Association of Critical-Care Nurses (AACN-West) members responding to a survey reported that they were colleagues with physicians and administrators and that they believed this was among the most important elements in creating a healthy work environment (Morton & Fontaine, 2009). At the heart of being a colleague is the ability not only to cooperate, but to *actively* collaborate. Collaboration is a multifaceted process of working together to accomplish a common goal; it involves a mix of differing viewpoints to better comprehend a challenging issue. Arising between true colleagues, collaboration is the ability to be innovative in achieving consensus to optimize shared goals.

According to Gardner there are 10 lessons in collaboration: (1) know thyself; (2) learn to value and manage diversity; (3) develop constructive conflict resolution skills; (4) use personal power to create win-win situations; (5) master interpersonal and process skills; (6) recognize that collaboration is a journey; (7) leverage all multidisciplinary forums; (8) appreciate that collaboration can occur spontaneously; (9) balance autonomy and unity in collaborative relationships; and (10) remember that collaboration is not required for all decisions (Gardner, 2005, Section 3).

Interprofessional collaboration is a vital aspect of plans designed to increase the effectiveness of delivery of health care (Morton & Fontaine, 2009). According to Dorrie Fontaine, RN, PhD, FAAN, former president of the AACN-West, "Escalating financial pressures and alarming workforce shortages make it imperative that physicians and nurses actively work together to establish new patient-focused practice models. The combined efforts of the AACN-West and the American College of Chest Physicians will establish a strong leadership force in effecting meaningful change in our hospitals and health systems on behalf of the critically ill patients we serve" (Morton & Fontaine, 2009). From initiatives to promote interdisciplinary education in health care to institutes focusing on fostering dynamic and intentional international collaboration involving nursing, medical and allied health researchers, clinicians, academics, and quality managers, collaboration among colleagues has emerged as vital to professional nursing.

An example of an important new arena for collaborative practice for nursing is the rapid advance of telehealth as a critical vehicle for health care delivery, especially in rural, underserved communities. Telehealth is the exchange of medical and other health information via electronic communications from one site to another with the intent of addressing patient needs. Through telehealth, colleagues provide medical, nursing, or other health care to a remote location. The remote site usually requires a nurse to be present with the patient to present the history and physical, provide clinical interventions, offer health education, and ensure follow-up. This is collaborative practice in its highest form, because the role of the nurse in this setting is to leverage technology and nursing expertise to provide quality health care (Cattell-Gordon, 2009).

Manager—Leading, Inspiring, Thinking Critically. Fundamental to nursing practice—whether it is an individual nurse directing patient care, an administrator of a nursing unit, or a chief nursing officer for a health system—is the role of nurse leader as manager. In this role the nurse recognizes the identity of manager as the caregiver of the caregivers. In short, nurse manager is the role of pulling together people with the common goal of caregiving.

Although the role of manager or administrator of a nursing unit is not one that every nurse will assume, understanding managing as a primary nursing function is essential. All nurses essentially assume the role of manager every day in their work when they care for patients. The role of manager requires a systematic way of providing care, a precise tending to details, and working from a comprehensive assessment and plan, as well as engaging colleagues in a compassionate, collaborative, interdisciplinary practice. With the growing complexity of nursing and health care, the systems assessment and management becomes crucial for effective and safe, quality care.

A nurse, for example, in caring for a dying patient, needs to know the critical point at which the family should be called, how to manage the medications, when to touch and not to touch, when to be silent, and when not to do anything but be present. This role calls for the nurse to manage care and demonstrate leadership, seeing the whole and the parts of the whole simultaneously—the individual patient and the whole of the process of dying.

A leader is someone grounded in the core value of compassion with the capacity to inspire mentorship, collaboration, creativity, and critical thinking. To communicate this leadership, the leader must provide the framework from which complex problem solving evolves. A core element of managing and leading is understanding the nature of servant leadership and possessing emotional intelligence (Triola, 2007). Nurse leaders demonstrate these identity characteristics when they set priorities based on the needs of those they are leading and are committed to the professional growth of others. Effective leadership is vital to creating healthy work environments that are conducive to promoting quality patient outcomes and health for staff. Authentic leadership, according to Kathleen McCauley (2005), former president of the AACN-West, is the "glue" needed to hold together a healthy work environment.

In some settings, a nursing culture with a focus on task orientation, rigid hierarchical structures, and the possible disempowerment of staff is an impediment to delivery of compassionate patient-centered care. As a nurse leader, if one sets the tone of joining with the patient in a process of compassionate collaboration, outcomes in health will be more optimally achieved (Jonsdottir, Litchfield, & Dexheiner, 2004).

Educator—Learning and Guiding. The role of the educator is essential to the overall function and identity of the nurse. In the complex world of contemporary health care, as patients seek to understand and manage their disease and cope with illness, the nurse assumes the primary role of educator. At every level the patient educator role exists within the scope of practice because it significantly affects a patient's health and quality of life. The process of providing education parallels the nursing process, with the first step being an assessment of the learner's needs, readiness to learn, and learning style, followed by an individually designed intervention, and completed only when the outcome has been evaluated (Bastable, 2007). The ability of nurses to effectively provide health education is essential in addressing local and global health problems. The skill set of communication becomes the priority skill for effective teaching and evaluation of understanding. See Chapter 8 for further discussion of effective communication.

To be effective as a teacher requires a commitment to be a learner; to see teaching and learning as the act of guiding; and to understand the essence of the phrase "to educate." As John Dewey posits, learners grow in concert with others: "Every experience lives on in further experiences. Hence, the central problem of ... education ... is to select the kind of present experiences that develop fruitfully and creatively in subsequent experiences" (Dewey, Kilpatrick, Hartmann, & Melby, 1937, p. 45). The role of educator in the profession of nursing is based on the desire to help individuals and communities grow. The nurse educator is nurturing a relationship, sharing knowledge, and empowering individuals, families, and communities. The nurse in this role can actively teach and guide patients, families, and communities about health/wellness and illness—about living and dying.

This role of the nurse as educator is further optimized by fostering personal knowing. It is the ability to be empathetic, to see an event from the perspective of another, and to recognize the other as a subject rather as an object. Personal knowing is the discovery of self and others, which is arrived at through reflection, synthesis of perceptions, and connecting with that which is known (Kaminski, 2006, p. 14).

In addition to empathy, nurse educators strive to foster critical thinking skills in their students. Lemire (2002, p. 69) notes that in educating nurses for leadership, the educator must emphasize the cognitive and disposition aspects of critical thinking in order to promote active and sequential learning. Critical thinking, clinical reasoning, and problem-solving skills are acquired over time through lifelong learning and experience.

From this place of learning and knowing comes the ability to be a caring person who seeks to collaborate to achieve a common purpose for health and wellness. This same posture applies to the role of nurse educator—whether it is within a school of nursing, a community college, or with fellow nurses on a unit or in a clinic. The critical pedagogy of nursing requires a fundamental understanding of the dyads, an ability to guide and teach others a whole understanding of the profession, and an evaluation of the sociopolitical context of learning and care. In short, professional nurse educators teach role and nurture identity.

Mentor—Sharing and Role Modeling. Mentoring refers to a formal or informal process in which a mentor and a mentee establish a relationship with the mutual goal of meeting the career goals of the mentee (Bally, 2007). One role of the mentor—to be true to oneself and guide another to greater personal awareness and skill—is crucial to retaining and encouraging nurses in the workplace. The evidence illustrates the initial 3 months of a newly graduated nurse's transition is vital to long-term success in the profession (Winfield, Melo, & Myrick, 2009). This initial transition involves an all-encompassing transformation of roles and responsibilities, an acceptance of the differences between the theoretical orientation of the nurse's education and the practical focus of professional work, and integration into an environment that emphasizes teamwork as opposed to individually based care provision. The role of the professional nurse as caregiver, leader, teacher, colleague, and mentor is a critical one in helping newly graduated nurses or any nurses who change roles to feel successful in their new environment (Schumacher & Meleis, 1994).

Because nursing excellence is embodied in the combined competency of skills and practice, the experienced mentor, grounded in the spirit of nurturing, is crucial to the development of careers, collaborative networks, and a contagious enthusiasm within the profession. For this enthusiasm to take hold, the mentor must be a person whom the mentee can trust. The mentor acts as a "role model and advocate to pass on life experiences and knowledge in order to motivate, support and enhance their mentee's personal and career development" (Kuhl, 2005, p. 9). Building on this, the key qualities in an effective nurse mentor reflect the identity characteristics of the role modeling and sharing.

The National League for Nursing (NLN), one of the membership organizations for nurse faculty and leaders in nursing education, states, "Experienced nurses everywhere have the opportunity to become mentors for other nurses. Mentoring another nurse is a professional means of passing along knowledge, skills, behaviors and values to a less experienced individual" (NLN, 2006). The NLN further asserts that in a positive sense, the act of mentoring provides nurses an opportunity to create a legacy. By sharing information and insights with members of their own profession, experienced nurses can enable others to maximize their potential, thereby improving patient care and ultimately strengthening the profession of nursing (Henk, 2005).

Researcher—Inquiring and Discovering.

Nothing in life is to be feared. It is only to be understood.

Marie Curie

The role of researcher in the nursing profession is vital for generating new knowledge to underpin nursing practice, clinical care, and public health. As both a caring art and scientific enterprise, nursing has an obligation to provide care that is continually examined through research (International Council of Nurses, 2009). Nurses working as independent investigators or in multidisciplinary research teams offer new insights and unique perspectives to the process. According to Patricia Munhall from the NLN, nurses change in "how" they believe in something rather than "what" they believe and states, "The sands of science itself are shifting, as more and more scientists, including nurse scientists, realize that science cannot be a field of absolute and final truth but is an endeavor focused on illuminating an ever-changing body of ideas" (Munhall, 2007, p. 12). Nursing research, in fact, is critical to the emergence of community-based participatory research, an approach in which the scientific process is applied to a collaborative process with the community of interest.

One way to illustrate the importance of the researcher role is to describe a misalignment between the role and identity of a nurse who works on an oncology unit who is not aware of research or curious about the discovery of new treatments for cancer. This dissonance in an area in which so many die from the disease is likely to cause frustration and burnout. Thus at the most basic level the role of the nurse requires a comfort with research and a curiosity with clinical investigation. At the next level the nurse applies research at the bedside by providing interventions that are based on current evidence. At an advanced level the role of nurse as a researcher is fundamental to improving patient care and public health by defining research questions and designing scientific studies to answer them. This process includes writing grants, analyzing data, and sharing findings with the larger health care community.

To be successful in the role of nurse researcher, the identity of the researcher must be grounded in curiosity and the desire for discovery driven by compassion for human suffering. This identity, in turn, empowers patients because it is not proprietary knowledge but rather is about sharing and inspiring new knowledge. Indeed, this scientific inquiry creates an interest in learning and guiding that helps break down barriers between cultures. The curious nurse researcher asks important "how" and "why" questions and builds essential stepping stones toward awareness, appreciation, and understanding of other cultures. Through curiosity people can gain new perspectives, unparalleled learning and growth, and an invitation for interesting conversation and reflection at every interaction (Kaminski, 2006).

Advocate—Passion and Vision.

An individual has not started living until he can rise above the narrow confines of his individualistic concerns to the broader concerns of all humanity.
                    Martin Luther King, Jr.

The purpose of advocacy is change, and true change requires vision, passion, and agitation. This role and spirit has been part of nursing since its inception, although it has not been without contention. Florence Nightingale, for instance, despite being a strong advocate for the improvement of care and conditions in British military hospitals, taught nurses to be unquestioningly obedient to doctors (Hewitt, 2002). References to nurses maintaining loyalty and obedience to doctors were not removed from the ICN's code until 1973 (Snowball, 1996).

Over the past two decades, the word *advocacy* has appeared in nursing literature with increasing frequency (Malik, 1997). Snowball (1996) speaks to the evolution of nurses as advocates. As nursing began to develop its professional identity in the late 1960s, it became more patient focused and less institution directed. Since then, with an emphasis on human rights, social justice, equality, and self-determination; the rise of nurse-led advocacy for the Patient's Bill of Rights; and the need for global and national health care reform, the role of nurse as advocate for patients, families, and communities has become essential to the future of health care.

Advocacy has become even more critical in our current high-technology health care environment. Patient autonomy may be limited by the imbalance of power and information in the physician-patient relationship and by the bureaucratic health care system with an emphasis on scientific and technological expertise. This may result in patients surrendering their independence and welfare to an institutional care system with tendencies toward opportunist behaviors such as overutilization of high-cost but low-benefit procedures or treatments. Tuxhill (1994) states patient advocacy as one of the roles that separates nursing ethics from medical ethics. Moral and ethical reasoning, autonomy, and patient empowerment have become inextricably linked with the triad of nurse, patient, and advocacy.

Benner and Wrubel (1988) state that advocacy is the base of nursing as a caring practice, arguing that to be with patients in such a way acknowledges a shared humanity because nursing is a discipline with an active compassion at its core. In the role of patient advocate, the nurse is demonstrating the value of other-centeredness to advance the health of an individual. In the University of Pennsylvania's Health System Nursing Annual Report (2005), Sharon Fitzpatrick, a critical care nurse, speaks to the difficulty of end-of-life care and her role as advocate for patients during stressful times: "Most relatives can't bring themselves to authorize the removal of life-sustaining equipment … in the meantime, however, they do not see the patient's suffering" (p. 11).

The role of nurse advocate is essential to ensure universal access to care and for the improvement of public health. Despite an exceptional health care system in the United States, there are well-documented disparities in access to care that result in needless suffering and death. To be a nurse grounded in the value of other-centeredness requires action to promote social justice and equal access to health care. As an example of advocacy in public policy, in May 2009, on the day after the anniversary of Florence Nightingale's birthday (May 12, 1820), a group of 30 nurses wearing red scrubs stood up in a Senate hearing on health care reform and turned their backs to reveal signs that read, "Nurses Say: Stop AHIP, Pass Single Payer." (AHIP stands for "America's Health Insurance Plans," a lobbying group for the health insurance industry.) After standing for a few minutes in silent protest, the nurses walked out of the hearing to applause. In the role of advocate for health for all, the nurse is demonstrating, for example, the characteristics of leading, caring, serving, and connecting (California Nurses Association, 2009).

PROFESSIONAL PRACTICE ROLES

The dyads previously discussed describe the common elements in professional nursing roles, but roles are also shaped by educational preparation and by the environments in which nurses practice. The mix of skills and knowledge among professional nurses and the diversity of nursing roles expand the profession's impact on health care. Nursing roles fluctuate with changes in the needs of individual patients, the systems of health care delivery, and availability of health care technology. For all nurses, other-centeredness remains the core, whereas the other role-identity dyads dictate the role functions and characteristics.

Educational Preparation

All nurses entering the profession must demonstrate competency by passing a state board examination. By passing this exam the nurse earns the title of registered nurse and demonstrates the ability to practice as a generalist nurse. Although the state board examination is the same for all persons entering the profession, there are several different educational programs that prepare nurses to sit for the state board examination and enter the practice of nursing. As discussed in Chapter 2, these educational programs include diploma, associate

degree (AD), bachelor of science in nursing (BSN), and master of science in nursing (MSN) programs, as well as clinical nurse leader (CNL) generalist track. Diploma programs are scarce today, and most of them are hospital based. Associate degree programs focus on nursing theory and skills and require 2 or 3 years of study. The bachelor's degree programs are 4 years in length, and the first 2 years are usually focused on general education at the collegiate level. Although AD-prepared nurses and BSN-prepared nurses often function with the same job descriptions, they bring unique skill sets that often complement each other in clinical practice. The greater focus on skills in AD preparation contrasts to the greater focus on evidence-based practice in BSN preparation, offering each the opportunity to contribute to the other's practice. Many programs are available today for AD-prepared nurses seeking to transition to BSN preparation.

In 2003 the American Association of Colleges of Nursing (AACN-East) introduced the CNL as a new generalist nursing role, requiring master's preparation. This role was a response to the nursing shortage, increasing complexity in the health care system, increased patient acuity, and a recognition that other members of the health care team were entering with postgraduate education. Although CNL graduates prepare for the same state board exam as AD- and BSN-prepared nurses, additional certification is available to CNL graduates through AACN-East. The CNL may be viewed as an advanced generalist role, because the master's degree emphasizes systems assessment and leadership skills with the intent of increasing nursing's involvement at a health care systems level. The educational focus of this role includes a quality and safety systems gap assessment and preparation to lead care for cohorts of patients based on available evidence in the clinical settings.

Nurses with specialty master's preparation or doctoral-level preparation often assume roles as advanced specialists. Although the dyads are the foundation for these nursing roles, advanced specialists offer additional skills and knowledge in a particular clinical area. For example, a community public health nurse designs and implements programs to address the health problems of a population, whereas a health systems specialist manages groups of nurses or other professionals within a health care system. The meta-dyad, other-centeredness, remains the focus of these roles, although the "other" is

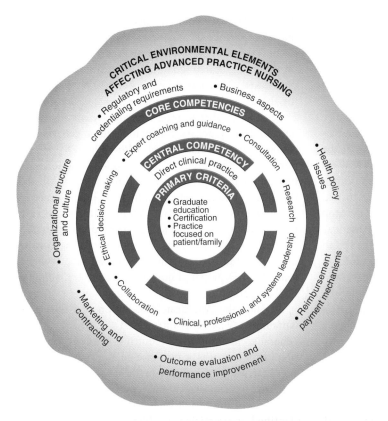

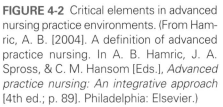

FIGURE 4-2 Critical elements in advanced nursing practice environments. (From Hamric, A. B. [2004]. A definition of advanced practice nursing. In A. B. Hamric, J. A. Spross, & C. M. Hansom [Eds.], *Advanced practice nursing: An integrative approach* [4th ed.; p. 89]. Philadelphia: Elsevier.)

not a single patient but an entire group, population, or system. Postgraduate education allows nurses in these roles to refine the application of the role-identity dyads to the population of concern.

Advanced practice nurses (APNs) are also categorized as advanced specialists. Figure 4-2 is taken from the leading text on advanced practice roles and shows the central aspects of clinical practice, certification, and master's preparation, along with seven core competencies (Hamric, Spross, & Hanson, 2008). The outer ring of the figure represents how the APN role interacts with the environment. All APNs apply the core competencies, but to varying degrees, and with particular emphasis on certain competencies over others depending on the setting in which they work. Currently four different roles of advanced practice nursing are recognized: the nurse practitioner, who provides a blend of nursing and medical care in primary or acute care settings; the clinical nurse specialist, who provides specialized nursing care to a selected population; the certified nurse midwife, who provides gynecological and obstetrical care;

and the certified registered nurse anesthetist, who provides anesthesia and monitoring of patients during surgery. Although these four categories are distinct, they share the model in Figure 4-2 as the foundation of their practice.

The 2004 Doctor of Nursing Practice (DNP) position statement sought a transformational change in the post-graduate education required for professional nurses who will practice with advanced degrees. The recommendation that nurses practicing at the highest level should receive doctoral level preparation was based on a number of factors, perhaps most significantly the need for improvement in health, quality, and safety outcomes. There was recognition of the need for expanded scientific reasoning for safe nursing practice, improved care quality, and increased application of systems theory to manage increasing complexity of care delivery. A definition was proposed by AACN-East (2004) that described the scope of advanced nursing practice as: "any form of nursing intervention that influences health care outcomes for individuals or populations, including the direct care of individual patients, management of care for individuals and populations, administration of nursing and health care organizations, and the development and implementation of health policy" (p. 2).

The AACN-East recognized the need for consistency in the degrees required for advanced nursing practice and detailed a position statement and doctoral practice essentials for advanced practice, recommending the DNP (AACN, 2006). In 2010, the Institute of Medicine report on the Future of Nursing moved this reasoning forward with the recommendations that nurses play a fundamental role in transforming the U.S. health care system. Recommendations specific to nursing education included: "1) Nurses should practice to the full extent of their education and training and 2) Nurses should achieve higher levels of education and training through an improved education system that promotes seamless academic progression" (IOM, 2010).

Work Environment

In 2008 the U.S. Department of Health and Human Services (USDHHS) estimated 2.5 million registered nurses (RNs) were employed in nursing, representing nearly 85 % of licensed RNs. This was the highest rate of nursing employment since the metric was first measured in 1977. Just over 62% of generalist nurses practice in hospitals, and the remaining 37% work in home care, outpatient clinics, or nursing homes (USDHHS, 2009).

The nursing workforce grew significantly after the year 2000, by nearly 25%. With the growth in new entrants, the number of nurses under the age of 30 increased, along with the aging of the current nurse population. Nearly one-third of nurses are over the age of 50 today. The diversity of the registered nursing workforce is slowly increasing (non-whites and men), and more than 65% of registered nurses are providing care in inpatient and outpatient settings in hospitals. The nursing pipeline is based on the number of individuals taking national licensing exams, and this number grew more than 100% from 2001 to 2011. There was a greater than 85% increase in the number of registered nurses earning bachelor's degrees from 2007 to 2011, and the number of graduate nursing degrees increased by 67% in the same time period (USDHHS, 2013).

The practice settings of the advanced specialist nurse are also diverse and may include schools of nursing, policy work groups, professional organizations,

outpatient clinics, state or local health departments, and acute care settings. Less than half of nurses with master's degrees work in hospitals; nearly 20% are in ambulatory care settings, and a little more than 10% are in academic education (USDHHS, 2009).

In every case nurses' roles are shaped by the environment in which they work. This occurs because of policies set in place by the administrators of the employing organization and the structure by which care is provided. For example, in the past a short supply of nurses lead hospitals to apply a team nursing model, in which one registered nurse (generalist) is assigned to care for a larger number of patients with the assistance of one or more unlicensed care providers. The tasks performed by that nurse are confined to those that require a license, such as medication administration and assessment, whereas all other tasks are performed by other members of the team under the nurse's supervision. In contrast, the primary nurse model of care assigns one nurse a smaller group of patients with the expectation that most of the required tasks are performed by that nurse (Kerfoot, 1997). In both cases the system of care shapes the implementation of the nursing role.

Many hospitals and health systems also differentiate nursing roles through a clinical ladder. Nurses are identified as practicing on different levels (or rungs) of the ladder and therefore face different role expectations (Fusilero et al., 2008). A new graduate from a BSN program is usually hired to the lowest level on the ladder and expected to demonstrate, within the first 1 or 2 years, the ability to practice at the next level and apply for promotion. Functioning as the charge nurse by applying the leader-managing and critical thinking dyad, precepting students or novice nurses by applying the mentoring-sharing and role modeling dyad, and participating in unit-based research projects by applying the researcher-inquiring and discovering dyad are all specific examples of activities associated with different levels in a clinical ladder. The work environment will also be explored later in this chapter in regard to how it relates to the creation of role stress.

ROLE DYNAMICS
Multiple Roles and Role Balance

As the role-identity dyads suggest, professional nurses assume multiple roles. Context dictates which of the role dyads are predominant. When caring for a patient who is grieving after hearing a terminal diagnosis, the caregiver-compassion dyad takes precedence, whereas caring for the same patient on the day he is being discharged may bring the educator-learning and guiding dyad to the forefront. Similarly, nurses may change their role because they have advanced their education or develop an interest in a different clinical setting; in these transitions, the same role-identity dyads are called on in new ways and to different degrees. In a given work setting, the professional nurse is cognizant of the role-identity dyads, selecting among them as the situation demands, and moving fluidly between them.

Professionals also assume roles outside the work setting, and nurses are no exception. In addition to professional roles such as the role of a health care provider, there are personal roles such as the role of partner, parent, team member, or friend. People also may participate in religious or civic organizations by assuming membership or leadership roles that demand a different set of role behaviors. Often, multiple roles are assumed within different contexts. For example, when a professional nurse is at home with family members, her primary role is clearly indicated by her physical location. When she walks through the doors of the hospital, a new physical environment invites a new role.

Balancing multiple roles occurs along a continuum that involves the dynamics of both segmentation and integration. Possessing clear boundaries between roles is referred to as *role segmentation*. Practicing strict role segmentation means avoiding any blending of personal and professional roles (Olson-Buchanan & Boswell, 2005). For instance, role segmentation includes avoiding checking an employment-related e-mail account from home or avoiding making a personal phone call at work. Role integration is the opposite of role segmentation. Practicing role integration means that the movement between multiple roles is fluid (Olson-Buchanan & Boswell, 2005). Such professionals might use a cell phone or pager to stay in touch with work during a day off, or they might do volunteer work with co-workers, incorporating both collegial and community roles.

Few people practice roles that are fully segmented or fully integrated; most are somewhere in the middle. The balancing of roles along this continuum fluctuates over time. For instance, a professional nurse's role may be highly segmented with days off to spend with friends and family and days working when the professional role takes precedence. However, during a work shift that same nurse may receive a call that a family member is ill or be asked to work overtime after making a commitment to attend a community event. In these instances juggling multiple roles is more challenging.

Role Stress

Role stress occurs when situations or aspects of the environment affect an individual's ability to carry out the perceived obligations of the role (Chen, Chen, Tsai, & Lo, 2007). In these situations the nurse may feel obligated to fulfill her professional role and also feel obligated to meet the needs of the sick family member or to follow through on the commitment made to the community event. Role strain refers to an emotional reaction when role stress is not resolved (Chen et al., 2007). Role stress is a common phenomenon that, if appropriately managed, can lead to increased role satisfaction. Unresolved role stress that leads to role strain contributes to professionals leaving a work setting. The terms *role stress* and *role strain* are sometimes used interchangeably, but understanding the difference is important. Role stress has a variety of forms; the causes are multifactorial and can be exacerbated when role functions collide with identity characteristics.

Role stress and role strain are not unique to nursing but can arise in any profession. The impact of role strain on health and well-being can be significant. One study found that depression and job strain were correlated; suggesting that job strain was responsible for mental health inequities (LaMontagne, Keegel, Vallance, Ostry, & Wolfe, 2008). Other research reveals that job strain has a modest effect on systolic blood pressure and that lower social support increases that impact (Guimont et al., 2006). In a survey of adults with personal roles as caregivers, Fredrikson and Scharlach (1997) found that those who worked shifts reported higher levels of role strain than those in salaried positions, perhaps because of conflicts between work and personal obligations that are not easily resolved in the face of rigid work schedules. This last study is particularly pertinent to nurses, who are likely to work shifts and also be looked to by friends and family to serve as caregivers outside the professional setting.

The meta-dyad of nursing, other-centeredness, may in part contribute to role stress. External elements shape the nurse's role, allowing for conflict, ambiguity, and differing expectations about specific role obligations to be likely to arise. In a review of international literature, Lambert and Lambert (2001) noted that the phenomenon of role strain occurs in nurses throughout the world. This review identified factors in the work environment that were consistently correlated to higher levels of role stress in nurses across a wide variety of cultures and settings. These factors included poor relationships with colleagues, perceived lack of control over the job, time demands, and lack of support from the employing organization.

In a national survey in the United States, Ulrich, Buerhaus, Donelan, Norman, and Dittus (2005) examined registered nurses' views on the work environment and compared their results with findings from a similar survey conducted 2 years earlier. Overall job satisfaction was slightly higher in the more recent survey. Nurses in 2004 reported greater satisfaction in relationships with colleagues than did those surveyed in 2002, suggesting that some improvement in work environments has occurred. The authors note three areas still to be improved: nurses in both surveys reported low decision-making authority, a lack of time to form relationships with patients, and inadequate respect and support from employing organizations. These factors, which represent an imbalance in the dyads, may continue to contribute to role stress among nurses. The USDHHS's Health Resources and Services Administration (USDHHS, 2009) reports nearly 30% of RNs were "extremely satisfied" and more than an additional 50% of RNs reported being "moderately satisfied" with their principal nursing position. This is slightly higher than 2004 rates of satisfaction.

Role Conflict. **Sources:** *Role conflict* refers to role stress that occurs when an individual feels required to meet the obligations of two different roles at once. Role conflict can occur between professional and personal roles. For example, consider the nurse who also is a parent or a primary caregiver to an aging relative. Attending to the needs of the dependent while also meeting the professional expectation to be on time for a shift and free of personal distractions creates role stress and may progress to role strain. Nevidjon (2004) notes that some nurses work multiple shifts in a single day, waking up early to do household chores and coming home after the work shift to childcare or eldercare responsibilities. Similarly, the nurse who is actively involved in the community may face role stress when asked to rotate to different shifts, requiring a change in sleep pattern.

In a review of literature, Stanley (2006) notes role conflict occurring among nurses who provide direct bedside care and have managerial responsibilities. Although both roles place a high priority on patient care and safety, the obligations of the direct bedside role are determined by the needs of a particular group of patients, whereas the obligations of the managerial role are determined by the needs of the unit and the institution. In both cases other-centeredness provides the foundation for the role; the conflict comes from having two "others" with different expectations. Efforts to honor clinical obligations and provide service to patients while honoring administrative obligations and the institution's mission, leaves the individual feeling pulled in different directions.

Strategies: Nevidjon (2004) lists several strategies to help alleviate the role stress that results from conflict between professional and personal roles. These include combining efforts, or finding ways to meet the obligations of two roles simultaneously, such as including friends in work-related events or inviting co-workers to community-based activities. These periods of greater role integration can alleviate the stress that comes from having multiple obligations in different directions. This author also suggests taking short breaks during work, exercising, and getting enough sleep to help alleviate role strain caused by role conflict.

An innovative strategy for addressing conflict between personal and professional roles involves adjusting the hours of nursing shifts. Some institutions offer flexible work hours, identified by Young, Albert, Paschke, and Meyer (2007) as "the Parent Shift," to reduce the stress that can occur from family and work role conflicts. The stress of conflicting personal and professional roles is widely recognized within our society. In 1993, federal legislation in the form of the Family Medical Leave Act (FMLA) was passed by Congress to ensure that employees who need time off to provide care to family members are able to return to their existing employment. Although documentation is required for FMLA time, the act applies to any personal caregiving role—from driving a sick child to multiple doctors' appointments to staying home to care for a dying relative.

Role Overload. **Sources:** *Role overload* refers to situations in which the time and resources allotted for a given role are insufficient to meet the role expectations. Essentially, role overload occurs when there is too much to do and too little time in which to do it. As indicated in the description of the dyads, professional nurses often have multiple sub-roles, or separate sets of behaviors and expectations that make up the larger role. The wide range of activities that constitute a professional nursing role is very rewarding but can also become overwhelming, particularly because many nurses work in shifts, meaning that a set time interval is given to complete required tasks.

Role overload is documented as a source of role stress among nurses (Chang & Hancock, 2003) and advanced practice nurses (Chen et al., 2007). Given the increasing system and patient complexity, the efforts to make health care delivery more efficient and affordable, and the increase in health care technology, the workload of professional nurses continues to expand. Although role overload is a real and concerning phenomenon, strategies can be used to reduce the strain it causes.

Strategies: Delegation is an essential strategy to prevent the stress of role overload. *Delegation* is defined by the American Nurses Association (ANA) as "the transfer of responsibility for the performance of a task from one individual to another while retaining accountability for the outcome" (American Nurses Association, 2005, p. 4). In this strategy the nurse asks another member of the health care team to perform particular tasks, such as obtaining patients' vital signs. By delegating a task the nurse is not required to observe the task's completion and thus can attend to other tasks. However, the nurse retains responsibility for the result of the task, so follow-up action may be required. Appropriate delegation requires understanding the competency level and scope of practice of the person to whom tasks are delegated and effectively communicating with that person regarding the patient's needs, the time in which the task should be completed, and the follow-up action planned.

As an example of delegation, consider a staff nurse who is assigned to care for patients and simultaneously take the charge nurse role for her unit. At a given time during the shift, she may be called on to be a caregiver when one of her patients requires medication for pain and also called on to act in a managerial role to determine how to manage a staffing shortage on the next shift. To resolve this potential role overload, the charge nurse can delegate the task of providing the patient's pain medicine to a clinician colleague or contact the nursing supervisor to address the staff shortage as advocate for all.

Prioritizing is also essential when role overload emerges. Creating a list of the tasks required and numbering them according to their importance guides some nurses to negotiate a busy shift. Taking time to reflect can allow for a deepened awareness of required activities to be performed. Inviting present-moment awareness can improve system and clinician safety and reduce the potential for errors during procedures like medication administration.

Another strategy to address role overload involves appropriate changes to the physical environment. For instance, if supplies are kept at a distance from the site of care delivery, the time required for each task will be unnecessarily lengthened (Christmas, 2008). Providing input to a unit manager about changes to the physical environment or joining a task force to examine what supplies are most often needed and so should be kept in a closer location can help resolve role stress caused by role overload.

Role Ambiguity. **Sources:** *Role ambiguity* refers to role stress that occurs when the obligations and privileges of a given role are not clearly defined. This leaves the individual unsure how to act. There are two distinct periods in which role ambiguity is likely to occur: during role transition and in times of role extension. Role transition occurs when an individual enters a new role, and role extension occurs when the duties associated with a particular role expand. Ideally, both role transition and role extension are temporary causes of role stress that resolve when an individual achieves role mastery, a sense of clarity regarding the role expectations and a firm confidence in the ability to meet those expectations.

An example of role transition occurs when a new graduate begins a position as a professional nurse. The degree of stress that a new graduate nurse experiences with this transition will vary depending on the availability of mentoring, organizational support, and preparation from the educational experience. In a study of new graduate nurses, Chang and Hancock (2003) found a correlation between role ambiguity and lower ratings of job satisfaction, indicating that this is an important source of stress and strain. Similarly, in examining role stress among nurses working 8- and 12-hour shifts, Hoffman and Scott (2003) found significantly different levels among nurses based on years of experience. Regardless of the length of the shift worked, higher levels of stress were reported by newer nurses.

The potential for role stress caused by role ambiguity is not confined to the new graduate. In interviews with nurses at different career stages, Deppoliti (2008) noted that there were discrete periods or "passage points" in which nurses reaffirmed their professional identity. At certain stages, such as transitioning to the charge nurse role or the preceptor role, the participants experienced role ambiguity. Similarly, Chen et al. (2007) noted that experienced nurses in Taiwan experienced role ambiguity when they transitioned to advanced practice roles and when those roles were extended by their employing institution. Their survey results confirmed a significant correlation between role ambiguity and lower ratings of job satisfaction. As hospitals and clinics adapt to economic and technological changes, nurses at every career stage are likely to experience periods of role ambiguity owing to role extension.

Strategies: Essential in resolving the stress of role ambiguity is the development of a clear definition of the role. As described by Young, Stuenkel, and Bawel-Brinkley (2008), role ambiguity among new graduates is best prevented with a comprehensive structured orientation program. A combination of clinical and classroom activities provides new graduates with the chance to observe nursing expertise and an opportunity to discuss and validate their own expectations. Authors identify that support from peers is essential in the resolution of role ambiguity (Bally, 2007; Young et al., 2007; Young et al., 2008). Orientation sessions in which new graduates interact with each other encourage the development of supportive peer networks.

Mentoring is also a key strategy for addressing the stress of role ambiguity. *Mentoring*, as described in the dyads, refers to a formal or informal process in which a mentor and a mentee establish a relationship with the mutual goal of meeting the career goals of the mentee (Bally, 2007). Mentors are distinct from friends in that there is not an even give-and-take expected. Although both parties expect to gain from the mentorship, the benefits on each side are different. Seeking a mentor who is not the assigned clinical preceptor provides a transitioning nurse with a wider base of support. The mentor can validate or correct the mentee's expectations about the new or expanded role and review situations that the mentee encounters during the orientation process.

All professional roles have written job descriptions that can be reviewed to assist in the process of gaining role clarity. This can be especially helpful for transitions into roles that are newly created. In advanced specialist roles, nurses may be asked to write or edit the content of the job description. Review of existing descriptions for similar roles or advice from a mentor can guide the process of creating a role description. When role transition or extension occurs, a nurse can craft a simple

statement or inquiry response that reinforces "what I do in my current role." Recalling, repeating, or responding with a prepared statement is helpful in alleviating role ambiguity during times of role transition or extension. An exercise to consider when role transitions and extensions occur is developing a one- or two-sentence description of the role (Hamric, 2008). An example of such an exercise is provided in the Critical Thinking Exercises at the end of this chapter.

Role Discrepancy. **Source:** *Role discrepancy* refers to role stress that occurs when an individual's conception of a role is incompatible with the actual obligations of the role. This phenomenon is well documented in studies of nurses. In fact, the importance of this source of role stress is exemplified by the fact that some professional nurse authors define role stress and strain as role discrepancy (Hall, 2004; Lambert & Lambert, 2001). Past president of the ANA, Barbara Blackeney, referenced role discrepancy when she told a *New York Times* reporter, "Nurses love nursing. They just hate their jobs" (Corbett, 2003, para 20). This quote suggests that a predominance of nurses have a concept of what their role *ought* to be that is inconsistent with the content of their day-to-day work.

Results of a national survey of nurses working in the United States suggest that Blackeney's assessment is accurate. More than half of respondents reported spending too little time engaged in direct patient care and too much time on documentation (Buerhaus, Donelan, Ulrich, DesRoches, & Dittus, 2007). Several authors note that role discrepancy as a source of role stress for nurses contributes to job dissatisfaction and even to the intention to quit (Lambert & Lambert, 2001; Takase, Maude, & Manias, 2006). Hall (2004), in a small qualitative explorative study, confirmed what the national survey indicated: nurses identified the inability to meet their own expectations as an important source of stress and strain.

Strategies: Although role discrepancy is a significant source of role stress and strain among nurses, there are strategies for managing it. Debriefing, which involves reviewing the events of a particular situation with a colleague or group of colleagues, can allow for the articulation of the role expectations that came into conflict in a given situation. Often, role expectations are taken for granted, and simply verbalizing these thoughts allows the concerned nurse to move forward in understanding the source of her stress. Additionally, colleagues who are present during a debriefing session can validate the concerned nurse's views and share similar experiences and expectations. In this way debriefing builds positive relationships within the clinical settings, a key factor in reducing role stress (Lambert & Lambert, 2001). Finally, debriefing is helpful in identifying the types of situations that contribute to role discrepancy so that strategies to prevent these situations can be implemented.

For example, consider a novice intensive care unit nurse whose elderly patient develops a change in his cardiac rhythm in the early morning hours. The doctor on call asks that the nurse to manage this change by calling a cardiology consult, an action usually taken by medical providers during daytime hours. On the same shift the charge nurse asks the novice ICU nurse to cover a break and give a report to the hospital's nursing supervisor if she calls. This nurse is at risk for role discrepancy in two directions. First, calling the cardiology team is not an expectation of the ICU nurse role in this institution. Second, having never been oriented to the charge role, this nurse did not expect to take responsibility for reporting to the supervisor.

In a debriefing session, the nurse in the aforementioned scenario describes the shift to the mentor and the mentor validates that the expectations placed on the nurse during that shift were not consistent with the nurse's own views of the role. Together they review possible ways of managing this kind of situation. First, the mentor suggests that the nurse politely but firmly refuse to call consults because this is not an appropriate expectation of the ICU nurse role. The mentor, who is a member of the unit leadership, also offers to write an e-mail to the unit's medical director to be forwarded to all medical providers, clarifying that ICU nurses are not expected to call consults. With regard to the charge nurse role, the nurse decides, with the support of the mentor, to speak with the manager about requiring charge nurses to seek coverage for breaks only from other nurses who are oriented to the charge role. In this way the nurse and the mentor take specific actions to change the expectations of others (the doctor and the charge nurse) so that the conflict with the nurse's own view of the role is resolved.

A second strategy to consider in situations of role discrepancy is investigating the role advancement program at the employing institution. Many institutions offer clinical ladders or advancement programs for registered nurses though which clinical experience,

requisite educational background, and demonstrated professionalism lead to promotion to a higher level (Fusilero et al., 2008). The benefits of promotion may include higher pay, input on shift assignment, and the opportunity to participate in additional professional development activities. Nurses who have not considered career advancement but are asked to perform in the charge role or to be clinical preceptors may experience role discrepancy because these sub-roles are not within the scope of a novice nursing role. If a nurse is comfortable assuming these roles, he or she ought to pursue career advancement in order to receive the full benefits of providing additional services to the institution.

A final strategy involves examining which tasks create role discrepancy and determining how these can be more efficiently completed (task analysis). For example, some nurses find that the time spent writing progress notes takes away from time interacting with patients, thus conflicting with their expectation that their primary role is to provide care. Approaching a manager, an advanced practice nurse, or unit leadership about strategies that make documentation more efficient can alleviate this source of role discrepancy. Is there a policy that could be changed to reduce the required documentation so that notes are written once every 24 hours rather than on every shift? Could a template for the required documentation be created so that this task can be completed more quickly? As in the example, in which the mentoring nurse sought to communicate with medical providers, actions that promote positive change can minimize and prevent role discrepancy.

***Role Incongruity.* Sources:** A final source of role stress for nurses is *role incongruity*. This term refers to situations in which the obligations of a role come into conflict with an individual's values. Although situations of role incongruity are similar to role discrepancy, they are likely to engender a more severe strain because values, unlike perceptions about a role, are personally determined and deeply revered. Values guide behavior, direct priorities, and determine how information is perceived (McNeese-Smith & Crook, 2003). Personal values are formed early in life through family, education, and religious and cultural experiences. Professional values develop through the process of professional socialization. Because values are deeply held, and a fundamental part of identity, they may be taken for granted and challenging to articulate (Raines, 1993). Related to role incongruity is **moral distress,** a phenomenon in which an individual feels compelled to act in a manner that she or he believes is morally wrong (Hamric, Davis, & Childress, 2006). Moral distress is discussed further in the chapter on ethics (Chapter 12).

Two recent studies describe role incongruity among nurses. Persky, Nelson, Watson, and Bent (2008) found that the nurses perceived by patients as most caring were also more likely to report frustration with the work environment. The authors explain these findings by noting that the high value placed on caring among these nurses was incongruent with the emphasis on efficient time management and judicious use of resources within the work environment. Similarly, in a national survey, Yarbrough, Alfred, and Martin (2008) identified the congruity of nurses' values across areas of practice (advanced practice, staff nurses, administrators, and educators) and suggested that dissonance with organizational values contributes to poor retention, or resigning. Their respondents identified privacy, respect for dignity, and accountability as top priorities that they felt were not highly valued by their institutions.

A striking example of role incongruity comes from studies of nurses working in New Orleans in 2005, after Hurricane Katrina. Nurses who valued their ability to provide care to vulnerable patients were required to do so without appropriate resources, without adequate rest, and in isolation from their families. Nurses interviewed about their experiences became tearful as they described making decisions about evacuating with their families or staying at the hospital, because both options engendered distress because of conflicting values (Giarratano, Orlando, & Savage, 2008).

Strategies: An essential starting point in managing role incongruity is values clarification, an exercise in which an individual practices articulating existing values. A variety of exercises are available for values clarification; but all of them encourage participants to become aware of how their choices, behaviors, and perceptions are determined by deeply rooted beliefs. By undergoing values clarification, a nurse will better articulate the role incongruity being experienced and begin to seek needed changes to the work environment. Values clarification is discussed further in the chapter on ethics (Chapter 12).

A second strategy in addressing role incongruity is empowerment. Manojlovich (2007) observes that empowerment develops when nurses are competent in their clinical practice, are providing nursing care

autonomously, and are represented on hospital committees and at administrative decision-making levels within an institution. Nurses can seek empowerment through connections with those in leadership positions and by recognizing their own ability to influence the work environment and control their nursing practice. Although caring and power may at first seem mutually exclusive, in fact, nurses are empowered by the care that they uniquely provide to patients (Manojlovich, 2007).

In situations in which role incongruity occurs repeatedly to the extent that the work environment is unsafe, the nurse may consider a whistle-blowing approach. *Whistle-blowing* refers to situations in which unethical or illegal conduct by an organization is reported to an outside authority by a member of that organization. An example of whistle-blowing includes when members of the U.S. Army reported the treatment of war criminals in prison camps to federal authorities (Shenon, 2004). Despite their lack of authority within the Army structure, the soldiers reporting this recognized they were part of an unethical environment and took steps to make a change. Lachman (2008) observes that nurses have a similar ethical obligation to act when a lack of organizational accountability threatens patient safety. Box 4-1 lists five recommendations for an ethical organizational culture. In an ethical organizational culture, nurses and all members of the health care team are benefited. In such an environment, role incongruity is seldom a source of role stress, because mechanisms for addressing values conflicts are firmly in place. Box 4-2 summarizes the stepwise approach to a role-related problem.

BOX 4-1 Recommendations for an Ethical Organizational Culture

- Develop a code of conduct that corresponds to the organization's values and that cannot be compromised.
- Develop an ethics committee whose mission is to create infrastructure to support organization's values.
- Provide educational forums on organizational ethics.
- Avoid passivity (the "bystander effect" and "diffusion of responsibility").
- Establish and publish an internal procedure for individuals to employ when they believe organizational values and "principles of care" are being violated.

Lachman, V. D. (2008). Whistleblowing: Role of organizational culture in prevention and management. *MEDSURG Nursing, 17*(4), 265–267.

BOX 4-2   Summary of a Stepwise Approach to Role-Related Problems

1. Identify the cause. Acknowledging and anticipating sources of role stress is the first step.
2. Develop internal role clarity. Use the following questions to assist in developing a clear definition of the role:
   What are the primary obligations of the role?
   What tasks are prioritized by persons in the role?
   What percentage of time is appropriate for each of the tasks above?
   What are the values of the organization in which you are employed?
   What personal values relate to this role?
3. Identify the key stakeholders. Role problems may create a sense of isolation and can affect family, co-workers, patients, and friends. Consider who else might be affected by this problem and who can facilitate the resolution. Identify the best time and manner in which to communicate with those involved; some co-workers may rely on e-mail and others may prefer face-to-face contact. Often, a unit manager or advanced practice nurse can provide guidance and support.
4. Develop specific interventions, based on the source of role stress. Consider the following specific strategies for different sources of role stress:

Role conflict: Seek opportunities for integrating personal and professional roles; adjust the work schedule for personal needs.

Role overload: Delegate, prioritize; make changes to the physical work environment.

Role ambiguity: Identify and form relationships with mentors. Consider adjusting your job description and develop a one- or two-sentence statement that describes your role.

Role discrepancy: Debriefing. Seek out support from co-workers and offer support to others. Identify strategies for making work processes more efficient.

Role incongruity: Values clarification. Repeated role incongruity may indicate the need for a whistle-blowing approach or a change in roles.

5. Select a course of action and take it!
6. Evaluate. What impact did the action have on your satisfaction with your role?
7. Reflect. With a deepened awareness regarding the assessment of the role-related challenge and evaluation of the intervention, allow time for an introspective invitation to inquiry.

SUMMARY

Nursing's contribution to health care is illustrated by the nature and diversity of nursing roles. At its core, the nursing profession requires a renewed vision for patient wellness and a passion for a society in which health and wellness is a right for all. Nursing demands a role identity to preserve the relationship at the individual level and for humanity at a societal level. We have reached a critical transformation point for both the nursing profession and the U.S. health care system. It is no longer sufficient simply to advocate for policy change or ensure the care of an individual patient. Massive system change and practice paradigm shifts are required in both health care delivery and nursing education and practice. The integration of nursing roles into a nurse's core identity and practice is necessary. That work begins in a renewed examination of the central role of nursing's other-centeredness (meta-dyad) and of all of the role-identity dyads (functions and characteristics) to ensure they are woven into a "single quilt" that is *nursing*. Although the roles described in this chapter do not constitute an exhaustive list, they are representative of the roles nurses commonly assume. As the health care system continues to change, it is anticipated that new nursing roles will emerge. According to the Future of Nursing (IOM) report (2010), nurses should be full partners, with physicians and other health care professionals, in redesigning health care in the United States. The 2010 Affordable Care Act mandates the creation of a National Health Care Workforce Commission and a National Center for Workforce Analysis to anticipate need for health care workers and support data collection and analysis. Nurses have an opportunity to play important leadership roles in decision making for the future of the United States health care system and are clearly being invited to this call to action.

SALIENT POINTS

- The practice of nursing involves assuming a number of diverse roles that have corresponding identity elements.
- Central to nursing is "other-centeredness" because all nursing roles are focused on addressing the needs of a specific person or population.
- Culture and history shape the way nursing roles are interpreted by society, whereas education and work environment affect how nursing roles are implemented.
- The need to assume multiple roles in nursing can result in role stress and strain.
- Strategies to modify role stress and strain are situation-specific and essential to effective nursing practice.

CRITICAL REFLECTION EXERCISES

The following statements are affirmative reflection principles to adopt to negotiate role balance and reduce role stress:

- Reflection and processing are critical for removing oversimplification.
- Examine where you might not have been intentional or contributed deliberate effort.
- Remain open to adaptation during examination and inquiry.
- Consider rationale for opinions that others hold. Empathize. Appreciate and try to understand. Try to evaluate all options prior to coming to a conclusion.
- Recognize the value in examining issues from all angles. Welcome different views.
- Explore positions that are different from yours. How might these positions have been shaped?
- Attempt to discover and apply meaning to what is seen, heard, and read. Be purposeful, informed, outcome-focused, and systematic.

Given these statements, explore your personal response to the following questions:

1. How do you make decisions and solve problems?
2. Is there a process that you follow? What is that process?
3. Consider what strategies you might use to reduce role stress and strain.
4. Do you ask pertinent questions and analyze multiple forms of evidence? What forms of evidence might you look for?
5. Consider how role stress and strain feels in your body when you are able to notice it. How can you begin to modify the role stress and strain? What works for you?

REFERENCES

American Association of Colleges of Nursing. (2004). Doctor of Nursing Practice position statement. Retrieved December 11, 2013, from http://www.aacn.nche.edu/publications/position/DNPpositionstatement.pdf.

American Association of Colleges of Nursing. (2006). The essentials of doctoral education for advanced nursing practice. Retrieved December 11, 2013, from http://www.aacn.nche.edu/publications/position/DNPEssentials.pdf.

American Nurses Association. (2005). *Principles of delegation.* Silver Spring, MD: American Nurses Association.

Armitage, G. (Director). (1971). *Private Duty Nurses* [Television series]. United States: New World Pictures.

Bally, J. M. G. (2007). The role of nursing leadership in creating a mentoring culture in acute care environments. *Nurse Economics, 25*(3), 143–148.

Bastable, S. (2007). *Nurse as educator: Principles of teaching and learning for nursing practice.* Sudbury, MA: Jones & Bartlett Publishers.

Benner, P., & Wrubel, J. (1988). *The primacy of caring, stress and coping in health and illness.* Menlo Park: Addison Wesley.

Biddle, B. J. (1979). *Role theory: Expectations, identities and behaviors.* New York: Academic Press.

Brackett, C. (Producer), & Wilder, B. (Director). (1945). *The Lost Weekend* [Motion picture]. United States: Paramount Pictures.

Brixius, L., Dunskey, E., & Wallem, L. (Creators). (2009). *Nurse Jackie* [Television series]. United States: Showtime Networks.

Bruckheimer, J., & Bay, M. (Producers), & Bay, M. (Director). (2001). *Pearl Harbor* [Motion picture]. United States: Touchstone Pictures.

Buerhaus, P. I., Donelan, K., Ulrich, B. T., DesRoches, C., & Dittus, R. (2007). Trends in the experiences of hospital-employed registered nurses: Results from three national surveys. *Nursing Economics, 25*(2), 69–80.

Burns, T. (Producer), & Chulack, C. (Director). (1994). *ER* [Television series]. United States: Amblin Entertainment & Warner Bros: Television Production, Inc.

California Nurses Association. (2009). *Nurses and doctors call for Florence Nightingale Day*. Protest: Against Max Baucus and health insurers: May 12, 2009. Retrieved from http://www.calnurses.org/media-center/press-releases/2009/may/nurses-and-doctors-call-for-florence-nightingale-day-protest-against-max-baucus-and-health-insurers-may-12.html.

Cattell-Gordon, D. (2009). *(Personal interview). Telehealth and collaborative practice*. University of Virginia Health System. Retrieved from http://www.healthsystem.virginia.edu/internettelemedicine.

Chang, E., & Hancock, K. (2003). Role stress and role ambiguity in new nursing graduates in Australia. *Nursing and Health Sciences, 5*, 155–163.

Chen, Y., Chen, S., Tsai, C., & Lo, L. (2007). Role stress and job satisfaction for nurse specialists. *Journal of Advanced Nursing, 59*(5), 497–509.

Childs, A. (2006). The complex gastrointestinal patient and Jean Watson's Theory of Caring in nutrition support. *Gastroenterology Nursing, 29*(4), 283–288.

Christmas, K. (2008). How work environment impacts retention. *Nurse Economics, 26*(5), 316–318.

Corbett, S. (2003, March 16). *The last shift*. Retrieved January 19, 2009, from http://query.nytimes.com/gst/fullpage.html?res=9E00E5D8163EF935A25750C0A9659C8B63&sec=health&spon=&pagewanted=2.

Corn, R. (Director). (2005). *Grey's Anatomy* [Television series]. United States: ABC Studios.

Covington, H. (2005). Caring presence: Providing a safe place for patients. *Holistic Nursing Practice, 19*(4), 169–172. Retrieved from http://www.ncbi.nlm.nih.gov/pubmed/16006831.

Cramer, D. (Producer). (1988). *Nightingales* [Television series]. United States: Aaron Spelling Productions.

Deppoliti, D. (2008). Exploring how new registered nurses construct professional identity in hospital settings. *The Journal of Continuing Education, 39*(6), 255–262.

Dewey, J., Kilpatrick, W. H., Hartmann, G. H., & Melby, E. O. (1937). *The teacher and society*. New York: Appleton-Century.

Douglas, K. (2012). *Nurses: If Florence could see us now*. Retrieved December 5, 2013, from http://firstrunfeatures.com/nursesdvd.html.

Douglas, M., & Zaentz, S. (Producers), & Forman, M. (Director). (1975). *One Flew Over the Cuckoo's Nest* [Motion picture]. United States: United Artists.

dyad. (2013). In *Merriam-Webster Online Dictionary*. Retrieved September 15, 2013, from http://www.merriam-webster.com/dictionary/dyad.

Evans, J. (2004). Men nurses: a historical and feminist perspective. *Journal of Advanced Nursing, 47*(3), 321–328.

Fredrikson, K. I., & Scharlach, A. E. (1997). Caregiving and employment: The impact of workplace characteristics on role strain. *Journal of Gerontological Social Work, 28*(4), 3–22.

Fusilero, J., Lini, L., Prohaska, P., Szweda, C., Carney, K., & Mion, L. C. (2008). The career advancement for registered nurse excellence program. *The Journal of Nursing Administration, 38*(12), 526–531.

Gardner, D. (2005). Ten lessons in collaboration. *Online Journal of Issues in Nursing*. Retrieved September 15, 2009, from http://www.nursingworld.org/ojin/topic26/tpc26_1.htm.

Giarratano, G., Orlando, S., & Savage, J. (2008). Perinatal nursing in uncertain times: The Katrina effect. *The American Journal of Maternal Child Nursing, 33*(4), 249–257.

Guimont, C., Brisson, C., Dagenais, G. R., Milot, A., Vezina, M., & Masse, B. (2006). Effects of job strain on blood pressure: A prospective study of white-collar workers. *American Journal of Public Health, 96*(8), 1436–1443.

Hall, D. S. (2004). Work-related stress of registered nurses in a hospital setting. *Journal for Nurses in Staff Development, 20*(1), 6–14.

Hamric, A. B. (2008). A definition of advanced practice. In A. B. Hamric, J. A. Spross, & C. M. Hanson (Eds.), *Advanced practice nursing: An integrative approach* (pp. 75–94). St Louis: Elsevier.

Hamric, A. B., Davis, W. S., & Childress, M. D. (2006). Moral distress in health care providers: What is it and what can we do about it? *The Pharos, 69*(1), 17–23.

Heldens, L. (Creator). (2009). *Mercy* [Television series]. United States: Universal Media Studios.

Henk, B. (2005). *Mentoring: What's it all about? Notes from a Navy leadership presentation held in Bremerton*. WA: Unpublished manuscript.

Hewitt, J. (2002). A critical review of the arguments debating the role of the nurse advocate. *Journal of Advanced Nursing, 37*(5), 439–445.

Hoffman, A. J., & Scott, L. D. (2003). Role stress and career satisfaction among registered nurses by work shift pattern. *Journal of Nursing Administration, 33*(6), 337–342.

Hogg, M., & Terry, D. (2000). *Attitudes, behavior and social context: The role of norms and group membership*. Mahwah, NJ: Lawrence Erlbaum Associates.

Hornberger, R. H. (Producer). (1972). *M*A*S*H* [Television series]. United States: 20th Century Fox.

identity. (2013). In *Merriam-Webster Online Dictionary*. Retrieved September 15, 2013, from http://www.merriam-webster.com/dictionary.identity.

Institute of Medicine. (2010). *The Future of Nursing: Leading Change; Advancing Health*. Retrieved December 10, 2013, from http://iom.edu/~/media/Files/Report%20Files/2010/The-Future-of-Nursing/Future%20of%20Nursing%202010%20Report%20Brief.pdf.

International Council of Nurses. (2009). *International Council of Nurses: Mission Statement*. Retrieved September 15, 2009, from http://www.icn.ch/res netbul_00.htm.

Jonsdottir, H., Litchfield, M., & Dexheimer Pharris, M. (2004). The relational core or nursing practice as partnership. *Journal of Advanced Nursing, 29*(5), 1205–1212.

Kaminski, J. (2006, March 14). *Nursing through the lens of culture: A multiple gaze*. Unpublished PhD. Vancouver: University of British Columbia.

Kerfoot, K. (1997). Role redesign: what has it accomplished? *Online Journal of Issues in Nursing, 2*(4). Retrieved from http://www.nursingworld.org/MainMenuCatagories/ANAMarketplace/Periodicals/OJIN/TableofContents/vol21997/No4Dec97/RoleRedesign.aspx.

Kuhl, L. (2005). Closing the revolving door: A look at mentoring. *Chart: Journal of Illinois Nursing, 102*(2), 9.

Lachman, V. D. (2008). Whistleblowing: Role of organizational culture in prevention and management. *MEDSURG Nursing, 17*(4), 265–267.

Lambert, V. A., & Lambert, C. E. (2001). Literature review of role stress/strain on nurses: An international perspective. *Nursing and Health Sciences, 3*, 161–172.

LaMontagne, A. D., Keegel, T., Vallance, D., Ostry, A., & Wolfe, R. (2008). Job strain—Attributable depression in a sample of working Australians: Assessing the contribution to health inequalities. *BMC Public Health, 8*(Article 181). Retrieved June 5, 2009, from http://www.biomedcentral.com/1471-2458/8/181.

Lawrence, B. (Producer). (2001). *Scrubs* [Television series]. United States: ABC Studios.

Leininger, M. (1988). Leininger's theory of nursing: Cultural care diversity and universality. *Nursing Science Quarterly, 1*(4), 152–160.

Leininger, M., & McFarland, M. (1997). *Transcultural nursing: Concepts, theories, research and practice* (3rd ed.). New York: McGraw-Hill Professional.

Lemire, J. (2002). Leader as critical thinker. *Nursing Leadership Forum, 7*, 69–76.

Lucas, J. (2009). History of male nurses. *Male Nurse Magazine*. Retrieved September 15, 2009, from http://www.malenursemagazine.com/historyofmalenurses.html.

Malik, M. (1997). Advocacy in nursing—a review of the literature. *Journal of Advanced Nursing, 25*(1), 130–138.

Manojlovich, M. (2007). Power and empowerment in nursing: Looking backward to inform the future. *OJIN: The Online Journal of Issues in Nursing, 12*(1). Manuscript 1. Retrieved from http://www.nursingworld.org/MainMenuCategories/ANAMarketplace/ANAPeriodicals/OJIN/TableofContents/Volume122007/No1Jan07/LookingBackwardtoInformtheFuture.aspx.

Marcia, J. (1966). Development and validation of ego identity status. *Journal of Personality and Social Psychology, 3*, 551–558.

Masius, J. (2009). *Hawthorne Television Series*. United States: John Masius Productions.

McCauley, K. (2005). Doing the right thing. *AACN News, 22*(2).

McEwan, I. (2001). *Atonement*. New York: Random House.

McFadden, E. (2006). Moral development and reproductive health decisions. *Journal of Obstetric, Gynecologic & Neonatal Nursing, 25*(6), 507–512.

McNeese-Smith, D. K., & Crook, M. (2003). Nursing values and a changing nurse workforce. *Journal of Nursing Administration, 33*(5), 260–270.

Morton, P. G., & Fontaine, D. (2009). *Critical care nursing: A holistic approach* (9th ed.). Philadelphia: Lippincott-Raven.

Munhall, P. (2007). The landscape of qualitative research in nursing. In P. Munhall (Ed.), *Nursing: A qualitative perspective* (4th ed.). Boston: Jones and Bartlett.

National League for Nursing. (2006). Statement: Mentoring of nurse faculty. *Nursing Education Perspectives, 27*(2), 110–113.

Nevidjon, B. (2004). Managing from the middle: Integrating midlife challenges, children, elder parents, and career. *Clinical Journal of Oncology Nursing, 8*(1), 72–75.

Nightingale, F. (1860). *Notes on nursing: What it is and what it is not* (First American Edition). New York: D. Appleton and Company.

Olson-Buchanan, J. B., & Boswell, W. R. (2005). Blurring boundaries: correlates of integration and segmentation between work and nonwork. *Journal of Vocational Behavior, 68*, 432–445.

Persky, G. J., Nelson, J. W., Watson, J., & Bent, K. (2008). Creating a profile of a nurse effective in caring. *Nursing Administration, 32*(1), 15–20.

Raines, D. A. (1993). Values: A guiding force. *AWHONN's Clinical Issues, 4*, 533–541.

Reiner, R. (Director), & Reiner, R., Scheinman, A., Stott, J., Nicolaides, S. (Producers). (1990). *Misery* [Motion picture]. United States: Columbia Pictures and Castle Rock Entertainment.

Robinson, K. (2003). Technology can't replace compassion in health care. *Journal of Emergency Nursing, 29*(3), 199–200.

role. (2013). In *Merriam-Webster Online Dictionary*. Retrieved September 15, 2013, from http://www.merriam-webster.com/dictionary/role.

Saenz, M. (Director). (1988). *China Beach: U.S. war drama* [Motion picture]. Retrieved from http://www.museum.tv.archives/etc/C/htmlC/chinabeach/chinabeach.htm.

Schumaker, K. L., & Meleis, A. I. (1994). Transitions: A central concept in nursing. *IMAGE: Journal of Nursing Scholarship, 26*(2), 119–127.

Shenon, P. (2004). *Officer suggests Iraq jail abuse was encouraged* [electronic version]. New York Times. Retrieved from http://www.nytimes.com/2004/05/02/international/middleeast/02ABUS.html?scp=1&sq=may%202004%20iraq%20prisoner&st=cse.

Siefert, P. (2009). The ANA Code of Ethics and AORN. *Perioperative Nursing Clinics, 3*(3), 183–189. Retrieved from http://visiblenurse.com/nurseculture7.html.

Snowball, J. (1996). Asking nurses about advocating for patients: 'reactive' and 'proactive' accounts. *Journal of Advanced Nursing, 24*(1), 67–75.

Spielberg, S. (Executive Producer). (1994). *ER* [Television series]. United States: Amblin Entertainment Company and Warner Bros: Television, NBC.

Stanley, D. (2006). Role conflict: Leaders and managers. *Nursing Management, 13*(5), 31–37.

Stanley, D. J. (2008). Celluloid angels: A research study of nurses in feature films 1900–2007. *Journal of Advanced Nursing, 64*(1), 84–95.

Summers, S. (2001). *History of the truth about nursing*. Retrieved December 9, 2013, from http://www.truthaboutnursing.org/about_us/our_history.html.

Takase, M., Maude, P., & Manias, E. (2006). The impact of role discrepancy on nurses' intention to quit their jobs. *Journal of Clinical Nursing, 15*, 1071–1080.

Tenenbaum, N. (Producer), & Roach, J. (Director). (2000). *Meet the Parents* [Motion picture]. United States: Universal Pictures & Dreamworks Productions.

Triolo, N. (2007). Authentic leadership begins with emotional intelligence. *AACN Advanced Critical Care, 18*(3), 244–247.

Tuxhill, C. (1994). In B. Miller, & Burnard P (Eds.), *Critical care nursing*. London: Balliere-Tindall.

Ulrich, B. T., Buerhaus, P. I., Donelan, K., Norman, L., & Dittus, R. (2005). How RNs view the work environment. *Journal of Nursing Administration, 35*(9), 20–38.

United States Census Bureau. (2012). *Men in Nursing Occupations*. Retrieved October 13, 2014, from http://www.census.gov/newsroom/releases/pdf/cb13-32_men_in_nursing_occupations.pdf.

United States Department of Health and Human Services. (2009). The Registered Nurse population: Findings from the 2008 National Sample Survey of Registered Nurses. *Executive Summary*. Retrieved December 13, 2013, from http://bhpr.hrsa.gov/healthworkforce/rnsurvey2008.html.

United States Department of Health and Human Services. (2013). The U.S. nursing workforce. *Trends in supply and education*. Retrieved May 30, 2014, from http://bhpr.hrsa.gov/healthworkforce/reports/nursingworkforce/nursingworkforcefullreport.pdf.

University of Pennsylvania Health System. *Nursing Annual Report 2005*. Retrieved September 15, 2009, from http://pennhealth.com/nursing/annual_report_2005.pdf.

USA Today. (2013). *More men join the nursing field as stigma starts to fade*. Retrieved December 5, 2013, from http://www.usatoday.com/story/news/nation/2013/07/10/men-join-nursing-field-as-stigma-fades/2504803/.

Wells, J. (Producer). (1988). *China Beach* [Television series]. United States: ABC Studios.

Winfield, C., Melo, K., & Myrick, F. (2009). *Journal for Nurses in Staff Development, 25*(2), E7–E13. http://dx.doi.org/10.1097/NND.ob013e31819c76a3.

Wood, D. (2012). *Nurses and the media: A call to action*. Retrieved December 9, 2013, from http://www.nursezone.com/nursing-news-events/more-news/Nurses-and-the-Media-A-Call-to-Action-at-UCLA-Symposium_39802.aspx.

Yarbrough, S., Alfred, D., & Martin, P. (2008). Research study: Professional values and retention. *Nursing, 39*(4), 10–18.

Young, C. M., Albert, N. M., Paschke, S. M., & Meyer, K. H. (2007). The 'parent shift' program: Incentives for nurses, rewards for nursing teams. *Nurse Economics, 25*(6), 339–344.

Young, M. E., Stuenkel, D. L., & Bawel-Brinkley, K. (2008). Strategies for easing the role transformation of graduate nurses. *Journal for Nurses in Staff Development, 24*(3), 105–110.

Zaentz, S. (Producer), & Minghella, A. (Director). (1996). *The English Patient* [Motion picture]. United States: Mirimax Films.

CHAPTER 5

Theories and Frameworks for Professional Nursing Practice

Mary Gunther, PhD, RN

http://evolve.elsevier.com/Friberg/bridge/

OBJECTIVES

At the completion of this chapter, the reader will be able to:

- Distinguish among a concept, a theory, a conceptual framework, and a model.
- Identify and define the four central concepts of nursing theories.
- Compare the main precepts of selected theories of nursing.
- Examine criteria for evaluating the utility of a specific nursing theory for its relevance to practice, education, or research.
- Identify selected theories from related disciplines that have application to nursing.

PROFILE IN PRACTICE

Jacqueline Fawcett, PhD, RN, FAAN
College of Nursing, University of Massachusetts—Boston, Boston, Massachusetts

Much of my current work focuses on helping nurses understand the connection between research and practice (Fawcett, 2000). I am firmly convinced that all nurse clinicians are also nurse researchers because the nursing practice process (assessment, labeling, goal setting, implementation, evaluation) is similar to the nursing research process (collection of baseline data, statement of the problem and hypotheses, experimental and control treatments, data analysis). I also am firmly convinced that the parallels between the nursing practice process and the nursing research process are most readily understood when both nursing practice and nursing research are guided by a nursing discipline–specific conceptual model or theory. The challenge is to assist nurses in practice to recognize that clinical information is research data and to report the effects of nursing practice in ways that will help other nurses and other health professionals and policymakers understand how nursing practice benefits the health of humankind.

Theory is the poetry of science. The poet's words are familiar, each standing alone, but brought together they sing, they astonish, they teach (Levine, 1995, p. 14).

I earned my baccalaureate degree in nursing from Boston University in 1964 and worked as an operating room staff nurse during that summer. My first exposure to a nursing discipline–specific theory occurred during my nursing coursework at Boston University. I learned Orlando's theory of the deliberative nursing process and have continued to find this simple yet elegant nursing theory of great utility in assisting patients, colleagues, and students to express their immediate needs for help.

I began teaching in a small hospital-based diploma nursing program in Connecticut in January 1965. I have continued to teach nursing since that time, first at the University of Connecticut for 6 years, with interruptions for my master's degree in parent-child nursing and my doctorate in nursing, then at the University of Pennsylvania for 21 years, and now at the University of Massachusetts in Boston.

During my master's program at New York University, I was introduced to theory-guided nursing practice. The clinical courses in parent-child nursing emphasized the application of theory to the nursing of childbearing women and their families, well children, and children with acute and chronic illnesses. At that time knowledge about nursing discipline–specific conceptual models and theories was limited. The New York University nursing faculty, my classmates, and I worked hard to adapt crisis theory to nursing situations and to explore the applicability of developmental theories and family theories to nursing situations. I immediately recognized the benefit of using theories to guide nursing practice—I had finally found a way to organize my thinking and my practice. Indeed, I finally knew what to say and do and the reasons for what I was saying and doing when I interacted with a patient!

When I returned to the University of Connecticut after earning my master's degree in 1970, my faculty colleagues and I began to design and implement a new curriculum based on crisis theory. We extended the original theory to encompass physiological as well as psychological events (Infante, 1982; White, 1983).

I returned to New York University 2 years later and entered the brave new world of Martha Rogers' conceptual system, now called the science of unitary human beings, which was my first exposure to a comprehensive nursing discipline–specific conceptual model. Given my strong interest in theory-guided nursing practice, I was very attracted to Rogers' work. I rapidly immersed myself in the coursework that led to my dissertation research, which was based on my extension of Rogers' conceptual system to the family (Fawcett, 1975, 1977). My coursework sensitized me to the need to use nursing discipline–specific conceptual models and theories to guide not only nursing practice but also nursing research. Furthermore, the coursework sensitized me to the reciprocal relationship between research

and conceptual models and between practice and conceptual models. I realized that conceptual models inform research and practice and that research findings and the results observed in practice in turn inform revisions in the conceptual model.

I returned to the University of Connecticut in 1975 and completed all requirements for the doctoral degree in 1976. I began to teach nursing research courses and had the opportunity to develop courses in contemporary nursing knowledge and the relationship of theory and research. The latter two courses became the focus of my scholarly work and the underlying reason for my passion about nursing.

I was recruited by the University of Pennsylvania in 1978 and had the honor of teaching the subject matter of my scholarly work in a new nursing doctoral program. Throughout all the years at University of Pennsylvania and now at the University of Massachusetts in Boston, my teaching has informed my scholarly work and my scholarly work has informed my teaching. My books about analysis of nursing models and theories (Fawcett, 1989, 1993, 2000, 2005) and the relationship of theory and research (Fawcett, 1999) are the direct result of my students' requests for more information and more examples about the use of nursing discipline–specific conceptual models and theories.

Since 1979 I have used Roy's adaptation model to guide my empirical research, which has focused on women's responses to cesarean birth and on functional status in normal life transitions and serious illness. I have found Roy's model to be a very useful guide for my research and for the nursing practice that stems from the findings of the research.

INTRODUCTION

Nursing is both a science and an art. The empirical (relying on or derived from observation, experiment, or practical experience) science of nursing includes both the natural sciences (e.g., biology, chemistry) and the human sciences (e.g., sociology, psychology). The art of nursing is the ability to form trusting relationships, perform procedures skillfully, prescribe appropriate treatments, and morally conduct nursing practice (Johnson, 1994). Nursing is a knowledge-based discipline significantly different from medicine. Medicine focuses on the identification and treatment of disease, whereas nursing focuses on the wholeness of human beings (Fawcett, 1993). Nursing claims the health of human beings in interaction with the environment as its domain. *Knowledge* is commonly defined as a general awareness or possession of information, facts, ideas, truths,

or principles and an understanding of the same gained through experience or study (Encarta World English Dictionary, 2009). Nursing knowledge is the organization of the discipline-specific concepts, theories, and ideas published in the literature (both print and electronic media) and demonstrated in professional practice. Nursing's desire to be regarded as a profession (e.g., law, medicine) was the impetus for building a substantial body of discipline-specific knowledge. Many of the existing theories emerged from the response to the simple question, "What is nursing?"

Theories and conceptual frameworks consist of the theorist's words brought together to form a meaningful whole. Theories and frameworks provide direction and guidance for structuring professional nursing practice, education, and research. They act as a "tool for reasoning, critical thinking, and decision-making" (Alligood, 2005, p. 272).

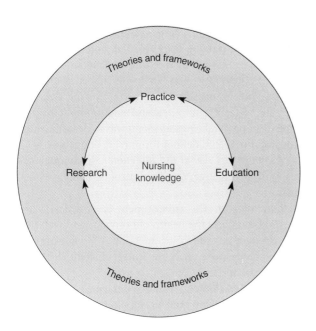

FIGURE 5-1 Relationships among theories and frameworks and nursing education, research, and practice.

In practice, theories and frameworks help nurses describe, explain, and predict everyday experiences. They also assist in organizing assessment data, making diagnoses, choosing interventions, and evaluating nursing care. In education, a conceptual framework provides the general focus for curriculum design. In research, the framework offers a systematic approach to identifying questions for study, selecting appropriate variables, and interpreting findings. The research findings may trigger revision and refinement of the theory. Figure 5-1 illustrates the relationships among theory, practice, education, and research.

Many nurse theorists have made substantial contributions to the development of a body of nursing knowledge. Offering an assortment of perspectives, the theories vary in their level of abstraction and their conceptualization of the client, health and illness, the environment, and nursing. From a historical perspective, nursing theories reflect the influence of the larger society and illustrate increased sophistication in the development of nursing ideas. The intent of this chapter is to provide a comprehensive overview of nursing theory to serve as a foundation for understanding how specific nursing theories relate to individual topics in subsequent chapters.

TERMINOLOGY ASSOCIATED WITH NURSING THEORY

The most fundamental building block of a theory is a concept, which is defined as "a word or phrase that summarizes ideas, observations, and experiences" (Fawcett, 2005, p. 4). For a theory to exist, concepts must be related to one another. Theoretical statements, also called *propositions*, describe a concept or the relationship between two or more concepts (Fawcett, 2005). One theoretical statement, or several theoretical statements taken together, can constitute a theory. A theory, then, is a statement or a group of statements that describe, explain, or predict relationships among concepts.

A nursing theory is composed of a set of concepts and propositions that claims to account for or characterize the central phenomena of interest to the discipline of nursing: person, environment, health/illness, and nursing. *Persons* are the recipients of nursing care and include individuals, families, and communities. *Environment* refers to the surroundings of the client, internal factors affecting the client, and the setting in which nursing care is delivered. *Health and illness* describe the client's state of well-being. *Nursing* refers to the actions taken when providing care to a patient. These concepts, taken together, make up what is known as the *metaparadigm of nursing* (Fawcett, 1997). Most nursing theories define or describe these central concepts, either explicitly or implicitly. Because a concept is an abstract representation of the real world, concepts embedded in a theory represent the theorist's perspective of reality and may differ from that of the reader without invalidating the theory.

Theories represent abstract ideas rather than concrete facts (Alligood, 2005) and may be broad or limited in scope, thus varying in their ability to describe, explain, or predict. Theories may be categorized by their level of abstraction as grand theories, midrange theories, or practice theories. Grand theories (also known as *conceptual models or frameworks*) are representations of the broad nature, purpose, and goals of the discipline. Concepts and their relationships are very abstract, not operationally defined, and not empirically testable. Midrange theories, which may be derived from grand theories, are less abstract with relatively concrete concepts that address specific phenomena across nursing settings and specialties. Relationships between and among concepts can be defined explicitly and measured.

Because they are narrower in scope, midrange theories appear more applicable to practice and remain abstract enough to allow a wide range of empirical research. Practice theories (sometimes called *situation-specific theories*) are limited further to a patient population or type of nursing practice (Im & Meleis, 1999; Meleis, 2005). Most practice theories are either descriptive (portraying an experience) or prescriptive (advocating specific nursing actions) in nature.

Descriptions of the theoretical perspectives presented in this chapter include a brief overview; the theory's basic assumptions about the individual and the environment; definitions of health and illness; a description of nursing, including the goal of nursing; and definitions of concepts and subconcepts specific to each theory. Some theories are more amenable to this scheme than others because of their degree of specificity or stage of development. When the needed information is not explicitly detailed by the theorist, inferences are made on the basis of what seems to be implicitly stated. Direct quotes from the theorists are used whenever possible to ensure that such interpretations are valid and reliable. The reader is encouraged to consult the primary source to gain a full appreciation of the depth, scope, and extent of the relationships put forth.

OVERVIEW OF SELECTED NURSING THEORIES

Theories and frameworks selected for inclusion in this chapter are those that exemplify the different definitions of nursing along varying levels of abstraction.

Exploring a variety of nursing theories ought to provide nurses with new insights into patient care, opening nursing options otherwise hidden, and stimulating innovative interventions. But it is imperative that there be variety—for there is no global theory of nursing that fits every situation.

(Levine, 1995, p. 13)

GRAND THEORY

Nightingale's Environmental Theory

Florence Nightingale conceptualized disease as a reparative process and described the nurse's role as manipulating the environment to facilitate and encourage this process. Her directions regarding ventilation, warmth, light, diet, cleanliness, variety, and noise are discussed in her classic nursing textbook *Notes on Nursing*, first published in London in 1859 and in America in 1860.

Brief Overview. The environment is critical to health, and the nurse's role in caring for the sick is to provide a clean, quiet, peaceful environment to promote healing. Nightingale's intent was to describe nursing and provide guidelines for nursing education.

Assumptions About the Individual. Individuals are responsible, creative, and in control of their lives and health.

Environment. The environment is external to the person but affects the health of both sick and well persons. As a chief source of infection, the environment must include pure air, pure water, efficient drainage, cleanliness, and light.

Health and Illness. Health is described as a state of being well and using one's powers to the fullest. Illness or disease is the reaction of nature against the conditions in which human beings have placed themselves. Disease is a reparative mechanism, an effort of nature to remedy a process of poisoning or of decay.

Nursing. Nursing is a service to humanity intended to relieve pain and suffering. Nursing's role is to promote or provide the proper environment for patients, including fresh air, light, pure water, cleanliness, warmth, quiet, and appropriate diet. The goal of nursing is to promote the reparative process by manipulating the environment.

Key Concepts. *Environment* refers to conditions external to the individual that affect life and development (e.g., ventilation, warmth, light, diet, cleanliness, noise). Nightingale (1860/1946) identified three major relationships: the environment to the patient, the nurse to the environment, and the nurse to the patient. Examples of these follow:

- The need for light, particularly sunlight, is second only to the need for ventilation. If necessary, the nurse should move the patient "about after the sun according to the aspects of the rooms, if circumstances permit, [rather] than let him linger in a room when the sun is off" (Nightingale, 1860/1946, p. 48).
- Nursing's role is to manipulate the environment to encourage healing. Nursing "ought to signify the proper use of fresh air, light, warmth, cleanliness, quiet, and the proper selection and administration of diet" (Nightingale, 1860/1946, p. 6).

- The sine qua non of all good nursing is never to allow a patient to be awakened, intentionally or accidentally: "A good nurse will always make sure that no blind or curtains should flap. If you wait till your patient tells you or reminds you of these things, where is the use of their having a nurse?" (Nightingale, 1860/1946, p. 27).
- Variety is important for patients to divert them from dwelling on their pain: "Variety of form and brilliancy of color in the objects presented are actual means of recovery" (Nightingale, 1860/1946, p. 34).

Rogers' Science of Unitary Human Beings

First presented in *An Introduction to the Theoretical Basis for Nursing* in 1970, Martha Rogers' conceptualizations, dating back to the 1960s, evolved into the current science of unitary human beings. She posited that human beings are dynamic energy fields who are integral with the environment and who are continuously evolving. She viewed nursing as a science and an art that focus on the nature and direction of human development and human betterment.

Brief Overview. The individual is viewed as an irreducible energy field, integral with the environment. The nurse seeks to promote symphonic (harmonious) interactions between human beings and their environments (Rogers, 1970).

Assumptions About the Individual. The individual is a unified, irreducible whole, manifesting characteristics that are more than, and different from, the sum of his or her parts and continuously evolving, irreversibly and unidirectionally along a space–time continuum. Pattern and organization of human beings are directed toward increasing complexity rather than maintaining equilibrium. The individual "is characterized by the capacity for abstraction and imagery, language and thought, sensation and emotion" (Rogers, 1970, p. 73).

Environment. The environment is an irreducible, pandimensional (pertaining to and across all dimensions of reality) energy field identified by pattern and integral with the human energy field (Rogers, 1994). The individual and the environment are continually exchanging matter and energy with one another, resulting in changing patterns in both the individual and the environment.

Health and Illness. Health and illness are value-laden, arbitrarily defined, and culturally infused notions. They are not dichotomous but are part of the same continuum. Health seems to occur when patterns of living are in harmony with environmental change, whereas illness occurs when patterns of living are in conflict with environmental change and are deemed unacceptable (Rogers, 1994).

Nursing. As both a science and an art, nursing is unique in its concern with unitary human beings as synergistic phenomena. The science of nursing should be concerned with studying the nature and direction of unitary human development integral with the environment and with evolving descriptive, explanatory, and predictive principles for use in nursing practice. The new age of nursing science is characterized by a synthesis of fact and ideas that generate principles and theories (Rogers, 1994). The art of nursing is the creative use of the science of nursing for human betterment (Rogers, 1990). The combination of art and science enhances the effect (outcomes) of nursing actions. The goal of nursing is the attainment of the best possible state of health for the individual who is continually evolving by promoting symphonic interactions between human beings and environments, strengthening the coherence and integrity of the human field, and directing and redirecting patterning of both fields for maximal health potential.

Key Concepts. The concepts describe the individual and environment as energy fields that are in constant interaction. The nature and direction of human development form the basis for the following principles of nursing science:

- *Energy field.* The fundamental unit of the living and nonliving. Energy fields are dynamic, continuously in motion, and infinite. They are of two types:
  - Human energy field: More than the biological, psychological, and sociological fields taken separately or together; an irreducible, indivisible, pandimensional whole identified by pattern and manifesting characteristics that cannot be predicted from the parts.
  - Environmental energy field: An irreducible, indivisible, pandimensional energy field identified by pattern and integral with the human field.
- *Openness.* Continuous change and mutual process as manifested in human and environmental fields.
- *Pattern.* The distinguishing characteristic of an energy field perceived as a single wave.
- *Principles of nursing science.* Principles postulating the nature and direction of unitary human development; these principles are also called principles of homeodynamics:

- Helicy: According to Rogers, helicy is "the continuous, innovative, probabilistic, increasing diversity of human and environmental field patterns characterized by repeating rhymicities" (1989, p. 186). Change occurs continuously.
- Resonancy: Rogers describes resonancy as "the continuous change from lower to higher frequency wave patterns in human and environmental fields" (1989, p. 186). Change is increasingly diverse.
- Integrality: Replacing the earlier concept of complementarity, integrality is "the continuous mutual human and environmental field process" (Rogers, 1989, p. 186). Field changes occur simultaneously.

Orem's Self-Care Deficit Theory

The foundations of Dorothea Orem's theory were introduced in the late 1950s, but the first edition of her work *Nursing: Concepts of Practice* was not published until 1971. Five subsequent editions (1980, 1985, 1991, 1995, 2001) show evidence of continued development and refinement of the theory. Orem focuses on nursing as deliberate human action and notes that all individuals can benefit from nursing when they have health-derived or health-related limitations for engaging in self-care or the care of dependent others. Three theories are subsumed in the self-care deficit theory of nursing: the theory of nursing systems, the theory of self-care deficits, and the theory of self-care (Orem, 2001).

Brief Overview. The individual practices self-care, a set of learned behaviors, to sustain life, maintain or restore functioning, and bring about a condition of well-being. The nurse assists the client with self-care when he or she experiences a deficit in the ability to perform.

Assumptions About the Individual. The individual is viewed as a unit whose functioning is linked with the environment and who, with the environment, forms an integrated (unified), functional whole. The individual functions biologically, symbolically, and socially.

Environment. The environment is linked to the individual, forming an integrated system. The environment is implied to be external to the individual.

Health and Illness. Health, which has physical, psychological, interpersonal, and social aspects, is a state in which human beings are structurally and functionally whole or sound (Orem, 1995). Illness occurs when an individual is incapable of maintaining self-care as a result of structural or functional limitations.

Nursing. Nursing involves assisting the individual with self-care practices to sustain life and health, recover from disease or injury, and cope with their effects (Orem, 1985). The nurse chooses deliberate actions from nursing systems (see later) designed to bring about desirable conditions in persons and their environments. The goal of nursing is to move a patient toward responsible self-care or to meet existing health care needs of those who have health care deficits.

Key Concepts. The concepts focus on self-care in terms of requisites, demands, and deficits and delineate the nurse's role in client care in the following manner:

- *Self-care.* This refers to "activities that individuals initiate and perform on their own behalf to maintain life, health, or well-being" (Orem, 1995, p. 104).
- *Dependent care agent.* A person other than the individual who provides the care; "the provider of infant care, child care, or dependent adult care" (Orem, 1991, p. 117).
- *Self-care requisites.* Actions that are known or hypothesized to be necessary to regulate human functioning. Three types exist:
  - Universal: Common to all human beings; concerned with the promotion and maintenance of structural and functional integrity. These include air, water, food, elimination, activity and rest, solitude and social interaction, prevention of hazards, and promotion of human functioning.
  - Developmental: Associated with conditions that promote known developmental processes; occurring at various stages of the life cycle.
  - Health deviation: Genetic and constitutional defects and deviations that affect integrated human functioning and impair the individual's ability to perform self-care.
- *Therapeutic self-care demand.* Based on the notion that self-care is a human regulatory function; the totality of self-care actions performed by the nurse or self to meet known self-care requisites.
- *Self-care agency.* Acquired ability to know and meet requirements to regulate own functioning and development.
- *Self-care deficits.* Gaps between known therapeutic self-care demands and the capability of the individual to perform self-care.
- *Nursing systems.* Systems of concrete actions for persons with limitations in self-care. These actions are of three types (Orem, 1995):

- Wholly compensatory: The nurse compensates for the individual's total inability to perform self-care activities.
- Partly compensatory: The nurse compensates for the individual's inability to perform some (but not all) self-care activities.
- Supportive-educative: With the individual able to perform all self-care activities, the nurse assists the client in decision making, behavior control, and the acquisition of knowledge and skill.
- Subsystems of each nursing system:
  - *Social:* The complementary and contractual relationship between the nurse and the client.
  - *Interpersonal:* The nurse-client interaction.
  - *Technological:* According to Orem, the "diagnosis, prescription, regulation of treatment, and management of nursing care" (1985, p. 160).

Roy's Adaptation Model

Sister Callista Roy has continuously expanded her model from its inception in the 1960s to the present, building on the conceptual framework of adaptation (dynamic evolutionary process of change). She focuses on the individual as a biopsychosocial adaptive system and describes nursing as a humanistic discipline that "places emphasis on the person's own coping abilities" (Roy, 1984, p. 32). The individual and the environment are sources of stimuli that require modification to promote adaptation.

Brief Overview. The individual is a biopsychosocial adaptive system, and the nurse promotes adaptation by modifying external stimuli.

Assumptions About the Individual. The individual is in constant interaction with a changing environment, and to respond positively to environmental change, a person must adapt. The person's adaptation level is determined by the combined effect of three classes of stimuli: focal, contextual, and residual. The individual uses both innate and acquired biological, psychological, or social adaptive mechanisms and has four modes of adaptation.

Environment. All conditions, circumstances, and influences surrounding and affecting the development and behavior of persons and groups constitute the environment. Having both internal and external components, the environment is constantly changing.

Health and Illness. According to Roy (1989), "health and illness are one inevitable dimension of a person's

life" (p. 106). Health is "a state and process of being and becoming integrated and whole" (Roy & Andrews, 1999, p. 31). Conversely, illness is a lack of integration.

Nursing. As an external regulatory force, nursing acts to modify stimuli affecting adaptation by increasing, decreasing, or maintaining stimuli. The goal of nursing is to promote the person's adaptation in the four adaptive modes, thus contributing to health, the quality of life, and dying with dignity (Roy, 2009).

Key Concepts. The following concepts describe and define adaptation in terms of the individual's internal control processes, adaptive modes, and adaptive level:

- *Adaptation.* The individual's ability to cope with the constantly changing environment.
- *Adaptive system.* Consists of two major internal control processes (coping mechanisms):
  - Regulator subsystem: Receives input from the external environment and from changes in the person's internal state and processes it through neural-chemical-endocrine channels.
  - Cognator subsystem: Receives input from external and internal stimuli that involve psychological, social, physical, and physiological factors and processes it through cognitive pathways.
- *Adaptive modes.* The four ways a person adapts:
  - Physiological: Determined by the need for physiological integrity derived from the basic physiological needs.
  - Self-concept: Determined by the need for interactions with others and psychic integrity regarding the perception of self.
  - Role function: Determined by the need for social integrity; refers to the performance of duties based on given positions within society.
  - Interdependence: Involves ways of seeking help, affection, and attention.

Adaptive level. Determined by the combined effects of stimuli:

- Focal stimulus: That which immediately confronts the individual.
- Contextual stimuli: All other stimuli present in the environment. These stimuli influence how the individual deals with the focal stimulus.
- Residual stimuli: Beliefs, attitudes, or traits that have an indeterminate effect on the present situation.

Neuman's Systems Model

Betty Neuman developed her systems model in 1970 in response to student requests to focus on breadth rather than depth in understanding human variables in nursing problems. First published in 1972 (Neuman & Young, 1972), the model was refined to its present form in *The Neuman Systems Model* (Neuman, 1995; Neuman & Fawcett, 2002). The Neuman systems model "is an open systems model that views nursing as being primarily concerned with defining appropriate actions in stress-related situations" (Neuman, 1995, p. 11). Neuman believes that nursing encompasses a wholistic (body, mind, and spirit) client systems approach to help individuals, families, communities, and society reach and maintain wellness. Neuman's focus on the *whole* system explains her use of the term *wholistic* rather than holistic (alternative healing practices).

Brief Overview. This theory offers a wholistic view of the client system, including the concepts of open system, environment, stressors, prevention, and reconstitution. Nursing is concerned with the whole person.

Assumptions About the Individual. In this model, the client is a whole person, a dynamic composite of interrelationships among physiological, psychological, sociocultural, developmental, and spiritual variables: "The client is viewed as an open system in interaction with the environment" (Neuman, 1989, p. 68). The client is in "dynamic constant energy exchange with the environment" (Neuman, 1989, p. 22).

Environment. Both internal and external environments exist, and the person maintains varying degrees of harmony between them. The environment includes all internal and external factors affecting and being affected by the system (Neuman, 1995). Emphasis is on all stressors—interpersonal, intrapersonal, extrapersonal—that might disturb the person's normal line of defense.

Health and Illness. Neuman (1995) asserts that "health and wellness is defined as the condition or degree of system stability" (p. 12). Disharmony among parts of the system is considered illness: "The wellness-illness continuum implies that energy flow is continuous between the client system and the environment" (Neuman, 1989, p. 33).

Nursing. Nursing is a "unique profession in that it is concerned with all of the variables affecting the individual's response to stress" (Neuman, 1982, p. 14).

The major concern of nursing is in "keeping the client system stable through accuracy in both the assessment of effects and possible effects of environmental stressors and in assisting client adjustments required for an optimal wellness level" (Neuman, 1989, p. 34). Nursing goals are determined by "negotiation with the client for desired prescriptive changes to correct variances from wellness" (Neuman, 1989, p. 73). This means that nursing interventions designed to improve health are accepted and approved by the individual client during communication with the nurse before implementation.

Key Concepts. The nurse is concerned with all the following variables affecting an individual's response to stressors:

- *Stressors.* Tension-producing stimuli that may alter system stability (Neuman, 1995):
  - Intrapersonal: Internal stressors (e.g., autoimmune response).
  - Interpersonal: External environmental forces in close proximity (e.g., communication patterns).
  - Extrapersonal: External environmental forces at distant range (e.g., financial concerns).
- Concepts related to client system stability:
  - Flexible line of defense: Outer boundary that ideally prevents stressors from entering the system.
  - Normal line of defense: A range of responses to environmental stressors when the flexible line of defense is penetrated; usual state of wellness (Neuman, 1995).
  - Lines of resistance: Protect the basic structure of the client and become activated when the normal line of defense is invaded by environmental stressors.
- *Interventions.* Purposeful nursing actions that help clients retain, attain, and/or maintain system stability. Three levels of intervention exist:
  - Primary prevention: Reduces the possibility of encounter with stressors and strengthens the flexible lines of defense.
  - Secondary prevention: Relates to appropriate prioritizing of interventions to reduce symptoms resulting from invasion of environmental stressors; protects the basic structure by strengthening the internal lines of resistance.
  - Tertiary prevention: Focuses on re-adaptation and stability. A primary goal is to strengthen

resistance to stressors by reeducation to help prevent recurrence of reaction or regression: "Tertiary prevention tends to lead back, in a circular fashion, toward primary prevention" (Neuman, 1989, p. 73).

Watson's Philosophy and Science of Caring

Jean Watson's theoretical formulations focus on the philosophy and science of caring as the core of nursing. With the aim of reducing the dichotomy between nursing theory and practice, Watson's original theory draws from multiple disciplines to derive carative factors that are central to nursing and describes concepts as they relate to the pivotal theme of caring: "Caring is acknowledged as the highest form of commitment to self, to others, to society, to environment, and, at this point in human history, even to the universe" (Watson, 1996, p. 146). Watson (2007) states: "I consider my work more a philosophical, ethical, intellectual blueprint for nursing's evolving disciplinary/professional matrix, rather than a specific theory per se" (para 8).

Brief Overview. Caring, which Watson sees as a moral ideal rather than a task-oriented behavior, is central to nursing practice and includes aspects of the actual caring occasion and the transpersonal caring relationship. An interpersonal process, caring results in the satisfaction of human needs.

Assumptions About the Individual. Individuals (i.e., both the nurse and the client) are nonreducible and are interconnected with others and nature (Watson, 1985).

Environment. The client's environment contains both external and internal variables. The nurse promotes a caring environment, one that allows individuals to make choices relative to the best action for themselves at that point in time.

Health and Illness. Health is more than the absence of illness, but because it is subjective, it is an elusive concept: "Health refers to unity and harmony within the mind, body, and soul" (Watson, 1985, p. 48). Conversely, illness is disharmony within the spheres of the person.

Nursing. The practice of nursing is different from curing. From my emerging perspective, I tried to make explicit nursing's values, knowledge, and practices of human caring that are geared toward subjective inner healing processes and the life world of the experiencing person, requiring unique caring healing arts and

a framework called "carative factors," which complemented conventional medicine but stood in stark contrast to "curative factors" (Watson, 2007).

Nursing is a transpersonal relationship that includes but is not limited to the 10 carative factors described in the following Key Concepts. The goal of nursing is to help persons attain a higher degree of harmony by offering a relationship that the client can use for personal growth and development.

Key Concepts. The caring relationship forms the core of nursing and the caritas processes (evolved from the original carative factors) delineate the domain of nursing practice:

- *Transpersonal caring.* An intersubjective human-to-human relationship in which the nurse affects and is affected by the other person (client). Caring is the moral ideal of nursing in which the utmost concern for human dignity and preservation of humanity is present (Watson, 1985).
- *Caritas processes* (Watson, 2007):
  - Embrace altruistic values and practice loving kindness with self and others within the context of caring consciousness.
  - Instill faith and hope and honor others.
  - Being authentically present, and enabling and sustaining the deep belief system and subjective life world of self and the one-being-cared-for. Be sensitive to self and others by nurturing individual beliefs and practices.
  - Develop helping, trusting, and caring relationships.
  - Promote and accept positive and negative feelings as you authentically listen to another's story.
  - Creative use of self and all ways of knowing as part of the caring process; to engage in the artistry of caring-healing practices. Use creative scientific problem-solving methods for caring decision making.
  - Engaging in genuine teaching-learning experience that attends to unity of being and meaning attempting to stay within other's frame of reference. Share teaching and learning that addresses the individual needs and comprehension styles.
  - Creating a healing environment at all levels, physical as well as nonphysical, subtle environment of energy and consciousness, whereby wholeness, beauty, comfort, dignity, and peace are potentiated. Create a healing environment

for the physical and spiritual self which respects human dignity.

- Assisting with basic needs, with an intentional caring consciousness, administering "human care essentials," which potentiate alignment of mind-body-spirit, wholeness, and unity of being in all aspects of care; tending to both embodied spirit and evolving spiritual emergence. Assist with basic physical, emotional, and spiritual human needs.
- Opening and attending to spiritual-mysterious, and existential dimensions of one's own life-death; soul care for self and the one-being-cared-for. Be open to mystery and allow miracles to enter.

MIDRANGE THEORY

Peplau's Interpersonal Process

Hildegard Peplau published *Interpersonal Relations in Nursing* in 1952. The book described the phases of the interpersonal process in nursing, roles for nurses, and methods for studying nursing as an interpersonal process. Over the years the theory evolved, and in 1991 she published *Interpersonal Relations in Nursing: A Conceptual Framework of Reference for Psychodynamic Nursing*.

Brief Overview. The focus of Peplau's model is the goal-directed interpersonal process: "Psychodynamic nursing is being able to understand one's own behavior to help others identify felt difficulties and to apply principles of human relations to the problems that arise at all levels of experience" (Peplau, 1952, p. xiii). The interpersonal relationship "has a starting point, proceeds through definable phases, and, being time-limited, has an end point" (Peplau, 1992, p. 4). Peplau believed that once the problem that prompts the client to ask for nursing help has been resolved, the relationship ends.

Assumptions About the Individual. The individual is an organism that lives in an unstable equilibrium and "strives in its own way to reduce tension generated by needs" (Peplau, 1952, p. 82).

Environment. Although the environment is not explicitly defined, it can be inferred that the environment consists of "existing forces outside the organism and in the context of culture" (Peplau, 1952, p. 163).

Health and Illness. Health is a "word symbol that implies forward movement of personality and other ongoing human processes in the direction of creative, constructive, productive, personal, and community living" (Peplau, 1952, p. 12). By implication, illness is a condition that is marked by no movement or by backward movement in these human processes.

Nursing. Nursing is a therapeutic interpersonal process because it involves the interaction between two or more individuals who have a common goal. For individuals who are sick and in need of health care, it is a healing art. Six nursing roles emerge in the various phases of the nurse-patient relationship: stranger, resource person, teacher, leader, surrogate, and counselor.

Key Concepts. The nurse-patient relationship consists of four phases:

- *Orientation.* The patient seeks professional assistance with a problem. The nurse and patient meet as strangers and recognize, clarify, and define the existing problem.
- *Identification.* The patient learns how to make use of the nurse-patient relationship and responds selectively to people who can meet his or her needs; the patient and nurse clarify each other's expectations.
- *Exploitation.* The patient takes advantage of all available services. The nurse helps the patient in maintaining a balance between dependence and independence and using the services to help solve the current problem and work toward optimal health.
- *Resolution.* The patient is free to move on with his or her life as old goals are put aside and new goals are adopted. The patient becomes independent of the nurse, and the relationship is terminated.

King's Theory of Goal Attainment

Although the foundation for Imogene King's theory was developed in 1964, she did not present her entire conceptual framework until the 1971 publication of her book *Toward a Theory for Nursing*. In it she identified the concepts of social systems, health, perception, and interpersonal relations. The midrange theory of goal attainment was refined in *A Theory for Nursing: Systems, Concepts, Process* (1981), in which King asserted that nursing is focused on people interacting with their environments. The goal of this interaction is a state of health, which King defines as the ability of people to function in their roles. The theory is derived from a systems framework and is concerned with human transactions in different types of environments (King, 1995a).

Brief Overview. The individual is viewed as an open system and as one component of a nurse-client interpersonal system whose interactions lead to the attainment of mutually agreed-upon goals.

Assumptions About the Individual. Human beings are open systems in transaction with the environment and are conceptualized as social, sentient, rational, perceiving, controlling, purposeful, action-oriented beings.

Environment. The theory implies that the open systems of the individual and the environment interact and that both the internal and external environments generate stressors.

Health and Illness. Health is described as an individual's ability to function in social roles. This implies optimal use of a person's resources to achieve continuous adjustment to internal and external environmental stressors. Illness is a deviation from normal, an imbalance in a person's biological structure, psychological makeup, or social relationships.

Nursing. In an interpersonal process of action, reaction, and interaction, the nurse and client communicate, set goals, and explore means to achieve those goals. According to King (1981), "the domain of nursing includes promoting, maintaining and restoring health, caring for the sick and injured and caring for the dying" (p. 4). Nursing's central goal is to help individuals maintain their health so that they can function in their roles. As King asserted, "The goal of the nursing system, as a whole, is health for individuals, health for groups, such as the family, and health for communities within a society" (King, 1995b, p. 24).

Key Concepts. Two sets of concepts are included in the theory, one relating to the parties involved in the nurse-client relationship and the other pertaining to the process of goal attainment, as follows:

- Concepts related to the nurse-client relationship:
  - Personal system: An individual.
  - Interpersonal system: Two or more interacting individuals.
  - Social system: Communities and societies.
- Concepts related to goal attainment:
  - Communication: The process of giving information from one person to another.
  - Interaction: The process of perception between the person and environment or one or more persons, represented by verbal and nonverbal behaviors that are goal directed.

- Perception: An individual's representation of reality.
- Transaction: Identification of mutual goals valued by persons interacting with each other.
- Role: A set of behaviors displayed by the individual, who occupies a given position in a social system.
- Stress: A dynamic state of interaction with the environment to maintain balance for growth, development, and performance.
- Growth and development: According to King (1981), these are "continuous changes in individuals occurring at molecular, cellular, and behavioral levels" (p. 148).
- Time: A duration between one event and another.
- Space: Defined by "gestures, postures, and visible boundaries erected to mark off personal space" (King, 1981, p. 148).

Leininger's Cultural Care Theory

Drawing from a background in cultural and social anthropology, Madeleine Leininger's contribution to nursing knowledge is related to transcultural nursing and caring. Her book *Transcultural Nursing: Concepts, Theories, and Practice* (1978) presented her conceptual framework for cultural care and health. She explicated the linkages between nursing and anthropology as she identified and defined concepts such as care, caring, culture, cultural values, and cultural variations (Leininger, 1984, 1991, 1995; Leininger & McFarland, 2002, 2006).

Brief Overview. Transcultural nursing focuses on a comparative study and analysis of different cultures and subcultures in the world regarding their caring behavior, nursing care, health-illness values, and patterns of behavior, with the goal of developing a scientific and humanistic body of knowledge from which to derive culture-specific and culture-universal nursing care practices (Leininger, 1978).

Assumptions About the Individual. Clients are caring and cultural beings who perceive health, illness, caring, curing, dependence, and independence differently. The social structure, worldview, and values of people vary transculturally.

Environment. The environment is a social structure, the "interrelated and interdependent systems of a society which determine how it functions with respect to certain major elements, namely: the political (including legal), economic, social (including kinship), educational, technical, religious, and cultural systems" (Leininger, 1978, p. 61). The environment is the totality of an event, situation, or particular experience that gives meaning to human expression and interaction.

Health and Illness. Perceptions of health and illness are culturally infused and therefore cannot be universally defined: "Health refers to a state of well-being that is culturally defined, valued, and practiced, and which reflects the ability of individuals (or groups) to perform their daily role activities in culturally expressed, beneficial, and patterned lifeways" (Leininger, 1991, p. 48). Worldviews, social structure, and cultural beliefs influence perceptions of health and illness and cannot be separated from them. For example, some cultures perceive illness to be largely a personal and internal body experience, whereas others view illness as an extrapersonal or cultural experience. Another example is that many clients of Asian descent believe that health is a personal responsibility, a result of the individual maintaining balance. In Western society, health may be defined by the medical profession. As the Report of the Surgeon General (U.S. Department of Health and Human Services, 1999) noted: "Ten years ago a serum cholesterol of 200 was considered normal. Today, this same number alarms some physicians and may lead to treatment."

Nursing. Nursing is a learned humanistic and scientific profession that focuses on personalized (individual and group) care behaviors, functions, and processes that have physical, psychocultural, and social significance or meaning. The goal of nursing is to assist, support, facilitate, or enable individuals or groups to regain or maintain their health in a way that is culturally congruent or to help people face handicaps or death (Leininger, 1991).

Key Concepts. Among the core concepts of transcultural nursing theory are the following:

- *Care.* Phenomena related to assistive, supportive, or enabling behavior toward or for another individual with evident or anticipated needs to ease or improve a human condition.
- *Caring.* Actions directed toward assisting, supporting, or enabling an individual (or group) to ameliorate or improve the human condition or "lifeway" (Leininger, 1991, p. 48).
- *Culture.* Values, beliefs, norms, and lifeway practices of a particular group that guides thinking, decisions, and actions in patterned ways.

- *Cultural care.* The cognitively known values, beliefs, and patterned lifeways that assist, support, or enable another individual or group to maintain well-being; improve a human condition or lifeway; or deal with illness, handicaps, or death.
  - Cultural care diversity: The variability of meaning, patterns, values, lifeways, or symbols of care that are culturally derived for health or to improve a human condition.
  - Cultural care universality: Common, similar, or uniform care meanings, patterns, values, lifeways, or symbols that are culturally derived for health or to improve a human condition.
- *Cultural-congruent care.* Assistive, supportive, facilitative, or enabling acts or decisions that fit individual, group, or institutional cultural values, beliefs, and lifeways (Leininger, 1995).
  - Cultural care preservation or maintenance: Professional actions and decisions that help people of a particular culture to retain and preserve relevant care values.
  - Cultural care accommodation or negotiation: Professional actions and decisions that help people of a designated culture adapt to or negotiate with others for a beneficial or satisfying health outcome.
  - Cultural care repatterning or restructuring: Professional actions and decisions that help a client change or modify his or her lifeway to improve health while still respecting the client's cultural values and beliefs.

PRACTICE THEORY

Being clinically specific, practice theories (also known as *situation-specific theories*) incorporate and reflect the actual provision of nursing care (McEwen, 2007), thus allowing the "incorporation of nurses' clinical wisdom" (Im & Meleis, 1999). They may be derived from existing theories, arise from practice, or emerge from research findings. The purpose of these theories is to describe or explain clinical problems or patient needs that nurses encounter daily within the boundaries of their specialty practices or settings. As such, they may prescribe specific nursing actions or lead to the in-depth analysis of such interventions. Practice theories may provide explanations about patient problems, describe therapeutic interventions, advocate specific approaches to a specified patient population, or identify nursing values that lead to a decision-making process (McEwen, 2007).

Examples of practice theories can be found in the nursing specialty–specific literature that discusses disease management and nursing interventions pertinent to a defined patient population. In an analysis of current trends in nursing theory, Im and Chang (2012) state that a "noticeable trend was nurses' trials to integrate theories into their practice…indicat(ing) that our discipline is now up to the stage that actually links theoretical basis to nursing care" (p. 161).

PRACTICE THEORY CHARACTERISTICS

- A lower level of abstraction: limited in scope and focus; not developed to transcend time or place.
- Focus on a single specific phenomenon of interest to nurses; developed to answer specific set of clinical questions.
- Specific sociopolitical, cultural, and/or historical context.
- Readily recognizable connection to both daily practice and clinical research.
- Apparent respect for diversity, complexity, and context reflected in decreased generalizability (Im & Meleis, 1999; McEwen, 2007).

APPLICATION TO NURSING PRACTICE

The nursing theories and frameworks discussed here offer a variety of perspectives for application to clinical practice. For example, some are process oriented and dynamic, such as Peplau's interpersonal process, King's theory of goal attainment, and Rogers' science of unitary human beings. Others are more outcome oriented, such as Roy's adaptation model and Orem's self-care deficit theory. The models of Rogers and Neuman focus on the wholeness of the individual and conceptualize nursing as one component of the individual's life process. King's theory is directed toward the interaction between the nurse and the client, who are inseparable (meaning that the roles are interdependent and undividable). Nightingale and Leininger developed humanistic perspectives, focusing on personalized, individualized care for all, and Roy conceptualizes the nurse as an external regulator whose function is to promote system balance or adaptation. Orem views the nurse as a person who assists the individual with

self-care practices when the individual is unable to effectively care for himself or herself. A comparison of the theoretical perspectives discussed in this chapter is presented in Table 5-1.

Many (if not all) of the nursing theories and frameworks presented in this chapter are too broad and abstract to be used in their entirety in any one nursing care situation. For example, Orem describes three types of nursing systems, but for a client who is in the intensive care unit and on life support, only the wholly compensatory nursing system is relevant. Similarly, with Neuman's three levels of prevention, only clients with symptoms resulting from invasion of environmental stressors are appropriate recipients of secondary prevention. Despite these limitations, the theories can guide nursing assessment in terms of what questions to ask and what areas to assess. The type of client, the setting in which care is delivered, and the goal of nursing are what influence the selection of an appropriate theoretical framework for practice. The more specific theories can be readily adapted for use in a practice setting. The more global theories may better serve as frameworks for research, the findings of which can then be applied to practice. Practice theories may best serve in the development of evidence based nursing practice by providing valid and reliable substantiation of clinical guidelines. Furthermore, use of specific theories to guide nursing practice facilitates the development of core competencies identified by the Institute of Medicine (2003) as necessary in the provision of quality care by interdisciplinary teams working to assure patient safety.

Evaluating the Utility of Nursing Theories

Not all theories and frameworks are equally comprehensive or equally useful in every situation, and they are not meant to be. The definition of the client and the setting in which care is delivered limit the usefulness of some of the theories and frameworks presented. To be useful in practice, a theory must work in a specific setting: "A nursing theory should structure the work, giving the practicing nurse a frame of reference from which to view patients and from which to make patient care decisions" (Barnum, 1998, p. 80). Its concepts must be operationalized in ways that promote application and facilitate nursing activities in that setting. Examination of a theory's usefulness for its intended purpose and the consistency of its internal structure is important. The

TABLE 5-1   Comparison of Theoretical Perspectives

THEORY/MODEL	NURSING	ENVIRONMENT	HEALTH	PERSON
Nightingale's Environmental Theory	Intended to relieve pain and suffering and restore health by manipulating the environment	Conditions external to the person that affect both sick and well persons	State of well-being; using an individual's power to the fullest	An individual who is in control of his or her own life and health and desires good health
Peplau's Interpersonal Process	Therapeutic interpersonal process	Existing forces outside the organism	Forward movement of ongoing human processes and personality	An organism that lives in an unstable equilibrium and strives to reduce tension generated by needs
Rogers' Science of Unitary Human Beings	Science and art; the art of nursing is the creative use of science for human betterment	Pandimensional energy field integral with the human energy field	Patterns of living in harmony with the environment	A unified irreducible whole; more than and different from the sum of parts
Orem's Self-Care Deficit Theory	Involves assisting individuals with self-care practices	Linked to the individual, forming an integrated system	State in which human beings are structurally and functionally whole	A unity who functions biologically, symbolically, and socially and whose functioning is linked with the environment
King's Theory of Goal Attainment	Process of action, reaction, and interaction	Interactive with the individual	Ability to function in social roles	An open system in transaction with the environment who is social, sentient, rational, perceiving, controlling, purposeful, and action oriented
Roy's Adaptation Model	An external regulatory force that modifies stimuli affecting adaptation	Internal and external conditions that surround and affect individuals	State and process of being and becoming an integrated and whole person	A biopsychosocial adaptive system that is in constant interaction with a changing environment
Neuman's Systems Model	Concerned with variables affecting the individual's response to stress	Internal and external factors affecting and affected by the individual	Optimal system stability	A whole person; a dynamic composite of physiological, psychological, sociocultural, developmental, and spiritual variables
Leininger's Cultural Care Theory	Culturally congruent care behaviors, functions, and processes that have physical, psychocultural, or social significance	The interrelated, interdependent systems of a society	State of well-being that is culturally defined	Caring, cultural beings who perceive health, illness, caring, curing, dependence, and independence differently
Watson's Philosophy and Science of Caring	Transpersonal caring relationship that includes use of 10 caritas processes	Internal and external variables	Unity and harmony within mind, body, and soul	An entity that is nonreducible and is interconnected with others and nature

value and logical structure of a theory can be evaluated by asking questions proposed by Fawcett (2005) and Barnum (1998), such as the following:

1. Are the assumptions inherent in the theory clearly stated?
2. Does the model provide adequate descriptions of all four concepts (person, environment, health, nursing) of nursing's metaparadigm?
3. Are the relationships among the concepts of nursing's metaparadigm clearly explained?
4. Is the theory stated clearly and concisely?
5. Does the structure of the theory contain conflicting views?
6. Can relationships between concepts be tested in research (i.e., observed and measured) and applied to practice?
7. Does the theory lead to nursing activities that meet societal expectations (social congruence)?
8. Does the theory lead to nursing activities that are likely to result in favorable client outcomes (social significance)?
9. Does the theory include explicit rules for use in practice, education, or research (social usefulness)?

Theories from Related Disciplines

Many nursing theories derived their conceptual basis from theories and frameworks developed by scholars from related disciplines and adapted to specific situations. Many of these theories are useful and relevant to nursing in their original form. A brief synopsis of selected theories from related disciplines follows.

One of the theories with wide applicability, general system theory, proposes that a system is a set of interrelated parts or subsystems that are in constant interaction with the environment working together toward a common goal (von Bertalanffy, 1956, 1968). Systems take in matter, information, and energy from the environment (input), process it (throughput), and release it back to the environment (output). Some of the output returns to the system as feedback in an attempt to return the system to a steady state (equilibrium) or, in the case of living systems, a condition of balance within the range of normal (homeostasis). A system is more than and different from the sum of its parts and, over time, becomes increasingly complex. The nurse who uses systems theory assesses the individual, family, or community as an aggregate and simultaneously considers the relationships among the subsystems, keeping in mind that a change in one part of the system changes the system as a whole.

Theories of change have been proposed by Lewin (1951) and expanded by Lippitt (1973) that view change as a goal-directed process. Lewin's theory includes three concepts: force field (driving and restraining forces for or against change), motivators (stimuli indicating the need for change), and stages of change (unfreezing, moving, refreezing). Lippitt focuses on the activities of the change agent to bring about the change. These theories provide a systematic method of planning, implementing, and evaluating change in individuals, organizations, and social systems.

Among the several theories of coping is one developed by Lazarus (1976) that views coping as a process that leads to adaptation. The major concepts in Lazarus' theory are stress caused by a lack of resources to cope with an environmental event, cognitive appraisal of the stressor to determine the perceived level of threat, and problem-focused coping (management of the stressor) or emotional-focused coping (management of the response) (Lazarus & Folkman, 1984). For clients experiencing an intense level of stress, nursing interventions designed to alter the perception of the threat level and promote and support the coping process can be derived from the relationships specified by this theory.

Aguilera (1998) provides a theory and framework for successful resolution of a crisis situation. She identifies three balancing factors (the perception of the event, the availability of situational supports, and usual coping mechanisms) that prevent an adverse reaction to a stressful situation. When a crisis or psychological disequilibrium occurs, the nurse can assess the balancing factors to establish a nursing diagnosis. Nursing interventions can then be designed to facilitate the return to equilibrium by assisting the client to establish a realistic perception of the event, providing situational supports, and identifying coping mechanisms.

Both coping and adjustment are embedded in Duvall's (1977) stages of family life and developmental tasks, which can serve as the framework for delivering age-specific or situation-specific nursing interventions to the family. Developmental stages are also specified in Erikson's theory (1963, 1982), which encompasses three major concepts: sequential developmental stages, developmental conflicts, and identity formation. Developmental tasks are associated with each stage, and a developmental conflict occurs if the tasks cannot be successfully accomplished. Identity formation is viewed as an ongoing process throughout the life span. Erikson's theory is useful as a framework for assessing an individual's psychosocial development and intervening when developmental conflicts are identified.

Selye's general adaptation syndrome, a theory of adaptation to stress, describes three phases of reaction to stress: stage of alarm, or immediate reaction to the stressor; stage of resistance, or adaptation to the stressor over time; and stage of exhaustion, or inability to adapt to the stressor (Selye, 1974, 1982). This theory can be applied to clients who are suffering not only psychological or social stress but physiological stress as well.

Maslow's theory of the hierarchy of needs is illustrated as a pyramid containing five broad layers of needs upon which human functioning is based. The bottom or first-level needs are physiological followed by safety and security, love and belonging, self-esteem, and self-actualization (Maslow, 1970). The theory contends that basic needs, such as air, water, food, and safety, must be met before meeting higher-level needs such as self-esteem or self-actualization. The application of this theory to nursing practice can provide a framework for client assessment and assist in identifying nursing care priorities.

These theories are only a sample of those developed by related disciplines that have uses in nursing. Indeed, with the drive toward teamwork and collaboration in health care these theories are relevant to all disciplines.

Others, such as Rotter's locus of control (1954) and Bandura's self-efficacy theory (1986), can be found in various chapters in this text. One or more of these theories can serve as a framework for designing interventions for clients throughout the life cycle, developing and implementing research studies, and framing educational curricula. In combination with nursing theories, a wide array of theoretical perspectives in various stages of development is available from which to choose.

SUMMARY

Nursing is a knowledge-based discipline that is significantly different from medicine and focused on the wholeness of human beings. Nursing knowledge is the organization of discipline-specific concepts, theories, and ideas published in both print and electronic media and demonstrated in professional practice. Theories and frameworks provide direction and guidance for structuring professional nursing practice, education, and research. They provide a way to educate nurses; describe, explain, predict, organize, assess, diagnose, intervene, and evaluate nursing practice; and question, study, and interpret research. This chapter provides a historical perspective and a comprehensive overview of some of the many nursing theorists who have made substantial contributions to the development of a body of nursing knowledge. The remainder of this text will introduce additional nursing theories that also contribute to the body of nursing knowledge.

SALIENT POINTS

- A theory is a group of statements that describe the relationship between two or more concepts.
- The main components of nursing theories are person, environment, health/illness, and nursing (nursing's metaparadigm).
- Nightingale's theory focuses on nursing's role in manipulating the environment.
- Peplau's theory centers on the interpersonal process in nursing.
- According to Rogers, the nurse seeks to promote coherence between individuals and their environments.

- As specified by Orem, when a client has a deficit in his or her ability for self-care, the nurse assists the individual with self-care practices.
- King conceptualizes the nurse and the client as components of an interpersonal system who seek to attain mutually agreed-upon goals.
- Roy's theory describes the client as a biopsychosocial adaptive system and the nurse as one who modifies stimuli to promote adaptation.
- Three levels of nursing intervention—primary, secondary, and tertiary prevention—are specified in Neuman's systems model.

- Leininger's theory centers on providing culturally congruent nursing care.
- Watson identifies the caring relationship and caritas processes that form the core of nursing.
- The more specific theories, in whole or in part, can be readily adapted for use in any practice setting.
- The more global theories may better serve as frameworks for research, the findings of which can then be applied to practice.

- Theories from related disciplines also have relevance to nursing practice, education, and research.
- All theories have the potential to make substantial contributions to the nursing profession by enhancing the development of a unique body of nursing knowledge.

CRITICAL REFLECTION EXERCISES

1. What is your personal philosophy of nursing? Which of the theoretical perspectives of nursing presented in this chapter is most closely aligned with your philosophy of nursing? Reflect on your most recent patient encounter and discuss how the chosen theory would guide your care of the patient.
2. How do Florence Nightingale's ideas apply to nursing practice in the current culture of patient safety and quality?

3. Identify the nursing theory or model that would be most useful to you in your practice and explain why.
4. Compare the definitions of health and illness in two nursing theories, citing similarities and differences. Which one is the most reflective of your own definitions of health and illness? Why?
5. Defend or refute the following statement: "We should have only one nursing theory, rather than several, to guide education, practice, and research."

REFERENCES

Aguilera, D. C. (1998). *Crisis intervention: Theory and methodology* (8th ed.). St Louis: Mosby.

Alligood, M. R. (2005). Nursing theory: The basis for professional nursing. In K. K. Chitty (Ed.), *Professional nursing concepts and challenges* (4th ed.) (pp. 271–298). Philadelphia: Saunders.

Bandura, A. (1986). *Social foundations of thought and action: A social cognitive theory*. Englewood Cliffs, NJ: Prentice Hall.

Barnum, B. S. (1998). Nursing theory *Analysis, application, evaluation*. Philadelphia: Lippincott.

Duvall, E. M. (1977). *Marriage and family development* (5th ed.). New York: Lippincott.

Encarta World English Dictionary. (2009). New York: Bloomsbury Publishing.

Erikson, E. H. (1963). *Childhood and society* (2nd ed.). New York: Norton.

Erikson, E. H. (1982). *The life cycle completed*. A review. New York: Norton.

Fawcett, J. (1975). The family as a living open system: An emerging conceptual framework for nursing. *International Nursing Review, 22*, 113–116.

Fawcett, J. (1977). The relationship between identification and patterns of change in spouses' body images during and after pregnancy. *International Journal of Nursing Studies, 14*, 199–213.

Fawcett, J. (1989). *Analysis and evaluation of conceptual models of nursing* (2nd ed.). Philadelphia: Davis.

Fawcett, J. (1993). *Analysis and evaluation of nursing theories*. Philadelphia: Davis.

Fawcett, J. (1997). The structural hierarchy of nursing knowledge: Components and their definitions. In I. M. King, & J. Fawcett (Eds.), *The language of nursing theory and metatheory* (pp. 11–17). Indianapolis: Sigma Theta Tau International.

Fawcett, J. (1999). *The relationship of theory and research* (3rd ed.). Philadelphia: Davis.

Fawcett, J. (2000). *Analysis and evaluation of contemporary nursing knowledge: Nursing models and theories*. Philadelphia: Davis.

Fawcett, J. (2005). *Analysis and evaluation of contemporary nursing knowledge: Nursing models and theories* (2nd ed.). Philadelphia: Davis.

Im, E., & Chang, S. J. (2012). Current trends in nursing theories. *Journal School of Nursing, 44*, 156–164.

Im, E., & Meleis, A. I. (1999). Situation-specific theories: Philosophical roots, properties, and approach. *Advances in Nursing Science, 22*(3), 11–24.

Infante, M. S. (1982). *Crisis theory: A frame-work for nursing practice*. Reston, VA: Reston Publishing.

Institute of Medicine (IOM). (2003). *Health professions education: A bridge to quality*. Washington, DC: National Academies Press. Retrieved from http://www.iom.edu/Reports/2003 /Health-Professions-Education-A-Bridge-to-Quality.aspx.

Johnson, J. L. (1994). A dialectical examination of nursing art. *Advances in Nursing Science, 17*(1), 1–14.

King, I. (1971). *Toward a theory for nursing.* New York: Wiley.

King, I. (1981). *A theory for nursing: Systems, concepts, process.* New York: Wiley.

King, I. (1995a). A systems framework for nursing. In M. A. Frey, & C. L. Sieloff (Eds.), *Advancing King's systems framework and theory of nursing* (pp. 14–22). Thousand Oaks, CA: Sage.

King, I. (1995b). The theory of goal attainment. In M. A. Frey, & C. L. Sieloff (Eds.), *Advancing King's systems framework and theory of nursing* (pp. 23–34). Thousand Oaks, CA: Sage.

Lazarus, R. S. (1976). *Patterns of adjustment* (3rd ed.). New York: McGraw-Hill.

Lazarus, R. S., & Folkman, S. (1984). *Stress appraisal and coping.* New York: Springer.

Leininger, M. (1978). *Transcultural nursing: Concepts, theories and practice.* New York: Wiley.

Leininger, M. (1984). *Care: The essence of nursing and health.* Thorofare, NJ: Slack.

Leininger, M. (1991). *Culture, care, diversity and universality. A theory of nursing.* New York: National League for Nursing. (NLN Publication No. 15–2402).

Leininger, M. (1995). *Transcultural nursing: Concepts, theories, research, and practice.* Columbus, OH: McGraw-Hill.

Leininger, M. M., & McFarland, M. R. (2002). *Transcultural nursing: Concepts, theories, research, and practice.* New York: McGraw-Hill.

Leininger, M. M., & McFarland, M. R. (2006). *Culture care, diversity and universality. A worldwide nursing theory.* Sudbury, MA: Jones & Bartlett.

Levine, M. E. (1995). The rhetoric of nursing theory. *Image Journal of Nursing Scholarship, 27,* 11–14.

Lewin, K. (1951). Defining the field at a given time. In D. Cartwright (Ed.), *Field theory in social science: Selected papers by Kurt Lewin.* New York: Harper and Brothers.

Lippitt, G. L. (1973). *Visualizing change.* LaJolla, CA: University Associates.

Maslow, A. (1970). *Motivation and personality* (2nd ed.). New York: Harper & Row.

McEwen, M. (2007). Application of theory in nursing practice. In M. McEwen, & E. M. Wills (Eds.), *Theoretical basis for nursing* (2nd ed.). Philadelphia: Lippincott Williams & Wilkins.

Meleis, A. I. (2005). *Theoretical nursing: Development and progress* (3rd ed). Philadelphia: Lippincott Williams & Wilkins.

Neuman, B. (1982). *The Neuman systems model: Application to nursing theory and practice.* Norwalk, CT: Appleton-Century-Crofts.

Neuman, B. (1989). *The Neuman systems model* (2nd ed.). Norwalk, CT: Appleton-Century-Crofts.

Neuman, B. (1995). *The Neuman systems model* (3rd ed.). Norwalk, CT: Appleton-Century-Crofts.

Neuman, B., & Fawcett, J. (2002). *The Neuman systems model* (4th ed.). Upper Saddle River, NJ: Prentice Hall.

Neuman, B. M., & Young, R. J. (1972). A model for teaching total person approach to patient problems. *Nursing Research, 21,* 264–269.

Nightingale, F. (1860–1946). *Notes on nursing: What it is and what it is not.* New York: Appleton Century.

Orem, D. E. (1971). *Nursing: Concepts of practice.* New York: McGraw-Hill.

Orem, D. E. (1980). *Nursing: Concepts of practice* (2nd ed.). New York: McGraw-Hill.

Orem, D. E. (1985). *Nursing: Concepts of practice* (3rd ed.). New York: McGraw-Hill.

Orem, D. E. (1991). *Nursing: Concepts of practice* (4th ed.). St Louis: Mosby.

Orem, D. E. (1995). *Nursing: Concepts of practice* (5th ed.). St Louis: Mosby.

Orem, D. E. (2001). *Nursing: Concepts of practice* (6th ed.). St Louis: Mosby.

Peplau, H. (1952). *Interpersonal relations in nursing: A conceptual framework of reference for psychodynamic nursing.* New York: Putnam.

Peplau, H. (1991). *Interpersonal relations in nursing: A conceptual framework of reference for psychodynamic nursing.* New York: Springer.

Peplau, H. (1992). Interpersonal relations: A theoretical framework for application in nursing practice. *Nursing Science Quarterly, 5,* 13–18.

Rogers, M. E. (1970). *An introduction to the theoretical basis of nursing.* Philadelphia: Davis.

Rogers, M. E. (1989). Nursing: A science of unitary man. In J. P. Reihl-Sisca (Ed.), *Conceptual models for nursing practice* (2nd ed.). Norwalk, CT: Appleton & Lange.

Rogers, M. E. (1990). Nursing Science of unitary, irreducible, human beings. In E. A. Barrett (Ed.), *Visions of Rogers' science-based nursing* (pp. 5–11). New York: National League for Nursing. Update 1990.

Rogers, M. E. (1994). Nursing science evolves. In M. A. Madrid, & E. A. Barrett (Eds.), *Rogers' scientific art of nursing practice* (NLN Publication No. 15-2610) (pp. 3–9). New York: National League for Nursing.

Rotter, J. B. (1954). *Social learning and clinical psychology.* Englewood Cliffs, NJ: Prentice Hall.

Roy, C. (1984). *Introduction to nursing: An adaptation model* (2nd ed.). Englewood Cliffs, NJ: Prentice Hall.

Roy, C. (1989). The Roy adaptation model. In J. P Reihl-Sisca (Ed.), *Conceptual models for nursing practice* (3rd ed.). Norwalk, CT: Appleton & Lange.

Roy, C. (2009). *The Roy adaptation model* (3rd ed.). Upper Saddle River, NJ: Prentice Hall.

Roy, C., & Andrews, H. A. (1999). *The Roy adaptation model* (2nd ed.). Stanford, CT: Appleton & Lange.

Selye, H. (1974). *Stress without distress.* Philadelphia: Lippincott.

Selye, H. (1982). History and the present status of the stress concept. In I. A. Goldberger, & S. Breznitz (Eds.), *Handbook of stress: Theoretical and clinical aspects* (pp. 7–20). New York: Free Press.

U.S Department of Health and Human Services. (1999). *Mental health: A report of the Surgeon General. Substance Abuse and Mental Health Services Administration.* Rockville, MD: U.S. Department of Health and Human Services. Center for Mental Health Services, National Institutes of Health, National Institute of Mental Health.

von Bertalanffy, L. (1956). General systems theory. In B. D. Ruben, & J. Kim (Eds.), *General systems theory and human communication* (pp. 7–16). Rochelle Park, NJ: Hayden.

von Bertalanffy, L. (1968). *General systems theory*. New York: Braziller.

Watson, J. (1985). *Nursing: Human science and health care*. Norwalk, CT: Appleton-Century-Crofts.

Watson, J. (1996). Watson's theory of transpersonal caring. In P. Hinton Walker, & B. Neuman (Eds.), *Blueprint for use of nursing models* (pp. 141–184). New York: NLN Press.

Watson, J. (2007). *Theory of human caring* (pp. 141–184). Denver: Watson Caring Science Institute. Retrieved 11/1/2013 from http://watsoncaring science.org/images/features/library/T HEORY%20OF%20HUMAN%20CA RING_Website.pdf/.

White, M. B. (1983). *Curriculum development from a nursing model: The crisis theory framework*. New York: Springer.

Health Policy and Planning and the Nursing Practice Environment

Debra C. Wallace, PhD, RN, FAAN and L. Louise Ivanov, PhD, RN, FAAN

ⓔ http://evolve.elsevier.com/Friberg/bridge/

OBJECTIVES

At the completion of this chapter, the reader will be able to:

- Identify political, legislative, social, and economic factors affecting health policy and nursing.
- Describe the legislative, budgetary, and regulatory processes for developing, implementing, and evaluating policy.
- Discuss selected health programs mandated by federal health policy.
- Evaluate health policies for their impact on nursing practice, education, research, and the practice environment.
- Discuss strategies for nurse participation in health policy.

👤 PROFILE IN PRACTICE

Eileen Kohlenberg, PhD, RN, NEA-BC, ANEF
Professor, University of North Carolina at Greensboro

As a faculty member and organization leader, I promote student awareness and involvement in the policy process, including knowledge of current issues, participation in professional nursing organizations, and advocacy for clients. Instilling a belief in students' own capacity for influencing nursing practice and health care is crucial to sustained participation. Preparing future professionals to contribute to the development and implementation of effective health policy and an effective practice environment is a privilege and responsibility.

My professional career has spanned several decades and many professional opportunities and challenges, including critical care or medical surgical staff nurse, faculty member, education administrator, and National League for Nursing Accreditation Commission evaluator. As is the case with many professionals, questions and concerns regarding access to care, delivery systems, and the impact of health policy on nursing and patients were formulated as the result of

encounters with the variety of experiences for professional practice. Clinical practice, doctoral studies, educational leadership, and nursing organization participation promoted an in-depth understanding and appreciation of the social, economic, political, policy, and global factors that affect nursing education, practice, and research.

A most important framework for understanding and contributing to health policy has been active participation in professional nursing organizations. Serving as President of the North Carolina Nurses Association, President of the North Carolina Foundation for Nursing, and a delegate to the American Nurses' Association has provided avenues to identify state and national needs, communicate nursing priorities, and collaborate with legislators to pursue agendas beneficial to patients, nurses, and the health care community. The policy work for the ANA Congress on Practice and Economics and collaborating as an author on the ANA Nurses' Bill of Rights and the ANA Principles of

Nurse Staffing created a remarkable opportunity for contribution to quality of care and health policy initiatives at the national level. I have served as a member of the NC Healthcare Information Communication Alliance and the NC Nurses Scholars Commissions, and an elected member of the ANA delegation, as well as a member of coalitions of nursing professionals focused on policy issues to address the workforce shortage, quality and access to nursing education, and provision of continuing competence for nurses in the state.

INTRODUCTION

Why should nurses be concerned with legislation regarding health? Health policy affects nursing at all levels of preparation, in all settings and specialties, and across all client groups. Policy decisions, allocations, and regulation dictate where care is delivered, to whom care is delivered, who delivers care, how care is delivered, and who pays for care. Specifically policy determines or assists in decisions of every aspect of health care, including delivery modalities, settings of care, quality of care provider qualifications, payment level and mechanisms, type of services, and access to care. Additionally practice environment, workplace safety, licensure, certification, accreditation, and educational funding are influenced by health policy and related regulation. Thus it is important for each nurse to have a working knowledge of health policy development, regulation, and evaluation so as to understand how members of the largest health care profession can influence policy to improve the health and well-being of society.

Before the 20th century, health care was typically an individual or private sector responsibility in most countries. Many health care facilities were affiliated with religious and civic organizations and groups or educational institutions. Physicians had private office practices with direct fee for service and out-of-pocket payment. The federal government in the United States became involved in the regulation, provision, and financing of health care primarily during the early 1900s. Government involvement, scientific developments, technology, social pressure, and increased costs associated with health care have resulted in the development of a health care industry that exceeds manufacturing and agriculture industries. The health care industry is often divided into subsystems that serve populations on the basis of payment decisions and condition specialties.

In industrialized countries in many parts of the world, such as the United Kingdom and Canada, centralized systems of care have been developed through socialized medicine models. In these countries the infrastructure controls the number and location of health care delivery sites and the training, distribution, and reimbursement of providers, both physicians and nurses. The nursing practice environment is hospital and community based and is regulated by the types of services offered, payment decisions, and access points. Regardless of the nation, multiple factors affect the development, implementation, and evaluation of health policy, as well as its influence on nursing and health care. Chapter 1 discusses the impact of these health industry shifts on the profession of nursing.

POLITICS

One of the major factors influencing health policy is politics. Individuals, organizations, agencies, state, and federal processes are involved in developing health policy, the regulations for implementation, and the evaluation of outcomes. For example, a citizen writes a member of Congress and argues that certain needs are not being met for technology-dependent children. An organization such as the American Nurses Association (ANA) may be involved by writing, visiting, and lobbying state and congressional representatives for new and continuing needs of nurses and patients. The need for educational and program grants in the Nurse Reinvestment Act is one example of a law that was passed to support nurses. Federal agencies such as the National Institutes of Health (NIH) and the Food and Drug Administration (FDA) invite members of Congress to attend administrative hearings and provide input on priority setting, program development, budgetary needs, and evaluation reports. For example, the Veterans Administration sought additional funding for care and research to improve care, resulting in the Veterans Mental Health and Other Care Improvements Act of 2008, which addressed post-deployment mental health and the Department of Veterans Affairs Expiring Authorities Act of 2013, which extends veterans services to veterans hospitals and clinics, including homeless and disabled veterans.

In addition, political leaders and legislators bring health-related agendas to congressional committees based on their constituents' values and priorities, as well as their own.

Organizations

Nurses are members of many organizations involved in and influencing the development of health policy and health care–related legislation. Nonlegislative citizens also play a political role in health policy development and implementation through participation in and support of civic organizations and activities, such as the American Association of Retired Persons (AARP), Mothers Against Drunk Driving (MADD), American Diabetes Association (ADA), the March of Dimes, the National Organization of Women (NOW), and the National Rifle Association (NRA). Most professional organizations (e.g., American Medical Association [AMA], American Hospital Association [AHA], American Academy of Nursing [AAN], Coalition for Patients' Rights [CPR]) develop legislative agendas, support political candidates, and employ lobbyists at state and federal levels. (See Box 6-1 for a list of government and health care organizations referred to in this chapter.) In 2004, the ANA moved its headquarters from Kansas City to Washington, DC, to increase visibility and access to federal agencies and Congress. State nursing associations often have lobbyists to ensure state laws for advanced practice licensure, Medicaid benefits and coverage, and work environment protections. Lay, civic, and professional organizations, whether or not associated with a political party—such as the AARP, the National Association for the Advancement of Colored Persons (NAACP), the NRA, the ANA, the National Home Care Association (NHCA), and the America's Health Insurance Plans (AHIP)—use grassroots activity, paid lobbyists, campaign support, advertisements, and organized rallies to make an impact on health policies affecting their members and special interest groups. Most health care professional organizations, including the ANA, have a paid lobbyist in each state capital and at least one in Washington, DC. Because these organizations fund political and lobbying activity, a proportion of membership dues to these organizations are not tax deductible. For example, the ANA uses approximately 25% of its dues for lobbying activities and has a full-time lobbyist in Washington. Many state nursing associations have their own lobbyist or contract for this work in their state legislature.

Political Parties

Three major political parties have been involved in legislation: the Republican National Committee (RNC), the Democratic National Committee (DNC), and the Independent Reform Party (IRP). More recently, the Libertarian Party (LP) has become more involved. Political parties set forth the major issues of concern through party platforms during presidential conventions, website postings, and paid media advertisements. The party platforms consist of "planks" that delineate the party's philosophy and stand on issues of the day. Platforms are a consensus of the convention delegates, but they also mirror the presidential candidate's stand and arguments to be used during the campaign. Platform issues, then, often become the agendas for state legislatures and the U.S. Congress. Many of the issues during the 20th century were health related, such as gun control, abortion, and Medicare. In the early part of the 21st century, issues surrounding stem cell research, prescription drug coverage, bioterrorism, and electronic health records have emerged. The most recent platforms and priority issues can be reviewed on party websites or received from each party's national or state offices. The ANA has traditionally supported more of the Democratic Party's health issue planks.

Political Action and 527 Committees

Registered *political action committees* (PACs) can be established independently or as a part of a formal organization to (1) raise, spend, and contribute money; (2) assist with campaigns; and (3) lobby on behalf of special interest groups, industries, or segments of society. Political action committees initiate much of the legislative activity or inactivity on both the state and federal levels. For example, *Roe v. Wade*, which legalized abortion, continues as a major PAC focus. Political action committees pay for television advertisements, hold public rallies and demonstrations, distribute literature, and invite political and other famous figures to events supporting their positions. Originally PACs represented persons with specific needs who had been overlooked or not protected by society (e.g., those with AIDS, older adults, the homeless, poor children). In the late 1990s PACs became more commonly representatives of particular groups of persons that banded political, human, and financial resources to get policies initiated, funded, extended, or terminated for social and corporate agendas. For example, the ANA has a PAC to address issues related to the health and nursing workforce, including

BOX 6-1   Important Health Care Terms and Organizations

Accreditation Commission for Education in Nursing (ACEN)
Administration on Aging (AOA)
Advanced Education Nursing Grants (AENP)
Advanced practice registered nurse (APRN)
Agency for Healthcare Research and Quality (AHRQ)
American Academy of Nursing (AAN)
American Association of Colleges of Nursing (AACN)
American Association of Critical-Care Nurses (AACCN)
American Association of Retired Persons (AARP)
American Dental Association (ADA)
American Diabetes Association (ADA)
America's Health Insurance Plans (AHIP)
American Hospital Association (AHA)
American Medical Association (AMA)
American Nurses' Association (ANA)
American Nurses Credentialing Center (ANCC)
American Nurses Foundation (ANF)
American Public Health Association (APHA)
American Red Cross (ARC)
Association for Women's Health, Obstetrical and Neonatal
    Nursing (AWHONN)
Bureau of Census (BOC)
Bureau of Health Professions (BHP)
Centers for Disease Control and Prevention (CDC)
Centers of Excellence (COE)
Centers for Medicare and Medicaid Services (CMS)
Certified registered nurse anesthetist (CRNA)
Children's Health Insurance Programs (CHIP)
Coalition for Patients' Rights (CPR)
Colorectal cancer (CRC)
Commission on Collegiate Nursing Education (CCNE)
Comprehensive Geriatric Education Program (CGEP)
Congressional Budget Office (CBO)
Consolidated Budget Resolution (CBR)
Coordinating Office for Terrorism Preparedness and Emergency
    Response (COTPER)
Council for the Advancement of Nursing Science (CANS)
Culturally and Linguistically Appropriate Services (CLAS)
Democratic National Committee (DNC)
Department of Agriculture (DA)
Department of Education (DE)
Department of Homeland Security (DHS)
Department of Labor (DL)
Department of Veterans Affairs (DVA)
Diagnostic related groups (DRG)
doctorate of nursing practice (DNP)
Evidence Based Practice (EBP)
Federal Elections Commission (FEC)
Food and Drug Administration (FDA)
General Accounting Office (GAO)

Gross Domestic Product (GDP)
Health Care Financing Administration (HCFA)
Health Insurance Portability and Accountability Act (HIPAA)
Health Resources and Services Administration (HRSA)
Homeland Security Act (HSA)
Independent Reform Party (IRP)
Institute of Medicine (IOM)
Interdisciplinary Nursing Quality Research Initiative (INQRI)
Internal Revenue Service (IRS)
Kaiser Family Foundation (KFF)
Libertarian Party (LP)
Licensed Practical Nurse (LPN)
Magnet Nursing Services Recognition Program (MNSRP)
Mothers Against Drunk Driving (MADD)
National Academies of Science (NAS)
National Advisory Council (NAC)
National Advisory Council on Nurse Education and
    Practice (NACNEP)
National Association for the Advancement of Colored
    Persons (NAACP)
National Center for Chronic Disease Prevention and Health
    Promotion (NCCDPHP)
National Center for Health Statistics (NCHS)
National Center for Minority Health and Health Disparities (NCMHD)
National Center for Nursing Research (NCNR)
National Center on Minority Health and Health Disparities (NCMHD)
National Council Licensure Examination (NCLEX)
National Council of State Boards of Nursing (NCSBN)
National Database of Nursing Quality Indicators (NDNQI)
National Home Care Association (NHCA)
National Institute on Aging (NIA)
National Institute of Child Health and Human Development (NICHD)
National Institute of Mental Health (NIMH)
National Institute of Nursing Research (NINR)
National Institute of Occupational Safety and Health (NIOSH)
National Institutes of Health (NIH)
National League for Nursing (NLN)
National League for Nursing Accreditation Commission (NLNAC)
National Office of Public Health Genomics (NOPHG)
National Organization of Women (NOW)
National Rifle Association (NRA)
North Carolina Association of Nurse Anesthetists (NCANA)
Nurse Education, Practice and Retention (NEPR) program
Nurse Faculty Loan Program (NFLP)
Nurse Practitioners (NPs)
Nursing Care Quality Initiative (NCQI)
Nursing Home Quality Initiative (NHQI)
Nursing Research Initiative (NRI)
Nursing Workforce Diversity (NWD) grants
Nursing's Agenda for Health Care Reform (NAHCR)

Continued

BOX 6-1 **Important Health Care Terms and Organizations—cont'd**	
Obstetrical and Neonatal Nursing (ONN)	Senior Community Service Employment Program (SCSEP)
Occupational Health and Safety Administration (OSHA)	Sigma Theta Tau International (STTI)
Office on Management and Budget (OMB)	Social and Rehabilitation Services (SRS)
Office of Public Health and Science (OPHS)	Social Security (SS)
Omnibus Budget Reconciliation Act (OBRA)	Society of Gastroenterology Nurses and Associates (SGNA)
Oncology Nursing Society (ONS)	State Children's Health Insurance Program (SCHIP)
Pew Charitable Trusts (PCT)	Substance Abuse and Mental Health Services Administration
Pew Health Professions Commission (PHPC)	(SAMHSA)
political action committees (PACs)	Surgeon General (SG)
Preadmission Screening and Resident Review (PASRR)	Sustainable Growth Rate (SGR)
prescription drug plan (PDP)	Tennessee Bureau of TennCare (TBOT)
Presidential Election Campaign Fund (PECF)	Tennessee Department of Health (TDH)
Republican National Committee (RNC)	Templeton Foundation (TF)
Registered Nurse (RN)	United States Department of Health and Human Services (USDHHS)
Robert Wood Johnson Foundation (RWJF)	Vocational Nurse (VN)
Safe Staffing Saves Lives (SSSL)	Women's Health Initiative (WHI)

staffing, mandatory overtime, and supervision and delegation. Also, the pharmaceutical industry has multiple PACs to lobby Congress.

These focused activities, as well as financial support for and against politicians who have voted or will vote on bills relating to an issue, make PACs some of the most powerful entities influencing health policy decisions, especially those related to regulation and allocation of funds. The large amount of funding used for and against campaigns has changed how legislation is formed, what is passed, and the amount and type of appropriations approved. Legislators are finding it more difficult to meet the needs of one special interest group and not offend another group. For example, when political power shifts in state and federal legislatures, the influence of PACs change. The passage or failure of bills to protect the environment, reauthorize labor union and workers' rights and safety, change gun control, revise tort reform, cut or raise taxes, or increase the minimum wage may depend on which party is in power. One result of legislators trying to remain supportive of their funding sources is that a higher number of bills pass that require additional federal monies or require states to increase dollars allocated to programs or allow elected officials to vote for or against an issue with no simultaneous action. The No Child Left Behind legislation is an example of one unfunded mandate in which federal legislation required action but did not result in federal funding to states.

Financing

A major concern over the past two decades has been the influence of money on campaigns, resulting in increased access to legislators and greater influence on legislation by PACs and financial contributors. The Federal Elections Commission (FEC) regulates the type, amount, and reporting of such funds. State commissions handle funds within state, county, and municipal governments. Each candidate, political party, and PAC is required to register and submit quarterly, monthly, or annual financial reports. This is traditionally referred to as *hard money*. *Soft money* is less regulated and refers to funds given to the party but for no specific purpose. Soft money is often used to support campaign activities but under a different guise. For example, instead of giving money to a senatorial campaign for travel to a state capital, the party supports a high school student workshop on a topic that invokes the candidate's position, thus averting the campaign finance rules constraining usage. Campaign finance reports, as well as documentation of PACs, corporate, and other large contributors to each party and candidate, are required by the FEC and are available to the public (see www.fec.gov). Monies spent on media, travel, and food by campaigns have increased tremendously in the past decade. Many of the organizations noted in the preceding section—as well as many nurses, doctors, physical therapists, and patients—donated to these campaigns. In federal campaigns in 2013 and 2014, individual contributions were limited to $2600 per candidate and $32,400 per national party, or a total of $48,600 to all candidates combined and $74,600 to all PACs or committees combined. In contrast, national, state, or local party committee contributions were limited to $5000 per candidate per election, unlimited to political parties yearly, and limited to a maximum of $45,000 to a U.S. Senate candidate per campaign (FEC, 2013a). However, in January 2010, the U.S. Supreme Court in *Citizens United v. Federal Election Commission* (559 U.S. 310) ruled that certain limits on campaign contributions were an unconstitutional denial of free speech. This case focused on the airing of a political advertisement within a previously limited time frame during an election cycle. Lawsuits to limit campaign financing continue to be filed in state and federal courts.

Many state political contribution limits are similar to national levels or are based on population and candidate numbers each election cycle. In addition to funds raised by candidates, the government provides funds from the taxpayer-supported Presidential Election Campaign Fund (PECF). These monies are designated on federal income tax forms and then distributed to candidates after they raise a specified amount. A cap of $45.6 million is placed on what can be spent on primaries or preconvention efforts for presidential candidates who choose to accept these funds. In 2008 $103 million in federal funds were used in the presidential primaries and campaign. During the 2012 election President Obama and Mr. Romney chose not to accept federal dollars (FEC, 2013b). As was true in 2004 and 2008, both candidates benefited greatly from the amounts the parties or PACS spent on advertisements and other media to support them. In the 2004 election, presidential candidates raised more than $298 million for their respective campaigns, and more than $1 billion was used by parties, candidates, and federal funds combined. This is more than the initial year of spending for the Medicare Prescription Drug Plan (PDP). During the 2012 election cycle, more than $3 billion was raised (FEC, 2013b), though final amended reports for some candidates and organizations have not been submitted as of December 2013.

Two new modes of funding appeared in the 2004 presidential campaign. Howard Dean, MD, was the first candidate to formally use the Internet to solicit and receive contributions. A new type of committee called *527 political groups* arose and altered political fundraising and campaign activities. These groups can engage in voter mobilization efforts, issue advocacy, and other activity short of expressly advocating the election or defeat of a federal candidate. There are no limits to how much they can raise. These organizations are regulated by the Internal Revenue Service (IRS), but not necessarily the FEC if they do not explicitly advocate for an individual's election or defeat or do not directly subsidize federal elections. Thus this is a major loophole to raising and using soft money. Swift Boat Veterans for Truth, Progress for America, MoveON.org, and Voices for Working Families are just a few of the organizations that provided significant media coverage and had a considerable impact on the election. In 2008 organizations ran advertisements that showed candidates' positions in a very demonstrative and stark manner. For example, John Kerry was portrayed as unpatriotic even though he volunteered and served in Vietnam. George W. Bush was portrayed as supporting child labor because of the large deficits, even though child labor laws were not changed during his term. In 2012 Romney was portrayed as a rich millionaire out of touch with most of America and Obama was portrayed as not being an American citizen.

Additionally lobbyists often provide for expenses incurred in "program-related" trips. These payments have caused scandals for national congressional representatives as well as state legislators and governors in the past decade, resulting in calls for and changes to ethics rules so that all persons have access to legislators regardless of socioeconomic means. The same issue has been found at state levels, and recently some officials have been found criminally responsible for taking bribes or inappropriately using their governmental positions to influence policy based on financial donations and arrangements.

Understanding the Legislative Process

An important process to understand is illustrated in *How Our Laws Are Made* (U.S. House of Representatives, 2003; U.S. Senate, 2003), which explains how a bill proceeds through the U.S. Congress. Steps, processes, facilitators, and barriers to enacting legislation at the federal level from introduction of a bill through its enrollment to the president are detailed (Figure 6-1). This illustration also identifies the House and Senate procedures, including leadership roles and responsibilities, committee assignment, readings on the chamber floor, and resolution between the two chambers. Many of the steps and processes, such as the House "hopper" and the system of bells and lights, originated in the late

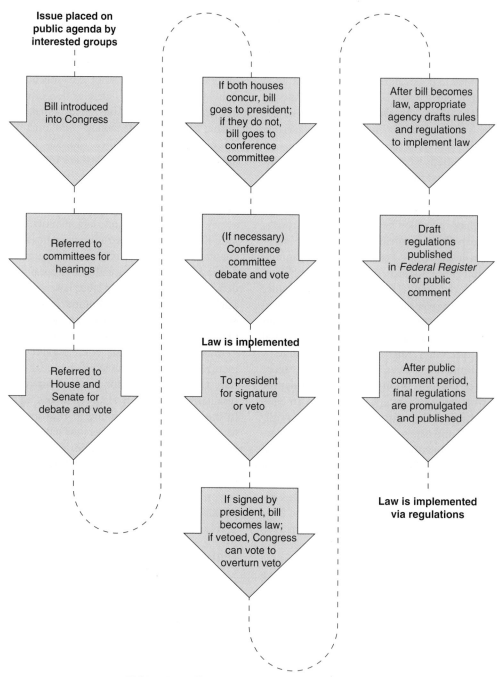

Issue placed on public agenda by interested groups

Bill introduced into Congress

Referred to committees for hearings

Referred to House and Senate for debate and vote

If both houses concur, bill goes to president; if they do not, bill goes to conference committee

(If necessary) Conference committee debate and vote

Law is implemented

To president for signature or veto

If signed by president, bill becomes law; if vetoed, Congress can vote to overturn veto

After bill becomes law, appropriate agency drafts rules and regulations to implement law

Draft regulations published in *Federal Register* for public comment

After public comment period, final regulations are promulgated and published

Law is implemented via regulations

FIGURE 6-1 Formal health care policy process.

19th century. The hopper is the box in which representatives initially place a piece of legislation they wish to be brought to the House for action. A system of bells and lights is in place throughout the Capitol building to notify senators and representatives of pending votes and other actions. Also discussed in this document is how to "bury" or "kill" a bill, and how the majority party ideas prevail even in the most sacred workings of our democracy. Many state legislatures follow similar protocols and procedures. It is incumbent upon nurses to know the major committees and legislators that deal with health and nursing issues in their own state, as well as the major pitfalls or bridges where nurse and health-focused legislation may be delayed or strengthened. The state nursing association can assist with identifying those persons, committees, barriers, and facilitators.

Administration and Committees

In addition to the constitutionally mandated process and structure, each Congress or state legislature establishes its own rules for administration and governance that affect how policies are made and which issues are considered. Rules include the number, type, and focus of committees where most of the legislative work takes place. In fact, committee chairpersons, assigned because of seniority, develop the calendar of issues and legislation to be discussed. In the past, and probably continuing into the future, bills that are brought forth for discussion and passage are not necessarily the purview of the particular committee. Rather, these issues may be germane to the constituents of the ranking majority or minority leader, based on the leader's personal beliefs and experience, or related to financial support received from individuals, organizations, and corporations.

Committee structure is also determined for each Congress, with the exception of several mandated committees by U.S. or state constitution. In Congress, committee structure was fairly stable from the 1960s through the early 1990s, years during which the Democrats controlled the House of Representatives and often the Senate. During that time, the Committee on Labor and Human Resources had primary responsibility for health care legislation and issues. With a new Republican majority in the House of Representatives beginning in 1994 and that party's control over the Senate and White House from 2001 to 2008, committee structure was altered and updated. Similar changes occurred in 2009 to 2010 when the Democrats controlled all three branches. Several

committees were terminated, and names and jurisdictions were changed. A new Health, Education, Labor, and Pensions Committee in the Senate was charged with primary health policy jurisdiction. However, many committees develop health-related bills and send forth authorizations and appropriations for those bills, such as the Senate Agriculture, Nutrition, and Forestry Committee (nutrition bill) and the House International Relations Committee (American Red Cross bill).

Congressional Sessions

Each U.S. Congress has two sessions for developing legislation. The 113th Congress began in January 2013 with the first session; the second session began in January 2014. Legislation that has passed both Houses, been resolved in conference committee, been enrolled to the president, and is signed, becomes public law. Laws are signified by the Congress in which they are passed, as well as their chronological order of passage (e.g., PL 110-361: law number 361 passed the 110th Congress). Financial allocations—more precisely, appropriations—are included in bills and usually include funding for 3 to 5 years. However, appropriations depend on the budget bills passed for each calendar year and thus can be revised, reauthorized, repealed, or not funded by subsequent congressional action. In addition, there are unofficial "lame duck" congresses, whereby little is accomplished, as everyone is waiting for the election result turnover of political parties in control of congressional houses or majorities.

Chamber Responsibilities

A constitutional directive mandates that all budget bills, including an increase in federal income taxes, originate in the U.S. House of Representatives. Thus the Senate cannot initiate an income tax increase, but it can increase spending limits and develop new programs that may result in the need for increased taxes. Either chamber can be the origin of bills that establish or increase funds through other means, such as airport, gasoline, or Medicare fees and taxes. The Ways and Means, Appropriations, and Finance committees have input to the budget and review legislation originating in other committees that require new or continuing appropriations. Any legislation that includes appropriations, whether continuing or new, is required to be submitted by committees and subcommittees to the chamber budget committees for calculation, inclusion in the fiscal year appropriations bills, and estimations of spending in the outlying years. On most occasions the budget committees change or alter the recommended allocations and refer these changes to the committee charged with a specific piece of legislation as well as to the committee of primary responsibility for that specific area (e.g., health care, education, transportation). The Senate has primary responsibility for approval of political appointments, such as judges, ambassadors, the surgeon general, cabinet members, and federal agency directors. In the 1990s the approval hearings were contentiously political and philosophical. Health-related issues such as sexual harassment, sex education, family planning, refugee support, and immigration laws served as litmus tests for appointee approval. Two other health issues, abortion and the death penalty, continue to be major points for discussion that affect health policy and the appointment of judges to state, appellate, and federal courts and the U.S. Supreme Court. More recently, universal health care, terrorism, and environmental issues have resulted in enthusiastic legislative discussions and often, a lack of legislative agreement and passage.

State Activities

Many state legislatures have two chambers, and leadership is similar to that of the national Congress in that a speaker of the house, a senate majority leader, and party leaders provide day-to-day administration of the legislative body. Chamber and committee leadership is determined by seniority, past party leadership, respective party caucuses, and persons who aspire to the party ideology and philosophy in setting legislative agendas. State legislatures play a large role in the budgetary decisions and health policy and nursing practice, including Medicaid services, health department auspices, certification of hospitals and nursing homes, and nursing licensure and prescriptive privileges within the state. Many state constitutions require a balanced budget submitted by the governor and approved by the legislature. Thus, even in states, health programs and nursing services can be advanced or be in jeopardy depending on annual budgetary decisions. Several states have instituted lotteries or video gambling to increase revenues directly tied to education or specific health programs. Public health initiatives, such as adolescent tobacco use reduction, drunk driving prevention, and school health programs, may be funded with these nonrecurring funds. Public education may also be supported by this type of fund or by recurring income tax funds. In that case, state-supported community colleges, universities,

and public schools (e.g., medical, nursing, pharmacy) can increase enrollment and faculty or offer more online and alternate-schedule courses. Similarly hospitals and health departments are supported by state and local allocations that affect bed capacity, working environment, salaries, and services provided.

State legislation also may include mandated overtime or nurse staffing levels in health care facilities. Most recently, states have passed bills that do not allow mandatory overtime for nurses. Another route to the same result is for nursing boards or other licensing boards to develop regulations concerning appropriate and safe working hours or limitations on overtime. Approximately one third of states have such statutes. This is where nurses can actively participate in the policy decisions to ensure a quality working situation and maximal patient safety and care. The ANA National Database of Nursing Quality Indicators (NDNQI) and Safe Staffing Saves Lives (SSSL) Initiatives, as well as research by Peter Buerhaus, Linda Aiken, and Susan Letvak and their colleagues, provide a foundation for those efforts. Press Ganey acquired the NDNQI® in June 2014 (http://pressganey.com/press-Room/2014/press-ganey-acquires-national-database-of-nursing-quality-indicators-(ndnqi-).

BUDGET PROCESS

Appropriation of Funds

Appropriation bills are required to approve funding for running the federal government each fiscal year (October 1 to September 30). Bills, which represent spending by each cabinet department (e.g., Treasury, Labor, Commerce, Health and Human Services, Defense), require congressional approval and presidential signature no later than the beginning of each fiscal year. Near the end of each congressional session, appropriation bills often are combined into one general appropriation bill, which before 1997 was called the *Omnibus Budget Reconciliation Act* (OBRA) and is now known as the *Consolidated Budget Resolution* (CBR). In the early 2000s, legislation titles began to be focused on social or financial priorities, such as the Taxpayer Relief Act. Specific bills for the 15 cabinet-level governmental agencies are titled, for instance, the Homeland Security Act.

Through the president's proposed budget, with input from the Administration's Office on Management and Budget (OMB), this process begins in Congress. After consideration of the proposed budget submitted by the White House, each chamber develops a budget resolution bill by April of each year. Additionally, all legislation under consideration that includes funding recommendations or appropriations is required to be submitted by committees to the Congressional Budget Office (CBO). The CBO reviews and calculates the actual costs to the federal government and considers how a particular appropriation fits into the proposed budget or *reconciliation bill.* One important issue at both state and federal levels is that revenue and expenditure estimates by varying interested parties are calculated with similar factors such as inflation, economic growth, gross domestic product (GDP), and consumer price index.

In the late 20th and early 21st centuries, state and federal budgets often were achieved through crisis management. This may have been because of a lack of clarity about legislation, large amounts of legislation to consider and act on, political strife, or budget shortfalls or surpluses. For example, in the late 1990s and early 2000s, disagreements and animosity caused a delay in the mandated federal budget approval in Congress. The lack of approval for a reconciliation or consolidation bill caused the federal government to shut down on more than one occasion. This type of crisis management resulted in special amendments being added to bills at the "11th hour" in order to convince certain representatives and senators to agree to vote for the final bill. This deal-making and "pork barrel" special interest spending added to what may have been appropriate legislation and allocations in an earlier version of a bill. Many bills were delayed in the early 2000s primarily because of discussions regarding terrorism funding or major disagreements on appropriations. In October 2008, the president signed a continuing resolution (PL. 110-329), and again many times over the next 4 years, which was necessary to keep the government running. In December 2013, a continuing budget resolution bill titled the Bipartisan Budget Act of 2013 was passed by the House and Senate. Also, this bill contained the Pathway for SGR Reform Act of 2013, which addressed Medicare payments to physicians and hospitals, special needs populations, long-term care, and repeals the ACA changes to hospital disproportionate care (Medicaid).

Another type of spending, *emergency spending,* may not be included in the fiscal year reconciliation bill but can be approved through supplemental appropriation bills. For example, after, Hurricane Katrina in 2005, Super Storm Sandy in 2012, and the terrorist attacks on September 11, 2001, special funds and Federal Emergency Management Agency increases were approved to provide disaster relief. Multiple *supplemental bills* have been passed to increase homeland security (Transportation Safety Administration) and defense spending (the war in Iraq) or to deal with other expenses not approved through the traditional congressional budget processes. This is less likely at the state level because of balanced budget statutes.

Authorization of Programs

Authorization and reauthorization bills (with funding requests) are required to establish or continue programs as well as to fund those mandates. The initial authorization is usually a separate bill named for the issue or program being established, for example, the Older Americans Act, the Ryan White AIDS Act, and the Public Health Service Act. New governmental agencies may be initiated or established, as was the case with the Administration on Aging in 1965 and the Department of Homeland Security (DHS) in 2002. Future authorization and reauthorization bills are required to make changes in governmental agencies, to expand programs, and to continue or alter funding levels. However, some authorization bills that are passed do not contain any funding levels. Rather, these bills are used to establish programs that are to be funded by governmental departments within present allocations or by individual states, or they are *unfunded mandates.* For example, the Brady Bill gun control legislation requires background checks on gun purchasers before a license is issued. This 1993 act was named after James Brady, who was shot and paralyzed during an attempted assassination of President Reagan in 1981. The federal law contained no continuing funds; thus states must provide funds or be in violation of the law, and as a result often suffer loss of government monies for law enforcement. The No Child Left Behind bill is similar in federal mandate and state funding. Some authorization bills purposely contain no funding recommendations so that members of Congress can support the issue without providing funding. The congressional decision is unfunded (the actual bill has no funding) or underfunded. The regulatory body may not be provided funding to oversee state implementation of the act. Mandating the Culturally and Linguistically Appropriate Services (CLAS) standards is another example in which a federal law required states to implement statutes, but little or no funding was provided.

Fiscal Responsibility

Several efforts were made in previous decades to mandate a balanced budget at the federal level. The Gramm-Rudman-Hollings law was passed in 1985 (PL 99-177), but the U.S. Supreme Court subsequently found this law to be unconstitutional. During the 104th Congress, a major effort by the newly Republican-controlled House of Representatives was launched to pass an amendment to the U.S. Constitution to require a balanced federal budget. This attempt failed in Congress; thus citizens did not vote on the constitutional amendment. Congress passed a Balanced Budget Act in 1997. The next year, Congress passed the Taxpayer Relief Act of 1998 as the reconciliation bill that included additional child-care exemptions and capital gains tax reform. In 1999, the reconciliation bill was the Taxpayer Refund and Relief Act. Although it passed both chambers of Congress, President Clinton vetoed the bill. Similar actions occurred with President Bush and the 110th Congress, and congressional divisions in the 112th Congress.

Appropriation or budget bills are required for the functioning of the federal government or other legislation, and thus specialized "pet" programs are often attached to the budget bills to get them enacted. For example, several times the Nurse Education Act's appropriation bills were tacked on to the budget to ensure that they were passed during that fiscal year before Congress adjourned. Much of the time, *pork-barrel* amendments are approved to gain the votes of specific members of Congress. Even though the spending will benefit constituencies, the programs often are not federal mandates or related to the responsibilities of the government. Because many of these amendments are added at the 11th hour and at times in conference committee to resolve the House and Senate differences, the public and some legislators are often not aware of these expenditures until they have been approved. The president does not have *line-item veto authority* and therefore must accept or veto each appropriation bill in its entirety to enact the fiscal year budget. Similar actions occur in state legislatures for appropriation bills for services such as museums, bypass highways, and new post offices.

Economics

A majority of the budget for the U.S. Department of Health and Human Services (USDHHS) is for *entitlement programs*, which means that only one third or less of the amount appropriated by Congress for this department can be controlled or used in discretionary ways. The NIH, the Centers for Medicare and Medicaid Services (CMS), and the Bureau of Health Professions (BHP) are included in the USDHHS budget. Nursing leaders and others have continually worked to increase these budgets, and these efforts resulted in budget increases during the late 1990s and early 2000s. More recently, those appropriations have been more stagnated. In calendar year 2012 CMS expenditures totaled more than $995.2 billion, with federal Medicaid obligations totaling $428.5 billion and federal Medicare obligations totaling $553.9 billion (CMS, 2013). The NIH fiscal year 2012 budget was $30.86 billion, and the National Institute of Nursing Research (NINR) budget was $144.77 million (NIH, 2012). Overall health care spending grew 3.6% in 2013 averaging $9,255 per person. The health care portion of the gross domestic product (GDP) was 17.4% in 2013 (Hartman et al., 2013; CMS, 2014). This is continued slow growth, but hospital care still provided for one-third of all expenditures. Various agency heads make budget requests to congressional committees each year through letters, hearings, and routine budgetary processes.

In 1999, a federal surplus of $170 billion resulted from a thriving economy, a leaner governmental structure, and the Balanced Budget Act of 1997. However, Congress has been borrowing from the Social Security (SS) Trust Fund since the early 1980s to meet annual operating costs and appropriations across the government. The retirement income and Medicare programs that are funded by current worker payroll taxes do not contain enough money to fund those same workers when they reach 65 years of age. The General Accounting Office (GAO) estimates that the SS Trust Fund will be unable to meet its obligations starting in the year 2040. Debate continues over how a government with a large national debt and a large tax base can best serve its citizens, given the promises made to citizens regarding retirement and health insurance in old age. In 2005 major efforts were proposed to change SS through decreased benefits to younger workers, initiation of private health savings accounts, gradually increasing the salary cap for paying SS taxes, and a means-tested eligibility for full benefits. The financial crisis of 2008 provided minimal change to SS retirement income and Medicare. The Affordable Care Act passage in 2010 revised Medicare, Medicaid, and access to care, but the implementation of all titles was delayed because of political and budgetary decisions during the 112th and 113th Congresses. State legislators dealt with budget shortfalls and used hiring freezes, layoffs, program cuts, new fees, and increased taxes to meet needs. Local agencies and school boards are often the most successful in dealing with budget shortfalls because they have not had—or have not chosen to use—the ability to borrow funds, incur long-term debt, or move costs from one budget year to another. More detail on the budget and health care costs can be found in Chapter 7.

HEALTH PROGRAMS

Two main types of federal health care programs exist, discretionary and entitlement. *Discretionary programs* are subject to annual appropriations by Congress and are considered controllable budgetary items. For this discussion, these programs primarily consist of categorical health services, training, and research programs. Categorical health services are services for somewhat narrowly defined categories of problems, such as programs for communicable diseases and family planning services. An example of a training program is the Nurse Reinvestment Act (PL 107-205), and an example of a research program is the National Institute of Nursing (NINR) at the National Institutes of Health.

Entitlements are those health care programs in which budgetary expenses are more difficult to control. Citizens who benefit from these programs are "entitled" to the benefits by law because of a specified age, disability, economic status, or prepayment. The federal government is obligated to pay these benefits regardless of the number of enrollees or the costs. The only major avenue to cut costs is by changing either the authorization or eligibility criteria through legislation. Costs cannot be limited by appropriating less money for expenditures. Social Security, veterans' compensation, and pensions are examples of income entitlement programs. Health care entitlement programs are Medicare, Medicaid, and State Children's Health Insurance Programs.

The enactment of the Social Security Act (SSA) in 1935 marked the first major act of government involvement in health. The act provides federal grants to the states for public health; maternal and child health; services for disabled children; and public assistance for the aged, blind, and families with dependent children. The role of the federal government in the provision of health care was expanded with the 1965 passage of Title XVIII and XIX amendments to the SSA, creating Medicare and Medicaid. These two programs have changed the face of health care and continue to have a large role in the provision of health care services. The addition of disabled persons and those with end-stage renal disease to Medicare in the 1970s increased costs and care. In 1997, Title XXI, the State Children's Health Insurance Program, was added, which dramatically increased the number of children now covered by federal and state legislations and budgets. Much of the discussion in the 105th through the 112th Congresses was related to how to deal with the increasing costs for these entitlement programs as well as to propose strategies for reforming the programs. The Affordable Care Act, the Bipartisan Budget Bill of 2013, and the Pathway for Sustainable Growth Rate Reform Act of 2013 legislate access to care, entitlement payment changes, and national budget cuts. Medicare and Social Security are major entitlements for budgetary expenses, but because they affect more than half of Americans, cutback revisions are difficult.

Implementation and Regulation

Multiple governmental agencies plan, implement, and evaluate health policy in the United States. The major agencies are headed by political appointment cabinet officials, directors, and administrators but are staffed by career civil servants. For example, the U.S. House of Representatives has 435 elected members, but 10,000 staff members are employed for duties such as cleaning, moving, painting, preparing and serving food, providing mail and phone services, and staffing the infirmary. Congressional legislation and presidential executive orders and mandates can alter workings across staff divisions of the executive, judicial, and legislative branches of government. The last major revisions occurred in 1996 after the Republican Congress and the Democratic vice president requested and mandated streamlining and reorganization of the government. The Balanced Budget Act of 1997 also mandated changes in the administration and implementation of federal programs. Before the 1990s most federal departments or regulatory oversight had changed very little. The Government Performance and Results Act of 1993 was a major effort to enhance accountability of agencies. The Federal Funding Accountability and Transparency Act of 2006, signed by President Bush, was another attempt to clarify governmental action and spending to the public. Several years passed, however, before actual changes occurred. In the

110th Congress, Senator Obama introduced a revision titled the Strengthening Transparency and Accountability in Federal Spending Act of 2008, but the bill died when that congressional session ended. Similar bills were introduced in 2013 (S. 1217: Housing Finance Reform and Taxpayer Protection Act) but remained in committee. However, several states have passed laws to increase transparency, access to government spending documents, and streamlined governmental structure.

The USDHHS is charged with protecting and ensuring the health of the nation and is headed by the Secretary of Health. Multiple agencies and divisions are included in the USDHHS, and several assistant secretaries are responsible for administrative aspects. The Surgeon General (SG) is an Assistant Secretary of Health and heads the Office of Public Health and Science (OPHS). An Assistant Secretary for Aging heads the Administration on Aging (AOA) and the Administration for Children and Families (ACF). Other agencies are headed by a commissioner (e.g., FDA) or director (e.g., NIH). Agencies include several sections or divisions. For example, the NIH has 27 institutes or centers, including the NINR, the Eunice Kennedy Shriver National Institute for Child Health and Human Development (NICHD), and the National Institute on Mental Health (NIMH). In Atlanta and other regional offices, the Centers for Disease Control and Prevention (CDC) houses 14 centers, institutes, and offices, including the National Center for Chronic Disease Prevention and Health Promotion (NCCDPHP), the National Office of Public Health Genomics (NOPHG), the National Center for Health Statistics (NCHS), and the Office for Public Health Preparedness and Response (PHPR) (CDC, 2013). Most federal government agencies and state agencies have civil rights, legal, public relations, and budget sections staffed by career employees. These agencies have public Internet sites for consumers and professionals to obtain program and contact information. Many political, professional, and health-related agencies and organizations also house websites for rapid and wide public access and dissemination of information.

Each federal agency has specific auspices or sponsorship, although these are not always consistent with the appropriation focus. The Department of Agriculture (DA) directs the commodity distribution program (e.g., nonfat dry milk, cheese products), the national school lunch program, farm programs, and food inspection. The CMS directs Medicare, Medicaid, and Children's Health Insurance Programs; the Department of Labor houses the Occupational Safety and Health Administration (OSHA); and the CDC houses the National Institute of Occupational Safety and Health (NIOSH). Most states have similar agencies and auspices to manage public programs. For example, the Tennessee Department of Health (TDH) houses the Bureau of TennCare (BOT) to administer the Medicaid waiver program, and Kansas has a State Secretary for Social and Rehabilitation Services (SRS).

Whereas laws are written in broad language, the *rules and regulations* to implement these laws are very specific and often can be revised without changing the original law. Agencies are charged with implementation, financial oversight, legislative interpretation, and the development of regulations and rules governing their respective programs. Often agencies are required to interpret the purpose and intent of congressional or state legislation to implement such laws. The perceptions, political savvy, and experiences of the agency's director, staff, and proponents have an impact on this interpretation of the issue under consideration. For example, former USDHHS Secretary Tommy Thompson reworded family planning regulations to include abstinence-only programs, President Clinton used presidential directives for regulations to allow stem cell research on embryos not used by couples who went through in vitro fertilization procedures, and President Bush wrote executive orders to allow only currently available stem cell lines to be used rather than new embryonic lines and vetoed bills to allow federal funding for certain research. In 2009, President Obama used executive orders to lift the ban on federal funding for "promising" embryonic stem cell research. Interpretations and changes in regulations can be related to the number and types of citizens served in a particular program, the increase or decrease in appropriations, the social or ethical values of directors and department heads, political climate, and societal crises.

In some instances the auspices and appropriations are not consistent. The DA receives appropriations for elder nutrition programs, but these are administered under the AOA through state, regional, and local agencies. The Department of Labor (DL) has administrative responsibility for the Senior Community Service Employment Program (SCSEP), which is under the auspices of the AOA. The Bureau of Census (BOC) collects vital data, but the NCHS and the DL analyze those data for developing policy and allocation decisions. Thus some health-related policy legislation and appropriations require extra effort to determine the auspices, regulation, and implementation and whether duplication or omission occurs.

As the health care industry evolves with new emphases, programs, and services, the governmental agencies must develop new strategies for evaluation of their implementation. Evaluation for specific policies and their implementation only recently began at the federal level. This evaluation of process, structure, and outcomes has become an emphasis, especially for the SS, Medicare, and Medicaid programs. Process and structure are often difficult to change in large, bureaucratic organizations of state and federal government. Annual performance plans now required of agencies should assist in more clearly evaluating program effectiveness and efficiency. The recent emphasis on outcomes should lead to changes in process and structure to meet the objectives set forth. Two such health-related efforts are the *Healthy People 2020* and national objectives and the initiatives to eliminate racial and ethnic disparities at the USDHHS. As these two efforts are revised to reflect new targets and new census health data, they will guide federal, state, and local efforts to improve the health of our community through system, policy, and funding decisions. Nursing has a vested interest in those efforts.

LEADERSHIP

During the 20th century, several persons and organizations provided leadership to ensure the passage of major health policies and regulation. Surgeon Generals C. Everett Koop, Jocelyn Elders, and David Satcher have supported efforts to deal with chronic diseases, prevent and reduce health risks through education, and target efforts based on *Healthy People* initiatives. Dr. Richard H. Carmona (formerly a nurse), who served as Surgeon General from 2002 to 2006, was a less visible leader partially because of the focus on bioterrorism and the overshadowing of the White House leadership related to stem cell research and abstinence education. There was no Surgeon General from 2006 to 2008, although Steven K. Galson served as Acting Surgeon General for part of that period. David Kessler, Commissioner of the FDA from 1990 to 1997, worked to protect consumers through regulation of nutritional and dietary supplements. He also argued for regulation of tobacco. The Tobacco Master Settlement Agreement was reached in 1998 within the Justice Department between the four largest tobacco companies and 46 state attorneys general, but not under the purview of the FDA. The lawsuit was brought by state departments of justice suing for repayment of public dollars (Medicare and Medicaid) spent on providing health care to those with tobacco-related illnesses. The $360 billion settlement agreed to by the tobacco industry is to be paid over a 25-year period. Activities associated with the agreement were the termination of soliciting adolescent smokers, bans on tobacco advertisements within specific distances of schools, and further supplementation of education and prevention programs across the country. However, money in most states is not being used for the purposes noted. This is an example of the judicial branch of government playing a role in health policy and planning. Another highly visible leader in health care regulation was Dr. Julie Gerberding, the former director of the CDC, from 2002 to 2009, whose tenure was marked by multiple national occurrences of food-borne illnesses. Dr. Kathleen Sebelius, the former Secretary of the DHHS, was active in the implementation of the Affordable Care Act.

Legislators

Senators Edward Kennedy (D-MA), Barbara Mikulski (D-MD), Paul Simon (D-IL), and Nancy Kassenbaum (R-KS) led health-related legislative efforts during the 1980s, 1990s, and early 2000s in the U.S. Senate. In the House of Representatives, efforts were led by Henry Waxman (D-WI), John Lewis (D-GA), Joseph Kennedy (D-MA), and Lois Capps (D-CA). Legislative efforts during this time were focused on programs for vulnerable populations such as children, the elderly, and low-income persons, as well as appropriations for new and continuing programs. During 1999, Senators John Breaux (D-LA) and Bill Frist (R-TN), a heart surgeon, headed the National Bipartisan Commission on the Future of Medicare. Additional health policy efforts in early 2000 were related to managed care (both private and public sector) and consumer rights regarding their health care coverage, use of personal information, the Health Insurance Portability and Accountability Act (HIPAA), and competency of providers. Representative Lois Capps (a nurse) led the initial Nurse Reinvestment Act effort in 2002 and continues to work with colleagues in both chambers to ensure funding. The issues of medical liability and welfare reform were led by Republicans in the House of Representatives and passed in 2003 and 2005. In 2007 Senator Brownback led efforts to develop electronic medical records (EMR) and Senator Akaka worked to block the establishment of electronic records unless privacy could be ensured. In 2008 Medicare, Medicaid, and the Children's Health Insurance Program (CHIP) were a major focus by both parties, with Senators Edward Kennedy and Hillary Clinton and minority whip James Clyburn in the House leading the efforts. In January 2009 the 111th Congress passed new State Children's Health Insurance Program (SCHIP) legislation that expanded coverage. During the 110th Congress, Senators Brownback (R-KS), Casey (D-PA), Inhofe (R-OK), Spector (R-PA), and Coleman (R-MA), along with Representative Watson (D-CA), introduced the compassionate care ACCESS Act to provide for physician and patient FDA options for experimental treatments. Most recently, Senators Mikulski and Collins (R-ME) and Representative Capps (D-CA) are leading supporters of increasing Nursing Workforce Development funds, HRSA nursing education funds, and extension of the Health Care and Education Reconciliation Act (P.L. 111-152). Representatives Walden (R-OR), Schwartz (D-PA), Bonnamici (D-OR), Noem (R-SD), Peterson (D-MN), Cramer (R-ND), and Daines (R-MT), and Senators Moran (R-KS), Thune (R-SD), and Tester (D-MT) sponsored legislation that allows nurse practitioners, clinical specialists, and midwives to receive federal payments (Medicare) for home health, primary care, and rural services. In 2013 six nurses served in the US House of Representatives (Bass, D-CA; Black, R-TN; Capps, D-CA; Ellmers, R-NC; Johnson, D-TX; McCarthy, D-NY).

Nurses

Many nurses have provided leadership at the national level to contribute to health policy and ensure that its influence on nursing is positive. Former ANA presidents Virginia Trotter Betts and Beverly Malone were instrumental in setting the original Nursing's Agenda for Health Care Reform (NAHCR). These two nurses also assisted the ANA Council on Practice and various professional practice organizations to promote the passage of third-party reimbursement changes for advanced practice nurses, accreditation of home health agencies, and provision of childhood immunizations. Betts and Malone later were appointed Assistant Secretaries of Health at USDHHS. Debbie Gettis, a registered professional nurse, served as the AIDS advisor to President Clinton. Dorothy Brooten, a nurse researcher, was

elected in 1991 to the Institute of Medicine (IOM), which advises Congress on health matters. In 1987 Ada Sue Hinshaw was appointed the first director of the National Center for Nursing Research (NCNR), and Patricia Grady is the current director. Nancy Bergstrom and Thelma Wells have provided leadership in the development of guidelines for practice for the Agency for Healthcare Research and Quality (AHRQ, formerly the AHCPR), and Nancy Fugate-Woods and Ora Strickland have spearheaded a national focus on women's health. Peter Buerhaus (an economist), Cheryl Jones, and Linda Moody have served as scientists at the national level to develop recommendations and projections for nursing workforce, staffing, and economic needs. Janet Allan, Lucy Marion, and Carol Loveland-Cherry have served on the U.S. Preventive Services Task Force, and Audrey Nelson has led patient safety and quality of care efforts at the Department of Veterans Affairs (DVA). Martha Hill serves as President of the American Heart Association, and Terry Fulmer served as President of the Gerontological Society of America. Nurses have been appointed to formal policy-level impact positions. Dr. Debra Barksdale (2010, 2012) was the only nurse appointed to the Board of Governors for the Patient-Centered Outcomes Research Initiative (PCORI) housed in the U.S. Governmental Accountability Office. Dr. Beth Collins Sharp serves as senior advisor for Women's and Gender Health, as well as Nursing, at AHRQ. Dr. Mary Wakefield is the Administrator of the Health Resources and Services Administration (2009) and Marilyn Tavenner is the Director of the Centers for Medicare and Medicaid (2013).

Think Tanks, Foundations, and Organizations

Other sources of health policy and planning encompass private or public "think tanks," philanthropic foundations, and policy centers that directly affect nursing. Several large foundations, such as the IOM, the Robert Wood Johnson Foundation (RWJF), and the Pew Charitable Trusts (PCT), play an important role in policy planning and evaluation. The PCT provides grants for health care demonstration and research activities and supports studies of the health care industry. One example is the Pew Health Professions Commission (PHPC), formed to study the future needs of the health care system in the United States. Multiple reports have been issued by this commission over the past 20 years. The reports delineate the nature of health care work, the restructuring of health care professional regulation, the number and types of professionals needed, and the training and education of professionals. Much of the discussion is, by necessity, in the context of an evolving health care system with dynamics not yet known. Although widely heralded, the commission's recommendations are slowly being enacted. The RWJF funds large demonstration projects to address varying health issues and populations. Priorities are reset every few years. In 2010 the RWJF established the Initiative on the Future of Nursing, Nurse Faculty Scholars, New Careers in Nursing Scholarship Program, the Interdisciplinary Nursing Quality Research Initiative (INQRI), Disparities Research for Change, and Public Health Law Research. The John A. Hartford Foundation partners with universities to improve nursing education for elder care through Centers, student fellowships and development of best practice guidelines. The Institute of Medicine (IOM), one of the National Academies of Science (NAS), advises Congress on health matters through position papers, expert witnesses, and recommendations for legislative initiation, approval, and funding.

NURSING

Nursing currently has three main issues. First are the workforce needs; that is, the qualifications and types of roles nurses will be required to fill. The American Association of Colleges of Nursing (AACN), the PHP, and the IOM (2010) recommend an increase in the number of registered nurses at the baccalaureate level and advanced practice nurses with master's and doctoral-level preparation (AACN, 2012a,b; IOM, 2010). A second issue is that of programs for nurse educators at the doctoral level to prepare nurses for the workforce needs. Although many doctoral programs have opened in the past three decades, the number of doctoral-prepared nurse educators available for appropriate training and education of the projected workforce has not kept pace with market need (AACN, 2012a,b). This lag can be attributed partly to the large number of nurses retiring in the early 2000s and partly to a lack of incentives to stay in public-rather than private-sector positions. A third nursing issue is that of competency-based education and practice, in which nurses demonstrate critical thinking, judgment and decision-making skills, and cultural competence, and engage in transdisciplinary practice. Curricular, regulation, and certification changes have been

implemented. In the mid-1990s, the National League for Nursing Accreditation Commission (NLNAC) for baccalaureate and master's degree programs placed an increased emphasis on critical thinking and community-based care. The AACN, in 2008 and 2012, revised essentials of baccalaureate, master's degree, and practice doctorate education, which includes health care delivery, ethics, and competency-based education. The Commission on Collegiate Nursing Education (CCNE) and Accreditation Commission for Education in Nursing (ACEN), the professional accreditation bodies, require that undergraduate programs target their mission to local and regional health rather than taking a "cookie cutter" approach to curriculum. Master's programs were standardized for clinical and role competence, as well as mastery of the health care delivery system and economic knowledge and skills. This standardization has resulted in an increase in nurses with specialty certification. The American Association of Critical-Care Nurses (AACCN), the Association for Women's Health (AWH), Obstetrical and Neonatal Nursing (ONN), and the Oncology Nursing Society (ONS) offer certification for master's-prepared nurses. The American Nurses Credentialing Center (ANCC) provides both specialty role (e.g., case management, nurse practitioner, clinical specialist) and population (e.g., psychiatric mental health, adult, pediatric) certifications. Recent changes that may impact the workforce include changes to certification for advanced practice nurses in both education and practice requirements. These changes increase in the number of clinical practice hours for doctoral-level advanced practice nurses, the elimination of stand-alone gerontological nurse practitioner certification, requirements for pharmacology, and physical assessment and pathophysiology for nurse educators at the master's level, and the emphasis on doctor of nursing practice programs. Several organizations have a major impact on health policy and nursing. The IOM is often involved in discussions of, and decisions for, auspices and allocations for the Division of Nursing and nurse education acts in Congress. In fact the Higher Education Opportunity Act of 2008 (PL 110-803) required the USDHHS secretary to negotiate with the IOM to conduct a study on the capacity of nursing schools to meet the needs of the nation. More important, *The Future of Nursing* landmark report (IOM, 2010) details multiple strategies to ensure a competent and adequate nursing workforce to meet future health needs.

The ANA, American Public Health Association (APHA), the AMA, the Gerontological Society of America, and the American Dental Association (ADA) all provide expert testimony to state and federal agencies and decision-making bodies on topics from product development and liability to school lunch programs, immunizations, disaster relief, bioterrorism, domestic violence and lesbian, gay, bisexual, transgender, and queer or questioning (LGBTQ) health.

HEALTH POLICIES

Health policies, or decisions regarding the health care system, are developed and implemented through several avenues. Congressional and state legislation; federal, state, and local rules and regulations for agencies; and appropriation decisions are methods to develop health policy. Some health policies are reached only through legislation, whereas others are developed by multiple avenues. All these avenues are affected by public opinion, the economy, societal demographics, professional expertise, technology, and knowledge about health.

Health Policies Before 1990

Three of the most influential health policies have been the SSA of 1935 and the amendments that established Medicare and Medicaid in 1965. Many of our national concerns with health and welfare have been addressed by amendments to these policies. Issues such as abortion, family planning, nutrition, and disability, as well as those related to *vulnerable populations* (the chronically ill, mentally ill, elderly, poor, and minorities), are included as major concerns and foci of programs and payments. These are also the largest programs in terms of population covered and dollars spent. With the aging of the population, technological and pharmaceutical advances, and changes in the racial/ethnic face of society, the original intent and expected costs of these programs have been far exceeded. A major issue today is how to continue these programs as a *safety net* for society. Many bills and acts have been passed that directly and indirectly affect the health of society (Table 6-1). In the 1960s the Hill-Burton Act funded for hospital construction. Legislation for payment to nurses was included in the Rural Health Clinics Act of 1977 and

---

TABLE 6-1   Selected Policies Affecting Nursing and Health Care Before 1990

YEAR	TITLE	CONTENT/PURPOSE
1935	Social Security Act (SSA)	Established the Social Security Administration and pension income
1938	Food, Drug, and Cosmetics Act	Provisions of safe and effective drugs through labeling; 1984 amendments applied to generic drugs
1941	Nurse Training Appropriations	Established to assist nursing schools in increasing enrollments and improving programs
1944	Public Health Service Act	Established the U.S. Public Health Service under one statute (Title 42, U.S. Code)
1964	Nurse Training Act	Initial federal act for professional nurse training
1965	Medicare (SSA amendment)	Established health coverage for the elderly
	Medicaid (SSA amendment)	Established health coverage for the indigent
1965	Older Americans Act	Established the Administration on Aging, which provides a broad network of services to elders
1970	Title X Public Health Service Act	Established family planning grant programs aimed at low-income women
1973	Health Maintenance Organization Act	Established alternative to fee-for-service for government-subsidized employers
1982	Omnibus Budget Reconciliation Act (OBRA)	Added the prospective payment system (diagnosis-related groups) to Medicare hospital admission payment
1986	Protection and advocacy of Mental Health Illness Act	Established agencies to investigate and pursue legal action against abuse and neglect of persons with mental illness
1987	Nursing Home Reform Act (OBRA)	Standardized the types of services nursing homes must provide; established standards of quality and patients' rights
1989	Amendments to Nursing Home Reform Act	Allowed nurse practitioner/clinical nurse specialist to certify need for nursing homes
1989	OBRA	Medicaid direct payment for pediatric and family nurse practitioners

extended with OBRA of 1989. In the 1970s and 1980s increased emphasis was placed on disease prevention, risk reduction, and research on the leading causes of death (cardiovascular disease, cancer). The OBRA of 1982 established the diagnostic-related groups (DRGs), which resulted in a prospective payment system (PPS) for Medicare hospitalization. Legislation regarding mental health, school lunch programs, disease research, rural manpower, and end-stage renal disease and disability were added to Medicare eligibility. The 1987 OBRA (PL 101-203) changed Medicare payments to hospitals, altered health maintenance organization (HMO) requirements, and authorized nurse practitioners and clinical nurse specialists to certify patient needs for nursing home care.

Health Policies 1990 To 2000

The 1990s were perhaps the most prolific decade for health policy reform and regulation for specific diseases, conditions, and vulnerable groups (Table 6-2). The Patient Self-Determination Act allowed persons to make decisions regarding their own health care. The Ryan White Act was passed to deal with issues related to HIV and AIDS. New NIH guidelines for inclusion of women and children in research altered past trends, the use of past findings, and subsequent health policies. As the number of homeless persons increased, private and public sectors had difficulty dealing with the costs and spectrum of services, and the McKinney Homelessness Act was passed with both funded and unfunded mandates. The Americans with Disabilities Act has affected

TABLE 6-2 **Selected Policies Affecting Health and Nursing Passed From 1990 to 2000**

YEAR	TITLE	CONTENT/PURPOSE
1990	Patient Self-Determination Act (PL 101-508)	Required all Medicare/Medicaid-paid health care institutions to provide or ask for advance directives
1990	Occupational Safety and Health Act, amended (PL 101-552)	Describes general working conditions, guidelines for handling blood and body fluids, prevention of infectious disease, and biohazard waste disposal
1990	Trauma Care Systems Planning and Development Act (PL 101-590)	Established guidelines for trauma care services; replaced 1973 Emergency Medical Services Act
1990	Americans with Disabilities Act (PL 101-336)	Prohibits discrimination against persons with disabilities in five specific areas
1992	Breast and Cervical Cancer Mortality Prevention Act (PL 101-354)	Provides grants to states for screening, referrals, educational programs, training, quality assurance programs, and research
1992	Mammography Quality Standards Act (PL 102-539)	Requires certification, accreditation, and inspection of centers, including equipment, technicians, and records
1993	Family and Medical Leave Act (PL 103-3)	Establishes leave (job security) for employees caring for an ill child or family member, experiencing childbirth or adoption, or experiencing own illness
1996	Welfare Reform Act (PL 104-93)	Limits adults to 5 years on welfare; must work within 2 years
1996	Health Insurance Portability and Accountability Act (PL 104-191)	Provides for portability when changing jobs, limits preexisting conditions, requires congressional reports to evaluate the impact
1996	Newborn's and Mother's Health Protection Act (PL 104-326)	Mandates medical decision for minimum 48-hour stay after delivery; *provider* includes midwife and nurse practitioner
1997	Balanced Budget Act (PL 105-33)	Medicare direct payment to advanced practice nurses; Children's Health Insurance program; welfare-to-work
1998	Health Professions Education and Partnership Act (PL 105-392)	Consolidated health professions education and training as well as minority health education and training; nursing education funding
1999	Healthcare Research and Quality Act (PL 106-129)	Changed name of Agency for Health Care Policy and Research (AHCPR) to Agency for Healthcare Research and Quality (AHRQ); mandates and funds quality and outcomes research
2000	Minority Health and Health Disparities Research and Education Act (PL 106-525)	Established the National Center on Minority Health and Health Disparities at NIH

health care as well as work and practice environments and the justice system.

Major changes in Medicaid occurred in 1996 with passage of the Personal Responsibility and Work Opportunities Act (Welfare) and Temporary Assistance to Needy Families, which replaced Aid to Families with Dependent Children. The 1997 Balanced Budget Act included SCHIP in the form of block grants to states to provide health care coverage to more low-income children. However, reports indicated that many children remained uncovered, resulting in the passage of the Children's Health Insurance Program Reauthorization Act (CHIPRA) in 2009 and continued authorization and appropriation through 2013.

Policies and new regulations in the 1990s also affected nurses and other health care workers. Parenting and caregiving concerns resulted in the Family and Medical Leave Act. Occupational Safety and Health Administration guidelines were developed regarding work-at-home employees. Reauthorization of programs and allocations for older Americans, children, and indigent care each year has an impact on nursing and health care. The Health Professions Education Partnerships Act included the Nursing Education and Practice Improvement Act, which established the National Advisory Council on Nurse Education and Practice (NACNEP) workforce needs. A major purpose of the Health Professions Education Partnerships Act was to consolidate health profession education, training, recruitment of minorities, and rural placements. Additionally, Health Care Financing Administration/CMS regulations were revised during the latter part of 1998 and 1999, which changed payment, diagnostic capabilities, and reimbursement for advanced practice nurses as a result of federal legislation. In 2000 the National Center on Minority Health and Health Disparities (NCMHD) was established as part of the NIH.

Health Policies 2001 To Present

Many new policies initiate, establish, or reauthorize nursing and health issues. The Nurse Reinvestment Act, the Medicare Prescription Drug Improvement and Modernization Act, and the Veterans' Health Care Authorization Act (Table 6-3) are such policies. The Medicare Modernization Act was an attempt to provide relief from high-cost prescriptions for the elderly and disabled. Drug discount cards were distributed

to qualified elderly and disabled persons to be used beginning in January 2006. As of December 2013, more than 36 million Medicare beneficiaries received Part D coverage with an additional 7.3 million eligible but using employer drug plans and 2013 expenditures of $69.2 billion (CMS, 2013), far greater than the $750 million per year estimated when Part D passed Congress. Consumers and vendors can update or change plans each year. The cost of this law is continually being updated. Medicare Part A is the traditional fee-for-service hospital insurance coverage and Part B is coverage for office visits and preventive care. Part C is an option to Part A, but allows persons to be in a managed care plan that may be less expensive, include wellness programs, not require prepayment, and may offset Part B premiums.

Mental health coverage has grown steadily over the past 15 years, culminating in the Paul Wellstone Mental Health and Addiction Equity Act of 2007 (PL 110-343). Politics was a factor even with this legislation, as it was tacked on to the Emergency Economic Stabilization Act of 2008 (which provided for the Troubled Asset Relief Program, or TARP). The growth of genomic medicine and the privacy issues regarding genetic information resulted in the Genetic Information Nondiscrimination Act of 2008 or GINA (PL 110-233), which prohibits discrimination or categorization of applicants or employees based on that information and mandates that genetic information be treated as confidential medical information. Many states have implemented similar laws for genetic protections. Other laws passed addressed Veterans health, domestic violence, premature birth, and nursing education. The Affordable Care Act health reform 2010 is addressed in a separate section that follows.

Managed Care

The rise in health care costs has contributed to the rise of managed care organizations and more policy focused on health care costs over the past three decades. Care provided under costs agreements has become the primary substructure for health care. Capitated costs under Medicare started in 1983 with diagnostic-related groups (DRGs). Formal Medicare Choice and Medicare Advantage managed care plans were established through care choice options in the mid- to late 1990s. The number of Americans participating in managed care plans increased steadily during the 1990s and 2005. In 1998

TABLE 6-3 Selected Policies Affecting Health and Nursing Passed From 2001 to Present

YEAR	TITLE	CONTENT/PURPOSE
2003	Nurse Reinvestment Act (PL 107-205)	Provides funding for nurse recruitment, retention, education, and care for special populations and underserved areas
2003	Medicare Modernization Act (PL 108-173)	Provides prescription drug benefit (Part D); enhances new Medicare Advantage regional health plan choices (Part C)
2004	Asthmatic Schoolchildren's Treatment and Health Management Act (PL 108-377)	Rewards states that require schools to allow students to self-administer medications for asthma or anaphylaxis
2007	Paul Wellstone Mental Health and Addiction Equity Act (PL 110-343)	Requires equity in the provision of mental health and substance-related disorder benefits under group health
2007	Food and Drug Administration Amendments Act (PL 110-85)	Extends the user-fee programs for prescription drugs and medical devices; enhances the postmarket authorities of the FDA with respect to the safety of drugs
2007	Conquer Childhood Cancer Act (PL 110-285)	Amends the Public Health Service Act to advance medical research and treatments into pediatric cancers; ensures patients and families have access to the current treatments and information regarding pediatric cancers
2007	National Breast and Cervical Cancer Early Detection Program Reauthorization Act (PL 110-18)	Established to provide waivers relating to grants for preventive health measures with respect to breast and cervical cancers
2007	Trauma Care Systems Planning and Development Act (PL 110-23)	Established to amend the Public Health Service Act to add requirements regarding trauma care and for other purposes
2007	Joshua Omvig Veterans Suicide Prevention Act (PL 110-110)	Developed to direct the Secretary of Veterans Affairs to develop and implement a comprehensive program designed to reduce the incidence of suicide among veterans
2007	Charlie W. Norwood Living Organ Donation Act (PL 110-144)	Established to amend the National Organ Transplant Act to provide that criminal penalties do not apply to human organ paired donation
2008	Genetic Information Nondiscrimination Act (PL 110-233)	Established to prohibit discrimination of applicants and employees based on genetic information
2009	Children's Health Insurance Program Reauthorization Act (PL 111-3)	Established to amend Social Security Act Title XXI to reauthorize the CHIP program through year 2013 at increased levels
2012	Child Protection Act (PL 112-206)	Penalties for child pornography, defines child witness protection, and establishes task force
2012	Safe Doses Act (PL 112-186)	Strengthening and Focusing Enforcement to Deter Organized Stealing and Enhance Safety Act of 2012
2013	Violence Against Women Reauthorization Act	Reauthorizes funds and enforcements
2013	Prematurity Research Expansion and Education for Mothers who deliver Infants Early (PL 113-55)	Authorizes the PREEMIE act through 2017, includes priority for telehealth services, prenatal and postnatal care, and establishes the Advisory Committee on Infant Mortality

approximately 80% of Americans with employer-sponsored health insurance had managed care plans. Initial Medicaid managed care plans were established through Health Care Financing Administration (HCFA) waivers to states in the early 1990s. By 2012 Medicaid eligibles number 66 million, managed care covers 39 million persons or 72% of enrolled recipients with $428 billion in expenditures annually. Almost 30% of Medicare beneficiaries were enrolled in managed care plans called Medicare Advantage programs. In addition Medicare Part D prescription drug plan had an enrollment of 36 million persons and spent more than $60 billion (CMS, 2013).

A presidential order required the USDHHS to enact regulations of consumer rights for Medicare and Medicaid beneficiaries with managed care options. However, the bipartisan debate continues over accountability and liability with managed care. State courts, and now the U.S. Supreme Court, deal with the issue of whether a patient has the right to sue a managed care organization for services provided or withheld based on economic rationale rather than clinical decision making. Individuals have the right to notification of denial, changes in benefits, provider network, and network institutions such as hospitals and pharmacies. In addition, some states provide the right to information—written and verbal—concerning the appeal or grievance processes, including a mechanism for arbitration over disputed denial of care. National- and state-level patient "bills of rights" are required to clarify these issues and ensure equitable care; several states have enacted this legislation. The Employment Retirement Income Security Act (ERISA) of 1974 and its reauthorizations also ensure certain worker rights regarding health care coverage as part of retirement benefits.

State Nurse Practice Acts

Legislation and related policies that directly affect nurses are addressed in *state practice acts*, or *other legislation governing health care professionals*. The nurse practice acts, or other legislation, and corresponding rules and regulations define educational preparation and programs, eligibility for licensure, and the scope of practice. All states require eligible nurses to pass the National Council Licensure Examination (NCLEX) for initial RN (registered nurse) licensure. Candidates for licensure must have graduated from a program approved by the state board of nursing, but the requirements for graduation from a nationally accredited school vary among states. Nursing practice in most states includes research, education, administration, counseling, and clinical practice or direct patient care. The new interstate RN and LPN/VN (licensed practical nurse/vocational nurse) licensure compact was developed through the National Council of State Boards of Nursing (NCSBN) in 1998, and the first states joined in 2000. In 2013 the compact had 24 member states. This compact may allow registered nurses to practice in member states without having a separate license,

especially for persons living near state borders. Nursing has found that it can often best manage its practice through rules and regulations that require only a state-recognized licensing board or committee to approve changes, rather than null legislative action. State nurse practice acts are discussed further in Chapter 11.

In addition to state boards of nursing, many national organizations play a role in defining practice. The NCSBN develops the licensure examination for nurses. The ANCC, as well as various national specialty organizations, determines eligibility, educational qualifications, experience, and examinations for national certification required in many states. This is especially true for advanced practice nursing. In some states, an advanced practice nurse can practice without certification but cannot have prescriptive privileges unless national certification is obtained. In other states, certification either is not required or is required for both.

State practice acts are statutes requiring legislative approval for establishment and amendment. In the past, the majority of changes occurred in the legislative arena. More recently, state boards of nursing have developed specific rules and regulations concerning practice that can be changed without legislative activity. This avoids the possibility of undesirable statute revisions that might occur when "opening" the practice act for legislative revision. Additionally, the rules and regulations allow the nursing profession to articulate the practice, roles, and responsibilities of nurses rather than having other entities define nursing. One example is that of anesthesia assistants or unlicensed personnel. For example, there is a national movement to allow anesthesia assistants and other unlicensed personnel to accept responsibilities and use titles traditionally reserved for RNs, LPNs, and certified registered nurse anesthetists (CRNAs).

NURSING AND HEALTH POLICY

Health policy, regulations, allocations, and care affect nursing and the practice environment and are in turn affected by nursing in several ways. The following sections focus on nursing practice, education, research, and the nursing discipline. The discipline requires professional nurses to conduct scholarly inquiry and participate in social and public policy through multiple avenues.

Practice

Today the health care arena requires nursing administrators and staff to be aware of economic, communication, and ethical issues to a greater extent than previously encountered. This entails knowledge of budgets and health payment, the use of community resources, product evaluation, technology, benchmarking, and outcomes accountability. Consumers are more educated and aware of their health needs and rights in today's world. Although the types of services may be different according to a particular agency, setting, or location, a standard level of competency, transparency, and accountability is required in all practice environments.

One effort to indicate quality and accountability by health care institutions is the magnet hospital program. The ANA, through the ANCC, developed the Magnet Nursing Services Recognition Program (MNSRP) in the late 1990s. This program is a voluntary external professional nurse peer review of the nursing practice and care environment of any hospital that wishes to participate. The review includes examination of the extent to which a hospital meets eight standards of care, which are incorporated within the model of professional practice at each site. The process of applying for magnet status involves both a written application and a site visit by a board of experts. Applicants are required to demonstrate nurse-sensitive quality at the unit or system level and to meet established state, regional, or national benchmarks. Governance, research, patient safety, and feedback processes are all part of magnet criteria. If a facility is designated as a magnet hospital, the effective practice environment and resulting quality of nursing care should be evident (ANCC, 2013; Steimpfel, Rosen, & McHugh, 2014; Kelly, McHugh, & Aiken, 2011).

For individual nurses, standards are provided by professional organizations, including the ANA's *Standards of Clinical Nursing Practice, Scope and Standards of Advanced Practice Registered Nurses*, and other specialty standards for practice, in response to both societal and professional requests for clarification of nursing. Identification of competencies, such as those for wound and ostomy care, cultural competence, and genetics may be required for nurses across practice settings. Studies examining nurse competence are also needed (Numminen, Mereroja, Isoaho, &

Leino-Kilpi, 2013; Starr & Wallace, 2009). Effectiveness studies that support competent and quality practice also have an impact on legislation. The Robert Wood Johnson foundation established the INQRI in 2005. Over the past decade Dunston, Boyle, and colleagues at the University of Kansas have led the effort to develop measures of acute care nursing through the ANA-supported National Database for Nursing Quality Indicators (NDNQI) now acquired by Press Ganey. Dr. Linda Cronenwett led the phased Quality and Safety in Education for Nursing (QSEN) initiative that has developed content and competencies to improve quality and safety in nursing curriculum. A literature search over a 2-year period found the need to continue researching the linkages between nursing and quality of patient care (Naylor, Volpe, Lustig, Kellye, Melichar, & Paulym, 2013). Beck, Weiss, Ryan-Wenger, Donaldson, Aydin, and Gardner (2013) support the need for continued research on nurses' impact on health care quality and as the population ages, the need for competent nursing with older adults is needed (Esterson, Bazille, Mezey, Cortes, & Huba, 2013). In addition, cultural competence and health literacy are needed to ensure quality of patient care as our population becomes more diverse. Using the Campinha-Bacote model, Ingram (2012) was able to show how to provide quality patient care to culturally diverse populations with low health literacy. These interventions and activities indicate to legislators and the public that nursing contributes to better health outcomes, quality care, and cost containment.

Self-development, continuing education, certification, and learning new skill sets (retooling) will be required as the health care delivery system continues to evolve. This learning must be of a transdisciplinary nature, including terminology and new taxonomy languages, client needs, treatment, and evaluation of outcomes, quality, and access. Hospitals and clinics will continue as major settings, but long-term care and alternative care settings and delivery methods that assist clients to achieve health must be initiated and embraced. Case management can assist in meeting the needs of specific populations. Homeless clinics, parish nursing, and collaborative efforts with physician practices and school systems are additional delivery methods that provide community-based care to vulnerable populations.

Education

Authorization for nursing education originated with the Nurse Training Act of 1964. Between 1965 and 1971, more than $380 million was spent on nursing education for both students and institutions. Doctoral nursing students and nursing doctoral programs received emphasis and support during the mid-1970s, and master's programs received larger allocations for increasing nurses in specific roles in the 1980s and 1990s. However, in the 1990s, with the onset of managed care and increased competition for health care dollars, the nursing education legislation was twice not enacted. Passage of the Health Professions Education Partnership Act in 1998 changed the tradition by which nursing was the only health profession to retain a separate funding law. Congressional funding for nursing education has increased and expanded to include baccalaureate, master's, and doctoral level, but enrollments have not increased to meet the projected needs in most areas of the country (AACN, 2012a,b).

To address the major shortages specific to nursing, the Nurse Reinvestment Act and subsequent legislative versions have been passed. The focus of these efforts was on funding and implementing strategies for nurse recruitment and nurse retention. Scholarships (Nursing Loan Repayment and Scholarships) are available to those nurses willing to work in health care facilities with a critical nursing shortage. Special grants are provided for schools of nursing to develop and implement programs focused on geriatrics through the Comprehensive Geriatric Education Program (CGEP). Grants and contracts are awarded to schools of nursing that expand their programs by increasing enrollment in 4-year programs, provide internships and residency programs for nursing students, and provide new programs such as distance learning by new technologies. This Nurse Education, Practice, and Retention (NEPR) program fosters the area of practice by providing funding for nurses caring for underserved populations and populations in noninstitutional settings, as well as for nurses interested in developing cultural competencies. Low-interest-rate loans—for instance, through the Nurse Faculty Loan Program (NFLP)—are available to master's and doctoral students who agree to work full-time in a school of nursing or nursing department after graduation. Nursing Workforce Diversity (NWD) grants provide educational funds to persons from disadvantaged backgrounds. The HRSA nursing workforce FY 2012 funding

was $148 million, down from $156 million in 2008. Federal dollars are the largest source of external funding for nursing education, primarily provided through the USDHHS BHP. Most of these federal dollars provide program funding; however, available funding for nursing students themselves is often inadequate. Various foundations provide scholarships for nursing workforce development. The Jonas Foundation has established a center for nursing and veteran's health care that provides leadership training, scholarship funds, and innovative models of nursing education. The John A. Hartford Foundation has funded the Gerontology Centers for the past decade. Recently DHHS provided $200 million in funding for demonstration projects to rapidly increase the number of nurse practitioners trained in medical centers. Partnerships with medical centers, accountable care organizations and payers, such as the University of Kentucky and the Norton Healthcare Institute for Nursing to increase the number of RN-BSN graduates, provide additional avenues to develop and grow the nursing workforce.

The National League for Nursing (NLN) initiated accreditation of nursing programs. Policies relative to accreditation came under scrutiny by the U.S. Department of Education in the 1990s, and the NLNAC was established as a freestanding entity. In 1999 CCNE, which evolved from the AACN, gained recognition from the Department of Education and now accredits most baccalaureate and graduate programs. In 2013 because of several years of litigation and financial disagreements, the NLNAC was dissolved, and a new body, the Accreditation Commission for Education in Nursing (ACEN) was created. This organization accredits associate, baccalaureate, and graduate-degree programs. These accrediting bodies understand the importance of the Pew Commission Report, the Kellogg sponsored Sullivan Commission USDHHS priorities, and congressional requirements, and thus encourage schools to initiate new curricula, develop creative teaching methods, stimulate lifelong learning, establish competency-based educational programs, focus on *Healthy People 2020*, address health disparities and diversity issues, and evaluate care delivered at all levels. The AACN "Essentials" for baccalaureate, master's, and practice doctorate education, the Consensus Model for APRN (Advanced Practice Registered Nurse) Regulation: Licensure, Accreditation, Certification, and Education, and the quality indicators for clinical and research doctoral education (www.aacn.nche.edu) are excellent beginning guidelines that will need to be evaluated and revised as the health care industry changes. Clinical doctorate programs, including DNP (Doctorate of Nursing Practice), are now funded by the Health Resources and Services Administration (HRSA) through Advanced Education Nursing Program (AENP) grants. In addition, workforce, staffing, and quality of care studies, such as those being conducted by Letvak, Ruhm, and Gupta (2013), Letvak (2013), Staiger, Auerbach, and Buerhaus (2012), Stimpfel and Aiken (2013), and NIH- and AHRQ-funded work (Aiken, Cimiotti, Sloane, Smith, Flynn, & Neff, 2011; Tubbs-Cooley, Cimiotti, Silber, Sloane, & Aiken, 2013) are becoming germane to nurses at the local and state levels as nurses lobby for continued authorization of funding programs and reimbursement and demonstrate quality-of-care benchmarks.

Successful efforts to foster collaboration and improve evidence-based practice (Fowler, Stern, 2014; Mann-Salinas, Hayes, Robbins, Sabido, Feider, Allen, & Yoder, 2013) and to provide effective education (Fogg, Carlson-Sabelli, Carlson, & Giddens, 2013) are needed. These studies and the directions they lead have an impact on the practice environments by identifying appropriate staffing, quality, and effective workforce development.

Research

The establishment of the NINR at the NIH in 1993, and its reauthorizations, have affected nursing research. First established as the National Center for Nursing Research in April 1986, with the purpose of providing a strong scientific base for nursing practice, it became the National Institute of Nursing Research (NINR) in 2000 and serves as an integral part of the NIH. The NINR National Advisory Council for Nursing Research (NACNR) participates in setting the NIH agenda, budget priorities, and funding recommendations. The NINR has led the NIH efforts to include the elimination of health disparities in their strategic plan. The program areas at the NINR in the 1990s were consistent with the national priorities set by the NIH and *Healthy People 2020*. The priority areas of science identified by the NINR in 2012 were symptom science, wellness, self-management, end of life and palliative care, and technology and training.

The NINR funds investigators who are not nurses; likewise, nurses receive funding from institutes other than the NINR. An interdisciplinary focus of projects is emphasized across program areas shared with many institutes, including the National Institute on Aging (NIA), the NIMH, the NICHD, the NIMHD, and the AHRQ. Agencies such as the NIOSH and CDC have provided funds to support nurse-directed studies on health in agricultural workers (Marcum, Browning, Reed, & Charnigo, 2011) and mental health of truck drivers (Shattell, Apostolopoulos, Collins, Sonmez, & Fehrenbacher, 2012; Shattell, Apostolopoulos, Sonmez, & Griffin, 2010). The AHRQ supports evidenced-based practice (EBP) centers (http://www.ahrq.gov/research/findings/evidence-based-reports/overview/index.html). The Eunice Kennedy Shriver NICHD supports studies related to the Best Pharmaceuticals for Children Act, and the NIMHD funds Centers of Excellence (COE) in Health Disparities Research. Nurses serve as nurse principal investigators of the NIMHD Centers.

The Substance Abuse and Mental Health Services Administration (SAMHSA) has supported demonstration projects to develop tools for Preadmission Screening and Resident Review (PASRR) Screening for Mental Illness in Nursing Facility Applicants and Residents (see www.samhsa.gov). The newest form of interdisciplinary study is the Patient-Centered Outcomes Research Initiatives (PCORI). Dr. Debra Moser, nursing professor, leads the team comparing heart health interventions among underserved in Appalachia. The new Clinical and Translational Science Awards efforts and activities have been led by nurses such as Drs. Cornelia Beck, Catherine Gillis, and Teresa Kelechi.

Nurses provide leadership in many ways. For example, Dr. Martha Hill, former dean of The Johns Hopkins University School of Nursing, co-chaired the committee to develop the IOM's *Unequal Treatment* report, which guides much of the system and disparities interventions. Dr. Hill also leads multidisciplinary and multinational intervention studies to prevent or control hypertension in African Americans and Africans. Dr. Audrey Nelson, as director of the VA Patient Safety Center of Inquiry in Tampa, leads efforts to improve patient safety and quality of care through the Veterans Administration. Dr. Cornelia Beck, Distinguished Professor at the University of Arkansas Medical Sciences, provides leadership in the national efforts to alleviate suffering from Alzheimer's disease. In addition, HIV/AIDS work has been led by Dr. William Holzemer and by Dr. Nancy McCain with an emphasis on biobehavioral interventions.

Research directions have been guided by foundations such as the RWJF and the W. K. Kellogg Foundation, which have funded community and rural health initiatives. Findings from nursing investigations and experience have resulted in input to the development of practice guidelines. Nancy Bergstrom and her colleagues' work on decubitus ulcers and Jean Wyman and Thelma Wells' work on incontinence influenced the AHRQ practice guidelines in the 1990s. More recently, nurse researchers have investigated factors related to differing health concerns in U.S. and international populations (Amireshani & Wallace, 2013; Bartlett & Shelton, 2010; Ivanov, Hu, & Leak, 2010; Stacciarini, Shattell, Coady, & Wiens, 2011; Wallace & Bartlett, 2013), as well as the effectiveness of interventions for vulnerable populations (Bellury, Ellington, Beck, Pett, Clar, & Stein, 2013; Hu, Wallace, & Tesh, 2010; Thomson, Berry, & Hu, 2013; Walton-Moss, Samuel, Nguyen, Commodore-Mensah, Hayat, & Szanton, 2013). In addition, Elaine Larson, Patricia Stone, and colleagues at Columbia Medical Center have built knowledge to prevent infections in hospitals and provided a cost analysis of those interventions.

The NINR, Sigma Theta Tau International (STTI), the four regional nursing research societies (Southern, Midwest, Eastern, and Western), specialty organizations, Friends of NINR, and the National Nursing Research Roundtable meet annually to discuss and plan for the direction, implementation, and funding of nursing research. Regional and national conferences and the Council for the Advancement of Nursing Science (CANS) State of the Science Congress highlight nursing research findings that have an impact on health care delivery, costs, access, and outcomes. Congressional members and persons from local, state, and regional political and legislative arenas are invited to attend these meetings to discuss nursing and health care efforts and needs. Additional research activities include the Veterans Administration Nursing Research Initiative (NRI), the American Nurses Foundation (ANF) awards, and nursing fellowships and grants by the AHRQ, the RWJF, the W. K. Kellogg Foundation, and the Templeton Foundation (TF). Nurses also fill positions as clinical researchers in medical centers across the country and conduct ongoing studies.

Outcomes and Quality

Outcomes research is now required to determine the effectiveness and accountability of practice. Much effort is directed at defining what constitutes outcomes and how to measure them. Outcomes research is a priority in the area of health services research. One policy initiative was the enactment of the Healthcare Research and Quality Act of 1999, which changed the name of the Agency for Health Care Policy and Research (AHCPR) to the AHRQ. This emphasis provides that research on outcomes and quality will provide a foundation for future policy, regulation, and allocation decisions for health care. National health indicators, *Healthy People 2020*, and the USDHHS initiative to eliminate racial and ethnic disparities provide another set of outcomes and measures of quality. Examining system outcomes is one avenue of research. System outcomes are those related to direct and indirect material and financial costs, length of stay, manpower, provider qualifications, and provider and payer satisfaction. For example, a hospital-based intervention improved nurse retention and quality of care provided to patients (Blake, Leach, Robbins, Pike, & Needlemann, 2012; Stichler, 2013).

Client outcomes such as consumer satisfaction, health status outcomes, adaptation, and function require study. Examples include nurses' perception of their work environment and its effect on patient satisfaction. Boev (2012) found a direct relationship between how nurses perceived their work environment and how satisfied their patients are with the care provided in adult critical care units. Other studies have found a relationship between nurses' satisfaction with work and patient outcomes (Bae, Mark, & Fried, 2010; Chevalier, Hudson, Thompson, & Constantine, 2011; Lange, Wallace, Gerard, Lovanio, Fausty, & Rychlewicz, 2009). A final issue to be addressed is how outcomes and quality relate to and affect one another. This will be a specific area for nursing to address in future practice, education, and research efforts. Future nursing efforts will be guided by the ANA's health policy analyses, position and principle statements, and ethics and practice guidelines to set forth priorities for workforce development, quality care, health access, and evolving practice environments.

NURSE PARTICIPATION IN HEALTH POLICY

Nurses have increasingly become active participants in the health policy arena as advocates and activists and in writing health policies at the state and federal levels. Nursing has progressed through several stages in its political development and involvement in the policy arena. Nursing is currently at the "leadership" stage, where it is recognized as a political entity with a recognizable agenda that guides health policy. The ANA has been consulted for advice and has offered recommendations on health care reform and on health policies, such as the Women's Health Initiative (WHI). A prime example occurred during the debate about health care reform in 2010 and subsequent years. The Affordable Care Act (ACA) implementations discussions resulted in ANA issuing briefs, position papers, and principle statements on access to care for immigrants, nursing workforce development, use of unlicensed personnel, expanding nurse practitioner practice, staffing guidelines, and measuring quality of care. These documents have been developed and shared with leaders of organizations representing health care providers, insurers, policy makers, employers, labor unions, and consumers. However, nursing often misses opportunities for input, such as with the Oral Health Initiative, partially because nurses fail to recognize or champion one another as experts.

In 2013 six nurses served as legislators in Congress. Representative Capps was instrumental in writing the initial Nurse Reinvestment Act. The original intent has been accomplished primarily through HRSA funding for graduate programs, nurse scholarships, grants to health care facilities to improve nurse retention and patient safety, faculty loan repayment, and funding for new undergraduate programs. Reauthorization was accomplished in 2008, 2010, and 2012. In addition, the Affordable Care Act (PL 111-148) and the partnering Health Care and Education Reconciliation Act of 2010 (P.L. 111-152) established the Graduate Nurse Education Demonstration program to develop a system of payments to hospitals for the costs of clinical training for advanced practice nurses, reauthorized the Nursing Workforce Development programs, and created a National Health Care Workforce Commission. However, funds have decreased over the past decade and appropriation of adequate support continues to be a concern.

Nurses have been instrumental in the policy arena, advocating for change in policies that affect nurses and health. Nurses are involved in numerous legislative efforts such as the National School Health Program (NLSP). Long, Luedicke, Dorsey, Flore, and Henderson (2013) analyzed the impact of the NLSP on schools voluntarily eliminating unhealthy competitive foods. They found support for implementation of NLSP standards for improving students' learning and health by providing healthier food alternatives for lunch. In another example, nurses who were members of Virginia's Old Dominion Society of Gastroenterology Nurses and Associates (SGNA) initiated the introduction of legislation to promote insurance payment for colorectal screening. This effort began when a nurse working at a gastroenterology unit in Virginia became concerned about the number of patients who were diagnosed with late-stage colon cancer because they did not get early screening. The President of SGNA contacted Virginia State Senator Emily Couric, sharing the group's concern for the lack of colorectal screening and asking her to write a legislative mandate for insurance coverage of colonoscopies. Through these efforts, Virginia became the first state to pass legislation mandating insurance coverage for colonoscopies to all individuals, including those covered by Medicaid. As of December 2013, the CDC reported that 29 states have enacted legislation mandating insurance coverage for at least one type of colorectal cancer (CRC) screening, and 11 states had introduced legislation that would cover some type of CRC screening (www.cdc.gov/cancer/colorectal/pdf/colorectal_cancer_activities.pdf).

In other areas, nurse practitioners (NPs) have been active in passing state laws dealing with prescription drug rights (Sampson, 2010). Nurse anesthetists have also been active in legislation dealing with their practice. The North Carolina Association of Nurse Anesthetists (NCANA) has been active in fighting to preserve the authority of CRNAs in North Carolina and against legislation that would allow licensing of anesthesiologist assistants (AAs). Julie Ann Lowery, president of the NCANA, reached out to grassroots groups and North Carolina residents in an effort to get them involved in legislation that would jeopardize CRNAs' practice in North Carolina.

These are only a few examples of nurse activism in the policy arena. As nurses become more informed, passionate, and committed about their leadership role in the policy arena, legislation at the state and federal levels will require input from nurses to advocate for patients, the public, and themselves.

HEALTH CARE REFORM 2010—2014

The historic health care insurance reform law, Patient Protection and Affordable Care Act (PPACA) of 2010 (Public Law 111-148) was signed into law by President Obama on March 23, 2010, and its companion Health Care and Education Affordability Reconciliation Act (PL 111-152) was signed into law on March 30, 2010. Bills are typed in a particular format that greatly expands the number of pages, and the complexity of the current health care system required that many interconnections be addressed. The federal government website for the Affordable Care Act (http://www.hhs.gov/healthcare/rights/index.html) provided details for titles, dates for implementation, summary of changes, and a link to the final law.

The government website (http://healthcare.gov/) provides useful information about specific aspects of the law and includes a section that addresses the law's impact by specific population or issue, including a map that allows the public to see the impact at a specific state level. Table 6-4 provides a summary of the 10 titles included in the PPACA Act, including the elements of the companion Reconciliation Act. The Office of Consumer Information and Insurance Oversight (OCIIO) is created within the DHHS to implement many of the provisions of the legislation that address private health insurance. Some provisions were enacted in 2010, and other provisions were enacted over the past few years. The full act was anticipated to be fully implemented by 2014; however, legislative, regulatory, and political issues have delayed some provisions. For example, the individual mandate to purchase health insurance was delayed because of website access problems, then by legislation in December 2013. The business mandate was delayed to allow time for regulations and consideration of cost levels, mostly by Executive Orders of President Obama in January and February 2014. As of October 2014, 23 states were not expanding Medicaid programs. Wisconsin is already providing Medicaid eligibility to adults up to the poverty level under a Medicaid waiver. The remaining 22 states are: Alabama, Alaska, Florida, Georgia, Idaho, Indiana, Kansas, Louisiana, Maine, Mississippi, Missouri, Montana, Nebraska, North Carolina, Oklahoma, South Carolina, South Dakota, Tennessee, Texas, Utah, Virginia, and Wyoming. The ACA Medicaid expansion was designed to address the high uninsured rates among adults living below poverty by providing coverage options for individuals with limited access to employer coverage and/or limited income to purchase coverage in the individual insurance market. Additionally, the expansion was designed to end categorical eligibility for Medicaid. With many states opting out of Medicaid expansion, millions of adults remain outside of reach of this health insurance reform initiative. Within the insurance gap, they do not qualify for publicly-financed coverage in their state; do not have access to employer-sponsored coverage; or cannot afford to purchase insurance on their own. The majority of these people are the 'working-poor'; employed either part-time or full-time but still living below the poverty line. Based on the state specific population characteristics, these decisions not to expand disproportionately affect people of color, particularly Black Americans. This has implications for efforts to address health disparities in health coverage, access, and outcomes among people of color (Kaiser Family Foundation, 2014). Box 6-2 lists the strategic provisions that will be addressed initially. The OCIIO has published several interim final rules for public comment on www.regulations.gov.

The Affordable Care Act (ACA) has been enacted and allows persons less than 26 years of age to remain or return to their parent's insurance coverage if certain conditions are met, removes lifetime limits on health coverage, and removes the use of preexisting conditions as a reason to deny or terminate coverage. Many discussions in the media, in Washington, DC, and in state legislative bodies occurred because of the new ACA insurance marketplace website access problems. In addition, diverse political and economic issues have taken place since the ACA became law. The web portal was made public in October 2013, but many problems arose and the site was taken off line until November 2013. Fewer than 500,000 persons were able to sign up in the first 2 months. States have made decisions regarding developing their own insurance exchanges or allowing the federal government to develop an exchange within the state. In 2014 at least 16 states ran their own exchanges and six states ran the state partnership exchange with the federal government. Decisions were

TABLE 6-4 Patient Protection and Affordable Care Act (PPACA) of 2010 (PL 111-148) and Health Care and Education Reconciliation Act of 2010

Act summary with designation of new and existing authorities.

Title I: Quality Affordable Health Care for All Americans	This Act allows individuals, families, and small business owners to make decisions about their health care. Premium costs are reduced for millions of working families and small businesses by providing hundreds of billions of dollars in tax relief—the largest middle class tax cut for health care in history. Out-of-pocket expenses are capped, and preventive care must be fully covered without out-of-pocket expense. For many Americans, their insurance coverage is not expected to change. Qualified health plans have been defined and exchange pools have been established for Americans without insurance coverage so they can choose their insurance coverage. The insurance exchange pools buying power and gives Americans choices of private insurance plans that have to compete for their business based on cost and quality. Small business owners may choose insurance coverage through this exchange as well as receive a tax credit to help offset the cost of covering their employees.
	The Act bans insurance companies from denying insurance coverage because of preexisting medical conditions and provides consumers new power to appeal insurance company decisions that deny doctor- ordered treatments covered by insurance.
	The USDHHS Secretary (Secretary) has the authority to implement many of these new provisions to help families and small business owners have the information they need to make the choices that work best for them.
Title II: The Role of Public Programs	The Act extends Medicaid while treating all states equally. It preserves CHIP, the successful children's insurance plan, and simplifies enrollment for individuals and families.
	Community-based care for Americans with disabilities is enhanced and states will have opportunities to expand home care services to people with long-term care needs.
	The Act gives flexibility to states to adopt innovative strategies to improve care and the coordination of services for Medicare and Medicaid beneficiaries.
	The Secretary has the authority to work with states and other partners to strengthen strategic public programs.
Title III: Improving the Quality and Efficiency of Health Care	The Act closes the Medicare prescription coverage gap called the "donut hole." In addition, the Act provides incentives for doctors, nurses, and hospitals that improve care and reduce errors.
	The Act enhances access to health care services in rural and underserved areas. Funding is provided for school-based and nurse- managed centers to assist in providing this care.
	Another change is the addition of a group of doctors and health care experts, rather than only members of Congress, who identify ideas to improve quality and reduce costs for Medicare beneficiaries.
	The Secretary has the authority to take steps to strengthen the Medicare program and implement reforms to improve the quality and efficiency of health care.
Title IV: Prevention of Chronic Disease and Improving Public Health	The Act directs the creation of a national prevention and health promotion strategy that incorporates the most effective and achievable methods to improve the health status of Americans and reduce the incidence of preventable illness and disability in the United States. Included in this title are the availability of science-based nutrition information and waiving co-payments for America's seniors on Medicare for prevention and health screenings.
	The Secretary has the authority to coordinate with other departments, develop and implement a prevention and health promotion strategy, and work to ensure that more Americans have access to critical preventive health services.
Title V: Health Care Workforce	The Act funds scholarships and loan repayment programs to increase the number of primary care physicians, nurses, physician assistants, mental health providers, and dentists in the areas of the country that need them most. In addition, funds are provided to expand, construct, and operate community health centers, with specific funding for nurse-managed health centers.
	Expansions are also noted for the advanced education nursing programs, the Nurse Faculty Loan Program, the Nurse Loan Repayment and Scholarship Program, and the Nursing Student Loan Program.
	The Secretary has the authority to take action to strengthen many existing programs that help support the primary care workforce.

Continued

TABLE 6-4 Patient Protection and Affordable Care Act (PPACA) of 2010 (PL 111-148) and Health Care and Education Reconciliation Act of 2010—cont'd

Title VI: Transparency and Program Integrity	The Act includes the Nursing Home Transparency program so that consumers can compare facilities. The Act protects whistleblowers, and it requires staffing accountability and disclosure.
	Finally the Act imposes rigorous disclosure requirements to identify high-risk providers who have defrauded the American taxpayer. It gives states new authority to prevent providers who have been penalized in one state from setting up in another and the flexibility to propose and test tort reforms for improving health care.
	The Secretary has new and improved authority to promote transparency and ensure that every dollar in the Act and in existing programs is spent wisely and well.
Title VII: Improving Access to Innovative Medical Therapies	The Act extends drug discounts to hospitals and communities that serve low-income patients and creates a pathway for the creation of generic versions of biological drugs.
	The Secretary of Health and Human Services has the authority to implement these provisions to help make medications more affordable.
Title VIII: Community Living Assistance Services and Support Act (CLASS)	The Act provides Americans with a new option to finance long-term services and care in the event of a disability.
	It is a self-funded and voluntary long-term care insurance option. Workers will pay premiums to receive a daily cash benefit if they develop a disability. Need will be based on difficulty in performing basic activities such as bathing or dressing. The benefit is flexible—it could be used for a range of community support services, from respite care to home care.
	Safeguards will be put in place to ensure that its premiums are enough to cover its costs.
	The Secretary has the authority to establish the CLASS Program.
Title IX: Revenue Provisions	The Act provides new tax credits that will reduce health premium costs for middle class families and allow them exchange pools for insurance purchase. Families making less than $250,000 are the primary targets of these provisions.
	This title will be implemented by the U.S. Department of the Treasury.
Title X:	The Act reauthorizes the Indian Health Care Improvement Act (IHCIA), which provides health care services to American Indians and Alaskan Natives.
	The Secretary, in consultation with the Indian Health Service, has the authority to implement the Indian Health Care Improvement Act.

Modified from Healthcare.gov and http://www.hhs.gov/healthcare/rights/index.html, accessed December 19, 2013 and Government Printing Office [DOCID: f: publ148.111, Page 124 STAT. 119], accessed December 19, 2013.

BOX 6-2 Key Provisions of PPACA 2010 That Have Taken Effect as of February 2014

1. Provides small business tax credits
2. Ensures no discrimination against children with preexisting conditions
3. Helps uninsured Americans with preexisting conditions until the exchange is available (Interim High-Risk Pool)
4. Guarantees renewable coverage
5. Prohibits discrimination against individual participants and beneficiaries based on health status
6. Begins to close the Medicare Part D Donut Hole for eligible persons
7. Provides free preventive health screenings under Medicare
8. Extends coverage for young people up to their 26th birthday through parent's insurance by certain eligibility
9. Provides reinsurance for early retirees
10. Bans lifetime limits on health insurance coverage
11. Bans restrictive annual limits on insurance coverage
12. Requires free preventive care under new private plans
13. Provides a new, independent appeals process
14. Ensures value for premium payments
15. Expands community health centers
16. Increases the number of primary care practitioners
17. Prohibits discrimination based on salary
18. Expands and requires certain health insurance consumer information
19. Monitors insurance companies for fair health insurance premiums
20. Affords availability of Health Insurance Exchanges to purchase insurance
21. Expands Medicaid

Source: Patient Protection and Affordable Care Act (PPACA) of 2010 (P.L. 111-148) and Health Care and Education Reconciliation Act of 2010 Act Summary with Designation of New and Existing Authorities. Modified from Healthcare.gov and http://www.hhs.gov/healthcare/rights/index.html, accessed on December 19, 2013 and Government Printing Office [DOCID: f: publ148.111, Page 124 STAT. 119], accessed December, 19, 2013.

made through governor choice or legislative approval. Twenty-seven states have chosen not to develop their state insurance or partnership exchanges but to allow federal entities to develop and manage the exchanges (Center on Budget and Policy Priorities, 2013). In addition, the ACA allowed expansion of Medicaid, which many states declined to enact, as noted prior. The decisions were logistical, political, and financial in nature. It is not known whether the federal or state exchanges will meet expectations for enrollment, access to care, and improved health, or whether states may expand Medicaid at a later date. As with any legislation, the ACA titles will be revised, removed, or implemented in future years. In addition, courts will be involved in decisions regarding the ACA in the future, similar to the 2013 US Supreme Court decisions on the ACA that the individual mandate is required and that Medicaid expansion could not be required by the states.

SUMMARY

As members of the largest group of health professionals and major providers of care, nurses can influence health care policy as individuals and as professionals. Consumers of health care, including nurses, desire affordable, accessible, and high-quality care. Nurses are obligated to ensure that the public has access to quality health care at controlled costs. Identifying and prioritizing client needs with sensitivity to culture and diversity, acquiring and demonstrating a knowledge of treatments and interventions (both nursing and interdisciplinary), maintaining a focus on outcomes (client, system, and provider), and ensuring safe, quality care in multiple environments are basic responsibilities of professional nursing in the 21st century.

Armed with information on how to influence health care policy, nurses serve as advocates for patients and active participants in the formation of effective health care policy. Organizational membership in regional, state, or national organizations and letter writing are two traditional activities for nurses involved in policy making. More focused involvement can be achieved through collective actions as members of PACs and political parties. Social, civic, professional, and lay organizations with interest in specific populations and concerns also provide a mechanism by which nurses can influence legislation and allocation decisions. Another avenue is to run for elected office or sit on boards, committees, councils, or commissions, especially those that make policy and funding decisions that affect health care. Opportunities exist and can be developed to share expertise and communicate nursing needs through consultation to elected officials, health agencies, foundations, educational institutions, and funding agencies. Policy decisions regarding financial resources influence the type of nursing staff, the number of nurses, the amount and type of management and support services, and the extent of educational program and research funding—all of which affect the practice environment and quality of nursing and health care. The settings and payment of care affect access and the spectrum of services available to the most vulnerable populations. Through professional and personal knowledge, expertise, and experience, nurses can take action in research, practice, and education areas. Politics, legislation, and economics provide ample opportunity and challenge for nursing involvement. Taking advantage of these opportunities and meeting the challenge of ensuring access to quality health care for all can be achieved through greater involvement in the health policy arena.

SALIENT POINTS

- Health policy is influenced by many factors, including politics, economics, demographics, and personal and societal priorities.
- Legislation is a complex process that includes multiple players, takes time, and involves political and special interests at local, state, and federal levels.
- A large portion of the federal budget and expenditures is directed at health programs, specifically Medicare, Medicaid, and Social Security entitlements.
- Federal and state legislation, as well as rules and regulations to implement policies, influence the availability, access, and spectrum of nursing practice and health care.

- New demographics and health needs will require changes in delivery of health care, to whom it is delivered, and the environment and practices of care.
- An outcomes and quality focus is required to ensure quality and useful nursing practice, education, and research.

- Nurses have a responsibility to participate in health policy and planning to ensure quality health care and an effective practice environment.
- Knowledge and involvement are keys to influencing health policy.

CRITICAL REFLECTION EXERCISES

1. What are the major health care issues in your community, state, and region? What are some solutions to these problems? How might you become involved in implementing these solutions?
2. Discuss how a practice, workplace, education, or research situation in your experience was directly affected by health policy decisions or allocations. What are the options for changing that policy? What are the barriers and facilitators to changing the policy?
3. Discuss how entitlements should be addressed with a health care provider, a health care economist or businessperson, and a client. Develop three strategies and share these with your state or national legislator and your professional organization.
4. Discuss your nursing practice and workplace environment and how these are affected by policy decisions at the local, state, and federal levels.
5. What are your responsibilities to ensure access to quality, timely, appropriate, and cost-effective care?
6. How does the Affordable Care Act impact your community?

REFERENCES

Association of Colleges of Nursing. (2012, August last revised). *Nursing shortage.* [Fact sheet]. Retrieved from http://www.aacn.nche.edu/media-relations/fact-sheets/nursing-shortage.

American Association of Colleges of Nursing. (2012, October, last revised). *Nursing faculty shortage.* [Fact sheet]. Retrieved from www.aacn.nche.edu/media-relations/fact-sheets/nursing-faculty-shortage.

American Association of Colleges of Nursing. (2012a). *Nursing Faculty shortage.* [Fact sheet]. Retrieved from www.aacn.nche.edu/media-relations/FacultyShortageFS.pdf.

American Association of Colleges of Nursing. (2012b). *Nursing shortage.* [Fact sheet]. Retrieved from www.aacn.nche.edu/media-relations/NrsgShortageFS.pdf .

American Nurses Credentialing Center. (2013). *2014 magnet® Application Manual Addendum.* Retrieved from http://www.nursecredentialing.org/2014-MagnetManualUpdates.

Aiken, L. H., Cimiotti, J. P., Sloane, D. M., Smith, H. L., Flynn, L., & Neff, D. F. (2011). The effects of nurse staffing and nurse education on patient deaths in hospitals with different nurse work environments. *Medical care, 49*(12), 1047.

Amirehsani, K. A., & Wallace, D. C. (2013). Tés, Licuados, and Cápsulas herbal self-care remedies of Latino/Hispanic immigrants for type 2 diabetes. *The Diabetes Educator, 39*(6), 828–840.

Bae, S. H., Mark, B., & Fried, B. (2010). Impact of nursing unit turnover on patient outcomes in hospitals. *Journal of Nursing Scholarship, 42*(1), 40–49.

Bartlett, R., & Shelton, T. (2010). Feasibility and initial efficacy testing of an HIV prevention intervention for black adolescent girls. *Issues in Mental Health Nursing, 31*(11), 731–738. Retrieved from http://ehis.ebscohost.com.

Beck, S. L., Weiss, M. E., Ryan-Wenger, N., Donaldson, N. E., Aydin, C., Towsley, G. L., & Gardner, W. (2013). Measuring nurses' impact on health care quality: Progress, challenges, and future directions. *Medical care, 51*, S15–S22.

Bellury, L., Ellington, L., Beck, S. L., Pett, M. A., Clark, J., & Stein, K. (2013, July). Older breast cancer survivors: Can interaction analyses identify vulnerable subgroups? A report from the American Cancer Society Studies of Cancer Survivors. *Oncology Nursing Forum, 40*(4), 325–336. Oncology Nursing Society.

Blake, N., Leach, L. S., Robbins, W., Pike, N., & Needleman, J. (2012). Healthy work environments and staff nurse retention: The relationship between communication, collaboration, and leadership in the pediatric intensive care unit. *Nursing Administration Quarterly, 37*(4), 356–370.

Boev, C. (2012). The relationship between nurses' perception of work environment and patient satisfaction in adult critical care. *Journal of Nursing Scholarship, 44*(4), 368–375.

Centers for Disease Control and Prevention. (2013). *CDC Health Disparities and Inequalities Report — United States.* Retrieved from www.cdc.gov/mmwr/pdf/other/su6203.pdf.

Centers for Medicare & Medicaid Services. (2013). *2013 CMS Statistics*. Retrieved from www.cms.gov/Research-Statistics-Data-and-Systems/Statistics-Trends-and-Reports/CMS-Statistics-Reference-Booklet/Downloads/CMS_Stats_2013_final.pdf.

Centers for Medicare & Medicaid Services. (2014). *National Health Expenditures 2013 Highlights*. Retrieved from www.cms.gov/Research-Statistics-Data-and-Systems/Statistics-Trends-and-Reports/NationalHealthExpendData/downloads/highlights.pdf.

Center on Budget and Policy Priorities. (2013). Status of State Health Insurance Exchange Implementation. Retrieved from www.cbpp.org/files/CBPP-Analysis-on-the-Status-of-State-Exchange-Implementation.pdf.

Chevalier, B. A., Hudson, S., Thompson, K., & Constantine, C. (2011). Patient outcomes, economic benefits associated with a heparin change in hemodialysis, and nurses' satisfaction. *Nephrology Nursing Journal: Journal of the American Nephrology Nurses' Association*, 38(4), 339.

Esterson, J., Bazile, Y., Mezey, M., Cortes, T. A., & Huba, G. J. (2013). Ensuring specialty nurse competence to care for older adults: Reflections on a decade of collaboration between specialty nursing associations and the Hartford Institute for Geriatric Nursing. *The Journal of nursing administration*, 43(10), 517–523.

Federal Elections Commission. (2013a). Contribution limits for 2013–14. Retrieved from December 18, 2013, http://www.fec.gov/pages/brochures/contriblimits.shtml.

Federal Elections Commission. (2013b). Campaign finance reports and data. Retrieved from www.fec.gov .

Fogg, L., Carlson-Sabelli, L., Carlson, K., & Giddens, J. (2013). The perceived benefits of virtual learning style, race, ethnicity and frequency of use on nursing students. *Nursing Education Perspectives*, 34(6), 390–394.

Fowler, S. B., & Stern, C. (2014). Evidence-based practice: The cochrane nursing care corner. *Clinical Nurse Specialist*, 28(1), 4.

Hartman, M., Martin, A. B., Benson, J., & Catlin, A. (2013). National Health Spending in 2011: Overall growth remains low, but some payers and services show signs of acceleration. *Health Affairs*, 32(1), 87–99.

Hu, J., Wallace, D., & Tesh, A. (2010). Physical activity, obesity, nutritional health and quality of life in low-income Hispanic adults with diabetes. *Journal of Community Health Nursing*, 27(2), 70–83. Retrieved from http://ehis.ebscohostcom.

Ingram, R. R. (2012). Using Campinha–Bacote's process of cultural competence model to examine the relationship between health literacy and cultural competence. *Journal of Advanced Nursing*, 68(3), 695–704.

Institute of Medicine. (2010). *The Future of Nursing: Leading Change; Advancing Health*. Retrieved December 10, 2013, from http://iom.edu/~/media/Files/Report%20Files/2010/The-Future-of-Nursing/Future%20of% 20Nursing%202010%20Report%20Brief.pdf.

Ivanov, L., Hu, J., & Leak, A. (2010). Immigrant women's cancer screening behavior. *Journal of Community Health Nursing*, 27(1), 32–45. Retrieved from http://ehis.ebscohostcom.

Kaiser Family Foundation. (2014, November). The Coverage Gap: Uninsured poor adults in states that do not expand Medicaid–An update. Retrieved from http://kff.org/health-reform/issue-brief/the-coverage-gap-uninsured-poor-adults-in-states-that-do-not-expand-medicaid-an-update/.

Kelly, L. A., McHugh, M. D., & Aiken, L. H. (2011). Nurse outcomes in Magnet® and non-magnet hospitals. *The Journal of Nursing Administration*, 41(10), 428.

Lange, J., Wallace, M., Gerard, S., Lovanio, K., Fausty, N., & Rychlewicz, S. (2009). Effect of an acute care geriatric educational program on fall rates and nurse work satisfaction. *Journal of continuing education in nursing*, 40(8), 371.

Letvak, S., Ruhm, C., & Gupta, S. (2013). Differences in health, productivity, and quality of care in younger and older nurses. *Journal of Nursing Management*, 21, 914–921. http://dx.doi.org/10.1111/jonm.12181.

Letvak, S. (2013). Managing nurses with health concerns. *Nursing Management*, 43(3), 7–10. http://dx.doi.org/10.1097/01.NUMA.0000412225.50350.bd.

Long, M. W., Luedicke, J., Dorsey, M., Fiore, S. S., & Henderson, K. E. (2013). Impact of Connecticut Legislation Incentivizing Elimination of Unhealthy Competitive Foods on National School Lunch Program Participation. *American Journal of Public Health*, 103(7), e59–e66.

Mann-Salinas, E., Hayes, E., Robbins, J., Sabido, J., Feider, L., Allen, D., & Yoder, L. (2013). A systematic review of the literature to support an evidence-based precepting program. *Burns*. Retrieved from http://dx.doi.org/10.1016/j.burns.2013.11.008.

Marcum, J. L., Browning, S. R., Reed, D. B., & Charnigo, R. J. (2011). Farmwork-related injury among farmers 50 years of age and older in Kentucky and South Carolina: A cohort study, 2002–2005. *Journal of Agricultural Safety and Health*, 17(3), 259.

National Institutes of Health. (2012). History of congressional appropriations, fiscal years 2000–2012. Retrieved from http://officeofbudget.od.nih.gov/pdfs/FY12/Approp.%20History%20by%20IC%292012.pdf.

Naylor, M. D., Volpe, E. M., Lustig, A., Kelley, H. J., Melichar, L., & Pauly, M. V. (2013). Linkages between nursing and the quality of patient care: A 2-year comparison. *Medical Care*, 51, S6–S14.

Numminen, O., Meretoja, R., Isoaho, H., & Leino–Kilpi, H. (2013). Professional competence of practising nurses. *Journal of Clinical Nursing*, 22(9–10), 1411–1423.

Sampson, D. (2010). The Idiosyncratic Politics of Prescriptive Authority. In E. Sullivan-Marx, D. McGiven, J. Fairman, & S. Greenberg (Eds.), *Nurse practitioners: The evolution and future of advanced practice* (pp. 149–158). New York, NY: Springer Publishing Company L.L.C.

Shattell, M., Apostolopoulos, Y., Sonmez, S., & Griffin, M. (2010). Occupational stressors and the mental health of truckers. *Issues in Mental Health Nursing*, 31(9), 61–568. Retrieved from http://dx.doi.org/10.3109/01612840.2010.488783.

Shattell, M., Apostolopoulos, Y., Collins, C., Sonmez, S., & Fehrenbacher, C. (2012). Trucking organization and mental health disorders of truck drivers. *Issues in Mental Health Nursing, 33*(7), 436–444. Retrieved from http://dx.doi.org/10.3109/01612840.2012.66516.

Stacciarini, J., Shattell, M., Coady, M., & Wiens, B. (2011). Community-based participatory research approach to address mental health in minority populations. *Community Mental Journal, Health Journal, 47*(5), 489–497. Retrieved from http://dx.doi.org/10.1007/s10597-010-9319-z.

Staiger, D. O., Auerbach, D. I., & Buerhaus, P. I. (2012). Registered Nurse Labor Supply and the Recession—Are We in a Bubble? *New England Journal of Medicine, 366*(16), 1463–1465.

Starr, S. S., & Wallace, D. C. (2009). Self- reported cultural competence of public health nurses in a Southeastern U.S. Public Health Department. *Public Health Nursing, 26*(1), 48–57.

Stichler, J. F. (2013). Healthy work environments for the ageing nursing workforce. *Journal of Nursing Management, 21*(7), 956–963.

Stimpfel, A. W., & Aiken, L. H. (2013). Hospital staff nurses' shift length associated with safety and quality of care. *Journal of Nursing Care Quality, 28*(2), 122–129.

Stimpfel, A. W., Rosen, J. E., & McHugh, M. D. (2014). Understanding the role of the professional practice environment on quality of care in magnet® and non-magnet hospitals. *The Journal of Nursing Administration, 44*(1), 10–16.

Thomson, W., Berry, D., & Hu, J. (2013). A church-based intervention to change attitudes about physical activity among black adolescent girls: A feasibility study. *Public Health Nursing, 30*(3), 221–230.

Tubbs-Cooley, H. L., Cimiotti, J. P., Silber, J. H., Sloane, D. M., & Aiken, L. H. (2013). An observational study of nurse staffing ratios and hospital readmission among children admitted for common conditions. *BMJ Quality and Safety, 22*, 735–742. Retrieved from http://dx.doi.org/10.1136/bmjqs-2012-001610.

U.S. House of Representatives. (2003). How our laws are made. Retrieved from January 29, 2009, http://thomas.loc.gov/home/lawsmade.toc.html.

U.S. Senate. (2003). How our laws are made. Document, 108–193. Retrieved from January 17, 2009, from http://www.senate.gov/reference/resources/pdf/howourlawsaremade.pdf.

Wallace, D., & Bartlett, R. (2013). Recruitment and retention of African American and Hispanic girls and women in research. *Public Health Nursing, 30*(2), 159–166.

Walton-Moss, B., Samuel, L., Nguyen, T. H., Commodore-Mensah, Y., Hayat, M., & Szanton, S. L. (2013). Community-based cardiovascular health interventions in vulnerable populations: A systematic review. *Journal of Cardiovascular Nursing*. Retrieved from http://dx.doi.org/10.1097/JCN.0b013e31828e2995.

PART II

Dimensions of Professional Nursing Practice

Economic Issues in Nursing and Health Care

Richard A. Ridge, MBA, PhD, RN, NEA-BC, CENP

http://evolve.elsevier.com/Friberg/bridge/

OBJECTIVES

At the completion of this chapter, the reader will be able to:

- Describe how the economic concepts of supply, demand, complements and substitutes, competition, and market failure apply to nursing and health care.
- Define and differentiate methods of cost evaluation.
- Discuss how the cost of care and quality of care are related.
- Compare and contrast the economic foundations of emerging models for health system reform.

PROFILE IN PRACTICE

Elizabeth E. Friberg, DNP, RN
Associate Professor, University of Virginia School of Nursing, Charlottesville, Virginia

While practicing in direct care for the first 15 years of my career in acute and community-based care, including private practice, I became interested in the production, delivery, and purchasing of health care services and the health care systems that delivered those services. Having a psych-mental health background and community-based focus, I was interested in the health-seeking behaviors of individuals, groups, organizations, and the larger delivery system, including the relationship of those behaviors to access, cost, and quality. Working with program-level budgets provided an education in the actual cost of producing and delivering health care services.

For the next 15 years, my practice was focused at a population level as I moved from community health to managed care and ultimately to the larger health insurance industry. I explored the use of incentives to guide behavior, health benefit design concepts, risk management, role of prevention, health system fraud and abuse, comparative effectiveness, professional guidelines, and the role of government to protect the public and at times correct behaviors that may negatively affect the public. This focus provided an education on the cost of purchasing health care services—from the varying perspectives of individuals, families, employers, unions, trust funds, and the government. Our system of health care in the United States is extremely complex and inefficient and often fails to produce the outcomes desired by most stakeholders. It tends to satisfy only the few. After 5 years of health care system consulting, I now teach nurs-

es at the undergraduate and graduate level about the complexity and realities of the cost and quality of our health care system.

Health care professionals need a working knowledge of topics such as delivery models, basic insurance principles, and the fissure between our public health and primary care system. One only needs to listen to recent media dialogue and "town hall meetings" or read op-ed pieces to understand the absolute confusion that exists in the public domain about our current public and private health care system. Nurses have an obligation to investigate and be familiar with the answers to the following questions: (1) How is the current system designed and how does it operate? (2) What are the drivers of quality health care? (3) What are the market forces that support or impede the delivery of quality health care? (4) What legitimate roles can the government play? and (5) Where are the opportunities to improve our health care system?

Is health care a legitimate right in our society, and if so, how can we provide it given the limitation of the health care dollar? What models exist that may inform our query, plus how can we adapt good ideas into a uniquely American approach? As our demographics shift, a solution is imperative because our current path is not sustainable. As nurses, we must be active and informed participants in the discussion, planning, implementation, and evaluation of a new way forward for all, for our patients/clients, and for the health and welfare of our nation.

INTRODUCTION

The importance of health care professionals' awareness and consideration of the economic impact of their decisions has been noted since the early years of cost control in the mid to late 1970s (Hyatt, 1975). Sovie (1985) identified the value of managing nursing resources in a constrained economic environment. Historically, managing costs and revenues had been separated from the clinical and management functions within health care organizations. However, the spiraling cost of health care as a portion of the nation's overall economy and the inefficient distribution and use of scarce resources within the health care sector (Goodell & Ginsberg, 2008; Institute of Medicine, 1999, 2011; Strickler, 2011) underscore the need for health care professionals to understand and incorporate economic principles in their clinical and management decision making.

With the number of registered nurses (RNs) estimated to be greater than 3 million as of 2012, RNs comprise the largest professional group in the health care workforce (Health Resources and Services Administration, 2013). Nurses are in a unique position to influence the efficient and effective use of scarce health care resources. More broadly an understanding of economic principles and the tools of economic evaluation enables nurses to demonstrate the contributions of nursing practice that improve resource use in the production of health care services. Nurses involved in clinical practice, administration, education, policy making, and research can use principles of economics to:

- Provide nursing care in the most cost effective manner.
- Protect the scope of nursing practice by demonstrating the quality and value of nursing services in relation to other professionals.
- Develop opportunities to expand settings for nursing practice by demonstrating the cost and quality of nursing interventions.
- Understand what purchasers and consumers want from nursing and take steps to satisfy these needs and demands.
- Promote health system change to expand access, improve the quality, and ensure more equitable distribution of health care resources (Buerhaus et al., 2012).
- Integrate nursing-specific quality measurement systems and concepts into larger organizational quality improvement initiatives that are largely controlled by nonnurses (Rutherford, 2008).

The purpose of this chapter is to introduce the reader to basic economic concepts that affect professional nursing practice and, more broadly, the delivery of health care services. The chapter is organized into three sections. The first section focuses on the economics of nursing with a particular emphasis on the nursing labor market. The next section addresses economic issues for advocacy to improve the quality and effectiveness of patient care and to inform system change. The third section focuses on health care reform, expanding insurance coverage, and consumerism. Common cost evaluation methods useful in demonstrating the economic effects of health care resource allocation decisions and skill development exercises are additionally presented.

HEALTH ECONOMICS

Economics is the study of the distribution of resources across a population (Sowell, 2011). *Health economics* is the study of the production and distribution of health care resources and their impact on a population (Santerre & Neun, 2013). Health care resources consist of *medical supplies*, such as pharmaceutical goods, latex gloves, and bed linens; *personnel*, including nurses, physicians, and other allied health professionals; and *capital inputs*, including hospitals and nursing home facilities, diagnostic and therapeutic equipment, and other items used to provide medical care (Santerre & Neun, 2013).

Health care resources are scarce; that is, there is a limit to the quantity that can be produced at a given time, although the demand for these resources can be limitless. Therefore economists are interested in how society makes important decisions regarding the *consumption, production, and distribution* of these goods and services within the health care sector and in relation to other societal needs, such as education, housing, and defense. As social scientists, health economists seek to answer four basic questions (Santerre & Neun, 2013):

1. What combination of nonmedical and medical goods and services should be produced in a general economy?
2. What particular medical goods and services should be produced in the health economy?

3. What specific health care resources should be used to produce the final medical goods and services?

4. Who should receive the medical goods and services?

Although economic theory is complex, it is guided by a relatively small set of principles and concepts. These concepts are presented in Box 7-1 and provide the foundation for a more detailed explanation of how economic principles underpin current health care issues discussed in this chapter (Henderson, 2012). Typically economists assume certain conditions to understand human behavior in relation to the production and distribution of resources. Unlike other industries, the health care sector violates a number of assumptions that support general economic theory (Rice, 1998).

Uncertainty

The need for health care services is irregular and cannot be predicted by either consumers or providers (Arrow, 1963; Glaser & Salzberg, 2011). Consumers who demand health care cannot predict when illness or catastrophe will strike, and health care providers cannot forecast the costs of the treatment(s) required. Health care professionals who provide health care interventions also face uncertainty regarding when patients will present themselves for treatment, as well as the extent

---

BOX 7-1   Ten Guiding Principles of Economics

1. The principle of scarcity and choice addresses the problem of limited resources and the need to economize. Not enough resources are available to meet all the desires of all the people, making rationing in some form unavoidable. We are forced to make choices among competing objectives—an inescapable result of scarcity.

2. The principle of opportunity costs recognizes that everything and everyone has alternatives. Time and resources used to satisfy one set of desires cannot be used to satisfy another set. The cost of any decision or action is measured in terms of the value placed on the opportunity forgone.

3. Marginal analysis is a way of thinking about the optimal use of resources. Decision makers weigh the tradeoffs of a little more of one thing and a little less of another. In this decision-making mode, consideration is given to the benefits and costs of one more unit of a good or service.

4. Self-interest is a primary motivator of economic decision makers. People respond to incentives and practice economizing behavior only when they as individuals can benefit from the behavior. In a just society, the pursuit of self-interest leads each individual to a course of action that promotes the general welfare of everyone in society.

5. Markets and pricing serve as the best way to allocate scarce resources. The market accomplishes this through a system of prices—everything has a price that a consumer is willing to pay for a good or service. Prices decrease if less is desired and increase if more is desired. The price mechanism enables a firm to gauge its output decisions in relation to consumer desires and buying behavior. When supply and demand are in balance, the market is in equilibrium.

6. Supply and demand serve as the foundation for all economic analysis. *Supply* refers to the amount of a good or service available to consumers in the market. *Demand* refers to a consumer's willingness to purchase a particular good or service. Goods and services are allocated among competing uses by striking a balance (equilibrium) between the consumers' willingness to pay and the suppliers' willingness to produce goods and ration those goods by the pricing mechanism.

7. Competition forces those who own resources to use their resources to produce the highest possible satisfaction for society—consumers, producers, and investors. Competition stimulates efficiency in a market environment by rewarding the resource owners who do well in producing a good or service with the best combination of available resources and penalizing those who are inept or inefficient in resource allocation decisions.

8. Efficiency in economics measures how well resources are being used to promote social welfare. Inefficient outcomes waste resources, whereas the efficient use of resources enhances social welfare. Resource allocation is considered efficient when no one can be made better off without making someone else worse off. This equalized allocation state is known as the *Pareto Optimum*.

9. Market failure arises when the free market fails to promote the efficient use of resources by producing either more or less than the optimal level of output.

10. Voluntary exchange in a free market environment promotes economic efficiency and ensures that all mutually beneficial transactions occur. Every transaction will benefit both a consumer and a provider. The market system is grounded in the concept of consumer sovereignty—what is produced is determined by what people want and what they are able to buy. No one individual or group dictates what must be produced or purchased.

From Henderson. *Health Economics and Policy (with Economic Applications)*, 5E. © 2012 South-Western, a part of Cengage Learning, Inc. Reproduced by permission. www.cengage.com/permissions.

to which patients will respond to prescribed treatment regimens. The unexpected and often costly nature of illness gives rise to the purchase of insurance as a safeguard against the cost of health care treatment in the event of illness (Folland, Goodman, & Stano, 2012).

Insurance and Third-Party Payment

Consumers buy insurance to guard against the risk and uncertainty of illness. Insurance introduces an intermediary between the consumer (person requiring health care) and the providers of care (health care professionals and organizations). Consumers do not pay the full price for their health care and are separated from making decisions about services based on the price of those services. In economic theory, *price* is the key measure used to determine what a consumer is willing to pay for a good or service and enables an organization to gauge its output in relation to consumer desires and buying behaviors (Folland et al., 2012). *Insurance* also changes the demand for care, and it potentially changes the incentives for providers to offer certain types of treatments that are reimbursed by insurance (Folland et al., 2012).

Problems with Information

Economic theory assumes buyers and sellers have equal information about the cost, price, and quality of goods and services. However, in health care markets, professionals (the sellers) typically have more information about treatment options than do clients (the buyers). In some instances information is unknown to both the professional and the individual. For example, when a person has cancer that has not yet been detected by regular screenings, a treatment course cannot be formulated because neither party knows health care services are needed. The lack of symmetrical information is a problem, because it distorts the basic mechanism of consumer sovereignty, in which consumers (clients) dictate what goods and services are produced because they know what they want and what they are willing to pay (Folland et al., 2012).

Large Role of Nonprofit Firms

Economists assume that organizations seek to maximize profits and that models of firm behavior explain how businesses allocate resources to increase profits. It is important to note that *all* businesses must take in more money than they spend (make a profit or surplus)

for continued operations. Many health care providers—including hospitals, nursing homes, and insurance companies—are operated as not-for-profits. As shown in Figure 7-1, 2894 or 50.57% of the nation's 5723 registered hospitals are organized as privately owned not-for-profit organizations (American Hospital Association, 2014). The nonprofit designation means the facility does not pay either state or local property taxes or federal income taxes because it is considered a charity, and instead provides community benefit, including uncompensated care, in accord with state and federal laws and tax codes (Medicare News Group, 2013). For-profit community hospitals comprise 18.66% of all hospitals, and state and government owned community hospitals comprise 18.12%. Nonfederal psychiatric hospitals comprise 7.22%. The federal government operates 3.69% of the hospitals, with the majority operated by the Veteran's

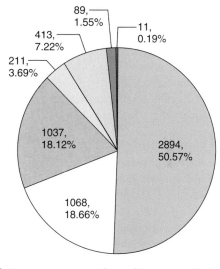

- ▨ Nongovernment not-for-profit community hospitals
- ☐ For-profit community hospitals
- ▨ State and local government community hospitals
- ☐ Federal government hospitals
- ☐ Nonfederal psychiatric hospitals
- ▨ Nonfederal long term care hospitals
- ▨ Hospital units of institutions

FIGURE 7-1 Distribution of U.S. acute care hospitals by type and ownership. (Data from American Hospital Association (AHA). (2014). *Fast facts*. Accessed on June 25, 2014 at http://www.aha.org/research/rc/stat-studies/fast-facts.shtml)

Administration. Nonfederal long-term care hospitals and others, which includes prison and campus hospital units comprise 1.6% and 0.2%, respectively.

Restrictions on Competition

Competition is a force that produces the most efficient allocation of resources because owners must use their resources to produce the highest satisfaction for society. Economists assume markets are perfectly competitive, consisting of numerous buyers and sellers, with no power over price, who have complete information, and can enter and exit the market freely by selling similar goods or services (Folland et al., 2012). Health care markets violate several of these assumptions. As described previously, health care markets are characterized by asymmetrical information and have weak pricing mechanisms because of third-party payment in the form of insurance. In addition, market entry is blocked by licensure for professional practice, advertising restrictions, and ethical standards that prevent providers from competing with one another. Because health care is considered to be a *public good*, organizations in the sector are subjected to regulation by state and federal government, as well as other outside entities, to ensure the quality of care and distribution of resources across geographic areas (Hoffman, Klees, & Curtis, 2007).

Role of Equity and Need

Economics is concerned with the distribution of scarce resources so that society receives the highest possible satisfaction from the combination of goods and services produced from these resources. *Distributive justice,* or *equity,* is the extent to which resources are allocated in a fair and equal manner to everyone involved (Baumrucker et al., 2012). In pure market economies, the price mechanism is used to strike a balance (equilibrium) between the price suppliers charge and the price purchasers are willing to pay. In pure egalitarian systems governments ensure everyone receives an equal distribution of resources (Folland et al., 2012).

The U.S. health care system is a mixed system in which goods and services are distributed both by markets and by government. The mixed system of markets and government is a factor in the inequitable distribution of health care resources, most notably in the lack of universal insurance or universal access to health care services in the United States. Advocates argue that in a just society people ought to get the health care they need, regardless of their ability to pay for these services (Daniels, Saloner, & Gelpi, 2009). We examine this topic in more detail in the section on health care reform.

Government Subsidies and Public Provision

The health care sector has more government intervention than other sectors of the national economy because of the uncertainty in the demand for, and provision of, services. In the United States, state and federal governments play major roles as financiers and payers of health care through the Medicare, Medicaid, and State Children's Health Insurance Programs (CHIPs). Medicare is the federal insurance program established in 1965 for persons older than 65 years of age, as well as for selected populations with severe and chronic disabilities. The Medicare program is divided into four parts (Medicare A, B, C, and D) and provides benefits for hospitalization, limited nursing home care, physicians' services, medical supplies, outpatient services, and most recently, prescription drugs. In comparison, Medicaid, also established in 1965, is a joint federal and state-funded insurance program that provides medical and health-related services to America's poorest people. Each state administers its own Medicaid program and sets eligibility requirements for program participation and the type of benefits and services covered. The CHIP was established in 1997 as part of the Federal Balanced Budget Act to extend health insurance benefits to children of families who do not qualify for the Medicaid program but are unable to buy private health insurance. Together, Medicare and Medicaid rose from 1.8 percent of Gross Domestic Product (GDP) in 1985 to 4.6 percent in 2012 (Congressional Budget Office, 2013; Topoleski, 2013).

ECONOMIC CONCEPTS SPECIFIC TO THE NURSING PROFESSION

The Supply and Demand for Nurses: The Cyclical Nature of the Nursing Workforce

In this section we examine the market for nurses to illustrate the concepts of supply and demand. The concepts of complements and substitutes are also presented to examine the use of advanced practice nurses (APNs) as an alternative to physicians as primary care providers.

Supply refers to the amount of a good or service available to consumers in the market and *demand* refers to a consumer's willingness to purchase a particular good or service (Santerre & Neun, 2013).

Economic theory predicts as demand increases, so will supply; the pricing mechanism, in the form of wages and other benefits, will create a balance (equilibrium) between firms in need of workers and individuals who are willing to work for the wage offered. When examining the market for labor, economists assume households have primary and secondary wage earners. Because a very high proportion of nurses are married, they are considered to be part of two-earner families and therefore have more flexibility to respond to employment opportunities as real wages change or in relation to the employment situation of their spouses (Santerre & Neun, 2013).

Nurses' decisions to enter the work force, as well as how many hours they work while employed, are cyclical in nature. In fact, there have been cyclical shortages and surpluses of nurses documented since the 1960s (American Nurses Association, 2011; Janiszewski Goodin, 2003). Data on the supply and distribution of nurses come from a variety of sources and are published primarily by the Bureau of Health Professions of the Health Resources and Services Administration (HRSA) and the Bureau of Health Professions' National Center for Health Workforce Analysis (Bureau of Health Professions, 2013a). Studies are usually published every 4 to 5 years, and usually are based on data that is 2 to 3 years old by the time it is published (Bureau of Health Professions, 2013a). The U.S. Health Workforce Chartbook (Bureau of Health Professions, 2013b) also provides data on a wide variety of other health workers, including, physicians, counselors, physical therapists, laboratory technicians, nursing assistants, and others.

The National Center for Health Workforce Analysis conducted the inaugural National Sample of Nurse Practitioners in 2012 (Bureau of Health Professions, 2012), which used a representative sample of 13,000 randomly selected nurse practitioners (NP) to establish national estimates of the NP workforce, with respect to education, certification, and practice patterns. There were an estimated 150,000 NPs with 132,000 practicing as NPs. Eleven thousand practiced in RN roles, and an equal number were not employed in nursing (Bureau of Health Professions, 2012).

The most recent study on the RN workforce is The U.S. Nursing Workforce: Trends in Supply and Education report, published by the National Center for Health

Workforce Analysis (Bureau of Health Professions, 2013c). The report is based on a 10-year span of data collected by the U.S. Census Bureau, using the American Community Survey 2008 to 2010 and the Census 2000 Long Form, and data on the nursing education pipeline from the National Council of State Boards in Nursing (NCSBN). The model used to project supply for clinicians in general is shown in Figure 7-2.

The RN nursing workforce increased by 24%, and outpaced the growth in the overall population during the same period. The number of RNs per 100,000 population (per capita) increased by 14%; the number of licensed practical nurses (LPNs) increased by 6%. Between 2008 and 2010, there were 2.8 million RNs and almost 700,000 LPNs working or seeking employment in nursing. Although the absolute number of RNs younger than 30 years of age increased, about one third of the nursing workforce is older than 50 years of age. The average age of nurses has increased over the past decade by almost 2 years for RNs and 1.75 years for LPNs, reflecting aging within the very large cohort of nurses aged 41 to 50 in 2000 (Bureau of Health Professions, 2013c).

The study draws from census demographic data to better describe the RN workforce population. The percentage of the RN workforce holding a bachelor's or higher degree increased from 50% to 55% over the past decade. The workforce has also become more diverse in race and gender. The proportion of non-white RNs increased from 20% to 25% during the past decade. The proportion of men in the RN workforce increased from 7.7% in 2000 to 9.1% in 2010 (p. 24).

The majority of RNs, 63%, provide inpatient and outpatient care in hospitals. Although the distribution of RNs across settings held steady over the past decade, the number of RNs working in hospitals increased by more than 350,000, or by 25%. In contrast to RNs, less than one third of LPNs, 29%, work in hospitals, and that proportion has declined slightly over the past decade (p. 25).

Significant positive growth has occurred in the nursing pipeline, as measured by the annual number of individuals who pass national nurse licensing exams. The number of RNs who passed the NCLEX-RN increased 108% between 2001 and 2011, and the number of LPNs who passed the NCLEX-PN increased 80%. In 2011, more than 142,000 new graduate RNs passed the NCLEX-RN as compared with 68,561 in 2001. The number of bachelor's prepared RN candidates taking

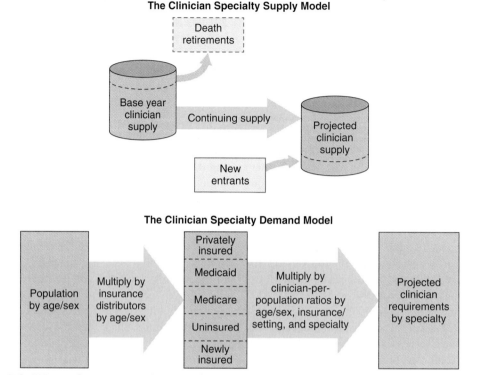

FIGURE 7-2 Basic models for forecasting supply and demand of health care profession-als in a dynamic market. (From Salsberg, E. (2013). *Projecting future clinical supply and demand: Advances and challenges.* National Center for Health Workforce Analysis Health Resources and Services Administration U.S. Department of Health and Human Services http://bhpr.hrsa.gov/healthworkforce/supplydemand/supplyanddemand.pdf)

the exam for the first time more than doubled, from 24,832 individuals in 2001 to 58,246 in 2011. Non–bachelor's prepared RN candidates taking the exam for the first time increased from 43,927 in 2001 to 86,337 in 2011. Non-bachelor's prepared RN candidates continue to constitute the majority of all RN candidates (60% in 2011) (p. 38).

The National Sample Survey of Registered Nurses (NSSRN), published every 4 years since 1980 by the Bureau of Health Professions' Division of Nursing, is the most extensive national source of RN statistical data. The survey uses a sample drawn from the State Boards of Nursing, and includes data from nurses whether or not they are practicing. The survey assesses the number of RNs, educational background, employ-ment setting, position, specialty areas, job satisfac-tion, and salary. In addition, the survey also identifies the geographic distribution of nurses throughout the

United States, as well as the personal composition of the U.S. nursing workforce in terms of gender, racial/ethnic background, age, and family structure.

The latest version, using data from 2008 and pub-lished in 2010, reinforces some of the findings from the Trends in Supply and Education report, but adds infor-mation regarding higher education, employment within and outside nursing, earnings, satisfaction, job changes, and future employment plans. In addition, the survey captures data from nurse faculty, nurse practitioners, nurse midwives, nurse anesthetists, and clinical nurse specialists. Further information is obtained regarding new graduates and those approaching retirement.

The Survey estimates a total of 3,063,162 licensed RNs, a net increase of 153,806 since 2004 (Bureau of Health Professions, 2013a). An estimated 444,668 RNs received their first U.S. license from 2004 through 2008, thus approximately 291,000 RNs allowed their U.S. licenses to lapse, possibly indicating the beginning of the expected substantial number of retirements.

The most common job title of RNs in the United States is "staff nurse" or equivalent (66%). Approximately 20% of nurses with graduate degrees hold staff nurse positions. The next most common job title in 2008 included management and administration titles (12.5%). Many RNs hold more than one job in nursing. Overall about 12% of RNs who have a full-time primary nursing position and 14% of those with part-time primary positions have additional nursing positions (Bureau of Health Professions, 2012).

Information on job changes and future employment plans provides insight on movement within and out of the profession. Among nurses who worked full-time in 2007, 11.6% changed to a different employer by 2008. Six percent of these RNs worked with the same employer, but held a different position. More than 73% of RNs reported they changed positions or employers owing at least in part to workplace issues, such as lack of good management or inadequate staffing. Personal career reasons, such as interest in another position or improved pay or benefits, were also identified as factors in job change decisions. The percentage of employed RNs under 55 years old who intended to leave nursing within 3 years is 3% or fewer (Bureau of Health Professions, 2012).

Among RNs age 55 and older who worked in nursing in 2008, 12.5% intended to leave the nursing profession within 3 years and another 9% intended to leave their current nursing jobs and were undecided about remaining in nursing. Of those who were employed in 2007 but not in 2008, 27.3% reported they stopped working because of retirement (Bureau of Health professions, 2012).

Studies generated from secondary analysis of publicly available data sets also provide useful information of nursing supply and demand. For example, Buerhaus and colleagues (2013) used publicly available data to provide regional-level projections to better inform policy and initiatives in specific regions. Key findings identify states whose RN workforce is expected to grow at slower rates relative to other states. The South and Midwest states have a greater supply of younger RNs to replace older RNs, and the Northeast and western states have fewer younger RNs compared with the number of older RNs. Understanding regional differences can lead

---

BOX 7-2   Supply and Demand: Estimating the Nursing Workforce

Determining the presence and severity of a nursing shortage, requires analysis of both the supply and demand of RNs within the health care labor market. It is generally accepted that there has been a looming nursing workforce shortage over the past 10 to 15 years owing primarily to (1) the aging of the nurse workforce, (2) insufficient nursing school enrollment and graduations, and (3) an increased demand for healthcare services due to the increased proportion of the elderly and the increased prevalence of chronic illness and disease. The National Center for Health Workforce Analysis within the Health Resources and Services Administration is the centralized agency that collects, analyzes, and publishes data related to the supply and demand of health care professions, including nursing.

Edward Salsberg (2013), Director of the National Center for Health Workforce Analysis, outlined the advances and challenges associated with projecting the supply and demand of the various health professions in a presentation at the 2013 National Health Policy Forum. Salsberg cautions that projections are not predictions. In fact, projections are based on a set of underlying assumptions, whereas predictions represent expectations of actual future events.

As shown in Figure 7-1, the basic supply model starts with data for a specific baseline period, and then projects deaths and retirements that reduce the end result and new entrants or graduates that increase the end result. The basic demand model focuses on population health needs as defined by age and gender, and then projects usage based on insurance coverage and clinician requirements by specialty.

Challenges in projecting supply and demand include:
- Availability of research and data to inform modeling
- Projecting the future based on the past
- Uncertainty of many possible changes in delivery and financing
- Extent of supply and demand interaction
- The unit of analysis is critical; (national) averages can mask enormous variations within the units being studied (communities)
- Resources needed for systematic assessment of each occupation/specialty (one size does not fit all)
- Identifying policy levers to influence future supply and demand

---

to better decision making related to nursing supply and demand. See Box 7-2 for more insight into estimating the nursing workforce.

Monopsony Power of Hospitals

In a well-functioning market, a shortage should be resolved by wage increases until a balance is restored (equilibrium) between organizations in need of workers and workers who are willing to participate in the labor force. One argument used to explain the chronic shortage of nurses is the notion that nurses are underpaid and it is the low wages, relative to other health professionals, as well as other job opportunities outside of nursing and health care, that keep individuals from participating in the workforce as RNs. From a purely economic perspective, linking the labor shortage to low wages is curious because it violates the basic assumptions of supply and demand. The monopsony model, which examines how employers set wages and make decisions about hiring workers, is used to explain this puzzle and provides a partial explanation as to why the market for RNs does not conform to the predictions of supply and demand. More specifically, the monopsony model explains the coexistence of high vacancy rates and lower-than-competitive wages for nurses (Folland et al., 2012).

Although nurses are employed in a number of community settings, hospitals are the main employer of nurses. Approximately 63% of RNs are employed in acute care hospital settings (National Center for Health Workforce Analysis, 2013). Therefore most of the information about the market for nursing labor is understood within the context of hospitals. The monopsony model is based on the assumptions that (1) the market has one dominant buyer (employer) or perhaps a few employers in a regional market who control the demand for workers, and (2) all persons who do the same work are paid the same wage. Because workers are paid the same wage, if the employer has to offer a higher wage to get additional workers, it must also raise the wages of the workers already employed. Eventually, all of the operating budget would go to paying salaries and the hospital would not be able to make a surplus or profit. As discussed previously, organizations need to make a surplus to stay in business.

The hospital using the monopsony model considers the cost of hiring one more nurse in relation to the amount of revenue it will gain from the productivity of that nurse. In effect, the hospital sets nurses' wages so it maximizes its ability to make a profit. In this situation, the wage level that satisfies the hospital's profit goal is lower than what nurses could be offered if there were more buyers in the market. Because nurses often have choices about participating in the labor force, they may decide the wage offered by a hospital is too low and

decide to forgo working for a particular hospital. Thus the hospital will continue to need nurses and the nurses' wages will be lower than other comparable workers.

In contrast markets with many hospitals competing for nursing labor conform more closely to the predictions of supply and demand. As noted previously the presence of multiple competitors (hospitals) in one market provides more favorable conditions for workers in terms of the wages employers will offer to satisfy their demand for labor. Under competitive market conditions, when faced with a shortage of nurses, some hospitals will move faster than others and offer a higher wage for nurses. The wage increase brings about two important outcomes that, taken together, help to alleviate the nursing shortage. In the short term, increased wages are incentives for nurses who are currently unemployed to join the workforce.

Additionally nurses who are currently employed may respond to the higher wages by working overtime hours, taking a second job, or changing from part-time to full-time employment. These responses typically increase the short-term supply of nurses participating in the workforce in RN roles. In the long term, the increased wages offered by hospitals and other organizations influence individuals' decisions to enter the nursing profession and are one mechanism to ensure an adequate supply of nurses (Buerhaus, 2008). Limited evidence suggests that increases in nurses' wages may have a positive impact on increasing the number of employed RNs. A study by the Institute for Women's Policy Research (2006) examined the relationship between hospital nurses' inflation-adjusted median weekly earnings and the number of nurses employed. Employment levels were flat from 1996 to 2001, but rose in 2002, following a wage increase in 2001. Employment growth continued in 2003, but decreased following the wage decrease in 2004 (pp. 9–10). More recent studies on the relationship between wages and nurse employment are not available. Buerhaus (2008) reports between 2002 and 2006 real wages for nurses in the United States increased an average of 6.9%, producing the expected drop in hospital RN vacancy rates from a national average of 13% reported in 2001 to 8.1% by 2006.

Although there have been reports in the popular media about hospitals' somewhat extravagant tactics to attract nurses—for instance, $100,000 annual salaries for experienced nurses and other incentives such as flat-screen TVs, gift certificates, and car leases in the past (Robert Wood Johnson Foundation, 2009)—there is no clear evidence that hospitals instituted wage controls in response to the national recession of 2008–2009. The Farlex Financial Dictionary (2012) defines wage controls as restrictions on wage or salary increases in a given year. Buerhaus (2008) warned against the use of wage controls to control nursing costs, which fails to recognize that any short-term savings would be vastly offset by the long-term costs associated with an exacerbated reduction in the nurse supply.

Given the changing population demographics in combination with the existing labor shortage, widespread use of wage controls may have destructive consequences for the nursing profession, patients, and hospitals.

It is important to note nurses' decisions to participate in the workforce are complex and are not fully explained by economic theory. Managerial and public policies targeting cost containment, such as efforts to reduce in-patient length of stay (LOS), have had a greater impact on the working conditions of nurses and have contributed to the duration of the current shortage (Aiken, 2008). Strong evidence suggests attributes of the organizational environment, also referred to as the *nursing practice environment*, factor into individual nurses' decisions to stay employed at a particular hospital or to participate in the workforce in the capacity as a registered nurse. Organizational factors such as work load, managers' leadership style, autonomy over nursing practice, promotion opportunities, and work schedules also contribute to nurses' decisions to work (Aiken, 2008; Brewer et al., 2006; Hayes et al., 2006).

Nurses as Complements and Substitutes for Physicians

Complements are products or services that are usually consumed jointly, so that an increase in the price of one decreases the demand for both (e.g., intravenous fluids and tubing) (Santerre & Neun, 2013). If nursing services are complements to physician services, then an increase in the price of physician services will decrease the demand for both physician and nursing services.

Substitutes, on the other hand, are goods or services that satisfy the same want or need, so an increase in the price of one will increase the demand for the other (Santerre & Neun, 2013). One example of substitutes in health care occurs when two medications have the same therapeutic effect. Another example is an obstetrician and a nurse midwife. If nursing services are substitutes

for physician obstetric services, then an increase in the cost of physician services will increase the demand for nursing midwife services.

In the physician arena an imbalance exists between generalists and specialists, resulting in a shortage of primary care physicians (Hauer et al., 2008; Mitka, 2007; National Center for Health Workforce Analysis, 2013). This disparity between consumer demand and physician supply creates favorable opportunities for APNs to practice in primary care centers as physician substitutes. Nurses are making arguments for their use as substitutes for more expensive providers of care for services that they have been formally trained to provide. For example, nurse practitioners work as primary care providers in hospital-based outpatient clinics or private practice. As the number of physicians in primary care practice falls short of the need, nurse practitioners and physician assistants will partially fill the gap between supply and demand. The nurse practitioners will likely increase in overall number and those employed in non-advanced practice roles will have the opportunity to shift to primary care roles (National Center for Health Workforce Analysis, 2013). Similarly, health care delivery organizations, in an effort to reduce input costs, are incorporating the use of unlicensed personnel as substitutes for nurses for those activities that do not require licensure. For example, hospitals and other delivery organizations have changed the nursing staff skill mix to include RNs, LRNs, and nursing assistants. Thus nurses are both substituting for some types of providers and being substituted by other types of providers.

Physicians have traditionally held a monopolistic power as primary care providers because regulations have prevented others from "practicing medicine." As alternative providers of health care services demonstrate their ability to provide comparable services, regulations are being changed to allow these substitutes to enter the market and compete with physicians. Such changes in regulation have come about because consumers have demanded more cost-effective providers, whereas organized physician interests have lost political power (e.g., the journal *Nurse Practitioner* for an annual legislative review governing advanced nursing practice).

With APNs working as physician substitutes, competition between these two providers can occur on the basis of cost effectiveness. Studies have demonstrated that the use of APNs as primary care providers can reduce costs of outpatient care, including laboratory costs, per-visit costs, per-episode costs, and long-term management costs (American Association of Nurse Practitioners, 2013; Brown & Grimes, 1993; Fulton & Baldwin, 2004; Schroeder, 1993; U.S. Congress, 1986). Nurse-managed services are typically those services offered by APNs (NPs, clinical nurse specialists, nurse midwives, and nurse anesthetists) based on the nursing philosophy emphasizing health promotion and preventative care—for example, chronic disease management, case management, or primary care. Researcher have documented that nurse-managed care, when compared with physician-managed care, reduces the frequency of hospitalizations, reduces the acuity of those admitted, reduces lengths of stay, reduces the cost of hospitalization, and results in equivalent ratings for patient satisfaction with service delivery (Brooten, Youngblut, Kutcher, & Bobo, 2004; Mundinger et al., 2000). Given the evidence for the efficacy of nurse-managed services, nurse leaders are developing arguments that move beyond comparing APNs as substitutes and complements to physician services and focus on the unique aspects and additional value of APNs in achieving optimal patient outcomes (Kleinpell & Gawlinski, 2005; Lin, Gebbie, Fullilove, & Arons, 2004; Mundinger, 2002; United Health Group, 2009). Newhouse et al. (2011) completed a systematic review of APN outcome studies from 1990 to 2008, and identified conclusive evidence that APNs provide effective and high quality care.

Retail clinics differ from urgent care clinics because they are located within discount stores, grocery stores, or drug stores; are staffed by either nurse practitioners or physician assistants; and offer a limited set of basic medical and preventative services. Retail clinics are an emerging trend whereby APNs act as substitutes for physicians to meet consumers' desire for more convenient and lower-cost medical care (The Advisory Board, 2013; PriceWaterhouseCoopers, 2013). Health care services typically offered at retail clinics include preventative care such as immunizations and blood pressure screening, as well as treatment for upper respiratory, sinusitis, ear, or urinary tract infections. Clients mainly pay for retail visits out of pocket, although in recent years many insurance companies, including Medicare and Medicaid, will pay for these visits (Mehrotra, Wang, Lave, Adams, & McGlynn, 2008; Pollack,

Gidengil, & Mehrota, 2010). Mehrotra and Lave (2012) in a Rand study, determined that retail clinic visits, usually to nurse practitioners, quadrupled from 2007 to 2009 (Figure 7-3). Retail clinics offer an alternative to urgent care clinics and emergency departments for simple acute problems. Despite the national shortage of primary care physicians, the emergence of these nurse-led clinics has drawn the ire of some medical societies, who question their quality and are asking for increased regulation. For instance, the American Medical Association, the American Academy of Family Physicians, and several state medical societies are recommending certain operating requirements, including limits on the scope of clinical services, the creation of referral systems with physician practices, and the use of electronic patient records (PricewaterhouseCoopers, 2013).

In an early evaluation comparing the client demographics of, and reasons for, visits to retail clinics, primary care physicians, and emergency departments, Mehrotra and colleagues (2008) found that retail clinics show signs of becoming *safety net providers* by offering services to a population that is currently underserved by primary care physicians. Clients seen at retail clinics were more likely to be young adults, between the ages of 18 and 44 years, who pay out of pocket for their care and are less likely to have an existing relationship with a primary care provider. Approximately 90% of retail clinic visits focus on treating 10 minor acute

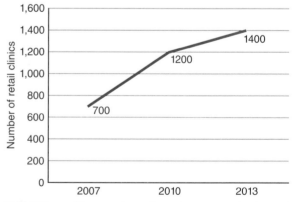

FIGURE 7-3 The number of retail clinics in the United States, 2007–2013. (Data from Mehrotra, A., & Lave, J. (2012). Visits to retail clinics grew fourfold from 2007 to 2009. *Rand Health.* http://www.rand.org/health/feature/retail-clinics.html)

conditions; these same conditions represent 13% of adult primary care physician visits, 30% of pediatric primary care physician visits, and 12% of emergency department visits. These early data suggest that nurse-led retail clinics serve an important role in expanding access to primary care services and relieve the stress on emergency departments. Whether there will be continued expansion and a widespread shift of uncomplicated acute care services from primary care physicians and emergency departments to retail clinics remains to be seen.

ECONOMIC CONCEPTS FOR ADVOCACY AND PROFESSIONAL PRACTICE

In this section we examine a number of economic concepts and how they affect health care delivery and professional nursing practice. We begin by examining the nature of health insurance markets and the relationship between insurance and access to health care. Next, we discuss relationships among cost, quality, and value and the role of technology as a key driver of health care costs. Finally, we examine the concepts of efficiency and effectiveness and present evaluation tools to assess the distribution and benefits of health care interventions.

Paying for Health Care: Insurance, National Health Expenditures, and Access to Care

This section begins with a brief overview of key concepts used to understand how health insurance affects the demand for medical care from the perspectives of consumers and providers. The discussion then turns to comparing the major types of health insurance and concludes by presenting current data on the rising financial burdens faced by U.S. consumers to pay for health care and the problems of the uninsured and underinsured.

Because medical care is costly and it is difficult to predict when one might need medical services, insurance functions as a buffer from the financial risks associated with treating illness or disease. People buy insurance as a way to avoid the *risks* and associated costs of illness and seeking medical treatment. A number of risks are associated with health. There is a risk to one's health or life associated with illness or disease. There is the additional risk that a given treatment course will not cure or alleviate the underlying disease. Also, there may be unavoidable harm from the treatment itself or

by the lack of skill or negligence on the part of the provider. There is a risk of incurring the costs that may be substantial to pay for any treatments. Individuals can take certain actions to reduce the risk of illness—getting vaccinations, avoiding dangerous environments, or leading a healthy lifestyle—but this considerable risk still remains largely uncertain (Folland et al., 2012; Santerre & Neun, 2013).

People buy health insurance to avoid the risk of having to pay for expensive medical care. Stated a different way, people are "risk averse" and try to safeguard their wealth or resources by buying insurance as protection from the financial consequences of an unpredictable event. Economists view risk aversion as a characteristic of people's utility functions (Folland et al., 2012). Marginal utility is the extra satisfaction, welfare, or well-being (utility) gained from consuming one more unit of a good or service. In the case of insurance, it is believed that people are more likely to buy insurance to cover low-probability events involving large losses than high-probability events associated with small losses (Kunreuther & Pauly, 2013).

Although it is difficult to predict when an individual will become sick or need expensive medical care, the risk for large numbers of people (or the expected value of all losses averaged over all people) is quite predictable. Insurance spreads risk across a group of people and involves a series of trades between people. This practice is known as *risk pooling*. Money is shifted between people who are healthy to people who are sick and in need to pay for expensive medical care. Insurance pools potential losses, but it does not eliminate or reduce the losses. That is, insurance companies specialize in *pricing* risks, not in taking risks. Insurance companies sell policies to large groups of people with predictable or average risks. Members pay a premium, which covers all losses across the group of policy holders as well as management fees (Getzen, 2004).

Moral hazard occurs when a person's behavior changes based on his or her insurance coverage. In the event of an illness or other adverse event, the insured person is offered medical care at a reduced price. Moral hazard in health insurance markets occurs to the extent that insurance increases the quantity of medical care used (Chernew, Hirth, Sonnad, Ermann, & Fendrick, 1998; Freeman, Kadiyala, Bell, & Martin, 2008; Johnson-Lans, 2006; Newhouse, 1992). One way insurance companies offset the risk of moral hazard is to require cost sharing with consumers. Deductibles and co-payments are two commonly used methods.

Co-payment is a sharing relationship between the consumer and the insurance company, as specified in a given policy. When consumers seek medical care, the insurance company pays for some of the costs and the consumer pays for the remainder (the co-payment). A *deductible* is a fixed amount that the consumer must pay toward a medical bill each year before any insurance payments are made. Deductibles are designed to generate more prudent care decisions on the part of the policy holder because they dissuade consumers from submitting claims to the insurance company for "small" losses or minor services (Getzen, 2004).

Consumers purchase health care depending on their perceptions of the impact of the care on their health (Kunreuther & Pauly, 2013). That is, consumers purchase health care, but their actual desire, with a few exceptions, is health. Thus the demand for health care "is derived from the more basic demand for health" (Feldstein, 1983, p. 81). The decision to purchase health care also depends on the cost of care to the consumer. Total consumer costs of health care include monetary costs (co-payment, deductibles, insurance premiums, out-of-pocket expenses, and lost time from wages and work), as well as nonmonetary costs (e.g., risk, pain, inconvenience).

The demand for health care also depends on the willingness of consumers to purchase services after weighing the expected benefits of the care against the costs of the care. If consumers carry insurance, their direct out-of-pocket expenses for the care will be less than if they are uninsured (Kunreuther & Pauly, 2013). Therefore the insurance status of consumers has an impact on the costs of care (to the consumers) and thus their demand for care.

Despite the fact consumers make co-payments and pay deductibles, they are generally insulated from the high costs of health care because insurance companies typically pay such a large portion of a bill. This separation of consumers from the price of health care resulting from health insurance coverage (either private or public) has dramatically increased demand for health care services. However, because demand is based on willingness and ability to purchase, demand for health care does not necessarily correlate with the need for health care. Demand for health care services changes over time as societal demographics and morbidity

patterns change. For instance, as baby boomers continue to age, the percentage of the population age 80 years and older will continue to increase proportionately. Their demands for health care will contribute to the already increasing demands of an existing elderly population (Redfoot, Feinberg, & Houser, 2013). Redfoot et al. identified the ratio of family caregivers to elder to be 7 to 1 in 2010. This ratio is expected to decrease to 4 to 1 by 2013 and 3 to 1 in 2050, when all baby boomers will be in the high-risk age group (p. 1).

Demand for specific services is also influenced by the recommendations and decisions of health care providers (Feldstein, 1983). Because providers of care possess more knowledge regarding treatment options than consumers do, the practice styles of providers, as well as how much information they share with consumers, can greatly affect the demand and consumption of services (Devers, Brewster, & Casalino, 2003; Felland, Grossman, & Tu, 2011). Similarly, the risk of litigation by consumers can result in a "defensive" practice style by providers. Fear of litigation can lead to overprescription of (often unnecessary) diagnostic tests or therapeutic interventions and ultimately result in higher health care costs.

The demand for health care services is not directly related to the amount or quality of services purchased as in other industries. This, in conjunction with the high levels of uncertainty and the unequal information among consumers, providers, and payers, leads to a situation called *market failure*. Market failure is characterized by the inability of buyers and sellers to strike a balance in the supply and demand of goods and services and ultimately fail to produce a socially desirable level of output (Santerre & Neun, 2013). For example, variation in the quality of care is an example of market failure arising from imperfect consumer information about physician practice patterns. This implies that some patients are getting too much treatment and some too little treatment. In fact, it is well documented that many Americans do not receive care that is based on the best scientific knowledge (Institute of Medicine, 2010a). More generally, supply-side drivers leading to market failure include the cost of care for hospital and physician services, access to care because of the prohibitive cost of health insurance, and medical outcomes and population health status in light of invested resources. Demand-side factors of market failure in health care include third-party insurance mechanism, in which the insurance company or government entity under the Medicare and Medicaid programs is the primary purchaser of health care services (Henderson, 2012).

Types of Insurance

There are four dominant methods consumers use to pay for their health care in the United States: out-of-pocket payment, private individual insurance, employer-sponsored group insurance, and public or government-sponsored individual or group insurance. Each of these payment modes can be viewed as a historical progression and as a categorization of current health care financing (Bodenheimer & Grumbach, 2012).

Out-of-Pocket Payment. Out-of-pocket payment for health care services is the simplest form of financing because the consumer directly pays the provider for services. This was the dominant model of paying for health care services in the 19th and early 20th centuries, when the technology and available interventions to cure disease or alleviate the symptoms of illness were relatively weak. However, out-of-pocket payment is a flawed way to pay for health care, especially because health care services have become more complex and increasingly expensive. Individuals cannot save or borrow enough money to pay for health care services.

Private Individual Insurance. This form of financing adds a third party (the insurance company) to the relationship between the consumer and provider. Payment for health care services is divided into two parts, a premium paid by the individual to the insurance company and a reimbursement payment to the provider from the insurance company. Indemnity insurance adds a third payment transaction: a reimbursement to the individual from the insurance company. Because of the administrative costs in managing these transactions, individual health insurance never became a dominant method of paying for health care (Starr, 1982). Currently individual policies provide health insurance for 9.8% in 2012, compared with only 3% of the U.S. population in 2008 (DeNavas-Walt, Proctor, & Smith, 2013; U.S. Census Bureau, 2013). Because of the growing burden of uninsurance and underinsurance, individual policies are gaining acceptance as a plausible way to expand insurance benefits, although their use remains limited (Claxton et al., 2007).

Health Savings Accounts. Health Savings Accounts (HSAs) were created by Congress in 2003 to allow individuals to pay for selected health care expenses with pre-tax dollars. Individuals pre-select the amount of money they have withheld from their gross income, and approved expenses are covered by this account. Thus individuals save the amount of money they would have incurred in income tax for these expenses (The Kaiser Family Foundation, 2006).

Employer-Sponsored Group Insurance. Employer-sponsored group insurance came into being during the Great Depression and expanded rapidly after World War II (Starr, 1982). The American Hospital Association first established the Blue Cross of California in 1939, offering hospital insurance to groups of workers. The first employer-based insurance plans were initiated by physicians and hospitals seeking a steady source of income, generous reimbursements, and protection from cost controls (Starr, 1982), all of which had declined during the Great Depression because people were not able to pay for their medical and hospital expenses out of pocket.

With employer-based insurance, the employer pays most of the premium to purchase health insurance on behalf of their employees (Fronstin, 2012). Thus in the United States, health insurance became a benefit of employment. The government treats employee health benefits as a tax-deductible business expense for employers (Fronstin, 2012). Because each dollar of employer-sponsored health insurance results in a reduction in taxes collected, the federal government is in essence subsidizing employer-sponsored insurance. This subsidy is estimated to be about $184 billion per year (Fronstin, 2012). Insurance increased the demand for, and cost of, medical services, which become difficult to control.

Public or Government-Sponsored Insurance. The U.S. government became involved in the financing of health care during the Great Depression (Starr, 1982). Individuals not participating in the labor force, especially the elderly and those with chronic conditions or low incomes, found it increasingly difficult to buy insurance on their own. This led to the creation of the government-sponsored Medicare and Medicaid programs in the mid-1960s, the State Children's Health Insurance Program in 1997, the establishment of health savings accounts in 2003, and the more recent Affordable Care Act (ACA) of 2010.

Government health insurance for the poor and elderly adds the taxpayer to the equation as the ultimate payer.

Much like private insurance, beneficiaries are required to make a contribution in order to receive benefits. Taxpayers need to contribute a certain amount to social security taxes to be eligible for Medicare (Santerre & Neun, 2012). In comparison, the state-funded Medicaid program is funded by taxpayer contributions, although not all taxpayers are eligible for Medicaid benefits. Because these programs are tax-funded, there is a double subsidy at play for taxpayers. As with private insurance, benefits are shifted from those who are healthy to those who are sick. The government-sponsored programs add an additional distribution of funds between the wealthy and the poor. That is, the healthy middle-income employees generally pay more Social Security taxes than they receive in health services (Bodenheimer & Grumbach, 2012). Unemployed, disabled, and lower-income elderly persons may receive more in health services than they contribute in taxes (Bodenheimer & Grumbach, 2012).

Trends in National Health Care Expenditures and Insurance Coverage in the United States

Health care costs in the United States have been rising for decades. Deemed "unsustainable" by many, the pressure to slow the steady rise of costs resulted in the passage of the Patient Protection and Affordable Care Act (PPACA) of 2010, addressed in detail elsewhere in this chapter and textbook (Chapter 6). It is important to understand the impact and trends in health care costs increases and the increasing burden of health insurance.

TRENDS IN HEALTH CARE COSTS

In 2012 U.S. health care spending reached $2.8 trillion, an increase of 3.7% from 2011 (Centers for Medicare & Medicaid Services, 2013a). This was the fourth consecutive year of low growth, although the overall GDP share comprised of health care expenditures decreased from 17.3% in 2011 to 17.2% in 2012. Health care expenditures have increased as a proportion of the overall economy over time, from 5% of the GDP in 1960, reaching double digits in 1980, and reaching its peak of 17.4% in 2010 (Centers for Medicare & Medicaid Services, 2013a). The gross domestic product (GDP) represents the total dollar value of all goods and services produced over a specific period of time. The GDP represents the total value of the economy, and now almost one dollar of every five is spent on health care.

The United States spends substantially more on health care than other developed countries (Organisation for Economic Cooperation and Development, 2013). Table 7-1 shows per capita health expenditures in 2011 U.S. dollars for select Organisation for Economic Co-operation and Development (OECD) countries with above-average per capita national income. According to OECD (2013) data, health spending per capita in the United States was $8508 in 2011. This amount was more than double the spending in the United Kingdom, Japan, and France, and almost twice the expense in Canada and Germany. Despite this relatively higher

TABLE 7-1 A Comparison of Key Health Care Statistics for Select Industrialized Nations, 2011

	CANADA	FRANCE	GERMANY	JAPAN	UNITED KINGDOM	UNITED STATES
Population (millions)	33.74	62.63	81.9	127.51	60.93	307.01
GDP (adjusted for purchasing parity, expressed in millions of U.S. dollars)	$40,643	$35,500	$39,779	$33,469	$36,223	$48,068
Health care spending per capita	$4552	$4118	$4495	$3213	$3405	$8508
Health care spending as percentage of GDP	11.2%	11.6%	11.3%	9.6%	9.4%	17.7%
Life expectancy at birth: females	83.3	85.7	83.2	85.9	83.1	81.1
Life expectancy at birth: males	78.7	78.7	78.4	79.4	79.1	76.3
Nurses (density per 1000 population)	9.3	8.7	11.4	10	8.6	11.1

Based on data from OECD (2013), *Health at a Glance 2013: OECD Indicators,* OECD Publishing. http://dx.doi.org/10.1787/health_glance-2013–en

level of spending, the United States does not appear to achieve substantially better health benchmarks as compared with other developed countries. As also shown in Table 7-1, the life expectancy for both males and females is less than in other industrialized nations.

Health care consumption in the United States is unevenly distributed (Office of the Actuary, 2013). A small share of people accounts for a significant share of expenses in any year. In 2009 almost half of all health care spending was used to treat just 5% of the population, which included individuals with health expenses at or above $17,402. Less than one fourth of health spending (21.8%) was consumed by the 1% of the population who had total health expenses above $51,951 in 2009. This pattern represents the emphasis on high technology hospital-based care in an environment with high levels of chronic illness, as opposed to a health care system based on health promotion and prevention.

The single greatest category of health care expense is hospital care. As shown in Figure 7-4, hospital care has decreased as a percentage of total expense since 1997, but it still accounts for 31.5% of total expenses. Physician expenses are the next highest category, and it has also decreased slightly as a percent of the total since 1997. Personal and other expenses have both increased since 1997, and are at 14.8% and 15.6%, respectively. Prescription expense decreased slightly between 2007 and 2011, but it still comprises almost 10% of the total.

More than half of all families report cutting back on some aspect of their medical care, as documented by the Kaiser Family Foundation (2012). For example, 33% reported relying on home remedies and over-the-counter drugs rather than visiting a doctor, and 28% postponed necessary care. Seventeen percent reported experiencing serious financial problems because of family medical bills. Seven percent reported being

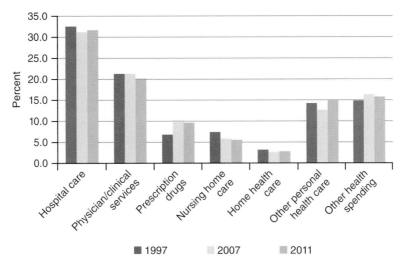

FIGURE 7-4 Distribution of health care spending by type of service, 1997, 2007, and 2011. Projections are for services delivered to individuals. Percentages may not total 100% because of rounding. "Other personal health care" includes, for example, dental and other professional health services, durable medical equipment. "Other health spending" includes, for example, administration and net cost of private health insurance, public health activity, research, and structures and equipment. (Adapted from "Distribution of National Health Expenditures, by Type of Service, 1997 and 2007," Kaiser Fast Facts, The Henry J. Kaiser Family Foundation, January 2009, and Kaiser Fast Facts, The Henry J. Kaiser Family Foundation, January 2009 (1997 and 2007 data) and Kaiser Fast Facts, The Henry J. Kaiser Family Foundation, March 2013 (2011 data). This information was reprinted with permission from the Henry J. Kaiser Family Foundation. The Kaiser Family Foundation is a non-profit private operating foundation, based in Menlo Park, California, dedicated to producing and communicating the best possible information, research and analysis on health issues.)

unable to pay for basic necessities such as food, heat, or housing because of health care costs. Forty percent reported being "very worried" about having to pay more for their health care or health insurance.

Recent evidence demonstrates that although health care spending continues to increase, the rate of growth has slowed down since 2009 (Centers for Medicare & Medicaid Services, 2013a). The Kaiser Family Foundation (2013) developed a model to explain and better understand the slowdown in health care spending growth. Overall spending increased, but the increase occurred at a much slower rate between 2009 and 2012. Inflation and an increase in the GDP explain most of the overall decline in the rate of growth. Specific mechanisms for the reduction include reductions by consumers as they used fewer services, an increase in the numbers of uninsured, and reductions in health benefits by employers.

THE INCREASING BURDEN OF HEALTH INSURANCE COSTS

Data regarding health insurance coverage is reported regularly by the U.S. Census Bureau (2013). As shown in Table 7-2, with a population of greater than 311 million people, approximately 85% were covered by some type of health insurance. Most of these were covered by private insurance, primarily employee based. Thirty-two percent were covered by a government health plan such as Medicare, Medicaid, or the Children's Health Insurance Program. Females have a slightly higher coverage rate, and a higher rate on government plans.

Significant disparities can be seen in terms of nativity (U.S. Census Bureau, 2013). Noncitizens had the lowest insured rate, followed by the foreign born. The rate for naturalized citizens was significantly higher than foreign born or noncitizens, but still less than the rate for native citizens (born in the United States). In terms of regional differences, the Southern and Western regions of the United States had the lowest rate of coverage, and also higher numbers of overall population. Thus the South and West are especially disadvantaged in terms of insurance coverage. Finally, the percentage of those with some type of insurance coverage is directly proportionate to household income. Households of less than $25,000 had a coverage rate of only 75.1%.

In a survey of the uninsured, the Kaiser Commission on Medicaid and the Uninsured (2013) identified some of the barriers preventing the uninsured from obtaining and keeping health insurance. As Figure 7-5 displays, insurance is deemed unaffordable by 33%, and 28% report losing their job as the primary reason. Approximately 9% left school and 2% report they do not have the need for insurance. A large percentage, 17%, reported their reason as other. Eleven percent of individuals reported that health insurance was "not offered".

Evaluating Health Systems: Cost, Quality, Value, and Technology

Costs. Costs are resources required by the provider of services to produce health care products and services, as well as the amount a consumer pays to purchase the products and services. The costs to produce health care are the actual costs of inputs incurred for production, whereas the costs to purchase health care services are what the health care economy will bear (i.e., what the consumers and financiers are able and willing to pay) (Folland et al., 2012). Thus costs depend on supply and demand. Costs may be monetary (pecuniary) or intangible (nonpecuniary). The pecuniary costs of care include salaries of health care providers, insurance premiums, the cost of supplies and equipment used during care, management overhead, pharmaceuticals, transportation, and lost salary of the consumer, as well as construction and maintenance costs and research. Nonpecuniary costs are those associated with the personal loss, pain, suffering, and other consequences associated with the consumption of health care services.

The costs of health care are affected by many factors, including the supply of services, the demand for services, and the use of medical technology. An increase in the input costs of providing a service increases health care expenditures, while the quantity and quality remain constant. Efforts are focused on reducing health care expenditures through reducing the input costs of care without sacrificing the quantity and quality of services (Folland et al., 2012). The resources consumed to produce or purchase a product or service are no longer available for the production or purchase of an alternative product or service. The value of the alternative product or service forgone is known as the *opportunity cost* (Pauly, 1993). The opportunity cost is therefore what is given up to obtain some good or service. A hospital that can afford to purchase only one of two diagnostic or therapeutic technologies must, in choosing one, give up known benefits of the other. The value

TABLE 7-2 Health Insurance Coverage by Sex, Nativity, Region, and Household Income (in thousands) 2012

	TOTAL COVERED	NOT COVERED AT ANY TIME DURING THE YEAR	COVERED BY SOME TYPE OF HEALTH INSURANCE DURING THE YEAR	PERCENT COVERED BY SOME TYPE OF HEALTH INSURANCE DURING THE YEAR	COVERED BY PRIVATE INSURANCE	COVERED BY EMPLOYMENT BASED	COVERED BY OWN EMPLOYMENT BASED	COVERED BY DIRECT-PURCHASE INSURANCE	COVERED BY GOVERNMENT HEALTH PLAN
Total Covered	311,116	47,951	263,165	84.6%	198,812	170,877	88,182	30,622	101,493
Sex									
Male	152,335	25,485	126,850	83.3%	97,428	84,821	48,049	14,190	46,927
Female	158,781	22,466	136,315	85.9%	101,383	86,056	40,133	16,432	54,565
Nativity									
Native	271,010	35,127	235,883	87.0%	178,877	153,544	77,266	27,551	91,506
Foreign-born	40,107	12,824	27,283	68.0%	19,934	17,332	10,915	3071	9987
Naturalized citizen	18,200	3322	14,879	81.8%	10,866	9386	6261	1776	5794
Not a citizen	21,906	9502	12,404	56.6%	9068	7946	4654	1295	4192
Region									
Northeast	55,135	5939	49,196	89.2%	37,781	32,944	16,608	5239	18,365
Midwest	66,422	7937	58,486	88.1%	46,403	39,365	19,911	7546	21,395
South	116,130	21,587	94,543	81.4%	69,426	60,079	32,172	10,489	38,222
West	73,429	12,488	60,940	83.0%	45,202	38,489	19,490	7348	23,510
Household Income									
Less than $25,000	58,332	14,512	43,821	75.1%	15,239	8719	5766	5516	35,277
$25,000 to $49,999	69,927	14,962	54,966	78.6%	35,389	27,633	16,601	7604	30,239
$50,000 to $74,999	56,776	8526	48,249	85.0%	40,129	35,039	18,674	5627	15,465
$75,000 or more	126,081	9951	116,130	92.1%	108,054	99,486	47,140	11,874	20,513

Note: The estimates by type of coverage are not mutually exclusive; people can be covered by more than one type of health insurance during the year. Data from U.S. Census Bureau. (2013). *Health Insurance Data.* http://www.census.gov/hhes/www/hlthins/data/incpovhlth/2012/tables.html

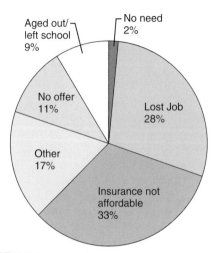

Aged out/
left school
9%

No need
2%

No offer
11%

Lost Job
28%

Other
17%

Insurance not
affordable
33%

FIGURE 7-5 Reasons for being uninsured among non-elderly adults, 2013. (Based on Kaiser Commission on Medicaid and the Uninsured. (2014). *Key Facts about the Uninsured Population.* The Kaiser Family Foundation. Retrieved from: http://files.kff.org/attachment/key-facts-about-the-uninsured-population-fact-sheet)

of the forgone benefits (revenue generated, lives saved) is the opportunity cost. The concept of opportunity cost can also be applied to personal economic decision making. In the case of RNs who decide to return to school full time to pursue advanced education, the opportunity cost of this career decision includes any lost earnings resulting from reducing work hours to complete the educational program.

Quality of Care. Nurses play a key role in quality improvement activities (Draper, Felland, Liebhaber, & Melichar, 2008). Manifest signs of quality of care problems in health care include medical errors, under-use of appropriate medical interventions, lack of integrated services, and poor allocation of resources across different parts of the health care system (Agency for Healthcare Research and Quality, 2013; Leape, 1994; Wallace, 2004). Other examples include health care outcome disparities by location, gender, race, and age (Agency for Healthcare Research and Quality, 2013). In their roles as clinicians, managers, researchers, and policy makers, nurses contribute in important ways to advancing the overall quality of health care service. For this discussion *health care quality* is defined as the degree to which health services for individuals and populations increase the likelihood of desired health outcomes and are consistent with current professional knowledge (Lohr, 1990). From an economic perspective, quality is the value gained from services for the amount of resources used in the production of those services. This section focuses on the contributions of professional nursing practice in quality improvement activities. Background information about systemic and organizational issues related to health care quality and its improvement can be found in the work of Shortell, Bennett, and Byck (1998), as well as the Institute of Medicine's companion reports, *To Err Is Human* (1999) and *Crossing the Quality Chasm* (2001), and the recent annual National Healthcare Quality Report, published by the Agency for Healthcare Research and Quality (2013).

Clinical Nurses. Within organizational settings, clinical nurses play an important role in ensuring the quality of care in three ways. First, clinical nurses act as interpreters among patients, families, physicians, and the system; they bear a responsibility for critical moment-to-moment decision making; and they spend more time than other health care providers in direct contact with patients. Clinical nurses have expertise in evaluating patients' responses to care. This expertise provides a platform to participate in projects that evaluate the costs and outcomes of new or different combinations of clinical interventions (Kennedy, Murphy, & Roberts, 2013).

Second, as consumers of nursing research, clinical nurses play a role in evaluating current practice patterns against best practices and integrating new knowledge into care pathways and unit-based nursing protocols and standards.

Finally as the interface between patients and an organization's care processes, clinical nurses play a role in providing managers with information regarding the extent to which systems and processes enhance or hinder clinical practice.

Nurse Managers. Nurse managers and executives play two key roles in quality improvement activities.

First, nurse managers, along with their peers, work to create a culture based on principles and practices of quality improvement and clinical excellence. Nurse executives shape the organization's vision and values associated with patient care service. Middle and first-line managers promote behaviors aligned with the organization's vision and values and work to implement the organization's quality improvement goals. Managers remove barriers between departments, lead evaluation activities, and keep the momentum of change going.

Second, nurse managers at all levels of an organization develop business cases for investing in technical and structural changes to promote clinical quality. *Business cases* are detailed arguments advanced by managers to allocate the organization's resources to achieve strategic goals. Senior managers integrate relevant investment proposals originating at the service or nursing unit level into the organization's budget and planning systems. Typical investments to support clinical quality improvement include training and skill development, information systems and electronic patient records, and consultations for data analysis and interpretation (Birken, Lee, & Weiner, 2012).

Nurse Researchers. Nurse researchers play a key role in advancing knowledge and sharpening understanding about nursing practice. To this end they have developed conceptual models and documented empirical evidence to articulate nursing's contribution to care quality, patient outcomes, and the costs of service delivery. Nurse researchers have contributed to the field of outcomes research by developing measures of functioning, well-being, and quality of life used to assess treatment effectiveness more comprehensively. Additionally, researchers working in the field of nursing administration have led the way in understanding phenomena such as the costs of nursing interventions or the relationships among leadership, staffing, and patient outcomes (Aiken, 2008). Nurses in policymaking roles work at the local, state, and national levels to translate research findings into regulations and laws for nursing and health care delivery (Institute of Medicine, 2010b).

Nurse Educators. Finally, nurse educators promote clinicians' understanding of the economic value of nursing and the profession's key role in providing cost-effective services. Within the higher education arena, nurse educators have developed innovations, such as simulations, to use limited teaching resources in a more creative and economical manner (Stevens, 2013). Further discussion about nursing roles can be found in Chapter 4.

Value. Value is the relationship between quality and cost. In the context of health care markets, *value* is defined as improved health outcomes in relation to the costs of producing services (Ginsberg, 2008). Stated more simply, value is the sum-total of the benefits a provider promises that a consumer will receive in return for purchasing goods or services. In comparison with other industrialized nations, the U.S. health care system suffers from a large value-gap. The United States spends more than any other industrialized country on health care as a percentage of GDP, yet we do not deliver the same levels of quality of care, patient outcomes, improvements in public health, or increases in life expectancy as other nations (Organisation for Economic Co-Operation and Development, 2013). As previously noted, Table 7-1 provides a comparison of the health spending patterns of the major industrialized nations (Organisation for Economic Co-Operation and Development, 2013). Although comparisons of U.S. health expenditures with those of other industrialized nations are helpful, they should be interpreted with caution. Henderson (2012) points out that differences in population demographics, per-capita income, disease incidence, and institutional features make direct comparisons difficult.

Rising health care costs and limited health care resources have created a call for documenting the value of professional nursing services and the impact of nursing care on organizational and hospital outcomes. An understanding of the relationship between the quality and the cost of care is paramount because these data inform decisions about the appropriateness and effectiveness of nurses in achieving desired levels of patient care quality (Henderson, 2012; Pappas, 2007; Rutherford, 2008). Under the diagnostic-related group (DRG) prospective payment system used by the Medicare program, hospitals are reimbursed a predetermined amount for services. Hospitals emphasize the daily costs of care, or the ratio of costs to charges for an episode of care, to align the expected reimbursement with profitability. Under this payment system, nursing services become vulnerable to cost-reduction efforts because nursing salaries and benefits make up a large portion of the per-day costs of hospital-based patient care. In an effort to reduce the daily costs of care, many hospitals responded by reducing nurse staffing levels or substituting RNs with unlicensed personnel. Reducing nurse staffing levels emphasizes the cost of nursing without considering how nurses contribute to the quality of patient care (Aiken, 2008).

Nursing research documented that the quality of patient care is sensitive to the intensity of direct nursing care. More specifically, evidence demonstrates that patients suffer from higher mortality rates and overall failure-to-rescue rates in hospitals where nurses cared for more (rather than fewer) patients (Aiken, Cimiotti, Sloane, Smith, Flynn, & Neff, 2011; Clarke & Aiken, 2003).

Failure to rescue is the inability of a clinician to save a patient's life when a complication arises. Additionally, higher hours of care from all nursing care providers in conjunction with a higher proportion of RN hours of care are associated with better outcomes for hospitalized patients (Aiken, 2008; Aiken, Shang, Xue, & Sloane, 2013; Pappas, 2007). This research establishes that nurses create value. That is, the costs associated with nursing services bring increased returns to the consumer through nurses' contribution to patient care quality and safety.

Newer approaches to describing the costs related to nursing services consider the process of care and how nursing care offsets the costs related to patient complications (Aiken, 2008; Rutherford, 2008). Methods for describing the costs, quality, and value of nursing services are used and well reported in the literature by nurse managers, researchers, and other leaders to communicate the value of nursing to hospital managers and the public at large. A number of economic evaluation techniques and examples are presented in Box 7-3; these techniques are useful in framing nursing services (as well as other health care services) in terms of their economic value, ultimately supporting increased investments in nursing services and the improved allocation of resources within the health care sector.

Technology. Health care technology has been cited as one of the significant drivers in the escalating costs of service delivery in the United States (Goodman & Norbeck, 2013). In its broadest sense, technology is the application of scientific knowledge used to transform inputs into outputs with the goal of improving productivity or economic growth (Henderson, 2012).

The expansion of health insurance since World War II has led to an interdependent relationship between health care technology and insurance and has had a dramatic effect on health care costs (Garber, 1994; Ginsberg, 2008; Goodman & Norbeck, 2013; Weisbrod, 1991). As the financing of services shifted from individuals to insurance companies, individuals became removed from, and insensitive to, the actual costs of health care technologies. Because of the retrospective payment system, in which all services rendered were reimbursed, health care providers (namely, physicians and hospitals) had financial incentives to use any and all technologies available regardless of cost. Research and development markets also had the financial incentives of reimbursement to continue to produce new health care technologies at any cost (Iglehart, 2001; Weisbrod, 1991). Consequently patient and provider demand for greater technology has heightened and become more widespread, as have soaring health care expenditures.

The abundant development and use of technologies have fueled the debate over the appropriateness of many disease-focused clinical interventions in improving health outcomes and overall health status. Because of how health technologies are financed, health care organizations have increased incentives to adopt new technologies, for many of which, the long-term effectiveness or costs are not fully known. Once a new technology is integrated into clinical practice routines, it is very difficult for an organization to disengage from using that technology. Studies suggest that newer technologies tend to complement, rather than replace, older technologies and that hospitals with constrained financial resources are likely to retain ineffective clinical technologies, creating a reverse access problem in which disadvantaged populations have access to ineffective, less effective, or harmful treatments at a higher rate than the population at large (Rye & Kimberly, 2007; Williams, 2011).

Technology assessment and outcomes research are intended to help decision makers deal with the development, acquisition, and use of health care practices and technologies. The goal is to improve patient health, efficiency, and value. Technology assessment, as a form of policy research, evaluates the safety, effectiveness, and costs of technologies to provide the basis for clinical and social policies, including resource allocation. A comprehensive technology assessment encompasses four aspects of the technology: safety, efficacy/effectiveness, costs-benefits, and social impact (Pillar, Jacox, & Redman, 1990).

Health technology assessment (HTA) has grown in popularity and use in response to cost containment pressures as a tool for evidence-based clinical and policy decision making. HTA has evolved from a technique of synthesizing best evidence for policy makers in national governments to disseminating information about the effectiveness of technologies to clinicians and

BOX 7-3 Methods to Evaluate Costs

The two predominant methods of evaluating the economic costs of a service or program are cost-benefit analysis and cost-effectiveness analysis. Other analytical methods used to assess the economic effects of new health care interventions or technologies include cost-minimization analysis, cost-consequence analysis, and cost-utility analysis (Rutherford, 2008; Stone, Curran, & Bakken, 2002).

Cost-Benefit Analysis

Cost-benefit analysis is an analytical technique for evaluating the necessary resources and benefits of producing a particular project, program, or technique. It requires assessment and evaluation of the costs and benefits of a program to determine whether the benefits of a project outweigh its costs. In a cost-benefit analysis all costs and benefits undergo valuation and are stated in monetary terms. This process places a dollar amount on both monetary and nonmonetary costs and benefits so that a comparison can be made between competing projects or programs. In doing so, value or worth is assigned to nonmonetary aspects of the project's costs and benefits.

Cost-benefit analysis is a useful and powerful tool to justify the investment in nurse-managed services to managers responsible for resource allocation decisions. In this era of resource efficiency and service change, a critical skill for nurses across practice settings and role descriptions is the ability not only to speak the language of economics, but also to demonstrate the unique value of nursing services in terms of cost, quality, and value. The widespread availability of personal computers and spreadsheet software makes cost-benefit analysis an accessible tool to a broad range of people. The calculations become effortless. Rather, quantification of the tangible and intangible costs is the difficulty of this method.

The comparative nature of cost-benefit analysis is an attractive feature of this analytical technique, but in determining the "worthiness" of a project, it is also a pitfall and a drawback. The major limitation of the application of cost-benefit analysis in health care scenarios is that the valuation of intangible costs such as pain or grief or premature loss of life varies not only from case to case, but also among analysts assigning the values. Specific criteria and arithmetic maneuvers have been suggested for determining the value of intangible costs and benefits, but these are controversial at best (Klarman, 1982; Pruitt & Jacox, 1991).

Cost-Effectiveness Analysis

Cost-effectiveness analysis is an analytical technique for comparing resource consumption between two or more alternatives that meet a particular objective (e.g., minimum quality of a product or production of a specific patient outcome). Cost-effectiveness analysis measures the costs involved with each alternative and determines the most cost-effective, or least costly, alternative (Kristen, 1983). In a cost-effectiveness analysis, only monetary costs of inputs into each alternative are considered. Because the objective (or outcome) of the alternatives is assumed to be the same, the valuation of benefits is not considered (Folland et al., 2012). Thus cost-effectiveness analysis avoids making valuations while providing empirical evaluation of costs of alternative health care interventions.

Cost-Minimization Analysis

A true cost-minimization analysis (CMA) compares the costs of alternatives. Interventions are assumed to offer equivalent outcomes so that it is possible to determine which intervention is the least costly. In clinical settings this method of analysis is rarely appropriate because different interventions yield different outcomes (Stone et al., 2002).

Cost-Consequence Analysis

In a cost-consequence analysis the consequences and costs of two or more alternatives are measured and evaluated. The cost-consequence analysis method separates the costs and consequences of comparable interventions so that decision makers can form opinions about the relative importance of findings. Brooten and colleagues' (1986) classic work on the early discharge of low-birth-weight infants whose care was managed by APNs compared with traditional care is an example of cost-consequence analysis.

Cost-Utility Analysis

Cost-utility analysis is a special type of cost-effectiveness analysis that includes measures for both quantity and quality of life. This analytical method includes an individual's preferences, or utilities, for different health outcomes. Preferences are ranked on a scale of 0 to 1, with perfect health represented by 1 and death represented by 0. Preference weights can be calculated for a variety of health states. The preference weights are then multiplied by the amount of time experienced in a health state to determine the number of quality-adjusted health years. Composite outcome analysis such as dollars per quality-adjusted health years is a superior method of assessing the economic effect of clinical interventions because both the quantity and quality of life are determined by using standardized measurements. Thus comparison of people within and across disease states may be possible (Stone et al., 2002).

Applied Examples

- Johnson and colleagues (2009) and identified the cost reductions and decrease length of stay associated with inserting PICC lines using portable ultrasound.
- Kang and colleagues (2011) examined the cost-effectiveness of active surveillance screening for *Methicillin*-resistant *Staphylococcus aureus*, and although the results were inconclusive, they established a valid model to study the problem.
- Melnyk and colleagues (2009) identified a savings of at least $4864 per infant admitted to a neonatal intensive care unit with an educational-behavioral intervention program aimed at empowering parents.

managers to influence the costs, safety, and quality of patient care. Early assessments tended to focus on large, expensive, machine-based technologies, the scope of which has expanded to include "softer" technologies, such as counseling and other process-oriented health care services (Banta, 2003).

Technology assessments are time consuming and costly. Traditional health care markets provide little incentive for investment in the process. During the 1990s technology assessment and the evidence-based practice movement gained importance as tools to inform policy, practice, and health care investment decisions. Nonetheless, these quality improvement methods are not without their limitations. Gilmartin, Melzer, and Donaghy (2004) assessed the extent to which HTAs produce recommendations that can and should affect clinical practice. In a sample of 53 therapeutic procedures and pharmacological interventions used in everyday medical practice, such as educational and psychosocial interventions for adolescents with diabetes or laxatives use for the elderly, the clinical effectiveness of 45% of these interventions was assessed as uncertain because of limitations of the pre-implementation data. Additionally, economic analyses of costs and benefits of these clinical technologies went largely unconsidered.

Huston (2013) identifies seven emerging technologies that will impact nursing and their associated benefits and challenges. Each of these technologies is likely to incur cost, and it will remain to be seen if the relative cost-benefit equation is positive. The seven technologies are: (1) genetics and genomics, (2) minimally invasive or noninvasive monitory tools, (3) three dimensional printing, (4) robotics, (5) biometrics, (6) electronic health care records, and (7) computerized provider order entry and decision support. Development and application of these technologies within patient care settings will require an expansion of current skill sets in nursing for optimal innovation adoption.

The growth of the evidence-based clinical practice and management movements has highlighted the role of the information gained from synthesizing research to improve the quality, safety, and effectiveness of patient care. Many groups have a stake in the outcome of HTAs. These include:

- *Policy makers:* Broad concern about technology and value for money

- *Insurers:* Overarching concern for controlling costs of care
- *Clinicians:* Mostly interested in quality of a technology with a lesser interest in the costs or the equitable distribution of technologies
- *Epidemiologists and other researchers:* Interested in the poor state of the primary research used in HTAs, with attention to improving research and the dissemination of HTA findings to clinicians and other decision makers
- *Industry:* Overriding concern for selling products with increasing pressures to demonstrate a given product's efficacy and cost-effectiveness
- *The general public:* Interested in access to health care that is of acceptable quality (Banta, 2003, 2009)

The Agency for Healthcare Research and Quality's (AHRQ) Technology Assessment program has conducted technology assessments for the Centers for Medicare & Medicaid Services (CMS) since 2009. The assessments address current and emerging technologies to guide CMS decision making in its national coverage decisions for the Medicare program. Private non-government insurance providers have access to this information as well (Technology Assessment Program, 2014).

Nursing practice, education, and administration are directly affected by the application of new medical and health care practices and technologies. However, nursing's participation in technology research has evolved significantly since 1990. Pillar, Jacox, and Redman (1990) noted nursing's relative absence in technology assessment at that time. In a systematic review of the literature, Ramacciati (2013) identified 70 technology assessment studies led by nurses. Nurses directly witness the individual, as well as societal, benefits and burdens that various practices and technologies bring and possess a wealth of clinical knowledge and expertise that could advance technology assessment. Nurses can play an important part on interdisciplinary technology assessment teams, developing clinical practice guidelines, leading to organizational change initiatives focused on integrating evidence into clinical practice routines, as well as advocating social policy regarding health care technologies. In today's marketplace payers are increasingly willing to pay only for those technologies that are cost effective and medically appropriate. Within this context the nursing profession has an

BOX 7-4 How to Read an Economic Analysis Paper

In the contemporary practice environment the allocation of limited resources in the production of health care services is a necessary component of clinical and policy decision making. As this chapter has illustrated, the economic cost of health care service delivery includes many tangible and intangible elements. A key skill for the professional nurse is the ability to analyze critically the quality of a study that reports the economic benefits of an intervention or new service. Greenhalgh (1997) presents the following 10-question checklist that is useful in judging economic analyses of a health care service:

1. Is the economic analysis based on a study that answers a clearly defined clinical question about an economically important issue?
2. From whose viewpoint are the costs and benefits being considered?
3. Have the interventions being compared been shown to be clinically effective?
4. Are the interventions sensible and workable in the setting in which they are likely to be applied?
5. Which method of economic analysis was used, and was it appropriate?
6. How were costs and benefits measured?
7. Were incremental (one unit/one more individual) rather than absolute (overall) benefits considered?
8. Was the "here and now" given precedence over the distant future?
9. Was a sensitivity analysis performed?
10. Were bottom-line aggregate scores overused?

From Greenhalgh, T. (1997). How to read a paper: Papers that tell you what things cost (economic analyses). *British Medical Journal, 315,* 596–599.

opportunity to develop and demonstrate the effectiveness of nurse-specific interventions and service technologies. The 10 question checklist provided in Box 7-4 is useful in judging an economic analysis of interventions or new health care services.

HEALTH SYSTEM REFORM: EMERGING MODELS, TRENDS, AND THE PATIENT PROTECTION AND AFFORDABLE CARE ACT 2010

The final section of this chapter introduces emerging trends shaping patient–provider relationships based on the principles of competition and consumer sovereignty.

The economic mechanisms and effects on health care delivery organizations and professional nursing practice are also considered. A summary and general overview of The Patient Protection and Affordable Care Act (PPACA) of 2010 and its economic implications provide an applied example of comprehensive health care reform. As with any complex and controversial law the specific details and probably even the overall intent and concepts of the law may in fact be eliminated, overturned, or drastically reduced via funding or administrative decisions at the national, state, and local levels. However, the following discussion provides a general overview.

The chapter concludes with a discussion of opportunities for professional nursing to achieve sustainable health system change.

Alternative Models of Organizing Provider–Consumer Relationships

Changes in U.S. health systems are subject to the principles of market competition. As described in the introductory section of this chapter, competition is a mechanism used to distribute resources in combinations that produce the highest possible satisfaction for society: consumers, producers, and investors. In health care, market approaches focus on improving the efficient allocation of resources to, and within, the sector to minimize the social cost of illness, including its treatment. Efficient resource allocation is achieved when the marginal dollar spent on health care produces the same value to society as the marginal dollar spent on education, defense, personal consumption, and other areas (Buchmueller, 2009; Enthoven, 1993).

Today the quality and economic performance of the health care sector remains a concern for citizens, health care professionals, employers, and policy makers. As health care reform continues to focus on access, quality, and cost, major changes will occur in health care delivery structures, processes, and outcomes. The Affordable Care Act of 2010, discussed in Chapter 6: Health Policy, is already having an extensive impact on health care delivery (Hooten & Zavadsky, 2014; Selby & Lipstein, 2014).

In the context of health care reform, competition, market mechanisms, and business practices are sometimes cited as the cause of the failing health care system. Economists and organizational theorists have developed a number of arguments for and against the use of market and other institutional forms to govern provider and consumer relationships in health care (Alexander & D'Aunno, 2003; Enthoven, 1988; Gilmartin & Freeman, 2002; Nichols, 2012; Rice, 1998).

From a conceptual perspective, two issues arise from the application of market-based models in health care. First is the appropriate application of economic theory. Rice (1998) argues that economic theory is based on a number of key assumptions that must be satisfied so the theory can accurately predict the behavior of consumers and providers. Health care markets violate most of these assumptions, thus reducing the predictive power of economic theory. Second, economic theory provides no support for the belief that competition, rather than government regulation and financing, will lead to superior social outcomes. On the basis of these analyses, competition clearly will not solve issues of social welfare, especially access to essential health care services. Ensuring the availability of, and access to, health care services is more likely to be a role played by government policy and regulation.

Nonetheless, as a resource allocation mechanism, particular models of competition can play a role in improving quality and efficiency in the health care system. In health care, competition has come to be associated with profit maximization, cost containment, and limited resources dedicated to patient care. Framed in this manner, competition has been practiced in a winner-takes-all, or zero-sum fashion. Organizational behaviors associated with *zero-sum competition* include (1) cost shifting rather than fundamental cost reduction; (2) pursuit of greater bargaining power between delivery organizations and insurance/managed care companies rather than efforts to provide better care; (3) restriction on choice and access to services instead of making care better and more efficient; and (4) the reliance on the court system to settle disputes among consumers, providers, and payers (Porter & Lee, 2013; Porter & Teisberg, 2004). Zero-sum competition hampers innovation and the adoption of new, more effective technologies, puts health care professionals and clients at odds with one another, and creates a practice environment in which more time is spent taking care of the system than the patient.

A more fruitful model of health care reform is based on *positive-sum competition*. Positive-sum competition recasts the relationships among providers, insurers, consumers and clients, and institutions,

with the specific goal of improving the quality and efficiency of health care service. A central goal of positive-sum competition is to create value, which is the economic relationship between cost and quality. Reframing competition in terms of value creation emphasizes the positive aspects of free markets such as invention, innovation, and entrepreneurship. Additionally, in well-functioning free markets consumers and clients play a role in shaping new or better services for themselves and their communities (Freeman, 2010; Gilmartin & Freeman, 2002; Porter & Lee, 2013).

Positive-sum competition draws on concepts from economics, systems theory, and ethics to reframe the nature and outcomes of market transactions between buyers and sellers. Positive-sum competition is based on the following four principles:

1. The principle of *stakeholder cooperation.* Value is created because consumers, employers, payers and financers, government, and communities can jointly satisfy their needs. The support of each group is necessary to sustain the activities of the organization. Over the long run, the interests of each group (as opposed to a particular issue) must be satisfied by the organization's activities.

2. The principle of *complexity.* Human beings are complex creatures and act based on many different values. Sometimes human beings act selfishly; sometimes they act for others. Competition works because of the complexity of values and perspectives of individuals and groups. Groups of people (some of whom share like values) will work together to create what they cannot do alone.

3. The principle of *continuous creation.* Managers and leaders cooperate with others to create value. Human creativity is the source of change and progress within well-functioning markets. One creation does not have to destroy another; rather, a continuous cycle of value creation raises the well-being of everyone.

4. The principle of *emergent competition.* Competition arises in a relatively free society so that stakeholders have options. Some forms of cooperation may well satisfy stakeholders' needs better than others, so in a free society stakeholders are free to form many different cooperative schemes (Freeman, 2010; Gilmartin & Freeman, 2002).

Using the principles of positive-sum competition, Porter & Teisberg (2004) describe a reformed health care system with the following attributes. There would be no restrictions to competition and choice including no preapprovals for referrals or treatments; no network restrictions; strict antitrust enforcements; and consumer incentives to seek good value through meaningful copayments and medicals saving accounts with high deductibles. Standardized information on treatments and alternatives, provider performance, and risk-adjusted outcomes are widely disseminated and easily accessible to support informed choices by patients. Pricing is set for a given treatment or procedure by the provider, provided in advance and transparent to the consumer. Billing processes are simplified and payers have the legal responsibility for medical bills of paid-up subscribers. Require health plan coverage, allowing insurers to create risk pools for those who need them while restricting re-underwriting of insurance. Establish a required standard for minimum benefit coverage while fostering expanded coverage through competition instead of litigation. Lawsuits address use of obsolete treatments and carelessness.

Consider the case of the single mother who returns home in the evening to a toddler having an asthma attack. The pediatrician's office is closed, so the mother has two options: She can either visit the local emergency department or the nurse-managed urgent care center at the mall. As an emergency department client she can expect to wait up to 5 hours, fill out a stack of insurance papers, pay a $250 co-payment for the visit, and possibly get a 10-minute consultation with the health care provider. Alternatively at the nurse-managed clinic, an NP is usually available within 15 minutes of arrival, and the consultation usually lasts 30 minutes. In addition to getting the immediate symptoms under control, the NP adjusts medication dosages and reviews administration and side effects, teaches symptom management techniques, and makes a referral to a local parent support group. The visit costs $85, and the registration process is simple. Moreover, an RN from the clinic calls the next morning to see how the mother and her child coped during the night and reinforces information on effective symptom management techniques.

Nurse-led clinics, like the one described in this scenario and the retail clinics profiled earlier, are examples of positive-sum competition based on the principles of stakeholder cooperation and emergent competition. Value is created because services are convenient and affordable and they fill an unmet market need. The nurses involved in these enterprises bring together clients, payers, and the community in a new combination to provide after-hours or expanded-hours primary care and urgent care services that complement overstretched physicians and hospital emergency departments. Additionally, the focus on chronic disease and symptom management distinguishes the nurse-led services from those offered by physicians. Kovner and Walni (2010) offer a comprehensive review of nurse managed health centers (NMHC) that identifies 200 NMHCs currently operating in 37 states with an estimated two million clinical encounters per year.

In effect, nurse-led services create a new standard of care that for some clients is superior to that of the traditional physician services. This model is not limited to the work of APNs. Nurse entrepreneurs, lawyers, and consultants working outside the hospital setting have identified gaps in the market between consumer demand and current provider offerings. Drawing on specialized knowledge, skills, and abilities, these nurses create new services to address an underlying problem associated with health care service.

Finally, magnet hospitals are an example of the power of positive-sum competition in organizational settings (American Nurses Credentialing Center, 2014). The magnet management and leadership philosophy focuses on developing cultures and systems of clinical excellence. Professionals work in a coordinated yet autonomous manner to deliver patient care services. These organizations emphasize expertise, collegiality, and performance, elements that in turn have a direct effect on the quality of care, patient outcomes, and patient and staff satisfaction ratings (Aiken, 2008; Aiken, Smith, & Lake, 1994; American Nurses Credentialing Center, 2014; Drenkard, 2013). In turn these clinical and service outcomes improve the reputation of the organization among consumers, payers, communities, and potential employees; as a result, all who are associated with the enterprise gain something.

Consumerism

The prolonged U.S. economic prosperity of the 1990s and early 2000s and the Internet revolution coincided with changing consumer expectations for goods and services. Across all sectors of the national economy, citizens expect immediate, low-cost products and services that are tailored to their specific needs.

Although many consumers have benefited from more affordable and often expanded health care coverage, restrictions on choice of primary care physicians and access to specialty care, emergency care, and inpatient admissions have led to a retreat from managed care and to a new emphasis on consumers as the central decision makers in U.S. health care (Robinson, 2001). Consumerism in health care can be traced to the women's liberation movement of the 1960s; the new wave of consumerism is squarely based on individual choice and self-responsibility to manage one's own health. The central idea underpinning the consumer movement is that health care belongs in the domain of personal rights and individual decision making (Robinson & Ginsberg, 2009).

As a mechanism to create socially optimal equilibrium, consumer-driven health care has the following limitations: (1) despite widespread dissemination of information, consumers will face significant obstacles in understanding the quality and true price of health insurance and services; (2) consumers vary enormously in their financial, cognitive, and cultural preparedness to navigate the complex health care system—the consumerism model most comfortably fits the educated, assertive, and prosperous and least comfortably fits the impoverished, meek, and poorly educated; (3) consumerism will complicate the pooling of risk between consistently healthy citizens and the chronically ill; and (4) consumerism will make transparent and render difficult the redistribution of income from rich to poor that otherwise results from the collective purchasing and administration of health insurance (Robinson, 2001; Starr, 2013).

Consumerism is a market-based mechanism in which individuals articulate what, when, and how they want health care service delivered. Advocates of consumerism emphasize the potential responses of consumers, employers, insurance companies, delivery organizations, and professionals to create new and better services. The hope is consumer-driven services will improve many of the problems and limitations that abound in health care. Opponents of consumerism emphasize that consumer choice is not an effective mechanism to allocate health care resources in a manner that will ensure equal access to a basic set of services for all citizens (Dayaratna, 2013).

In its original conception, the health care consumerism movement focused on the development of convenient, low-cost, high-quality services and client–health care professional relationships based on a partnership model (Dayaratna, 2013; Herzlinger, 2000, 2007). In this model, health care professionals provide guidance, education, and advice to patients/clients on a plan of care that ultimately is the individual's responsibility to purchase and carry out. The consumerism movement is now in its second decade and has evolved in ways that diverge from its original intent (Grob, Schlesinger, Davis, Cohen, & Lapps, 2013).

Most of the evolution of health care consumerism has taken place in the form of health insurance benefits, most notably the development of high-deductible health plans (HDHPs) with savings options. These plans function like true insurance in that they are designed to cover high-cost unpredictable needs, while leaving low-cost more predictable types of care to be paid out of pocket. The central idea of these plans is to reduce moral hazard by giving enrollees control over how and when they purchase "minor" health care services. The number of people with these high deductible plans has increased from 11.4 million in 2011 to nearly 15.5 million people in 2013, an average annual rate of 15% (Center for Policy and Research, 2013).

It is likely as consumerism evolves, insurance companies will develop programs seeking to improve the care of enrollees along the spectrum from full health to dire illness. These include preventative and wellness programs for healthy enrollees, service coordination for patients needing acute care, disease management for enrollees with chronic conditions, and intensive case management for enrollees with severe conditions. These services will likely be presented as options rather than mandates, possibly with higher cost-sharing for those who are eligible but choose not to participate (Center for Policy and Research, 2013; Robinson & Ginsburg, 2009).

In the context of the health consumerism movement, professional nurses occupy a unique position. Nurses advocate personal responsibility and knowledge to achieve an optimal level of health and wellness. In particular, nurses may play a role in promoting more choice for self-management among the seriously ill and vulnerable populations. Nursing's professional value system provides a foundation for important insights to shape new services, organizational strategies, and policies to balance the competing demands of consumerism.

HIGHLIGHTS OF THE PATIENT PROTECTION AND AFFORDABLE CARE ACT 2010

The PPACA was signed into law in 2010 by President Obama and is commonly referred to as Obamacare. The law addresses all three major aspects of health care policy and economics: Cost, Quality, and Access. There are four major provisions of the law, as organized in a Fact Sheet by the New America Foundation (2010).

1. The Act creates three main economic incentives for providers to accept payment structure that reward meeting cost and quality targets, rather than primarily fee-for-service arrangements that reward increased volumes. First, Accountable Care Organizations (ACOs) were created to allow for business relationships among providers, hospitals, and insurers for the purpose of maximizing quality and minimizing costs for a select population of patients. Second, Medical Homes (community-based health teams) are provided further support by increased funding for the creation of teams and networks, and for local providers to manage medications for the chronically ill. Third, the Act establishes a demonstration project to assess the use of bundled payments for Medicaid hospital and physician services. The Act also establishes a demonstration project to adjust the payment structure for safety-net hospitals from fee-for-service to capitated payments.

2. The Act establishes three new entities to oversee and evaluate the quality of care and cost of the health care system. First, the Center for Medicare and Medicaid Innovation was created to test innovative payment and delivery models to reduce costs while preserving or enhancing the quality of care for populations served by Medicare, Medicaid, and the Children's Health Insurance Program (CHIP). Second, The Independent Payment Advisory Board (IPAB) was created and empowered to make changes to Medicare payment rates and program rules. Previously, Congressional approval was required to make any changes. Third, the Patient-Centered Outcomes Research Institute (PCORI) was established as a nongovernment advisory entity comprised of patients, physicians, nurses, hospitals, drug makers, device manufacturers, insurers, payers, government officials, and health experts. PCORI examines the "relative health outcomes, clinical effectiveness, and appropriateness" of different medical treatments by evaluating existing studies and conducting its own. The PCORI then provides recommendations to the Centers for Medicare and Medicaid Services (CMS).

3. The Act encourages quality improvement through the development of reliable quality measurements and enforcing accountability. Numerous provisions include (1) development of quality measures for Medicaid patients, similar to core measures currently used for Medicare patients; (2) extends the physician quality reporting initiative; (3) further development of value based purchasing programs; and (4) new or enhanced quality reporting for physicians, long-term care hospitals, inpatient rehabilitation hospitals, inpatient psychiatric hospitals, hospice programs, and cancer centers. Specifically, the Act reduces payments to hospitals with 25th percentile or higher rate of hospital acquired infections.

4. The Act addresses patient empowerment in numerous ways. First, health insurance companies are required to justify and publicize rates and rate increases. The Act helps states strengthen or create rate review processes. The Health Insurance Marketplace is the primary vehicle for the flow of this information. Second, further consumer protection includes elimination of pre-existing conditions for denials of insurance coverage, elimination of lifetime dollar limits, and establishment of the right to appeal for private insurance recipients. Third, several programs created include (1) shared decision making by providers and patients, (2) home-based primary care for the chronically ill, (3) navigator systems to help patients overcome barriers, and (4) risk reduction programs for pre-Medicare populations.

ACCOUNTABLE CARE ORGANIZATIONS

The contemporary concept of Accountable Care Organizations (ACOs) is generally believed to been created at a public meeting of the Medicare Payment Advisory Commission (Medpac) in 2006. Dr. Fisher and colleagues (2007) addressed the formation of ACOs in a seminal article immediately following the consensus meeting. They argued that approaches to performance measurement and payment reform that focus on individual physicians risk reinforces fragmentation of care and lack of coordination experienced by patients with serious illness. Thus ACOs should be created on the basis of "extended hospital medical staff" that "work within and around" local hospitals.

The Medicare Shared Savings Program created by the Accountable Care Act, creates financial incentives for hospitals, physicians, and other health care providers to limit growth in health care costs through improved coordination of care (Centers for Medicare & Medicaid Services Medicare Learning Network, 2011). Before the Shared Savings program, financial incentives for combined physician and hospital entities were limited to a few pilot programs created to establish feasibility. Hospitals are now allowed to formally partner with physicians and other providers through the legal and financial entity of the ACO. The ACO is held accountable for improving the outcomes and experience for individuals and populations. Better coordinated care helps to ensure that patients receive the right care at the right time, with less duplication and fewer errors.

Accountable Care Organizations are similar to Health Maintenance Organizations (HMOs), yet there are key differences. HMOs are primarily insurance providers who assume the risk for a population of members within their service programs. First, ACOs generally are comprised of fewer enrollees; current regulations require a minimum of 5000 Medicare beneficiaries. Second, ACOs, at least as currently defined, bear less financial risk. ACOs are rewarded for high performance, but not accountable for 100% of the costs as in the HMO model.

The ACOs enrollees are tracked and monitored by the ACO and CMS. The ACO selects one of two options at the outset: (1) operate on a shared savings agreement, or (2) elect a higher risk option that allows the ACO to share savings and losses, thus attaining a higher share of any savings generated.

HEALTH INSURANCE MARKETPLACE

The Health Insurance Marketplace was created by the PPACA Act of 2010, as a mechanism for consumers to identify health insurance options, determine available subsidies, and select insurance with the desirable mix of coverage, out-of-pocket expenses, and monthly premiums (Collins & Garber, 2013). The consumer can also determine their eligibility for free or low-cost coverage available through Medicaid or the CHIP. The law requires individuals to secure insurance or face penalties that could be assessed by the Internal Revenue Service. Also called

Exchanges, health care marketplaces may be established at the state level, or users default to the federal version if their particular state has not created one. As of 2013, 18 states plus the District of Columbia have formed state-level marketplaces (Office of the Assistant Secretary, 2013). Massachusetts implemented their exchange in 2006, with a health care reform model commonly referred to as Romney Care, which also was based on universal access through public and private insurance coverage options.

MEDICAID EXPANSION AND THE SUPREME COURT DECISION OF JUNE 2012

The ACA initially had expanded Medicaid eligibility, scheduled to begin in 2014, to nearly all people under 65 years of age at or below 138% of the federal poverty level ($15,856 for an individual in 2013). To fund the expansion, the federal government will fund 100% of the costs through 2016, and then gradually decrease to 90% by 2020 and thereafter. However, in a lawsuit won by Florida and then joined by 25 other states, the Supreme Court ruled that states could not be required to expand Medicaid. As a result, as of December 2013, only 25 states and the District of Columbia have expanded Medicaid. Thus a significant policy provision for increasing the percentage of insured persons was eliminated from the ACA law.

Although many governors had argued that state expansion of Medicaid would cause significant financial burden on the states, the Congressional Budget Office (CBO) refutes this claim, estimating that the additional impact will be limited to 2.8% because federal funding would provide nearly 93% of the costs over the first 9 years (Angeles, 2012). In addition, the impact of 2.8% would be significantly decreased by the savings that state and local governments will realize in other health care spending for the uninsured.

The Urban Institute has estimated that overall state savings in these areas will total between $26 and $52 billion from 2014 through 2019 from savings in uncompensated care (Kenney et al., 2012).

HOSPITAL VALUE-BASED PURCHASING

The Medicare Prescription Drug, Improvement, and Modernization Act of 2003, and the Deficit Reduction Act of 2005 allowed the CMS to reward acute-care hospitals for the quality of care they provide to Medicare patients.

The ACA of 2010 builds on this incentive concept by rewarding hospitals with better patient outcomes with funds created by withholding portions of payments from hospitals with lower quality outcomes.

The Hospital Value-Based Purchasing (VBP) Program's primary purpose is to improve care through the use of economic incentives and disincentives. The funds to support VBP incentive payments to hospitals are generated through reductions in DRG payments (CMS, 2013b). Beginning in FY2013, 1.0% was withheld from hospitals' Medicare payments, with incremental annual increases culminating in 2.0% being withheld by 2017 and beyond. The CMS calculates payments based on Total Performance Scores (TPS) of Clinical Process of Care (quality measures) and Patient Experience of Care (HCAHPS-patient satisfaction). Beginning in 2013, the quality measures contribute 70% to the overall score, and patient satisfaction contributes 30%. These percentages are expected to equalize in subsequent years.

Quality measures include specific criteria for a set of common medical and surgical conditions such as anterior myocardial infarction, heart failure, pneumonia, and patients undergoing surgeries. Examples include patients receiving fibrinolytic therapy within 30 minutes of hospital arrival and receiving primary percutaneous coronary intervention within 90 minutes of hospital arrival. Other measures relate to discharge instructions for heart failure patients and prophylactic antibiotics before surgery. The patient experience domain relates directly to the Hospital Consumer Assessment of Healthcare Providers and Systems Survey (HCAHPS).

The HCAHPS is a national standardized survey used to measure CMS patients' perceptions of care. The survey asks questions about critical aspects of patients' hospital experiences, including communication with nurses and doctors, the responsiveness of hospital staff, the cleanliness and quietness of the hospital environment, pain management, communication about medicines, discharge information, overall rating of hospital, and whether they would recommend the hospital to others. The majority of measures are directly or indirectly related to nursing practice, nurses work environment, and workload.

To understand the financial impact at the hospital level, it is helpful to look at how the Medicare dollars are withheld and divided. According to the Medicare Payment Advisory Commission's (MEDPAC) 2013 Report to Congress, $158 billion was paid to 4800 acute care hospitals for approximately 10 million Medicare inpatient discharges. Thus the average hospital would have normally received approximately $33 million. Under VBP, 1% or $15.8 billion is withheld. The average hospital's Medicare revenue of $33 million is reduced by $330,000. The funds withheld from the lower performing hospitals will be used to fund rebates for the higher-performing hospitals. The average hospital will initially have $330,000 withheld, and half of the hospitals could receive up to two times $330,000, or $660,000.

Opportunities for Professional Nursing

In the face of the growing urgency for sustainable national health reform, professional nursing is poised to take a leadership role in defining the attributes of a socially just health care system and bringing about sustainable changes in the organization and delivery of health care services. The American Nurses Association (2011) advocates that nurses practice to the full extent of their education and license, and that all barriers such as limitations in state nurse practice acts or restrictive reimbursement rules should be eliminated. They also advocate expanding professional nursing roles and nurse-managed services to address the unmet demand for health care services, working toward universal access to health care services and organizational environments that value nursing's contributions to patient outcomes, care, and safety. Moreover, the profession's clinical expertise for health promotion, disease prevention, and chronic disease management will be integral in addressing the following manifest signs of the ailing U.S. health care system (Institute of Medicine, 2010b; Lavizzo-Mourey, 2008):

- Tens of millions are uninsured or underinsured.
- Variations in the quality, safety, performance, and treatment are endemic.
- Avoidable medical and hospital errors kill thousands each year.
- Access to care is declining, uneven, and unfair.
- Racial and ethnic disparities in health and health care delivery are pervasive.
- Adult and childhood obesity has become epidemic.
- Prevention is overlooked, and mental health is discounted.
- Public health suffers from years of political neglect.
- Spending trends are unsustainable.
- Resources flood specialty care; resource drought afflicts primary chronic care.
- Demands of profit and process marginalize patients.

Specifically, The PPACA provides numerous opportunities for nursing at the general and advance practice levels, within the care delivery and academic domains, to address issues and challenges related to health care cost, access, and quality.

Nurses at all levels will be in a prime position within hospitals to lead and participate in programs and projects that relate to Value Based Purchasing and associated initiatives that reward hospitals financially for improving outcomes (Capezuti, 2013). Nurses have the education preparation and the clinical background and experience to understand and address clinical outcomes that affect financial performance. Falls prevention, and reducing nosocomial infections, re-hospitalizations, and hospital throughput times are only a few of the financially at-risk areas that nurses are in a position to address.

As financial incentives shift the focus of care from hospitals to less expensive venues in the community, APNs and nurses in home and community nursing practice settings will likely be afforded significant opportunities to lead and implement change. Advanced practice nurses will likely assume greater responsibility in primary care as state Nurse Practice Acts and related legislation at the federal and state levels loosen restrictions on nursing practice and promote higher levels of fee equity between primary care providers of all disciplines.

SUMMARY

This chapter has provided an overview of the many economic issues that are shaping the national discussion about health care service, its effect on our society, and by extension, its effect on professional nursing practice. Professional nurses must have a basic understanding of economic forces and the ability to apply these principles if they are to participate in shaping a patient-centered, health-focused care delivery system. This chapter serves as a foundation on which to build knowledge and skills to participate in health system reform efforts. Keeping abreast of changes in the dynamic health care economy is one way in which new knowledge shapes the practice environment and professional decision making. Journalistic accounts, professional publications, and Internet resources dedicated to the presentation and discussion of issues in health and nursing economics are widely available. Table 7-3 lists a variety of websites that address economic issues related to health care. Professional nurses have the knowledge and expertise to create a socially just health care system. Nursing participation in decision-making activities will occur by placing nursing services within an economic context.

SALIENT POINTS

- Economics in health care represents the relationships among the supply, demand, and costs of health care.
- The supply of health care refers to the amount of health care facilities, personnel, and financing available to consumers. Supply levels are affected by technological discoveries, costs for services, consumer demands, the level of competition in the marketplace, and the effect of government regulations.
- The demand for health care indicates what health care the consumer is willing to purchase. The demand level revolves around consumer needs and desires, the costs of health care, treatment selections ordered by health care providers, and general societal needs.
- The costs for health care reflect any financial expenditures contributed by providers or consumers to deliver and receive health care, as well as the intangible costs of seeking and receiving care. Factors influencing the cost of health care are numerous, ranging from consumer demands to advancements in medical technology to the status of the nation's economy.
- Economic concepts relevant to nursing practice include opportunity cost, complements and substitutes, and competition. Nurses must be able to incorporate these economic concepts into their management and clinical decision-making processes.
- Cost-containment pressures require that clinicians, managers, and researchers be able to incorporate economic methods such as cost-effectiveness analysis and cost-benefit analysis into practice routines. Such economically and clinically based research can serve as the basis for policy decision making regarding regulatory reform, prioritization, and rationing of health care technologies and services, as well as reimbursement for APNs.

TABLE 7-3 Web Watch: Keeping Abreast of Economic Issues in Health Care

WEBSITE	DESCRIPTION	INTERNET ADDRESS
CDC-National Center for Health Statistics	Comprehensive site of U.S. health care statistics to inform policy and improve the health of the American people	http://www.cdc.gov/nchs/
Future of Nursing Campaign for Action at the Center to Champion Nursing in America	Information hub for all recommendations contained in the Institute of Medicine's "Future of Nursing Leading Change, Advancing Health Report"	http://campaignforaction.org/about-us
The Health System Measurement Project	Tracks government data on critical U.S. health system indicators, such as age, sex, income level, and insurance coverage status.	https://healthmeasures.aspe.hhs.gov/
Kaiser Family Foundation	Information and resources about health costs, reform, insurance and disparities at the federal and state levels	http://kff.org/
Medpac	Provides data, information, and recommendations to U.S. Congress regarding Medicare	http://www.medpac.gov/
National Center for Health Workforce Analysis	Estimates the supply and demand for health workers in the United States and develops tools and resources to inform decision making on health care workforce investments.	http://bhpr.hrsa.gov/healthworkforce/
National Committee for Quality Assurance	An independent not-for-profit organization that manages accreditation, certification, and physician recognition programs. Contains key provider quality data.	http://www.ncqa.org/
National Institutes of Health	Provides an overview of information on health, grants and funding, and research and education organized by 27 Institutes and Centers	http://www.nih.gov/
National Information Center on Health Services Research and Health Care Technology (NICHSR)	Provides data, information, and training related to health information technology and health services research	http://www.nlm.nih.gov/nichsr/
Nursing World	The official website of the American Nurses Association; provides access to the online journal *Issues in Nursing*	http://www.nursingworld.org/
RAND Corporation	Not-for-profit research institution advances understanding of health and health behaviors and examines how the organization and financing of care affect costs, quality, and access.	http://www.rand.org/topics/health-and-health-care.html
Robert Wood Johnson Foundation	Provides information on their initiatives that focus on "building evidence and producing, synthesizing and distributing knowledge, new ideas, and expertise" by funding research and demonstration projects primarily through partnerships.	http://www.rwjf.org/
U.S. Census Bureau	Provides statistics on population demographics and health insurance	http://www.census.gov/

From Henderson. *Health Economics and Policy (with Info Apps 2-Semester printed across card)*, 4E. © 2009 South-Western, a part of Cengage Learning, Inc. Reproduced by permission. www.cengage.com/permissions.

- Nurses can bring a unique perspective to the economic analysis of health care that can have an impact on health care delivery systems, health policy, and most important, patient care.
- The rising costs of health care necessitate the provision of more cost-effective ways to provide comparable services. Nurses must continue to demonstrate their accessibility, quality of services, and cost effectiveness to validate existing and expanding roles,

to broaden reimbursement policies for services that nurses are trained to render and are capable of providing, and to effectively compete with physicians and other providers of care.

- The Patient Protection and Affordable Care Act (PPACA, 2010) commonly called the Affordable Care Act (ACA) or "Obamacare" was signed into law in 2010, with many of its provisions and funding for these provisions to be phased in by 2017.

Many provisions and programs within the law have been challenged in the U.S. federal and supreme courts, and also in Congress, where opposition remains fierce.

It is important to understand the original intent and framework of the ACA and to keep apprised of its continually changing components.

CRITICAL REFLECTION EXERCISES

1. Discuss the economic concepts of supply, demand, and costs of health care as they relate to your nursing practice.
2. What are the implications for the nursing profession of the issues of:
   a. Access to health care
   b. Cost containment
   c. Quality of care
3. Selecting one of the ten guiding principles of economics from Box 7-1, and apply it to an analysis of health care delivery in your own organization.
4. Discuss the impact of the Affordable Care Act on access to care, cost, and quality of care.
5. Using the criteria presented in Box 7-4, critique a paper presenting an economic analysis of a nurse-managed service or intervention.
6. Estimating the nursing workforce in terms of supply and demand is a challenging and complex process.
   a. Discuss the impact on the demand for nursing by one of the following:

- A major genetic breakthrough that leads to early identification of 50% of cancer cases.
- A widespread outbreak of Ebola in the U.S.
- Advances in non-invasive medicine leads to a 75% reduction in cardiac surgery.

   b. Discuss the impact on the supply of nursing by one of the following:

- Implementation of a mandatory BSN for initial licensure.
- Mandatory overtime rules retsrict nurses from working over 40 hours per week or more than 3 consecutive days.
- Implementation of minimum staffing ratios in medical-surgical units.

7. Applying the principles of supply and demand, and data from the National Center for Health Workforce Analysis, determine the impact of the salary differential between Advanced Practice Registered Nurses, including Nurse Practitioners and Registered Nurses on the future short- and long-term supply of both nursing workforce subgroups.

REFERENCES

The Advisory Board. (2013). *From vaccinations to ACOs: Retailers expand health care services*. Daily briefing. Retrieved from http://www.advisory.com/Daily-Briefing/2013/05/08/Retailers-expand-into-primary-accountable-care

Agency for Healthcare Research and Quality. (2013). *National healthcare quality report*. Retrieved from http://www.ahrq.gov/research/findings/nhqrdr/nhqr13/2013nhqr.pdf

Aiken, L. H. (2008). Economics of nursing. *Policy, Politics and Nursing Practice, 9*(2), 73–79.

Aiken, L. H., Cimiotti, L., Sloane, D., Smith, H., Flynn, L., & Neff, D. (2011). Effects of nurse staffing and nurse education on patient deaths in hospitals with different nurse work environments. *Journal of Nursing Administration, 42*(10 Suppl.), S10–16.

Aiken, L. H., Shang, J., Xue, Y., & Sloane, D. (2013). Hospital use of agency-employed supplemental nurses and patient mortality and failure to rescue. *Health Services Research, 48*(3), 931–948.

Aiken, L. H., Smith, H., & Lake, E. (1994). Lower medicare mortality among a set of hospitals known for good nursing care. *Medical Care, 32*(8), 771–787.

Alexander, J. A., & D'Aunno, T. A. (2003). Alternative perspectives on institutional and market forces in the U.S. health care sector. In S. S. Mick (Ed.), *Advances in health care organization theory*. San Francisco: Jossey-Bass.

American Association of Nurse Practitioners. (2013). *Nurse practitioner cost-effectiveness*. Retrieved from http://www.aanp.org/images/documents/publications/costeffectiveness.pdf

American Hospital Association (AHA). (2014). *Fast facts*. Accessed on June 25, 2014 at http://www.aha.org/research/rc/stat-studies/fast-facts.shtml

American Nurses Association (ANA). (2011). *Backgrounder: Understanding the nursing shortage and what it means for patients*. Accessed on June 25, 2014 at http://www.nursingworld.org/FunctionalMenuCategories/MediaResources/MediaBackgrounders/Nursing-Shortage-Backgrounder.pdf

American Nurses Credentialing Center. (2014). *ANCC magnet recognition program*. Retrieved from http://www.nursecredentialing.org/magnet.aspx

Angeles, J. (2012). *How health reform's medicaid expansion will impact state budgets federal government will pick up nearly all costs, even as expansion provides coverage to millions of low-income uninsured Americans.* Center on Budget and Policy Priorities. http://www.cbpp.org/cms/?fa=view &id=3801

Arrow, K. (1963). Uncertainty and the welfare economics of medical care. *American Economic Review, 53*(5), 851–883.

Banta, D. (2003). The development of health technology assessment. *Health Policy, 63*(1), 121–132.

Banta, D. (2009). What is technology assessment? *International Journal of Technology Assessment in Health Care, 25*(Suppl. 1), 7–9.

Baumrucker, S., Stolick, M., Mingle, P., Oertli, K., Morris, G., & VandeKieft, G. (2012). The principle of distributive justice. *American Journal of Hospice & Palliative Medicine, 29*(2), 151–156.

Birken, S., Lee, S., & Weiner, B. (2012). Uncovering middle managers' role in healthcare innovation implementation. *Implement Science, 7*, 28. Retrieved from http://www.ncbi. nlm.nih.gov/pmc/articles/PMC337 2435/

Bodenheimer, T. S., & Grumbach, K. (2012). *Understanding health policy: A clinical approach* (6th ed.). New York: Lange/McGraw-Hill.

Brewer, C. S., Kovner, C. T., Wu, Y. -W., Greene, W., Liu, Y., & Reimers, C. W. (2006). Factors influencing female registered nurses' work behavior. *Health Services Research, 41*(3, Part 1), 860–866.

Brooten, D., Kumar, S., Brown, L. P., Finkler, S. A., Bakewell-Sachs, S., & Gibbons, A. (1986). A randomized clinical trial of early hospital discharge and home follow-up of very-low-birth-weight-infants. *New England Journal of Medicine, 315*(15), 934–939.

Brooten, D., Youngblut, J. M., Kutcher, J., & Bobo, C. (2004). Quality and the nursing workforce: APNs, patient outcomes and health care costs. *Nursing Outlook, 52*(1), 45–52.

Brown, S. A., & Grimes, D. E. (1993). *Nurse practitioners and certified nurse-midwives: A meta-analysis of studies on nurses in primary care roles.* Washington, DC: American Nurses Publishing.

Buchmueller, T. C. (2009). Consumer-oriented health care reform strategies: A review of the evidence on managed competition and consumer-directed health insurance. *Milbank Quarterly, 87*(4), 820–841.

Buerhaus, P. I. (2008). The potential imposition of wage controls on nurses: A threat to nurses, patients and hospitals. *Nursing Economics, 26*(4), 276–279.

Buerhaus, P. I., Auerbach, D., Staiger, D., & Muench, U. (2013). Projections of the long-term growth of the registered nurse workforce: A regional analysis. *Nursing Economics, 31*(1), 14–17.

Buerhaus, P. I., DesRoches, C., Applebaum, S., Hess, R., Norman, L. D., & Donelan, K. (2012). Are nurses ready for health care reform? A decade of survey research. *Nursing Economics, 30*(6), 318–329.

Buerhaus, P. I., Staiger, D., & Auerbach, D. (2008). *The future of the nursing workforce in the United States: Data, trends and implications.* Boston: Jones & Bartlett.

Bureau of Health Professions. (2012). *Highlights from the 2012 national sample survey of nurse practitioners.* Washington, DC: U.S. Department of Health and Human Services. Health Resources and Services Administration. Retrieved from http://bhpr.hrsa.gov/healthworkforce/s upplydemand/nursing/nursepractiti onersurvey/npsurveyhighlights. pdfa

Bureau of Health Professions. (2013a). *The registered nurse population: Findings from the 2008 national survey sample of registered nurses.* Washington, DC: U.S. Department of Health and Human Services. Health Resources and Services Administration. Retrieved from http://bhpr.hrsa. gov/healthworkforce/rnsurveys/ rnsurveyfinal.pdf

Bureau of Health Professions. (2013b). *The U.S. health workforce chartbook.* Washington, DC: U.S. Department of Health and Human Services, Health Resources and Services Administration. Accessed on June 25, 2014 at http ://bhpr.hrsa.gov/healthworkforce/sup plydemand/usworkforce/chartbook/i ndex.html

Bureau of Health Professions. (2013c). *The U.S. nursing workforce: Trends in supply and education.* Washington, DC: U.S. Department of Health and Human Services, Health Resources and Services Administration. Retrieved from http://bhpr.hr sa.gov/healthworkforce/reports/nur singworkforce/nursingworkforcefu llreport.pdf

Capezuti, E. (2013). The opportunity of the affordable care act. *Future of Nursing Campaign for Action at the Center to Champion Nursing in America.* http://campaignforaction. org/community-post/opportunity-affordable-care-act

Center for Policy and Research. (2013). Census shows 15.5 million people covered by health savings account/high-deductible health plans (HSA/HDHPs). *America's Health Insurance Plans.* http://www.ahip.org/ HSA2013/

Centers for Medicare & Medicaid Services. (2011). Medicare learning network. *Final Rule Provisions for Accountable Care Organizations under the Medicare Shared Savings Program. (2011).* http://www.cms.gov/ Medicare/Medicare-Fee-for-Service-Payment/sharedsavingsprogram/ Downloads/ACO_Summary_Factsheet _ICN907404.pdf

Centers for Medicare & Medicaid Services. (2013a). *National Health Expenditures 2012 Highlights.* Retrieved from http://www.cms.gov/Research-Statistics-Data-and-Systems/ Statistics-Trends-and-Reports/Nation alHealthExpendData/Downloads/hig hlights.pdf

Centers for Medicare & Medicaid Services. (2013b). *Hospital Value-based Purchasing.* http://www.cms.gov/Medicare/Quality-Initiatives-Patient-Assessment-Instruments/hospital-value-based-purchasing/index.html?redirect=/Hospital-Value-Based-Purchasing/

Chernew, M. E., Hirth, R. A., Sonnad, S. S., Ermann, R., & Fendrick, M. (1998). Managed care, medical technology and health care cost growth: A review of the evidence. *Medical Care Research and Review, 55*(3), 259–288.

Clarke, S., & Aiken, L. (2003). Failure to rescue: Needless deaths are prime examples of the need for more nurses at the bedside. *American Journal of Nursing, 103*(1), 42–47.

Claxton, C., Gabel, J., DiJulio, B., Pickreign, J., Whitmore, H., & Finder, B. (2007). Health benefits in 2007: Premium increases fall to an eight-year low, while offer rates and enrollment remain stable. *Health Affairs, 26*(5), 1407–1416.

Collins, S., & Garber, T. (2013). Enrollment in the affordable care act's health insurance options: An update. *The Commonwealth Fund.* http://www.commonwealthfund.org/Blog/2013/Nov/Enrollment-in-the-Affordable-Care-Act.aspx

Congressional Budget Office. (2013). *The 2013 Long Term Budget Outlook.* Retrieved from http://www.cbo.gov/sites/default/files/44521-LTBO2013_0.pdf

Daniels, N., Saloner, B., & Gelpi, A. (2009). Access, cost, and financing: Achieving an ethical health reform. *Health Affairs, 28*(5), w909–w916.

Dayaratna, K. (2013). Competitive markets in health care: The next revolution. *The Heritage Foundation.* Retrieved from http://www.heritage.org/research/reports/2013/08/competitive-markets-in-health-care-the-next-revolution

DeNavas-Walt, C., Proctor, B., & Smith, J. (2013). *Income, poverty, and health insurance coverage in the United States: 2012.* Washington, DC: U.S. Department of Commerce, Economics and Statistics Administration, U.S. Census Bureau. http://www.census.gov/prod/2013pubs/p60-245.pdf

Devers, K. J., Brewster, L. P., & Casalino, L. P. (2003). Changes in hospital competitive strategy: A new medical arms race? Longitudinal changes in communities' health care systems, 1996–2001: Analyses from the Community Tracking Study site visits. *Health Services Research, 38*(1), 447–471.

Draper, D., Felland, L., Liebhaber, A., & Melichar, L. (2008). The role of nurses in hospital quality improvement. *Center for Studying Health System Change.* Retrieved from http://www.hschange.com/CONTENT/972/

Drenkard, K. (2013). The value of magnet. *Journal of Nursing Administration, 43*(10 Suppl), S2–S3.

Employment Benefits Research Institute. (2008). *Fast facts: Tax expenditures and employment benefits.* Retrieved November 30, 2008 from http://www.ebri.org/pdf/publications/facts/0208fact.pdf

Enthoven, A. (1988). Managed competition of alternative delivery systems. *Journal of Health Politics. Policy and Law, 13*(2), 305–335.

Enthoven, A. (1993). The history and principles of managed competition. *Health Affairs, Supplement,* 24–48.

Feldstein, P. J. (1983). *Health care economics* (2nd ed.). New York: Wiley.

Felland, L., Grossman, J., & Tu, H. (2011). Key findings from HSC's 2010 site visits. *Center for Studying Health System Change,* Issue Brief No. 15(135). Center for Studying Health System Change. Retrieved from http://www.hschange.com/CONTENT/1209/

Fisher, E., Staiger, D., Bynum, J., & Gottlieb, D. (2007). Creating accountable care organizations: The extended hospital medical staff. *Health Affairs, 26,* 44–57. http://www.ncbi.nlm.nih.gov/pmc/articles/PMC2131738/

Folland, S., Goodman, A. C., & Stano, M. (2012). *The economics of health and health care* (7th ed.). Upper Saddle River, NJ: Pearson Prentice Hall.

Freeman, R. (2010). *Strategic management: A stakeholder approach.* New York: Cambridge University Press.

Freeman, J. D., Kidiyala, S., Bell, J. F., & Martin, D. P. (2008). The causal effect of health insurance on utilization and outcomes in adults: A systematic review of U.S. studies. *Medical Care, 46*(10), 1023–1032.

Fronstin, P. (2012). *The tax treatment of health insurance and out-of-pocket expenses.* Employee Benefit Research Institute. Retrieved from http://www.ebri.org/pdf/programs/policyforums/Fronstin0512.pdf

Fulton, J. S., & Baldwin, K. (2004). An annotated bibliography reflecting CNS practice and outcomes. *Clinical Nurse Specialist, 18*(1), 21–39.

Garber, A. M. (1994). Can technology assessment control health spending? *Health Affairs, 13*(3), 115–126.

Getzen, T. E. (2004). *Health economics: Fundamentals and flows of funds* (2nd ed.). New York: Wiley.

Gilmartin, M. J., & Freeman, R. E. (2002). Business ethics and health care: A stakeholder perspective. *Health Care Management Review, 27*(2), 50–65.

Gilmartin, M. J., Melzer, D., & Donaghy, P. (2004). Health technology assessment: More questions than answers for clinical practice? In M. Tavakoli, & H. Davies (Eds.), *Policy, finance and performance.* London: Ashgate.

Ginsberg, P. B. (2008). *High and rising health care costs: Demystifying U.S. health care spending.* (Research Synthesis Report No. 16). Princeton, NJ: Robert Wood Johnson Foundation.

Glaser, J., & Salzberg, C. (2011). *The strategic application of information technology in health care organizations* (3rd ed.) San Francisco, CA: Jossey-Bass.

Goodell, S., & Ginsberg, P. B. (2008). *High and rising health care costs: Demystifying U.S. health care spending.* (The Synthesis Project Policy Brief No. 16). Princeton, NJ: Robert Wood Johnson Foundation.

Goodman, L., & Norbeck, T. (2013). Who's to blame for our rising health-care costs? *Forbes.* Retrieved from http://www.forbes.com/sites/realspin/2013/04/03/whos-to-blame-for-our-rising-healthcare-costs/.

Greenhalgh, T. (1997). How to read a paper: Papers that tell you what things cost (economic analyses). *British Medical Journal, 315*(7108), 596–599.

Grob, R., Schlesinger, M., Davis, S., Cohen, D., & Lapps, J. (2013). The Affordable Care Act's plan for consumer assistance with insurance moves states forward but remains a work in progress. *Health Affairs, 32*(2), 347–356.

Hauer, K. E., Durning, S. J., Kernan, W. N., Fagan, M. J., Mintz, M., O'Sullivan, P. S., et al. (2008). Factors associated with medical students' career choices regarding internal medicine. *Journal of the American Medical Association, 300*(10), 1154–1164.

Hayes, L. J., O'Brien-Pallas, L., Duffield, C., Shaniar, J., Buchan, J., & Hughes, F. (2006). Nursing turnover: A literature review. *International Journal of Nursing Studies, 43*(2), 237–263.

Health Resources and Services Administration. (2013). *The U.S. nursing workforce: Trends in supply and education*. Health Resources and Services Administration Bureau of Health Professions National Center for Health Workforce Analysis. Retrieved from http://bhpr.hrsa.gov/healthworkforce/reports/nursingworkforce/nursingworkforcefullreport.pdf

Henderson, J. (2012). *Health economics and policy* (5th ed.). Cincinnati, OH: South-Western College Publishing.

Herzlinger, R. (2000). Market-driven, focused health care: The role of managers. *Frontiers of Health Services Management, 16*(3), 3–12.

Herzlinger, R. (2007). *Who killed health care? America's $2 trillion medical problem-and the consumer-driven cure*. New York: McGraw-Hill.

Hoffman, E., Klees, B., & Curtis, C. A. (2007). *Brief summaries of medicare and medicaid*. Washington, DC: Office of the Actuary, Medicare and Medicaid Services, Department of Health and Human Services.

Hooten, D., & Zavadsky, M. (2014). The 'patient experience' revolution. *Journal of Emergency Medical Services, 39*(2), 54–59.

Huston, C. (2013). The impact of emerging technology on nursing care: Warp speed ahead. *Online Journal in Nursing, 2*(18).

Hyatt, H. H. (1975). Protecting the medical commons: Who is responsible? *New England Journal of Medicine, 293*, 235–241.

Iglehart, J. K. (2001). America's love affair with medical innovation. *Health Affairs, 20*(5), 6.

Institute for Women's Policy Research. (2006). *Solving the nursing shortage through higher wages*. Retrieved from http://www.iwpr.org/publications/pubs/solving-the-nursing-shortage-through-higher-wages-1

Institute of Medicine. (1999). *To err is human: Building a safer health system*. Washington, DC: National Academy Press.

Institute of Medicine. (2001). *Crossing the quality chasm: A new health system for the 21st century*. Washington, DC: National Academy Press.

Institute of Medicine. (2010a). *Redesigning the clinical effectiveness research paradigm: Innovation and practice-based approaches*. Workshop summary. Retrieved from http://www.nap.edu/catalog.php?record_id=12197

Institute of Medicine. (2010b). *The future of nursing: Leading change, advancing health*. Retrieved from http://www.nap.edu/download.php?record_id=12956#

Institute of Medicine. (2011). *The healthcare imperative: Lowering costs and improving outcomes*. Workshop Series Summary.

Janiszewski Goodin, H. (2003). The nursing shortage in the United States of America: an integrative review of the literature. *Journal of Advanced Nursing, 43*(4), 335–343.

Johnson, M. A., McKenzie, L., Tussey, S., Jacobs, H., & Couch, C. (2009). Portable ultrasound: A cost-effective process improvement tool for PICC placement. *Nursing Management, 40*(1), 47–50.

Johnson-Lans, S. (2006). *Health Economics: A Primer*. Upper Saddle River, New Jersey: Prentice Hall.

The Kaiser Commission on Medicaid and the Uninsured. (2013). *Key facts about the uninsured population*. Washington, DC: Kaiser Family Foundation. Retrieved from http://kaiserfamilyfoundation.files.wordpress.com/2013/09/8488-key-facts-about-the-uninsured-population.pdf

Kaiser Family Foundation. (2006). *Health savings accounts and high deductible health plans: Are they an option for low-income families?* Retrieved from http://kff.org/health-costs/issue-brief/health-savings-accounts-and-high-deductible-health/

Kaiser Family Foundation. (2008). *Fact sheet: Women's health insurance coverage. #6000–07*. Menlo Park, CA: Kaiser Family Foundation.

Kaiser Family Foundation. (2012). *Health care costs: A primer. Key information on health care costs and their impact*. Retrieved from http://kaiserfamilyfoundation.files.wordpress.com/2013/01/7670-03.pdf

Kaiser Family Foundation. (2013). *Assessing the effects of the economy on the recent slowdown in health spending*. Retrieved from http://kff.org/health-costs/issue-brief/assessing-the-effects-of-the-economy-on-the-recent-slowdown-in-health-spending-2/

Kang, J., Mandsager, P., Biddle, A., & Weber, D. (2011). Cost-effectiveness analysis of active surveillance screening for methicillin-resistant *Staphylococcus aureus* in a tertiary hospital setting. *American Journal of Infection Control, 39*(5), E209.

Kennedy, R., Murphy, & J. Roberts, D. (2013). An overview of the national quality strategy: Where do nurses fit? *The Online Journal of Issues in Nursing, 18*(3).

Kenney, G., Zuckerman, S., Dubay, L., Huntress, M., Lynch, V., Haley, J., & Anderson, N. (2012). Timely analysis of immediate health policy issues. *Opting in to the Medicaid Expansion under the ACA: Who Are the Uninsured Adults Who Could Gain Health Insurance Coverage?* http://www.urban.org/UploadedPDF/412630-opting-in-medicaid.pdf

Klarman, H. E. (1982). The road to cost-effectiveness analysis. *The Milbank Memorial Fund Quarterly, 60*(4), 585–603.

Kleinpell, R., & Gawlinski, A. (2005). Assessing outcomes in advanced practice nursing practice: The use of quality indicators and evidence based practice. *AACN Clinical Issues, 16*(1), 43–57.

Kovner, K., & Walani, S. (2010). *Nurse managed health centers (NMHCs)*. Research Brief. Robert Wood Johnson Foundation: Nursing Research Network. Retrieved from http://thefutureofnursing.org/sites/default/files/Research%20Brief-%20Nurse%20Managed%20Health%20Centers.pdf

Kristen, M. M. (1983). Using cost-effectiveness analysis and cost-benefit analysis for health policy making. *Advances in Health Economics and Health Services Research, 4*, 199–224.

Kunreuther, H., & Pauly, M. (2013). *Insurance and behavioral economics: Improving decisions in the most misunderstood industry.* New York: Cambridge University Press.

Lavizzo-Mourey, R. (2008). *Road to reform: President's message from the 2008 Robert Wood Johnson Foundation Annual Report.* Princeton, NJ: Robert Wood Johnson Foundation.

Leape, L. L. (1994). Error in medicine. *Journal of the American Medical Association, 272*(23), 1851–1857.

Lin, S. X., Gebbie, K. M., Fullilove, R. E., & Arons, R. R. (2004). Do nurse practitioners make a difference in the provision of health counseling in hospital outpatient departments? *American Academy of Nurse Practitioners, 16*(10), 462–466.

Lohr, K. N. (1990). *Medicine: A strategy for quality assurance.* Washington, DC: National Academy Press.

Medicare News Group. (2013). *Medicare facts.* Accessed on June 25, 2014, from http://www.medicarenewsgroup.com/news/medicare-faqs/individual-faq?faqId=31a98723-ad91-4801-9bd8-1f968a7c0f1b

Medpac. (2013). *Report to the congress: medicare payment policy,* p. 41. Retrieved from http://www.medpac.gov/documents/Mar13_Entire Report.pdf

Mehrotra, A., & Lave, J. (2012). Visits to retail clinics grew fourfold from 2007 to 2009. *Rand Health.* http://www.rand.org/health/feature/retail-clinics.html

Mehrotra, A., Wang, M. C., Lave, J. R., Adams, J. L., & McGlynn, E. A. (2008). Retail clinics, primary care physicians, and emergency departments: A comparison of patients' visits. *Health Affairs, 27*(5), 1272–1282.

Melnyk, B., & Feinstein, N. (2009). Reducing hospital expenditures with the COPE (Creating Opportunities for Parent Empowerment) program for parents and premature infants: An analysis of direct healthcare neonatal intensive care unit costs and savings. *Nursing Administration Quarterly, 33*(1), 32–37.

Mitka, M. (2007). Looming shortage of physicians raises concerns about access to care. *Journal of the American Medical Association, 297*(10), 1045–1046.

Mundinger, M. O. (2002). Perspectives: Through a different looking glass. *Health Affairs, 21*(1), 163–164.

Mundinger, M. O., Kane, R. L., Lenz, E. R., Totten, A. M., Wei-Yann, T., & Cleary, P. D. (2000). Primary care outcomes in patients treated by nurse practitioners or physicians. *Journal of the American Medical Association, 283*(1), 59–68.

National Academy of Sciences. (2008). Retrieved December 10, 2008, from http://www.iom.edu/uninsured

National Center for Health Workforce Analysis. (2013). *The U.S. nursing workforce: Trends in supply and education.* Washington, DC: Health Resources and Services Administration. Bureau of Health Professions. http://bhpr.hrsa.gov/healthworkforce/reports/nursingworkforce/nursingworkforcefullreport.pdf

New America Foundation. (2010). *Fact sheet: The patient protection and affordable care act: Delivery system reform.* Retrieved from http://health.newamerica.net/sites/newamerica.net/files/profiles/attachments/dsr_provisions_final.pdf

Newhouse, J. P. (1992). Medical care costs: How much welfare loss? *Journal of Economic Perspectives, 6*(3), 3–21.

Newhouse, R., Stanik-Hutt, J., White, K., Johantgen, M., Bass, E., Zangaro, G., et al. (2011). Advanced practice nurse outcomes 1990–2008: A systematic review. *Nursing Economics, 29*(5), 230–250.

Nichols, L. (2012). Government intervention in health care markets is practical, necessary, and morally sound. *Journal of Law, Medicine & Ethics, 40*(3), 547–557.

Office of the Actuary in the Centers for Medicare & Medicaid Services. (2013). *National health expenditure projections 2012–2022.* http://www.cms.gov/Research-Statistics-Data-and-Systems/Statistics-Trends-and-Reports/NationalHealthExpendData/Downloads/Proj2012.pdf

Office of the Assistant Secretary for Planning and Evaluation. (2013). *Health insurance marketplace: November enrollment report.* Department of Health and Human Services. http://aspe.hhs.gov

Organisation for Economic Co-Operation and Development. (2013). *Health at a glance: OECD indicators.* Paris: OECD. http://www.oecd.org/health/health-systems/oecdhealthdata.htm

Pappas, S. H. (2007). Describing costs related to nursing. *Journal of Nursing Administration, 37*(1), 32–40.

Pauly, M. V. (1993). U.S. health care costs: The untold true story. *Health Affairs, 12*(3), 152–159.

Pillar, B., Jacox, A. K., & Redman, B. K. (1990). Technology, its assessment, and nursing. *Nursing Outlook, 38*(1), 16–19.

Pollack, C., Gidengil, C., & Mehrota, A. (2010). The growth of retail clinics and the medical home: Two trends in conflict? *Health Affairs (Millwood), 29*(5), 998–1003.

Porter, M. E., & Lee, T. (2013). The strategy that will fix health care. *Harvard Business Review, 91*(10), 50–70.

Porter, M. E., & Teisberg, E. O. (2004). Redefining competition in health care. *Harvard Business Review,* June 2004, 65–76.

PriceWaterhouseCoopers. (2013). *Medical cost trend: Behind the numbers. 2014.* Retrieved from http://www.pwc.com/en_us/us/health-industries/behind-the-numbers/assets/medical-cost-trend-behind-the-numbers-2014.pdf

Pruitt, R. H., & Jacox, A. K. (1991). Looking above the bottom line: Decisions using economic evaluation. *Nursing Economics, 9*(2), 87–91.

Ramacciati, N. (2013). Health technology assessment in nursing: A literature review. *International Nursing Review, 60*(1), 23–30.

Redfoot, D., Feinberg, L., & Houser, A. (2013). *The aging of the baby boom and the growing care gap: A look at future declines in the availability of family caregivers.* Washington, DC: AARP Public Policy Institute. Retrieved at http://www.aarp.org/content/dam/aarp/research/public_policy_institute/ltc/2013/baby-boom-and-the-growing-care-gap-insight-AARP-ppi-ltc.pdf

Rhoades, J. A. (2005). *The long-term uninsured in America, 2001 to 2002: Estimates for the U.S. population under age 65*. Rockville, MD: Agency for Health Care Research and Quality. Retrieved January 20, 2007, from http://www.ahrq.gov/about/cfact/cfactbib28.htm#Rhoadespg

Rice, T. H. (1998). *The economics of health reconsidered*. Chicago: Health Administration Press.

Robert Wood Johnson Foundation, Building Human Capital News Digest. (2009). *Hospitals offering extravagant incentives to attract nursing talent*. Retrieved January 12, 2009, from http://www.rwjf.org/humancapital/digest.jsp?id=9271&;c=EMC-ND137

Robinson, J. C. (2001). The end of managed care. *Journal of the American Medical Association*, 285(20), 2622–2628.

Robinson, J. C., & Ginsburg, P. (2009). Consumer-driven health care: promise and performance. *Health Affairs*, 28(2), 272–281.

Rutherford, M. (2008). The valuation of nursing begins with identifying value drivers. *Journal of Nursing Administration*, 40(3) 115–120.

Rye, C. B., & Kimberly, J. R. (2007). The adoption of innovations by provider organizations in health care. *Medical Care Research and Review*, 64(3), 235–278.

Salsberg, E. (2013). *Projecting future clinician supply and demand: Advances and challenges*. National Center for Health Workforce Analysis Health Resources and Services Administration U.S. Department of Health and Human Services. Retrieved from http://bhpr.hrsa.gov/healthworkforce/supplydemand/supplyanddemand.pdf

Santerre, R. E., & Neun, S. P. (2013). *Health economics: theories, insights and industry studies* (3rd ed.). Mason, OH: Thomson, South-Western College Publishing.

Schroeder, C. (1993). Nursing response to the crisis of access, cost, and quality in health care. *Advances in Nursing Science*, 16(1), 1–20.

Selby, J., & Lipstein, S. (2014). PCORI at 3 years-progress, lessons, and plans. *New England Journal of Medicine*, 370(7), 592–595.

Shortell, S. M., Bennett, C. L., & Byck, G. R. (1998). Assessing the impact of continuous quality improvement in clinical practice: What will it take to accelerate progress? *The Milbank Quarterly*, 76(4), 593–624.

Sovie, M. (1985). Managing nursing resources in a constrained economic environment. *Nursing Economics*, 3(2), 85–94.

Sowell, T. (2011). *Basic economics: A common sense guide to the economy*. New York: Basic Books.

Starr, P. (1982). *The social transformation of American medicine*. New York: Basic Books.

Starr, P. (2013). *Remedy and reaction: The peculiar American struggle over health care reform*. New Haven, CT: Yale University Press.

Starr, P. (2013). Law and the fog of health care: Complexity and uncertainty in the struggle over health policy. *St. Louis University Journal of Health Law and Policy*, 6, 213–228.

Stevens, K. (2013). The impact of evidence-based practice in nursing and the next big ideas. *The Online Journal of Issues in Nursing*, 18(2).

Stone, P. W., Curran, C. R., & Bakken, S. (2002). Economic evidence for evidence-based practice. *Image: Journal of Nursing Scholarship*, 34(3), 277–282.

Strickler, A. (2011). *Preventing a crisis of American health care costs by optimizing efficiency*. Policy brief. University of Virginia. Accessed on July 3, 2014, from https://pages.shanti.virginia.edu/allenstrickler/files/2011/04/Policy Brief.pdf

Technology Assessment Program. (2014). *Agency for healthcare research and quality*. Retrieved from http://www.ahrq.gov/research/findings/ta/index.html

Topoleski, J. (2013). *Federal spending on the government's major health care programs is projected to rise substantially relative to GDP*. Congressional Budget Office. Retrieved from http://www.cbo.gov/publication/44582

United Health Group. (2009). *Federal health care cost containment: How in practice can it be done? Options with a real world track record of success*. Retrieved from http://www.unitedhealthgroup.com/~/media/UHG/PDF/2009/UNH-Working-Paper-1.ashx

U.S. Census Bureau. (2013). *Health insurance data*. http://www.census.gov/hhes/www/hlthins/data/incpovhlth/2012/tables.html

U.S. Congress. (1986). *Nurse practitioners, physician assistants, and certified nurse midwives: A policy analysis*. Health Technology Case Study 37; Publication No. OTA-HCS-37. Washington, DC: U.S. Government Printing Office.

Wallace, P. (2004). The health of nations: A survey of health-care finance. *The Economist, July 17*, 3–18.

Weisbrod, B. (1991). The health care quadrilemma: An essay on technological change, insurance, quality of care, and cost containment. *Journal of Economic Literature*, 29(2), 523–552.

Williams, L. (2011). Organizational readiness for innovation in health care: Some lessons from the recent literature. *Health Services Management Research*, 4(24), 213–218.

Effective Communication

Katharine C. Cook, PhD, RN

e http://evolve.elsevier.com/Friberg/bridge/

OBJECTIVES

At the completion of this chapter, the reader will be able to:

- Describe and define the components of effective communication.
- Describe the levels of communication.
- Differentiate between effective and ineffective professional communication.
- Identify the three strategies that enhance interpersonal communication.
- Identify types of group behaviors.
- Identify the three types of organizational communication.

PROFILE IN PRACTICE

Jeanne Cupper Pryor, BSN, RN, CPN

Effective communication is quite challenging to practice in the workplace—especially in health care when it can affect the health and safety of your patient. I have been in the inpatient arena for several years working as a pediatric registered nurse. I am not an expert in workplace environment communication but I faced many challenging experiences with communication that were thought-provoking over the past few years. Whether talking with a resident physician about a medication or trying to explain discharge orders to a deaf patient and family, effective communication is crucial to providing efficient and high-quality hands-on care. When I first started as a new graduate nurse, I entered the hospital with very concrete thoughts. I focused on planning my day, administering scheduled medications, and other set tasks. I was not flexible as a nurse and I wanted everything to happen in a step-wise fashion. I worked in an intensive care unit (ICU) and with this novice mindset, I encountered situations in which I experienced problems with communication. I remember being focused on the needed patient-care tasks such that I missed cues my patient was becoming more ill. My ears and eyes were not attuned to subtle signals my patient was showing me. I was also unfamiliar with the role parents and families had in communicating changes or cues regarding their children. By taking the time to stop, look, and simply listen, I started to become aware of nonverbal cues. It finally dawned on me that thoughtful, high-quality communication was essential to the well-being of each patient. Although difficult to learn and even more difficult to practice, effective communication skills led to my growth and success as an experienced pediatric registered nurse.

I remained in the ICU for several years and faced several challenging times because of ineffective communication. The overall unit morale was down. Both nurses and physicians were under immense stress and a culture of bullying reigned. Open communication appeared to be unwelcomed, employee turnover was high, and patient and family satisfaction decreased, which was evident on our annual survey scores. As a hospital unit, the staff faced immense challenges voicing concerns and respect was at a minimum. I became burned out, like many others, and transferred to another impatient unit in the hospital.

There is an immense difference in the communication style and atmosphere in my new unit of hire. Employees make eye contact with other staff members, first names are remembered by physicians and employees feel proud about their line of work. My job satisfaction improved immensely after the transfer to a different unit where communication and morale were valued. It took me years, but I came to the realization that high-quality, efficient communication takes teamwork, dedication, and patience. Experiencing the many different elements of communication, whether negative or positive, has crafted me into a more reflective, flexible, open-minded staff nurse.

INTRODUCTION

We are healed of a suffering only by expressing it to the full.

Marcel Proust

Communication is universal yet parochial. All human beings and, as increasing evidence suggests, most living creatures share and try to understand one another's feelings and thoughts, even when not intending to do so. Such is the nature of the world; the deepest interaction is that of communication. Rudyard Kipling likened words to drugs and believed them to be even more potent than pills (1928). Although registered nurses are proficient in the administration of drugs and assessment of drug actions and reactions, most nurses do not understand the powerful actions and potential side effects of communication. Effective communication, like effective drug therapy, requires the five rights: right drug, right route, right dose, right time, and right person. This chapter discusses communication (right drug) in all its universality and in all its peculiarities concerning route, dose, timing, and personal interpretation. Exploring communication helps us to learn about ourselves and others; to be more empathetic and present to our patients and co-workers; and to more effectively change practice by the successful use of written and oral words.

What is communication? The *Merriam-Webster Online Dictionary* defines *communication* as an act of transmission from one person to another: "to transmit information, thought, or feeling so that it is satisfactorily received or understood" (2014).

The Latin root is *communicare*, meaning "to share." Thus, the key word in the definition is *exchanging*, which implies a giver and a receiver. The more powerful definition when exploring what one gives and what one receives from honest communication is an unusual take on the word as when two rooms connect (communicate) or open into each other. To open into each other is a courageous and generous act, far more potent at times than the strongest medicine. This chapter approaches concepts related to effective communication using classical, foundational, and current references to clearly reflect key principles and demonstrate relevant present-day applications.

Communication theory is based on this construct. Many early theories of human communication were built on a linear model, which assumed one person (sender) sent a message to another person (receiver). This conceptualization, however, simplifies a process that is very complex and makes static a process that is dynamic. Contrary to conventional wisdom, communication is complex. The message is created by a process of interacting components: the meanings people actively create, the time and place of the communication, the relationships established between the receiver and sender, the past experiences of both parties, the personalities involved, the purposes of the communication, and the effects of human communication on people and situations. Meanwhile, as all these components dynamically interact, communication is occurring on many levels: intrapersonal communication, which occurs within the individual; interpersonal communication, in which two people interact; small group communication; and organizational communication. Each level builds on another, and successful communication at all levels depends on success at *each* communication level (Patidar, 2012).

INTRAPERSONAL COMMUNICATION

The foundation of the communication pyramid is formed by intrapersonal communication. This level is within the communicator's internal environment, where the critical skills of communication begin. Personal translation processes allow the person to constantly encode or create messages and to decode or interpret messages. During translation, the person creates meanings of the messages given and received from an intensely unique perspective. No word, object, or thing has any inherent meaning. The individual brings to bear influencing factors such as past experiences, personality, and relationships to the interpretation of content (Patidar, 2012).

Context

The biggest influence on interpretation of content is the context in which the message is received. Context is much larger and richer than simply the time and place of communication: "It is more than background; it is the total frame that gives a message its meaning" (Maxwell, 1993, p. 1). Work by language theorists (Clifford & Marcus, 1986; Gergen, 1991; Maxwell, 1993) have led to the belief in a social construction of reality. Instead of one unmitigated universal external reality, what an individual thinks and understands is the result of interaction with others. Each person individually constructs reality; nothing is universal and neutral. All individuals do not necessarily share the same perceptions and conceptual frameworks. One readily given explanation for these phenomena is the traditionally understood differences in culture, but one must be careful not to fall into a static and unchanging viewpoint of culture. Cultural diversity is only a piece of what contributes to multiple understandings of the same word, object, or content. As Maxwell (1993) states, "Postmodern approaches instead stress how emergent such understandings are as people interact with others, especially in multicultural environments where people have access to interaction with such varied others" (p. 2). Culture and context both help and hinder communication. Language is ambiguous and depends on understanding implicit meanings and nuances of a situation. Returning to the drug metaphor, something as routine as receiving a message that a patient is in pain is ambiguous. Is the patient assigned to you? What kind of pain? Has the patient recently received pain medication? Did something happen that caused the pain? The list of questions is endless and automatic for an experienced nurse. It requires further communication, relying on shared meanings, and incorporating nuances of the situation. Linguists call this experienced communication response *pragmatic competence in communication* (Hearnden, 2008).

Self-Awareness

Given that communication is the underpinning that forms a person's reality, an understanding of the *self*—and how it is influenced by many external factors—is imperative. How does a person come to such an understanding of self?

Johari Window. One helpful framework is the Johari window (Table 8-1), a conceptual framework of the self that is named after its creators, Joseph Luft and Harry Ingham (Luft & Ingham, 1955). The metaphor in this theory is that of a window with four panes—one open, one blind, one hidden, and one unknown. The open pane represents what is personally known and also known to others. When interacting for the first time with a person, the size of this windowpane is small because each person knows little about the other person. This window becomes more open as a

TABLE 8-1   Johari Window

	KNOWN TO SELF	UNKNOWN TO SELF
Known to others	Open area	Blind area
Unknown to others	Hidden area	Unknown area

Adapted from Luft, J. (1969). *Of human interaction.* Palo Alto, CA: National Press.

relationship develops and people self-disclose. The second pane reveals what an outsider knows about another but is unknown to the self; therefore it is called *blind*. This might occur when nonverbal and verbal messages are incongruent and the receiver chooses to believe the nonverbal message, of which the sender may be unaware. The third pane is hidden. This is information that is known to the self but not known to the outsider. The last pane is the unknown, about which neither the person nor others know. This unconscious area can be revealed to one or both as conversation takes place.

The ideal for effective communication is to raise the shade on the open pane of glass so that the self is more transparent to others. However, one should use caution in deciding what information to share with others. In personal relationships it is often not desirable to reveal things that could undo the balance of power in the relationship (e.g., past indiscretions in sexual behavior, mental health problems, life-altering failures). In professional relationships self-disclosure needs to be in the best interest of the patient. Nurses can encourage reciprocal self-disclosure by revealing the nurse's self as open, honest, and human (Gordon & Edwards, 1995). Storytelling, for instance, is a powerful means of connection, allowing caregiver and patient to understand commonalities and differences (Heilker, 2007).

A good rule of thumb, however, is to withhold any unresolved information. Unresolved information can shift the focus from the patient to the professional and can become an undue burden. This can be especially tempting when interacting with someone who is close to one's own age. Even when teaching adults, the professional must be wary of sharing too much personal information. For example, consider a nurse who shared ongoing personal problems with the orientees she was coaching in a clinical setting. The new nurses tried to understand and be supportive but eventually asked for less self-disclosure from the mentor because it had become a source of worry and distraction.

BOX 8-1 Values Clarification Exercise

Below is a list of values that people commonly hold. Rank these values in order of the priority each holds for you, with 1 being your top priority and 10 being your last. After completing the list, share your top three values with your peers. Discuss how these priorities affect your interpretations and decisions.

_____ Achievement (sense of accomplishment)
_____ Advancement (promotions)
_____ Adventure (risk taking)
_____ Caring (love, affection)
_____ Economic security
_____ Family
_____ Time freedom
_____ Health
_____ Loyalty
_____ Spirituality

Modified from Simon, S., Howe, L., & Kirschenbaum, H. (1972). *Values clarification: A handbook of practical strategies for teachers and students.* New York: Hart.

The more self-aware you are, the more you can dwell in authentic presence bringing genuineness and honesty of self to the relationship (Watson, 2008).

Values Clarification. Another method for increasing self-awareness is values clarification. Simon, Howe, and Kirschenbaum (1972) set six criteria that must be met for full value development: freedom in choosing, awareness of alternatives, awareness of consequences for each alternative, happiness with the choice, acting with the choice, and consistently incorporating the choice in one's actions. Values evolve over a lifetime in response to changing circumstances. During values clarification the aim is not to change values but to become aware of what those values are and the priority assigned to each. Only then can the nurse separate his or her values from that of the patient. Box 8-1 provides a list of common values.

Personal values are an important influence on how meaning is assigned to interactions and therefore decisions. The inherent tension between time freedom and economic security is one example. If someone must work to make a living but highly values free time, the person is likely to choose a lower-paying job if it is more flexible than a job with assigned office hours.

INTERPERSONAL COMMUNICATION

The next level of communication takes place interpersonally between two individuals. Receiver and sender become both intra-related and inter-related. As one is encoding or creating messages to be sent, the other is already decoding or interpreting the messages being sent. Human beings have an ability to selectively perceive at any given time the information most important to them.

In everyday life, especially in the 21st century, people are barraged by constant external messages. To cope with this noisy environment, three strategies are inherent to the cognitive process. The first, selective attention, is reinforced and made possible by the process of habituation. During selective attention, the most important messages are given more cognitive space than less-important messages. Habituation enhances this adaptation by blocking out extraneous external and internal messages.

Both selective attention and habituation are constantly in a state of flux. What is important to a new nurse in conversation with a patient might be vastly different from the selective attention of an experienced nurse, who might be more attuned to subtle clues about the patient's health status. Both nurses, however, can be influenced by internal messages that interfere with their ability to listen actively. This is especially true in today's health care environment, in which fatigue from 12-hour shifts or too many patients can interfere with communication. To survive in such an environment, habituation allows the nurse to block out fatigue and problems at home to listen to critical messages sent by the patient (Kreps & Thornton, 1984).

One final skill inherent in human beings is the ability for closure. During closure, people make sense out of the messages to which they attended. Educated assumptions are made to fill in the gaps about the message based on the receiver's logic and past experiences. Thus reality is relative and inexorably connected to past experiences (Kreps & Thornton, 1984). The nurse needs to develop particular skills to avoid premature closure, the most important of which is active listening.

Active Listening

Active listening is a learned skill in which the nurse suspends personal beliefs and values, resists categorization, and stays in the present, minimizing the influence of past experiences and self-directed current and future problems. The focus is entirely on the patient. The nurse, however, is not passive but is actively examining the content of the patient's message, sorting the relevant from the irrelevant, and seeking clarification from the sender. Selective attention and habituation undergo change as the nurse identifies themes from the conversation and educated assumptions are voiced for patient validation. Often nurses perceive listening to clients as "doing nothing for them." Active listening properly done, however, provides care and can require as much energy as the nurse expends during physical care of the patient (Pagano & Ragan, 1992; Sheldon, 2004; Williams, 2004).

Silence is an inherent part of active listening. Most nurses are uncomfortable with the use of silence in communication, deeming a pause in conversation as a patient's need for reassurance and a cue for a nurse to "fill in the blanks," often bringing the interaction to premature closure. Silence serves a critical role in communication, allowing both nurse and client to reflect on the interaction and its meaning. Often, letting the patient break the silence is important because it indicates to the sender (patient) that the nurse is willing to listen to the patient's feelings, thoughts, and insights. Occasionally, however, the nurse will need to respond, either by performing a therapeutic technique, moving the conversation in a different direction, or concluding the conversation. The essential interpretation on the part of the nurse is to ascertain carefully whether the silence is uncomfortable for the patient or for the receiver (the nurse); that determination should guide the nurse's actions (Northouse & Northouse, 1998; Sheldon, 2004; Williams, 2004).

Therapeutic Responses

In addition to silence, active listening is enhanced by verbal communication strategies that help the listener accurately receive the sender's intended message. The names of verbal communication strategies vary from author to author. The principal focus should be on the rationale for using any one particular technique and the effectiveness of the response in keeping the receiver selectively attending to the message sent and keeping the communication open until closure is truly achieved.

Restatement is a communication approach that has been variously described as repeating verbatim the last few words a patient says or paraphrasing the patient's words. Regardless, the goals of restatement are to let the patient know he or she is being listened to and to encourage the patient to elaborate without asking direct questions. This response technique should be used sparingly because overuse leads to an air of insincerity

and could be misconstrued as parroting the patient (Arnold & Boggs, 2011; Sheldon, 2004). Box 8-2 provides an example of restatement.

Reflection is another type of communication nurses can use to let patients know they are attending to their underlying feelings. Often patients will not come out and say how they feel about something, especially to health care providers, where the balance of power is uneven. As nurses, we should actively listen to what patients are communicating, even if the content of the message does not include stated feelings, and then reflect perceptions back to them for validation. Box 8-3 provides an example of reflection.

Clarification is an ongoing strategy to ensure that the message received is the message that was sent. Human beings want to make sense of the world around them and will often move toward premature closure by filling in the gaps by using logic and past experience without checking the accuracy of their assumptions with the sender. This can be one of the most grievous mistakes in therapeutic communication, almost guaranteeing that the patient will feel misunderstood. In a concept analysis of feeling misunderstood, Condon (2008) found that consequences included "termination of activity, such as relationships" (p. 183). Thus the patient will become reluctant to engage. Therefore clarification should be used when the patient makes a

---

BOX 8-2   Restatement

Patient: I don't know when to schedule my surgery. The surgeon has offered me Monday or Tuesday.

   Nurse 1: Monday or Tuesday ...?

   Nurse 2: You are unsure of which day would be best to schedule surgery.

   Note that in both responses, the nurse is offering the patient an opportunity to discuss why deciding when to schedule surgery is difficult.

BOX 8-3   Reflection

Patient: I don't want to take this treatment anymore. It just makes me sicker than when I came into the hospital. How is this helping me?

   Nurse: You are afraid that the treatment we are giving you will not make you well.

   Note that the nurse identified an underlying fear the patient has about the effectiveness of the treatment.

vague statement or retroactively after the patient finishes a train of thought. Box 8-4 provides an example of clarification.

Minimal cues, leads, and touch are also useful in therapeutic communication. Minimal cues show that the nurse is interested and present for the patient without interrupting the patient's flow of thought. Leaning forward, giving short leads such as "yes," "uh huh," and "go on" convey a clear message that the nurse is actively listening. Touch is a basic sense and need that all human beings share. Intentionally touching the patient lightly on the arm or shoulder sends a message of comfort that is more powerful and deep than many words (Arnold & Boggs, 2011). The nurse should carefully discern when the patient would accept touch in the context of cultural influences and past experiences.

Summarization helps both the patient and the nurse integrate the meaning of the interaction by relating ideas and feelings expressed during the conversation in a short synopsis for review by both of the participants. The nurse is responsible for critically thinking about the material and offering a brief summation. In turn the patient's responsibility is to add to the nurse's observations or correct them. With summarization both nurse and client can move on to a different topic or terminate the interaction.

Questioning is a strategy that every nurse uses on a daily basis to obtain information about the client. Questions can be closed or open ended. Contrary to the belief that all close-ended questions must be answered with a yes or no response, the basic premise of a close-ended question is to compel a direct response from the patient. Examples include asking the patient's age, as well as inquiries that require the patient to answer yes or no. Open-ended questions, on the other hand, allow patients to respond in any direction they wish and give the nurse new information about their concerns and goals. Patients are given a general invitation to respond to when, where, and how they sought help in the health care system. Asking "why" is not a helpful strategy because it puts the patient on the defensive by asking reasons for behavior that even the patient might not understand (Arnold & Boggs, 2011; Williams, 2004).

Many nursing students, especially experienced RNs, get caught up in the minutiae and appear stilted and uncomfortable when trying to implement these communication strategies. The best approach is to be oneself and put specific, concrete strategies into a larger picture. There is tension among nursing professionals about the use of strategies, which some believe to be a task-based approach. The crux of intentional dialogue is to focus on creating ease in the relationship; to set aside "self-focus to be truly present and gather another's story about a health challenge" (Smith & Liehr, 2008, p. 176). A more comprehensive framework helps the nurse to draw together the whole and incorporates four of the rights mentioned at the beginning of the chapter: the right route, right dose, right time, and the right person.

Determining the Right Route

There is more to communication than talking and listening. A powerful alternative route to understanding the client is the use and interpretation of nonverbal behavior. The nurse gives and receives nonverbal cues that greatly influence the interaction. Important nonverbal behaviors include facial expression, eye contact, hand and arm gestures, posture, and use of personal space. Facial expressions are informative in terms of their congruence with the subject matter under discussion. If the patient is recalling a frightening event, is his expression serious and reflective of his feelings? A broad smile or laugh would indicate an inconsistency between the spoken and unspoken message that needs to be explored. One approach to this situation is to confront the patient directly with the incongruence by stating, "You are telling me about a very frightening experience, yet you are laughing about it."

The meaning of eye contact varies from person to person and from culture to culture. Looking someone in the eye can convey many things: a sense of respect and trustworthiness, confidence in oneself, a personal interest in the speaker, and conversely, hostility or insult. Culture is

---

BOX 8-4   Clarification

Patient: I cannot stand that other nurse. She comes in and only looks at the IV pump and then quickly leaves the room.

Nurse 1: Tell me more about what happened with the nurse this morning.

Nurse 2: You said earlier in the conversation that you were having trouble with one nurse. Can you give me an example?

Note that Nurse 1 immediately follows up to help the patient clarify what he perceives in the nurse's actions. Nurse 2 reminds the patient of an earlier remark and asks the patient to elaborate. In both cases, the nurses are asking for specifics to help both them and their client be clear about the situation.

the main influencing factor regarding the interpretation of eye contact. For example, Asians and Pacific Islanders understand a downward glance as a sign of respect, whereas Americans might interpret looking away as disinterest or boredom (Sheldon, 2004).

Arm and hand gestures inform the nurse during the interaction. Open gestures indicate a willingness to share and be open, whereas folded arms convey unwillingness to talk or vulnerability and a need for self-protection (Sheldon, 2004). Posture also reveals underlying feelings. Leaning forward conveys a sense of interest and active listening, whereas a rigid posture could imply, "I don't want to talk to you." In addition, the use of personal space is telling. Although different cultures use personal space in varying ways, Americans generally understand this distance to be 18 inches to 4 feet. These boundaries, which help people maintain a sense of identity and assert safety and control in a vulnerable situation, must be observed (Northouse & Northouse, 1998; Sheldon, 2004).

An appropriate setting, the use of understandable language, boundaries set with a clear contract, and the establishment of confidentiality are also routes to effective therapeutic communication. Although difficult in today's health care environment, a quiet, private setting to talk with a patient is fundamental, as is the use of language that the patient understands. A noisy public setting will cause distractions and fear of being overheard, and professional jargon confuses the patient, who will rarely ask for clarification. A clear contract gives the patient insight into the purpose of the interaction, how long the professional relationship is expected to last, and what the patient can expect of the health care provider. Confidentiality is an expectation that should be overtly stated; under Health Insurance Portability and Accountability Act (HIPAA) regulations, this should be given to the patient in writing.

The Right Dose

Although the nurse cannot precisely measure the dose of communication as is possible with drug therapy, several guidelines can help determine the intensity, the depth, and the content of a therapeutic interaction. Simply put, the client is the one person who directs the dose of the intervention. Mirroring the client depth or lack thereof during the interaction is important. If the client is exploring deeper feelings, then the nurse must go there with him or her. However, when the patient

gives a superficial response, responding with intensity is contraindicated. In addition, verbal responses need to match the patient's words without embellishment or minimization. Before the nurse can make assumptions, enough data must be available to warrant an interpretation (Arnold & Boggs, 2011).

The use of humor, reframing, presentation of reality, metaphors, and the sharing of personal information all must be given in the right dose. Humor is effective when purposely inserted into the conversation for a specific purpose. It can help reduce an overly intensive situation and allow the patient to appreciate the absurdities of life and humanity. Occasional use is more therapeutic than constant humor, which can minimize the seriousness of the patient's concerns. Another strategy, reframing, helps the patient see the larger reality and put things into perspective. One clue that reframing may be helpful is when the patient uses black-and-white phrases such as "always" or "never." Rarely in life, if at all, do such absolutes exist. Having the patient reexamine statements helps ameliorate feelings and opens the opportunity for a patient to move on. The use of metaphors can be overdone but is sometimes crucial to aid in the patient's understanding. Consider how this chapter uses a metaphor that equates the effective use of therapeutic communication with the correct method of drug administration in terms of how essential each task is to the patient's health. Finally, the right dose of personal information must be determined when interacting with a patient. A general guideline is to share only those issues that are fully resolved and pertinent to the conversation at hand to help the patient better understand himself or herself (Arnold & Boggs, 2011).

The Right Time

Timing is of the utmost importance when deciding how to respond in a therapeutic interaction. The first consideration is the stage of the relationship. Therapeutic relationships typically have four sequential phases: pre-orientation, orientation, working, and termination (Peplau, 1952). Pre-orientation takes place before the nurse even meets the client. During this phase the nurse reflects on professional roles and responsibilities, sets broad goals for the interaction, gets an overview of the patient's status, anticipates obstacles or difficulties, and thinks about the physical environment to maximize privacy and comfort.

The second stage, orientation, is when the therapeutic relationship begins. The main objective during this phase is to establish trust. The nurse is unfamiliar to the patient, who might be in new surroundings as well. To lay the groundwork for trust, the nurse needs to give the client basic information about himself or herself and explain why the nurse is there. The focus is the immediate problem that brought the patient to the health care system; deep exploration is avoided. Honesty and commitment are essential. If a nurse cannot keep an appointment, the patient deserves an explanation. Content is kept fairly superficial as the nurse bonds with the patient over everyday life interests; the nurse listens to the patient's story. Even seasoned registered nurses often ask how to begin a therapeutic conversation with a client they might be treating over a number of months. A helpful rule is to start a social conversation, perhaps asking about family pictures that may be on display or about something of interest to the client based on environmental clues (Smith & Liehr, 2008; Williams, 2004).

The third stage is when the work of the therapeutic relationship begins, thus the name *working phase*. During this phase rapport has been established and the interaction becomes more focused and intense for both the nurse and the patient. The nurse uses active listening and indirect verbal responses as the client reveals health care concerns. Because part of the relationship is more interactive, the importance of mirroring the client cannot be stressed enough. The nurse follows the client's lead, pursuing in-depth those issues that the client indicates a readiness to explore (Smith & Liehr, 2008). For example during gerontology courses, where students refine therapeutic communication, older adults will often tell students things they have never discussed with anyone.

The termination phase actually begins at the start of the relationship. During pre-orientation the nurse reflects on feelings about past experiences with endings. During orientation the nurse needs to be clear about the length of the contract, and the topic of termination needs to be revisited by the nurse and client during the working phase, when both parties have an opportunity to discuss what this ending might mean to them. Despite preparation, the client and even the nurse might resist termination. Behaviors that indicate resistance might be cancellation of appointments, anger, or an expressed disinterest in talking about important issues or termination itself. The responsibility of

the registered nurse student is to accept these feelings nonjudgmentally and help the client understand their meaning. If client issues need further intervention, the nurse should help connect the client to other resources.

Registered nurse students often become uncomfortable with the notion of leaving the client at a potentially important juncture in their work together and feel that they have "used" the client to further their own education at the client's expense. Students could be correct in that assumption if adequate preparation for termination has been ignored during the other phases of the relationship. Most often, however, this anxiety is part of student-centered issues around past losses that the student is reluctant to face.

The Right Person

The patient determines the right person to whom to entrust their deepest thoughts and concerns. The nurse can only prepare intra-personally (see beginning of chapter) and offer a safe and therapeutic environment for interpersonal interaction. If the patient is not ready or chooses someone else to confide in, the nurse should follow the patient's wishes and avoid taking the patient's decision personally.

ORGANIZATIONAL COMMUNICATION

An organization is by definition an interdependent entity whose members strive toward a common purpose of accomplishing stated goals: "Organizational communication refers to human communication between organization members (as well as between organization members and related others) during the performance of organizational tasks and the accomplishment of organizational goals" (Kreps & Thornton, 1984, p. 155). This discussion focuses on the basic understanding of the dynamics of organizational communication and group process.

Systems theory is a helpful way to understand the complexity of organizations. This theory posits that systems have both environmental inputs and outputs, which are vastly different by virtue of the synergy or added energy that occurs from the interactions among system parts. Therefore the product of the system is uniquely different from the mere summation of its parts or, as is often noted, the whole is greater than the sum of its parts. Think of the organization (hospital or health care system) as the system whose various patient and community health needs (inputs) are processed by the many levels of health team members, allowing its output to be flexible in providing health care services for many client groups (Kreps & Thornton, 1984). Figure 8-1 illustrates some of the influencing factors (throughput) on the product (output) of a health care organization. These influencing factors include upward, downward, and vertical or horizontal communication within the organization itself and the group process of its team members. Systems theory is also discussed in Chapter 5.

Types of Organizational Communication

Three types of formal organizational communication exist: upward, downward, and vertical. These formal networks follow the chain of command. Upward communication from subordinates to superiors usually takes on the form of reports. Downward communications from administration to workers on lower levels often are commands about decisions to be implemented, rules, and regulations.

Vertical communication, on the other hand, can be part of a formal or informal network. Formal ways of communicating horizontally are work groups and vertical connections among departments. Informal networks are formed by employees and are not controlled by management. These "grapevines" are faster than formal channels and are busy when employees feel insecure, are threatened, or are faced with organizational change. These communications are approximately 75% accurate and are the main source of practical job information (Baskin, 1984).

A key to successful outputs in a health care organization is professional-to-professional communication. Given the complexity of patient care problems, collaboration and cooperation are essential to deliver quality health care services. The nurse is often the coordinator of care and, as such, takes the lead in communication. This communication can be adversely influenced by three factors: role stress, lack of interprofessional understanding, and autonomy struggles (Northouse & Northouse, 1998).

Role stress is familiar to registered nurse and baccalaureate-degree students when roles are complicated by

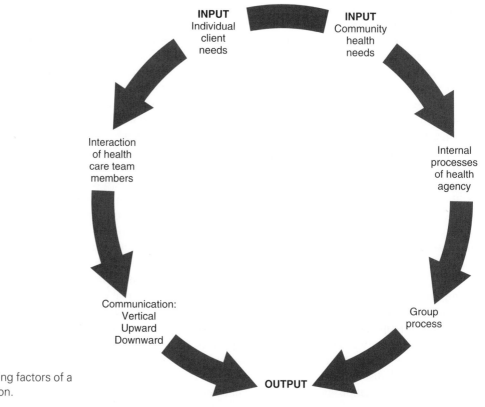

INPUT
Individual client needs

INPUT
Community health needs

Interaction of health care team members

Internal processes of health agency

Communication:
Vertical
Upward
Downward

Group process

OUTPUT

FIGURE 8-1 Influencing factors of a health care organization.

the addition of academic demands in already overscheduled lives. To better understand role stress, looking at two components is helpful: role conflict and role overload. Role conflict occurs when competing demands vie for attention in a limited time frame and the nurse is faced with choices that affect patient care. One example is the decrease in hospital days and the need to hurriedly discharge patients to open beds for other admissions. The new patient needs the hospital care, but the patient being discharged also needs teaching and planning for care outside the health care setting. Role overload is also common in settings, where the nursing shortage requires regular overtime and the responsibilities of the nurse increase as staffing decreases (Northouse & Northouse, 1998). These role challenges persist in today's rapidly changing health care environment and are discussed in more detail in Chapter 4. Additionally, the impacts of professional-to-professional communication are addressed in Chapter 20.

Lack of interprofessional understanding is cited as a significant impediment to communication. In a study by Laschinger and Weston (1995), groups of nursing and medical students were asked to describe their perceptions of one another's role. Not surprisingly, each group misunderstood the other group's expertise. The consequences of these misperceptions were profound and produced an inverse relationship in collaboration. The greater the gap in interprofessional understanding, the more negative the participants were toward shared decision making.

Autonomy struggles between health care professionals also disrupt professional-to-professional communication. Historically the nurse has been seen as the handmaiden of the physician. This perception has changed as physicians and nurses must work together in critical care settings, emergency departments, community-based practices, and long-term care of an increasingly aging population to achieve quality patient outcomes (Northouse & Northouse, 1998).

GROUP PROCESS

When considering organizational communication, it is important to understand group process and behaviors. Contrary to the popular notion of group inefficiency and ineffectiveness, groups tend to formulate effective solutions by building on one another's ideas, bringing different perspectives to the problem at hand,

and increasing commitment to a decision formed by consensus. To lead and participate in productive work groups, the nurse needs to understand group processes and behaviors. Two important dynamics are the life cycle of groups and group functions (Arnold & Boggs, 2011).

Group Phases

The typical group phases are forming, storming, norming, performing, and adjourning. When the group first forms, anxiety by group members is focused on acceptance. During this forming phase, group members are polite as they establish commonalities around goal setting, group identification, explicit norms of behavior, and methods of communication. As group comfort increases, members begin to challenge one another about boundaries, methods of goal achievement, group format, and discussion topics. This storming phase, although essential to deeper levels of group understanding, can be uncomfortable and thus sometimes not acknowledged. During this phase group members must acknowledge the tension and work toward developing group norms so that the group can progress to the next phase of group development (Arnold & Boggs, 2011).

During the next phase, norming, communication is more spontaneous and personal. Consensus is reached about group behavior that will increase the likelihood of the group achieving its goal. Members are more comfortable with divergent opinions but are able to agree on the best way to proceed. Consensus does not mean that all members must wholeheartedly agree on all the particulars, but rather each member supports group decisions enough to prevent conscious or unconscious undermining of their implementation. Group cohesiveness increases, and the members move on to the performing phase. An *esprit de corps* facilitates the accomplishment of group goals and group members feel a sense of both intellectual and emotional fulfillment. With the group's purpose realized, the group is no longer needed and the adjourning phase occurs. During this termination, members share feelings about group members and personal contributions to the group's work. Closing comments can help process previous interactions, integrate emotional and cognitive experiences, and "summarize the group experience" (Arnold & Boggs, 2011, p. 320).

Group Functions

More than a half-century ago, Bennis and Shepard (1956) separated group participant roles into three distinct functions: maintenance, task, and self-serving. Maintenance role functions help increase group satisfaction, whereas task role functions move the group toward goal accomplishment. Self-serving role functions serve individual needs that are unrelated to the group's purpose and thus interfere with group work toward a common mission (Arnold & Boggs, 2011; Northouse & Northouse, 1998).

Tables 8-2 to 8-4 give examples of task, maintenance, and self-serving behaviors. These behaviors occur in all groups. Therefore vital tasks include understanding, observing, and for task and maintenance behaviors, putting into practice group communication strategies that help move the group toward task accomplishment.

TABLE 8-2 Task Behaviors in Groups

TASK BEHAVIORS	DEFINITION	EXAMPLE
Initiator/contributor	Suggests new ideas	"Have you thought of …?"
Information seeker	Asks for clarification or information	"Do you mean …?"
Opinion seeker	Clarifies values	"What do you think …?"
Information giver	Offer facts or personal experiences	"I read in this research article …"
Opinion giver	States personal beliefs	"I think we should …"
Elaborator	Expands on ideas	"We could also …"
Coordinator	Pulls ideas together	"Sally suggested … and Tim's idea is similar …"
Orientor	Defines present position or raises questions about direction of group	"Where are we as a group on this?"
Evaluator-critic	Explores practicality and logic of discussion	"Given _____, will this idea work?"
Energizer	Urges group toward action	"Have we had enough discussion to move toward a decision?"
Procedural technician	Carries out routine tasks	Sets up chairs in a circle before meeting
Recorder	Writes down proceedings	E-mails group members a summary after each meeting

Modified from Northouse, L. L., & Northouse, P. G. (1998). *Health communication: Strategies for professionals.* Stamford, CT: Appleton & Lange.

TABLE 8-3 Maintenance Behaviors in Groups

MAINTENANCE BEHAVIORS	DEFINITION	EXAMPLE
Encourager	Praises and accepts others' contributions	"I really think that is a useful idea."
Harmonizer	Acts as a go-between	"I think you two are really saying the same thing."
Compromiser	Modifies position	"I see that some of the things I value are included so I can agree to …"
Gatekeeper	Regulates flow of group discussion	"We have 15 minutes left to discuss …"
Standard setter	Points out group goal	"I think we are getting off track …"
Group observer	Offers comments on group process	"Everyone seems to be much more comfortable offering different opinions on …"
Follower	Goes along with group	"If everyone else thinks …"

Modified from Northouse, L. L., & Northouse, P. G. (1998). *Health communication: Strategies for professionals.* Stamford, CT: Appleton & Lange.

TABLE 8-4 Self-Serving Behaviors in Groups

SELF-SERVING BEHAVIORS	DEFINITION	EXAMPLE
Aggressor	Verbally attacks others	"I think that idea is silly."
Blocker	Consistently disagrees with group ideas	"This situation is not going to change."
Recognition seeker	Calls attention to self	"I thought of that idea last night."
Self-confessor	Expresses unrelated personal feelings	"I felt awkward in that situation …"
Playboy/playgirl	Plays around and not involved	"Did you see on television last night …?"
Dominator	Interrupts other group members	"Before you finish, let me …"
Help seeker	Tries to elicit sympathy	"I just can't get this task done because …"
Special interest pleader	Champions positions of particular groups	"I know the union would …"

Modified from Northouse, L. L., & Northouse, P. G. (1998). *Health communication: Strategies for professionals.* Stamford, CT: Appleton & Lange.

SUMMARY

Effective communication can be analyzed using the processes developed for medication giving. Communication is dynamic and includes intrapersonal, interpersonal, and organizational communication. By using values clarification and other techniques, nurses can strive to improve their professional communication skills.

SALIENT POINTS

- Effective communication is conceptually similar to medication administration; it includes the right route, right dose, right time, and right person.
- Communication is the giving or exchanging of information signals or messages through gestures, writing, and talk.
- Communication occurs dynamically at many levels, including intrapersonal, interpersonal, small group, and organizational.
- Johari's window is a conceptual framework of the self expressed through a four-pane window metaphor. This framework is helpful in identifying boundaries for self-disclosure, depending on the intended form of communication.
- In professional relationships, self-disclosure is based on what is in the best interest of the patient.
- Values clarification is a method of developing self-awareness. Values clarification assists the nurses in separating their values from those of the patient.
- Strategies that enhance the cognitive processes involved in interpersonal communication include selective attention, habituation, and active listening.
- Nonverbal communication cues greatly influence interactions.
- Therapeutic communication is an important and effective intervention that is essential to a patient's health.
- The dynamics and complexity of organizational communication are best understood by using systems theory. Systems theory proposes that the environmental inputs and outputs of a system are greater than the sum of its parts because of the synergy of the interactions among its parts.
- A lack of interprofessional understanding among nursing and medical students of different disciplines has an inverse relationship on their ability to collaborate.

CRITICAL REFLECTION EXERCISES

1. Complete the value clarification exercise in Box 8-1 and discuss the results with your peers. Consider how your values could affect your ability to therapeutically communicate with patients.

2. Practice active listening by asking a peer to talk about her or his day. Lead with a broad statement such as "Tell me about your day." At various intervals use different responses to encourage the speaker to continue and to feel understood. Pay particular attention to reflecting feelings and content, restatement, and clarification. Have the speaker and a third person comment on your use of communication responses.

3. Reflect on your clinical/work experiences at various organizations and identify differences in upward, downward, and vertical communication patterns. Consider how the difference in organizational communication patterns affected the unit work environment (e.g., mentorship, staff morale, orientation processes).

4. Using Table 8-2, identify your role in group interactions. Obtain feedback from peers regarding their perceptions of your group communications and compare the feedback to your self-evaluation.

5. Visit http://empathy.colstate.edu/Exercises/sugar_test .htm to read about the Sugar Test by Thomas Endres (1998). Demonstrate the two sugar exercises and lead a class/group discussion on systems theory and the interdependence of group members.

REFERENCES

Arnold, A., & Boggs, K. U. (2011). *Interpersonal relationships: Professional communication skills for nurses* (6th ed.). Philadelphia: Elsevier-Saunders.

Baskin, O. W. (1984). *Interpersonal communication in organizations.* Glenview, IL: Scott Foresman.

Bennis, W., & Shepard, H. (1956). A theory of group development. *Human Relations, 9,* 415–437.

Clifford, J., & Marcus, G. (1986). *Writing culture: The poetic and politics of ethnography.* Berkeley, CA: University of California Press.

Condon, B. B. (2008). Feeling misunderstood: A concept analysis. *Nursing Forum, 43*(4), 177–191.

communication. (2014). Retrieved November 25, 2014, from In *Merriam-Webster Online Dictionary.* http://www.merriam-webster.com/dictionary/communicate.

Endres, T. G. (1998). *The sugar test: Demonstrating interdependence.* NCA Convention, November 1998 New York: Presented as part of the GIFTS program. Retrieved August 30, 2009, from http://empathy.colstate .edu/Exercises/sugar_test.htm.

Gergen, K. (1991). *The saturated self.* New York: Basic Books.

Gordon, T., & Edwards, W. S. (1995). *Making the patient your partner: Communication skills for doctors and other health care professionals.* Westport, CT: Auburn House.

Hearnden, M. (2008). Coping with differences in culture and communication in healthcare. *Nursing Standard, 23*(11), 49–59.

Heilker, D. (2007). Story sharing: Restoring the reciprocity of caring in long-term care. *Journal of Psychosocial Nursing and Mental Health Services, 45*(7), 20–24.

Kipling, R. (1928). *A book of words: Selections from speeches and addresses delivered between 1906 and 1927.* Manchester, NH: Ayer.

Kreps, G. L., & Thornton, B. C. (1984). *Health communication: Theory and practice.* New York: Longman.

Laschinger, H. K., & Weston, W. (1995). Role perceptions of freshman and senior nursing and medical students and attitudes toward collaborative decision making. *Journal of Professional Nursing, 11*(2), 119–128.

Luft, J., & Ingham, H. (1955). *The Johari window: A graphic model of interpersonal awareness.* Los Angeles: UCLA, Proceedings of the Western Training Laboratory in Group Development.

Maxwell, M. (1993). The authenticity of ethnographic research. *Journal of Childhood Communication Disorders, 13,* 1–12.

Northouse, L. L., & Northouse, P. G. (1998). *Health communication: Strategies for professionals.* Stamford, CT: Appleton & Lange.

Pagano, M. P., & Ragan, S. L. (1992). *Communication skills for nurses.* London: Sage.

Peplau, H. E. (1952). *Interpersonal relations in nursing.* New York: Putnam.

Patidar, A. B. (2012). *Communication and nursing education.* India: Pearson Education.

Sheldon, L. S. (2004). *Communication for nurses.* Thorofare, NJ: Slack.

Simon, S., Howe, L., & Kirschenbaum, H. (1972). *Values clarification: A handbook of practical strategies for teachers and students.* New York: Hart.

Smith, M. J., & Liehr, P. (2008). Theory guided translation: Emphasizing the human connection. *Archives of Psychiatric Nursing, 22*(3), 175–176.

Watson, J. (2008). *Nursing: The philosophy and science of caring* (rev. ed., pp. 281–288. Boulder, CO: University Press of Colorado.

Williams, C. (2004). *Therapeutic communication in nursing.* Thorofare, NJ: Slack.

CHAPTER 9

Think Like a Nurse: Essential Thinking Skills for Professional Nurses

Brenda C. Morris, EdD, MS, RN, CNE

http://evolve.elsevier.com/Friberg/bridge/

OBJECTIVES

At the completion of this chapter, the reader will be able to:

- Compare and contrast the concepts: critical thinking, clinical judgment, and clinical reasoning.
- Describe strategies to develop critical thinking and clinical reasoning.
- Apply the universal intellectual standards of thought to nursing practice.
- Describe the steps of the nursing process and the relationships among those steps.
- Discuss nursing activities associated with each step of the nursing process.
- Discuss the relationships among critical thinking, clinical judgment, clinical reasoning, and the nursing process.
- Apply critical thinking, clinical judgment, and clinical reasoning skills in nursing practice situations.

PROFILE IN PRACTICE

Elizabeth R. Lenz, PhD, RN, FAAN
Professor Emeritus, and Former Dean, College of Nursing, The Ohio State University, Columbus, Ohio

Critical thinking: it's recognizable when someone does it well and certainly evident when it is not happening. During the past three decades we have talked increasingly about critical thinking in nursing, but that wasn't always the case. In the early 1960s when I was entering the profession, serious efforts to change the "handmaiden" image of nursing were only just beginning. Clearly, if one's role is defined as handmaiden, rather than as colleague or independent decision maker, critical thinking is not deemed particularly important or even desirable. Rather, blind, noncritical obedience is the order of the day. Fortunately, as nursing has become more truly professional and nurses have functioned with increasing autonomy in increasingly complex situations, critical thinking has become a most important and valued competency.

What elements converge to produce a good critical thinker? Two essential types of learning provide the basis for critical thinking. The first is substantive. It is impossible to think critically about something you do not understand or about which you possess only partial information. Mastery of the theory and research findings that relate to the problem or issue to be addressed is essential to thinking critically.

The second type of learning involves the process of thinking critically. The skills of raising questions, using logic, and comprehensively considering alternative perspectives, explanations, and courses of action often can best be learned experientially within an environment that mandates thoughtful consideration, such as those that encourage discussion of diagnostic reasoning, facilitate debate, and challenge ideas. At first this type of candor can be frightening; however, the critical input of others, strengthens one's critical thinking abilities.

For me, the groundwork for critical thinking was laid early in my education. Fortunately, the faculty responsible for the BSN program I attended were forward-thinking and highly committed to the emerging definition of nursing as a true profession, with the requisite obligation to base action on scientific knowledge and clear and logical thinking. Without labeling the goal as such, we were consistently encouraged, groomed, and enabled to be critical thinkers. We were continually challenged by being asked to provide rationales for our decisions, to make explicit all of the alternative approaches and explanations we had considered and rejected, and to explain why.

The base hopefully having been laid during one's professional education, critical thinking depends not only on training, but also on an environment or context that enables, encourages, and rewards it. In clinical settings, time to engage in deliberative critical thinking is difficult to attain. Rather, it is expected that critical thinking occurs routinely without much cultivation. Benner's theory of novice to expert suggests that excellent clinical experience fosters the development of critical thinking, and that eventually critical thinking becomes almost automatic and intuitive. However, I assert that the level of critical thinking displayed by clinical experts needs to

be developed deliberately and strategically. The clinical environment in which I have seen critical thinking encouraged most effectively was one in which the expectations were explicit, critical thinking was measured routinely in the practice context, relevant learning and growth opportunities were provided, and critical thinking was taken into account in performance evaluation. In other words, the nursing leadership in that academic medical center truly valued critical thinking and was willing to assign it priority.

Nursing has reached the point in its evolution in which a consistent and continuous pattern of critical thinking by its practitioners is a mandate—a *sine qua non*. The assurance that critical thinking will be truly woven into the fabric of our profession will depend on our ability to recruit and retain intelligent, interested, and committed nurses; to provide challenging educational opportunities that develop the requisite competencies; and to provide and sustain the kinds of environments in which critical thinking is valued and demanded.

INTRODUCTION

To think like a nurse requires that we learn the content of nursing; the ideas, concepts and theories of nursing and develop our intellectual capacities and skills so that we become disciplined, self-directed, critical thinkers.

(Heaslip, 2008, retrieved from http://www.crit icalthinking.org/pages/critical-thinking-to-think-like-a-nurse/834)

Dramatic changes in the health care system and the practice of nursing have occurred during the past few decades as a result of changing population demographics, expanded access to health care, cost containment efforts, rapid technological advances, increased complexity of clients' health care needs, and a shift from acute care to community-based care. These changes have transformed nursing into a knowledge-based profession in which nurses routinely process information from multiple sources to make complex clinical judgments in planning, managing, delivering, and evaluating the health care of their clients (Huston, 2013). Nurses use critical thinking and clinical reasoning skills to make clinical judgments in the application of content specific knowledge to clinical practice (Heaslip, 2008, retrieved from http://www.criticalthinking.org/pages/critical-thinking-to-think-like-a-nurse/834). This chapter covers both classic and current sources to examine

the processes nurses use "to think like a nurse," including critical thinking, clinical reasoning, clinical judgment, and the nursing process.

WHAT IS CRITICAL THINKING?

Watson and Glaser (1964) described the concept of critical thinking as the combination of abilities needed to define a problem, recognize stated and unstated assumptions, formulate and select hypotheses, draw conclusions, and judge the validity of inferences. Scriven and Paul (1987) defined critical thinking as an intellectually disciplined process of conceptualizing, applying, analyzing, synthesizing, and evaluating information (retrieved from http://www.criticalthinking.org/pages/defining-critical-thinking/766). Ennis (1989) added the dimension of self-reflection, when he described critical thinking as "reasonable reflective thinking focused on deciding what to believe or do" (p. 4).

The American Philosophical Association (1990) Delphi research project produced the following consensus definition of critical thinking as:

Purposeful, self-regulatory, judgment which results in interpretation, analysis, evaluation, and inference, as well as explanation of evidential, conceptual, methodological, criteriological, or contextual considerations upon which that judgment is based. (American Philosophical Association, 1990)

BOX 9-1 Critical Thinking Cognitive Skills and Subskills

Interpretation	Inference
Categorization	Querying evidence
Decoding sentences	Conjecturing alternatives
Clarifying meaning	Drawing conclusions
Analysis	**Explanation**
Examining ideas	Stating results
Identifying arguments	Justifying procedures
Analyzing arguments	Presenting arguments
Evaluation	**Self-Regulation**
Assessing claims	Self-examination
Assessing arguments	Self-correction

Examples of the cognitive and metacognitive skills and sub-skills associated with critical thinking are presented in Box 9-1.

Facione and Facione (1996) recognized that critical thinking has two elements, including a disposition to think critically, as well as specific cognitive and metacognitive processes. Some characteristics consistent with the disposition to think critically include:

- *Inquisitiveness* is the demonstration of intellectual curiosity and a true desire for learning. Nurses who routinely ask, "I wonder why …" in the absence of a specific problem display inquisitiveness.
- *Systematicity* is the tendency toward organized, orderly, focused, and diligent inquiry.
  - Nurses who use a systematic approach to gathering data demonstrate systematicity.
- *Analyticity* is application of reasoning and the use of evidence to resolve problems. Nurses who use an analytic approach connect clinical observations with the theoretical knowledge to anticipate clinical events and intervene to prevent complications.
- *Truth seeking* is the desire to seek the best knowledge in a given context. Nurses who engage in truth seeking demonstrate courage in asking questions and strive to remain objective, and continually reevaluate new information.
- *Open-mindedness* is being tolerant of divergent views and being sensitive to one's own biases. Nurses who practice open-mindedness support the provision of culturally competent care to diverse populations.

- *Self-confidence* is trusting in one's own reasoning processes, and judgments. Nurses who demonstrate self-confidence are able to effectively present their clinical reasoning and judgments to improve client care.
- *Maturity* is the ability to approach problems, inquiry, and decision making with the understanding that some problems are ill defined, and that some situations have more than one plausible option. It is important for nurses to demonstrate maturity to facilitate ethical decision making in nursing.

Scheffer and Rubenfeld (2000) replicated the Delphi study with a panel of 55 nurse educators to obtain a consensus definition of critical thinking for nursing as:

> *An essential component of professional accountability and quality nursing care. Critical thinkers in nursing exhibit these habits of the mind: confidence, contextual perspective, creativity, flexibility, inquisitiveness, intellectual integrity, intuition, open-mindedness, perseverance, and reflection. Critical thinkers in nursing practice the cognitive skills of analyzing, applying standards, discriminating, information seeking, logical reasoning, predicting and transforming knowledge (p. 7).*

Elder and Paul (2010) defined critical thinking as self-directed, self-disciplined, and self-corrective thinking, implying that the individual applies intellectual standards to their thinking, and engages in a reflective thinking process. Critical thinkers are able to formulate clear and precise questions, gather information and assess its relevance, develop conclusions, think open-mindedly and explore alternative solutions to problems, and communicate effectively with others (Elder & Paul, 2010). It is important for critical thinkers to apply the Universal Intellectual Standards of clarity, accuracy, precision, relevance, depth, breadth, logic, and fairness to assess the quality of reasoning about a problem, issue, or situation (Paul & Elder, 2010, retrieved from http://www.criticalthinking.org/pages/universal-intellectual-standards/527).

Alfaro-LeFevre (2013) defines critical thinking in nursing as "purposeful, informed, outcome-focused thinking" (p. 8). Critical thinking applies logic, intuition, creativity, and reflective thinking to identify problems, issues, and risks and make judgments based on evidence. Critical thinking is guided by standards and laws, and incorporates elements of the nursing process, problem-solving, the scientific method, clinical reasoning, and clinical judgment (Alfaro-LeFevre, 2013).

There is consensus amongst most authors that critical thinking processes are generalizable and transferable across disciplines (Ennis, 1987; Facione, 1990; Paul, 1992; Watson & Glaser, 1964). However, the difference lies in the discipline specific context in which the critical thinking processes are applied. For example, professional nurses apply critical thinking to client care situations so as to make sound clinical judgments, whereas engineers apply critical thinking to business or industrial situations so as to make sound decisions. To effectively apply critical thinking to a discipline, the individual must have discipline specific knowledge, in addition to understanding how to use critical thinking processes.

Although a universally accepted definition of critical thinking has not emerged, agreement exists that it is a complex process. The variety of definitions helps provide insight into the myriad dimensions of critical thinking. The definitions presented earlier are summarized for comparison in Table 9-1.

INTELLECTUAL TRAITS OF CRITICAL THINKERS

Eight interdependent traits of mind are essential to becoming a critical thinker. These are presented in Box 9-2 (Elder & Paul, 2012):

- Intellectual integrity—the application of rigorous and consistent standards of evidence and the admission of errors when they occur
- Intellectual humility—an awareness of the limits of one's knowledge and sensitivity to the possibility of self-deception
- Confidence in reason—confidence in one's ability to think fairly
- Intellectual perseverance—willingness to seek intellectual insights continually over a period of time and in the face of difficulties
- Fair-mindedness—a consciousness of the need to treat all viewpoints alike, without reference to one's own feelings or vested interests
- Intellectual courage—a willingness to listen and examine all ideas, including those that trigger a negative reaction

TABLE 9-1 **Definitions of Critical Thinking**	
AUTHOR	**DEFINITION**
Watson & Glaser (1964)	The combination of abilities needed to define a problem, recognize stated and unstated assumptions, formulate and select hypotheses, draw conclusions, and judge the validity of inferences.
Scriven & Paul (1987)	An intellectually disciplined process of conceptualizing, applying, analyzing, synthesizing, and evaluating information.
Ennis (1989)	"Reasonable reflective thinking focused on deciding what to believe or do" (p. 4).
American Philosophical Association (1990) Delphi research project	Purposeful, self-regulatory, judgment which results in interpretation, analysis, evaluation, and inference, as well as explanation of evidential, conceptual, methodological, criteriological, or contextual considerations upon which that judgment is based.
Scheffer & Rubenfeld (2000)	"An essential component of professional accountability and quality nursing care. Critical thinkers in nursing exhibit these habits of the mind: confidence, contextual perspective, creativity, flexibility, inquisitiveness, intellectual integrity, intuition, open-mindedness, perseverance, and reflection. Critical thinkers in nursing practice the cognitive skills of analyzing, applying standards, discriminating, information seeking, logical reasoning, predicting and transforming knowledge" (p. 7).
Elder & Paul (2010)	Self-directed, self-disciplined, and self-corrective thinking, implying that the individual applies intellectual standards to their thinking, and engages in a reflective thinking process.
Alfaro-LeFevre (2013)	"Purposeful, informed, outcome-focused thinking" (p. 8).

- Intellectual empathy—imagining oneself in the place of others to better understand them; allows reasoning from the viewpoint of others
- Intellectual autonomy—having rational control of one's beliefs, values, and inferences

BOX 9-2   Intellectual Traits of Critical Thinkers

Intellectual Integrity
Application of standards of evidence and the admission of errors when they occur

Intellectual Humility
An awareness of the limits of one's knowledge

Confidence in Reason
Confident in one's ability to think fairly

Intellectual Perseverance
Seek intellectual insights continually over a period of time

Fair-Mindedness
Ability to treat all viewpoints alike, without reference to one's own feelings

Intellectual Courage
Willingness to listen and examine all ideas

Intellectual Empathy
Ability to reason from the viewpoint of others

Intellectual Autonomy
Have control of one's beliefs, values, and inferences

Adapted from Elder and Paul, 2012.

STRATEGIES TO BUILD CRITICAL THINKING SKILLS

Critical thinking is enhanced in environments that are caring, nonthreatening, flexible, and respectful of diverse points of view. Nurses who are familiar with the nursing process, the scientific method, evidence-based practice, and research methods already know much about critical thinking because they are based on some of the same principles.

Strategies to enhance critical thinking include fostering the development of critical thinking dispositions, the intellectual traits of critical thinkers, and taking time to reflect upon one's thinking and nursing practice. Becoming a critical thinker is a lifelong process; everyone can improve by working at it.

CLINICAL REASONING

Definitions of clinical reasoning are presented in Table 9-2. Alfaro-LeFevre (2013) defines clinical

reasoning as "ways of thinking about patient care situations" (p. 8). Clinical reasoning applies the thought processes associated with critical thinking, such as problem solving, diagnostic, ethical and moral reasoning, decision making, and evidence-based practice to make judgments about patient care situations.

Tanner (2006) defines clinical reasoning as the "processes by which nurses and other clinicians make their judgments, and includes both the deliberate process of generating alternatives, weighing them against the evidence, and choosing the most appropriate" (pp. 204-205).

Benner, Sutphen, Leonard, and Day (2010) define clinical reasoning as "ability to reason about a clinical situation as it unfolds, as well as the patient and family concerns and the context" (p. 46). Contextualization is important in developing clinical reasoning, as it allows the nurse to consider the multiple variables that impact the patient's situation, such as the patient's history, responses to the environment, interventions, and treatments: interrelationships between physiological systems, social interactions with others, and the presence/absence of a support system (Benner et al., 2010). Contextualization helps the nurse to apply clinical reasoning to a specific patient situation and make appropriate patient-specific clinical judgments.

Simmons (2010) defines clinical reasoning as a, "complex process that uses cognition, metacognition, and discipline-specific knowledge to gather and analyze patient information, evaluate its significance, and weigh alternative actions" (p. 1151). The attributes of clinical reasoning include analysis, deliberation, inference, metacognition, logic, cognition, information processing, and intuition. Nurses use clinical reasoning cognitive processes when applying the nursing process to client care situations. Many variables affect clinical reasoning, such as cognitive ability, life experience, professional expertise, and maturity (Simmons, 2010).

The cognitive and metacognitive thought processes used to develop critical thinking, and contextualization help the nurse develop clinical reasoning. For example, when assessing the patient, the nurse uses metacognition to reflect upon data collection to ensure that all essential information has been gathered; and that appropriate analysis and interpretation have occurred. The nurse uses contextualization to assess for cues to

TABLE 9-2   Definitions of Clinical Reasoning

AUTHOR	DEFINITION
Alfaro-LeFevre (2013)	"Ways of thinking about patient care situations" (p. 8).
Tanner (2006)	"Processes by which nurses and other clinicians make their judgments, and includes both the deliberate process of generating alternatives, weighing them against the evidence, and choosing the most appropriate" (pp. 204–205).
Benner et al. (2010)	"The ability to reason about a clinical situation as it unfolds, as well as the patient and family concerns and the context" (p. 46).
Simmons (2010)	"Complex process that uses cognition, metacognition, and discipline-specific knowledge to gather and analyze patient information, evaluate its significance, and weigh alternative actions" (p. 1151).

better understand the patient's specific situation and to guide the clinical reasoning process. Another helpful strategy to develop clinical reasoning is learning how to anticipate potential complications or outcomes, and how to respond to prevent the onset of the complications or untoward outcomes.

In summary, clinical reasoning is a complex cognitive process that involves metacognition, contextualization, and discipline specific knowledge to make decisions about client care. Clinical reasoning is similar to critical thinking in that many of the same cognitive and metacognitive processes are used. However, critical thinking is broader than clinical reasoning, and may be applied in both clinical and nonclinical situations.

CLINICAL JUDGMENT

Critical thinking and clinical reasoning are the processes used to make a clinical judgment, which is "the conclusion you come to, the decision you make, or the opinion you form" (Alfaro-LeFevre, 2013, p. 70). Tanner (2006) defines clinical judgment as "an

interpretation or conclusion about a patient's needs, concerns or health problems, and/or the decision to take action (or not), use or modify standard approaches, or improvise new ones as deemed appropriate by the patient's response" (p. 204).

To make good clinical judgments, the nurse must "understand the pathophysiological and diagnostic aspects of a patient's disease, but also the illness experience for the patient and family, and their physical, social and emotional strengths and coping resources" (Tanner, 2006, p. 205). Several factors influence a nurse's ability to make clinical judgments, including prior experience and knowledge, assessment of the situation, knowing the patient's typical pattern of responses, and understanding the political and social contexts in which the situation occurs. Nurses use one or more different types of reasoning to make clinical judgments. The analytical approach to reasoning involves breaking down a situation into its elements and comparing the elements to the desired clinical outcomes or textbook outcomes for a similar situation. Other reasoning approaches include the use of intuition or narrative thinking.

Tanner (2006) developed a four-step model that describes the major phases of clinical judgment (noticing, interpreting, responding, and reflecting) for use in rapidly changing clinical situations. The first step in the model is noticing; during this phase, the nurse assesses the clinical situation based on knowledge of the patient, including the patient's usual response patterns, and prior experience with similar types of situations. The nurse uses reasoning skills to interpret the meaning of the data and respond to the situation by determining the appropriate course of action during the interpreting and responding phases. The nurse reflects upon the situation during the final phase (reflection). The initial reflection-in-action occurs during the noticing, interpreting, and responding phases when the nurse evaluates the assessment of the patient, patient's response to nursing interventions, and outcomes (Lasater, 2007). After responding to the clinical situation, the nurse performs reflection-on-action, where the nurse retrospectively evaluates the overall situation, and connects nursing actions with outcomes. It is during the reflection-on-action phase, that new clinical learning occurs (Lasater, 2007; Tanner, 2006). Table 9-3 presents definitions of clinical judgment.

TABLE 9-3 Definitions of Clinical Judgment

AUTHOR	DEFINITION
Alfaro-LeFevre (2013)	Critical thinking and clinical reasoning are the processes used to make a clinical judgment, which is "the conclusion you come to, the decision you make, or the opinion you form" (p. 70).
Tanner (2006)	"An interpretation or conclusion about a patient's needs, concerns or health problems, and/or the decision to take action (or not), use or modify standard approaches, or improvise new ones as deemed appropriate by the patient's response" (p. 204).

THE NURSING PROCESS

The nursing process is a systematic, problem-solving approach that provides the framework for nursing practice in the United States and Canada (ANA, 2004; Carpenito, 2013). The nursing process has five steps including:

- *Assessment*—gathering and validating client health data, strengths, risks, and concerns
- Diagnosis—analyzing and processing client data to identify appropriate nursing diagnoses*
- *Planning*—developing interventions to solve identified problems and build on client strengths
- *Implementation*—delivering nursing interventions and documenting the planned care
- *Evaluation*—determining the effectiveness of the care delivered

The American Nurses Association (ANA), in its publication *Nursing: Scope and Standards of Practice* (2004), uses the nursing process as the framework for professional nursing practice. Outcome identification, which follows the nursing diagnosis phase and precedes the planning phase, is identified as a separate step in the ANA model.

---

* Outcomes identification may be included as part of the diagnosis phase, or it may be recognized as a separate step in the nursing process.

The nursing process is sometimes depicted as a systematic, linear model proceeding from assessment through diagnosis, planning, implementation, and evaluation. It is more appropriately conceptualized as a continuous and interactive model, thereby providing a flexible and dynamic approach to client care. This model can accommodate changes in the client's health status or failure to achieve expected outcomes through a feedback mechanism. The interactive nature of the model with its feedback mechanism permits the nurse to reenter the nursing process at the appropriate stage to collect additional data, restructure nursing diagnoses, design a new plan, or change implementation strategies. This model is consistent with the concepts of critical thinking and clinical reasoning as ways of processing thinking about client care issues. Further examination of the elements of the nursing process reveals the multiple activities embedded in each step.

Assessment

In the assessment phase, the nurse deliberately and systematically collects data to determine the client's health, functional status, strengths, and risk factors (Carpenito, 2013). Data collection centers on the use of multiple sources and types of data, a variety of data collection techniques, and the use of reliable and valid measurement instruments. All these elements are critical to building a comprehensive database.

Sources of Data. The primary source of data is the client, whether the client is defined as the individual, the family, or the community. Secondary sources of data include written records, other health care providers, and significant others (e.g., family members, friends). To strengthen the overall assessment and validate client data, it is important to use primary and secondary data sources.

Data Collection Techniques. Assessment techniques include measurement, observation, and interview. Measurement is used to determine the dimensions of a given indicator (e.g., blood pressure) or to ascertain characteristics such as quantity, size, or frequency. Measurement may require the use of specialized equipment (e.g., stethoscope, thermometer) or specialized assessment tools (e.g., pain scale, depression scale) to assess functional, behavioral, social, or cognitive domains. Data collection by observation requires the use of the senses, including visual observation and tactile (palpation) and auditory techniques (auscultation). Observation provides a variety and depth of data that may be difficult to obtain by other methods. A structured or unstructured interview may be used to obtain information such as a health history and demographic data. A structured interview is commonly used in emergency situations when the nurse needs to gather specific information. An unstructured interview is commonly used in situations in which the nurse wishes to elicit information from the client's perspective or gain insight to the client's understanding of a problem. The unstructured interview allows the nurse to use active listening skills while building rapport with the client through the use of an open-ended interview format. These communication techniques are discussed in more detail in Chapter 8.

Types of Data. To complete a comprehensive assessment, objective and subjective data are obtained. Objective data are factual data, usually obtained through observation or measurement. An example of objective data occurs when the nurse uses an otoscope to assess the client's tympanic membrane and observes that it is reddened and inflamed. Subjective data are based on the client's perception of the health problem. An example of subjective data occurs when the client states that he is having pain in his right ear. It is important to collect both objective and subjective data to complete a comprehensive assessment. Care should be taken to record data factually and to avoid personal or biased interpretations.

Data Collection Instruments. The use of selected data collection measures and instruments can assist the nurse in compiling a comprehensive database and organizing data into meaningful patterns. Assessment usually begins by taking a nursing history and conducting a physical examination. The nursing database should include the following categories of information:

- Demographic data
- Current and past medical problems
- Family medical history
- Surgical and (if appropriate) obstetrical history
- Childhood illnesses
- Allergies
- Current medications
- Psychological status
- Social history
- Environmental background
- Physical assessment

The amount of detail may vary; for example, a history obtained in an emergency department may be different from one taken in an extended care facility. The focus of the assessment and history also may vary on the basis of the type of client served. For example, on an oncology unit emphasis may be placed on assessment of pain, social support networks, and coping skills, whereas in a prenatal clinic the focus would be on assessment of fetal growth, knowledge of nutrition, and the need for community resources such as childbirth education classes. Beyond the areas of particular concern, however, all dimensions of the client, including physiological, psychological, sociocultural, developmental, and spiritual aspects, should be assessed (Carpenito, 2013).

To ensure appropriate identification of client health problems, it is important to perform a comprehensive assessment. The nurse may also use the assessment phase as a time to establish the nurse–client and nurse–family relationships and begin the discharge planning process. Completion of a comprehensive assessment lays the foundation for making effective clinical judgments and implementing appropriate nursing care to meet the client's identified health needs. To accurately assess a client, the nurse must apply the critical thinking skills of observing, distinguishing relevant from irrelevant data, validating the accuracy and completeness of the data, and organizing the data to provide the basis for subsequent analysis and diagnosis.

Analysis/Nursing Diagnoses

Analysis involves processing the data by organizing, categorizing, and synthesizing the information. The nurse uses critical thinking skills to make inferences in the data from which conclusions can be drawn. Analysis gives meaning to the data as client strengths, problems, and risks are identified. Client data may be compared against known norms, such as the stages of growth and development or disease-specific behaviors or expectations. Gaps or incongruities in the data are identified, and patterns of behavior are ascertained. Analysis occurs while the nurse is actively listening and questioning the client, and later, when the nurse processes the information to formulate a plan of care. Analysis is an ongoing process that is initiated when new information is obtained or changes in the client's health status occur. The end result of data analysis is the formation of a *nursing diagnosis*.

As noted in Carpenito (2013), the North American Nursing Diagnosis Association (NANDA) defines nursing diagnosis as a "clinical judgment about individual, family or community responses to actual or potential health problems/life processes. The nursing diagnosis provides the basis for selection of nursing interventions to achieve outcomes for which the nurse is accountable" (Carpenito, 2013, p. 20). Diagnosis involves using critical thinking and clinical reasoning skills to draw conclusions from identified patterns in the data. Diagnosis includes the elements of deliberation, inference, interpretation, and choice (Carpenito, 2013). The nurse uses inductive and deductive reasoning to determine an appropriate nursing diagnosis. A nurse uses *inductive reasoning* when making the observation that clients who underwent bowel resection surgery experience intense postoperative pain. From this observation, the nurse concludes that all clients who undergo bowel resection surgery will probably experience pain postoperatively and therefore will have the nursing diagnosis of acute pain. *Deductive reasoning* is used to draw specific conclusions from generalized data or facts. If the nurse accepts the premise that pain in the left arm and jaw is a cardinal sign of a myocardial infarction, then when a client presents to the emergency department complaining of left arm and jaw pain, the nurse uses deductive reasoning to suspect that the client is having a myocardial infarction until it can be proved otherwise. Diagnosis entails back-and-forth movement between these two modes of reasoning.

Nursing diagnoses reflect actual or potential health problems that can be treated within the scope of nursing practice (Carpenito, 2013). A nursing diagnostic statement differs from a medical diagnosis in both content and context. The medical diagnosis describes a pathological condition or symptom that requires treatment aimed at curing the disease or alleviating the symptom. The nursing diagnosis, on the other hand, describes the human response to the illness or life event.

It is important for the nurse to accurately identify the client's nursing diagnoses and to validate these nursing diagnoses with the client. If the nursing diagnoses are not validated with the client before nursing interventions are implemented, the nursing care plan may be ineffective and may not meet the client's health care needs. The client's nursing diagnosis guides the planning, implementation, and evaluation phases of nursing care.

Planning

During the planning phase of the nursing process, the nurse collaborates with the client to establish the priority nursing diagnosis or diagnoses, determine client outcomes, and identify nursing interventions to assist the client toward optimal achievement of outcomes (Carpenito, 2013). It is important to involve the client, family, and significant others in the planning process, when appropriate, to gain their support for implementing the plan of care.

Prioritizing nursing diagnoses consists of ranking them according to importance. In general, the highest-priority nursing diagnoses address basic survival needs, life-threatening client problems, and safety. Additional considerations in setting priorities are the need for early resolution of health problems that have the potential to impair functioning or normal growth and development; the client's individual needs, values, and overall health status; and constraints of time and resources. Ideally, the client and nurse mutually determine the priority nursing diagnoses; however, this is not always possible.

Once priorities are established, desired outcomes are identified. *Outcomes* are client centered, specific, realistic, and measurable, and they include a time frame. Outcomes are written to reflect attainment of an optimal level of health, alleviation or minimization of a health problem, or modifications of lifestyle. It is recommended to begin the outcome statement with the phrase "The client will …." This helps the nurse to write the outcome from the client's perspective rather than the nurse's perspective. It is helpful to use the following format when writing an outcome statement: "The client will (*insert action verb and behavioral criterion*) by (*insert time frame*)." An example of a well-written outcome is as follows: "The client will ambulate 50 feet with the assistance of a walker by the first postoperative day." In this example, the phrase "ambulate 50 feet with the assistance of a walker" includes the action verb and behavioral criterion; the phrase "by the first postoperative day" describes the time frame. In clinical situations a specific date and time (e.g., 9 AM on 10/10/2015) may be used. See Table 9-4 for another example of a well-written client outcome.

Each outcome must be accompanied by one or more *nursing interventions* aimed at helping the client achieve the outcome. Nursing interventions may be nurse- or physician-prescribed (Carpenito, 2013). All

TABLE 9-4   Example of a Measurable Behavioral Outcome

OUTCOME	CHARACTERISTIC
The client will walk	Performance
One half the length of the hall	Criterion
Unassisted	Condition
On the second postoperative day	Condition

nursing interventions require the use of critical thinking, clinical reasoning, and clinical judgment because the nurse is legally responsible for intervening appropriately (Carpenito, 2013). Nursing interventions may be performed by the nurse or delegated to assistive personnel as appropriate. It is important to select nursing interventions that are specific to the nursing diagnosis, acceptable to the client, feasible to implement, realistic, and supported with scientific rationale or evidence.

Nursing diagnoses, client outcomes, and nursing interventions are incorporated into a nursing care plan. *The nursing care plan* is used as a communication tool between nurses and other health professionals and serves as a guide for nursing care. Clinical agencies may use standardized care plans or care maps created by clinical experts, which contain common nursing diagnoses, client outcomes, and nursing interventions for clients experiencing common medical and surgical illnesses. Nurses customize the standardized care plans or care maps to meet the specific needs of their client.

Implementation

During the implementation phase, the nurse executes the previously identified plan of care by using intellectual, interpersonal, and technical skills to provide care that is client focused and outcome oriented and meets the needs of the client. Common nursing interventions initiated during the implementation phase include performing assessments to monitor client health status; providing or assisting the client with personal care; assisting the client to perform activities of daily living; administering medications or other prescribed treatments; teaching the client; or consulting with other health care professionals. During implementation, the nurse uses critical thinking, and clinical reasoning skills to apply knowledge to client care situations, reflect upon implementation of the plan of care by assessing for changes in the client's condition, evaluating the

effectiveness of the nursing interventions, and making changes to the plan of care based on this assessment.

The final step in the implementation phase is careful documentation. The system of documentation may be agency specific, but the content should reflect the client's concerns and the nursing process. It is important to include the following information in the record:

- A description of the nursing intervention that was performed
- The client's response to the intervention
- Any new data that may have emerged
- Progress (or lack of it) toward achievement of client care outcomes

Documentation should also include a description of any planned interventions that did not occur and the reasons why they were not implemented. It is very important to ensure that all information is documented correctly; therefore it is recommended that nurses review their documentation for errors prior to finalization.

Evaluation

Evaluation is an ongoing activity that occurs at each stage of the nursing process. The overall purpose of the evaluation phase of the nursing process is to determine whether the client met the identified outcomes. The nurse evaluates the attainment of outcomes by comparing the predicted outcome with the client's actual progress toward meeting the outcome.

Evaluation occurs within each step of the nursing process. During the assessment phase, evaluation focuses on the appropriateness and completeness of data collection. During the analysis and diagnosis phase, evaluation centers on whether the data are appropriately clustered; whether the nursing diagnoses reflect the data and the client's health concerns; and whether the nursing diagnoses are clear, concise, and relevant. During the planning process, evaluation activities are directed toward determining the appropriateness of the outcomes, nursing diagnosis priorities, and selected nursing interventions. During the implementation stage, evaluation focuses on the relevance and effectiveness of specific nursing interventions. The nurse and client continue to evaluate these components until the client's health concerns are resolved, the outcomes are achieved, or the episode of care ends.

Another way to focus evaluation activities is to judge the appropriateness, effectiveness, and efficiency of the plan of care and its implementation. The ideal plan of care is relevant to the client's health concerns and focuses on mutually desirable outcomes; is effective in achieving desired outcomes within the specified time frame; and is efficient in maximizing the use of client, provider, and agency resources.

Guidelines for Evaluation. As previously mentioned, evaluation includes comparing actual outcomes against predicted outcomes and evaluating the nursing care plan. If the outcomes are not met, the nurse and client must determine the reason. The following questions may be asked:

- Were the assessment data appropriate and complete?
- Were the data interpreted correctly?
- Were the nursing diagnoses appropriate?
- Were the outcomes realistic, attainable, and measurable?
- Was the nursing care plan directed toward resolution of nursing diagnoses?
- Was the implementation of the plan individualized in accordance with the client's strengths and limitations?
- Were both the nurse and the client working toward the same outcomes?

Based on the answers to these questions, the nurse will modify the plan of care.

The nursing process principles discussed in this chapter as they relate to nursing care for individuals and families can be applied to communities, populations, systems, and organizations to address health status, care environments, or delivery of services.

CRITICAL THINKING, CLINICAL REASONING, CLINICAL JUDGMENT, AND THE NURSING PROCESS: PUTTING IT ALL TOGETHER IN NURSING PRACTICE

What is the significance of critical thinking, clinical reasoning, and clinical judgment to professional nursing practice?

Nurses have become more autonomous in their practice and responsible for the outcomes of patient care during the past few decades. The use of technology in providing health care and the acuity of hospitalized patients has increased significantly requiring more complex nursing care management. The ongoing shift from acute care to community-based care requires nurses to become experts in coordinating complicated transitions of care with patients and families. Because of these fast paced changes in the health care environment, and the increased complexity of nursing practice, it is imperative for nurses to have strong critical thinking, clinical reasoning, and clinical judgment skills to provide safe, effective nursing care.

The American Association of Colleges of Nursing (AACN) establishes nursing program standards and defines entry-level competencies for baccalaureate-prepared nurses and recognizes the significance of producing nurse graduates who demonstrate strong critical thinking, clinical reasoning, and clinical judgment skills (AACN Baccalaureate Essentials, 2008). Baccalaureate nurse graduates are provided with a solid foundation for the development of clinical reasoning and critical thinking through the liberal arts coursework provided by baccalaureate education, and the resulting integration of concepts from the arts; behavioral, biological, and natural sciences. These courses provide the pre-requisite knowledge for understanding the dimensions of health and illness necessary for the development of clinical reasoning and critical thinking (AACN Baccalaureate Essentials, 2008).

Essential competencies for baccalaureate nurse graduates are to "practice from a holistic, caring framework; promote safe, quality patient care; demonstrate strong critical reasoning, clinical judgment, communication, and assessment skills" (AACN Essentials for Baccalaureate Nursing Education, 2008, p. 9). Baccalaureate nurse graduates integrate evidence from multiple sources "to inform practice and make clinical judgments" (AACN Essentials for Baccalaureate Nursing Education, 2008, p. 17). In addition, "the baccalaureate graduate demonstrates clinical reasoning within the context of patient centered care to form the basis for nursing practice that reflects ethical values" (AACN Essentials for Baccalaureate Nursing Education, 2008, p. 29).

Professional standards, such as the American Nurses Association's (ANA) *Code of Ethics for Nurses with Interpretive Statements (2004)*, the ANA's (2010) *Scope and Standards of Nursing Practice*, and state nurse practice acts further define required competencies for professional nursing practice. These professional standards use the nursing process as the framework for nursing practice. These standards recognize the importance of critical thinking and clinical reasoning as cognitive and metacognitive processes required to successfully implement the nursing process, and make sound clinical judgments.

The nursing process serves as a framework for applying critical thinking, clinical reasoning, and clinical judgment to nursing practice. The nurse uses the cognitive and metacognitive processes inherent in critical thinking and clinical reasoning throughout the nursing process to sort and categorize data; identify patterns in the data; draw inferences; develop hypotheses that are stated in the form of outcomes; test these hypotheses as care is delivered; and make criterion-based judgments of effectiveness. Therefore critical thinking and clinical reasoning can distinguish between fact and fiction, providing a rational basis for clinical judgments and the delivery of nursing care. Although the components of the nursing process are described as separate and distinct steps, they become an integrated way of thinking as nurses gain more clinical experience. A thorough understanding of the nursing process reveals that critical thinking, clinical reasoning, and clinical judgment are integral parts of its most effective use.

APPLICATION OF TANNER'S FOUR-STEP CLINICAL JUDGMENT MODEL AND CRITICAL THINKING TO A CLINICAL SITUATION

Clinical judgment is an interpretation or conclusion about a patient's needs, concerns or health problems, and/or decisions to take action (or not), use or modify standard approaches, or improvise new ones as deemed appropriate by the patient's response. (Tanner, 2006, p. 204)

Situation

Mr. Jones is a 78-year-old patient admitted to the Medical unit with diagnoses of Congestive Heart Failure, Chronic Obstructive Pulmonary Disease, and Diabetes. The patient's wife notifies the nurse that there is "something wrong with her husband" when he stops talking to her in the middle of a conversation and does not respond to her attempts to awake him.

Noticing. The nurse assesses the patient and obtains the following data. The patient is:

- Diaphoretic
- Skin is pale
- Nonresponsive to verbal stimuli
- Blood glucose = 25 mg/dL
- Blood glucose values have ranged from 120 mg/dL to 240 mg/dL for the past 48 hours
- Baseline mental status is alert and oriented to person, place, and time

Interpreting. The patient has diabetes and is displaying symptoms consistent with a severe hypoglycemic reaction (decreased blood glucose value, diaphoretic, nonresponsive).

Responding. The nurse reviews the standing orders for this patient and implements the orders for managing a severe hypoglycemic reaction in a nonresponsive patient. The nurse administers Dextrose intravenously per the standing order.

The patient becomes responsive to verbal stimuli and is able to follow simple commands within two minutes of the intravenous administration of Dextrose. The patient's blood glucose is 100 mg/dL following treatment.

Reflecting.

Reflecting in Action. The nurse uses reflecting-in-action to evaluate assessment findings, determine the patient's response to the nursing interventions implemented, and to evaluate the patient outcomes.

Reflecting on Action. The nurse uses reflection-on-action to retrospectively evaluate the overall clinical situation. The nurse uses the critical thinking skill, deductive reasoning, and the clinical judgment skill of contextualization to reflect upon why this patient may have experienced a severe hypoglycemic reaction, when the patient's most recent blood glucose levels have been in the normal to hyperglycemic range. Upon further evaluation, the nurse learns that the patient received his usual dose of insulin 30 minutes before the delivery of his lunch tray. However, he did not eat his lunch because he felt nauseous. The severe hypoglycemic reaction occurred 45 minutes after the insulin administration.

SUMMARY

It is crucial for the nurse to be able to think critically and apply clinical reasoning skills to provide a safe environment and deliver optimal client care. As nurses enhance their critical thinking and clinical reasoning skills, they will make sound clinical judgments based on evidence.

Today's health care environment requires nurses to solve complex problems, explore unique client situations, and evaluate the effectiveness of a wide range of interventions. Critical thinking and clinical reasoning are integral parts of effective nursing action. They are complex cognitive and metacognitive processes that nurses use to make clinical judgments. The conscious application of critical thinking principles and clinical reasoning can result in effective decision making and ultimately enhance the quality of care.

SALIENT POINTS

- Critical thinking incorporates thinking skills and a disposition to think critically.
- Critical thinking skills are transferable and may be applied across disciplines.
- Nurses use critical thinking and clinical reasoning skills throughout the steps of the nursing process.
- Nursing process is a systematic problem-solving approach used by nurses to manage client care situations.
- Clinical judgments are outcomes of critical thinking in nursing or clinical reasoning.

- Appraisal, problem solving, creativity, and decision making are interrelated concepts in critical thinking.
- Nurses with expert clinical judgment display characteristics of high-level critical thinking.
- To think critically, nurses must be able to see connections; use logic; differentiate fact, inference, and assumptions; evaluate arguments; consider many sides of an issue; be creative; and believe in their ability to think and reason.
- Becoming a critical thinker is a lifelong process that involves acquiring a set of skills and developing a disposition toward critical thinking.

CRITICAL REFLECTION EXERCISES

1. Compare and contrast the terms, *critical thinking, clinical reasoning, clinical judgment, problem solving,* and *decision making.*
2. Think about a patient care situation that you have recently encountered.
   a. Apply Tanner's (2006) four-step clinical judgment model to this situation.
   b. What did you learn from this situation?
3. Mr. Jones, 82 years of age, is admitted to your hospital unit. In conducting his initial assessment, you notice that he is somewhat confused. His admitting notes indicate that he takes Digoxin and Lasix. You suspect that the client may be experiencing side effects from his medications.
   a. What are the common side effects of Digoxin and Lasix?
   b. What assessment data will you gather?

4. Evaluate the nursing assessment instrument used in your current area of practice in terms of its adequacy for your clinical setting, usefulness in other clinical settings, and comprehensiveness. What additional data would be useful and how might you collect this information?
5. Describe the best and worst decision making you have seen by a nurse in a client care situation.
   a. Compare these two situations in terms of the thought process used, the underlying assumptions of the nurses, the accuracy of available information, the interpretation of information, and the soundness of the decision reached.
6. Describe strategies you can use to enhance critical thinking.
7. Discuss the inter-relationships between critical thinking, clinical reasoning, clinical judgment, and the nursing process.

WEBSITE RESOURCES

Foundation for Critical Thinking:
http://www.criticalthinking.org
Insight Assessment—Measuring Critical Thinking Worldwide:
http://www.insightassessment.com

National Center for Teaching Thinking: http://www.nctt.net
Teach smart: http://www.alfaroteachsmart.com/index.html

REFERENCES

Alfaro-LeFevre, R. (2013). *Critical thinking, clinical reasoning, and clinical judgment: A practical approach* (5th ed.). St. Louis: Elsevier.

American Association of Colleges of Nursing (AACN). (2008). *Essentials for baccalaureate nursing education.* Washington, DC: Author.

American Nurses Association. (2004). *Nursing: Scope and standards of practice.* Washington, DC: Author.

American Nurses Association. (2010). *Scope and standards of nursing practice.* Washington, DC: Author.

American Philosophical Association. (1990). *Critical thinking: A statement of expert consensus for purposes of educational assessment and instruction. The Delphi Report: Research findings and recommendations prepared for the Committee of Pre-college Philosophy.* Newark, DE: Author.

Benner, P., Sutphen, M., Leonard, V., & Day, L. (2010). *Educating nurses: A call for radical transformation.* Stamford, CA: The Carnegie Foundation for the Advancement of Teaching.

Carpenito, L. (2013). *Nursing diagnosis: Application to clinical practice* (14th ed.). Philadelphia: Lippincott Williams & Wilkins.

Elder, L., & Paul, R. (2010). Critical thinking: Competency standards essential to the cultivation of intellectual skills, part 1. *Journal of Developmental Education, 34*(2), 38–39.

Elder, L., & Paul, R. (2012). Critical thinking: Competency standards essential to the cultivation of intellectual skills, part 4. *Journal of Developmental Education, 35*(3), 30–31.

Ennis, R. (1987). Critical thinking and the curriculum. In M. Heiman, & J. Slomianko (Eds.), *Thinking skills instruction: Concepts and techniques.* Washington, DC: National Education Association.

Ennis, R. (1989). Critical thinking and subject specificity: Clarification and needed research. *Educational Researcher, 18,* 4–10.

Facione, P. (1990). Critical thinking: A statement of expert consensus for purposes of educational assessment and instruction (executive summary). In *The Delphi Report* (pp. 1–19). Millbrae, CA: California: Academic Press.

Facione, N. C., & Facione, P. A. (1996). Externalizing the critical thinking in knowledge development and clinical judgment. *Nursing Outlook, 44,* 129–136.

Facione, N. C., Facione, P. A., & Sanchez, C. A. (1994). Critical thinking disposition as a measure of competent clinical judgment: The development of the California Critical Thinking Disposition Inventory. *Journal of Nursing Education, 33,* 345–350.

Heaslip, P. (2008). Critical thinking in nursing and the health professions. In *The Critical Thinking Community.* Retrieved from http://www.criticalthinking.org/pages/critical-thinking-to-think-like-a-nurse.

Huston, C. (2013). The impact of emerging technology on nursing care: Warp speed ahead. *Online Journal of Issues in Nursing, 18*(2), 1–15.

Lasater, K. (2007). Clinical judgment development: Using simulation to create an assessment rubric. *Journal of Nursing Education, 46*(11), 496–503.

Paul, R. (1992). *Critical thinking: What every person needs to survive in a rapidly changing world.* Santa Rosa, CA: Foundation for Critical Thinking.

Paul, R. (1993). The art of redesigning instruction. In J. Willsen, & A. J. Binker (Eds.), *Critical thinking: How to prepare students for a rapidly changing world* (p. 319). Santa Rosa, CA: Foundation for Critical Thinking.

Paul, R. W. (1990). *Critical thinking: What every person needs to survive in a rapidly changing world.* Rohnert Park, CA: Center for Critical Thinking and Moral Critique.

Paul, R., & Elder, L. (2008). *The miniature guide to critical thinking concepts and tools.* Dillon Beach, CA: Foundation for Critical Thinking Press.

Paul, R., & Elder, L. (October 2010). Universal intellectual standards. In *The Critical Thinking Community.* Retrieved from http://www.criticalthinking.org/pages/using-intellectual-standards-to-assess-student-reasoning.

Scheffer, B., & Rubenfeld, G. (2000). A consensus statement on critical thinking in nursing. *Journal of Nursing Education, 39,* 352–359.

Scriven, M., & Paul, R. (1987, Summer). *National Council for Excellence in Critical Thinking: Critical thinking defined.* Paper presented at the Eighth Annual International Conference on Critical Thinking and Education Reform. Retrieved from http://www.criticalthinking.org/pages/defining-critical-thinking.

Simmons, B. (2010). Clinical reasoning: Concept analysis. *Journal of Advanced Nursing, 66*(5), 1151–1158.

Tanner, C. (2006). Thinking like a nurse: A research-based model of clinical judgment in nursing. *Journal of Nursing Education, 45*(6), 204–211.

Watson, G., & Glaser, E. (1964). *Critical thinking appraisal.* Orlando, FL: Harcourt Brace Jovanovich.

CHAPTER 10

Teaching and Learning in the 21st Century

Teresa Maggard Stephens, PhD, MSN, RN

http://evolve.elsevier.com/Friberg/bridge/

OBJECTIVES

At the completion of this chapter, the reader will be able to:

- Compare and contrast major teaching-learning theories.
- Discuss the principles and practices of effective teaching-learning experiences.
- Discuss the role of technology in teaching and learning.
- Discuss the concept of health literacy in relation to teaching and learning.
- Design teaching-learning experiences for both individuals and groups.

PROFILE IN PRACTICE

Robin Harris, PhD, ANP-BC, ACNS-BC
Clinical Director, Cardiovascular Associates, Kingsport, Tennessee

I have witnessed many changes in the delivery of health care during my career, especially considering the advances afforded via technology in recent years. My practice as a clinical director and advanced practice nurse in a busy cardiology practice involves both direct patient care and the precepting of nurse practitioner students. Technological advances have greatly affected the methods I use to teach and mentor these students. The use of smartphones or tablets is ideal to access credible and up-to-date information on medications, diagnoses, and disease management guidelines. Mobile technology enhances the learning experience for the student and allows me to provide the supplemental resources needed for real-time decision making. Several professional organizations provide resources via mobile technology related to disease or condition specific focus with educational resources for the professional, including printable resources, podcasts, webinars, and videos.

These are very useful when seeking appropriate, reliable information in a timely and efficient manner to provide current, evidence-based care to our patients.

More specifically, I spend time with nurse practitioner students in our outpatient heart failure clinic, where they learn to provide care for patients with heart failure and cardiovascular disease from an advanced practice perspective. I use mobile technology to help students learn about heart failure as a diagnosis, the physical assessment of patients with heart failure, current treatment guidelines, and important research findings to support evidence-based practice. The students are able to visualize many of the aspects of heart failure using the resources such as photos, videos, simulations, and/or podcasts. The use of mobile technology facilitates student learning in completing the history taking and physical assessment, as well as the critical thinking needed to develop a comprehensive plan of care.

INTRODUCTION

Teaching and learning in the nursing profession have rapidly evolved in recent years, offering both opportunities and challenges for nurses, teachers, and learners.

Vast advances in technology and the increased use of social media coupled with the demand for the transformation of nursing education have redefined the world of nursing. Although many embrace these changes and see the benefits to health care, others are reluctant to adapt and adopt the strategies that require a paradigm shift, and often involve a rather steep learning curve. Despite any misgivings or reluctance to embrace change, nursing's teaching and learning strategies must be adapted to meet the needs of the 21st-century learner, whether that learner is a student, a colleague, or a client. Several recent publications and initiatives have emphasized the need for this transformation, including the Institute of Medicine's Report, *The Future of Nursing: Leading Change, Advancing Health,* the Carnegie Foundation's *Educating Nurses: A Call for Radical Transformation,* and the Robert Wood Johnson Foundation's *Quality and Safety Education for Nurses (QSEN) Initiative.* These reports/initiatives reinforce the need to incorporate evidence-based practice, technology, interdisciplinary collaboration, and patient-centered care into education efforts. As we continue to look to the future and nursing's role in the transformation of health care, we must work together to effectively improve and enhance the education of providers, patients, and communities.

It can be said that those who practice nursing are not only nurses, but also teachers and learners. Nurses engage in teaching and learning while studying to become nurses, in their everyday practice, and as they further their professional development. Additionally, nurses are often sought for advice on health-related matters in their personal lives. As nursing professionals we are trusted to provide credible information. To do this we must be careful to base our responses on accurate, evidence-based information. It is much better to offer to obtain the information needed to provide a correct response, than to provide incorrect and potentially harmful information. This is especially important when posting in a public forum, such as social media. Remember, as a professional health care provider, your teaching and learning responsibilities extend beyond the bedside or formal education setting.

Clearly, readers of this text are experiencing some form of teaching and learning either through formal (course-required readings) or informal (professional development) methods of learning. Furthermore, readers either have already taught patients and colleagues or they will in the very near future. Most readers have encountered teaching situations similar to the following:

- A 16-year-old female inquires about the "morning-after pill" after reporting she might be pregnant

because she has felt nauseous every morning for 2 weeks.
- A 50-year-old wife accompanies her husband to the doctor. She states, "We have seen a lot of information on TV about personal health records. Can you help us get one started?"
- The mother of a 2-year-old boy recently diagnosed with insulin-dependent juvenile diabetes states, "There is no way I will be able to give him shots. I faint at the site of blood."
- A 54-year-old man newly diagnosed with hyperlipidemia states, "I would like to find some information on the Internet to help me manage this diagnosis. Which sites are the best?"
- A 46-year-old RN-BSN student in an online program asks, "We are required to post our final research presentation online. What are some ways I can do this that are free?"

Few nurses have had formal preparation or coursework in teaching and learning. With the increased focus on patient-centered care and the increasing complexity of health care, nursing professionals need to possess the knowledge and skills necessary to provide education in various contexts and to multiple populations. Nursing programs are integrating teaching and learning content into their curricula, which might very well be the reason you are reading this chapter. Whether you are a nurse working in a hospital, clinic, or community setting, an educator, an administrator, or a student, it is necessary to have basic knowledge of the teaching-learning process and the ways that technology influences teaching, learning, and information seeking. This chapter reviews the more commonly used learning theories in health education, discusses the ways technology influences teaching and learning practices, explores the benefits and challenges of the online learning environment, and presents effective teaching-learning practices with relevant supporting research, including similarities and differences between individual and group teaching-learning experiences.

TEACHING AND LEARNING THEORIES

Most commonly and simply stated, *teaching* is defined as the act or process of imparting knowledge (Merriam-Webster, 2014). This definition implies that those who teach present information and those who learn passively accept the knowledge. However, *learning* represents a change in meaning for the learner that is based on previous meaningful experiences (Merriam-Webster, 2014). More than 200 teaching and learning theories exist, and numerous Internet sites provide information about these theories (e.g., http://tip.psychology.org). Although it is unrealistic to review all of the theories in this chapter, this section compares and contrasts several viewpoints and reflects on the comparisons by presenting learning principles and teaching applications for each of the following theory viewpoints: behaviorism, cognitivism, change, and humanism. This chapter references the classical works of theorists to allow the reader the opportunity to explore teaching and learning principles in more depth.

Behaviorist Theories

Teaching based on a behaviorist model, known as *behaviorism* or *instructivism*, presents objectives and content in a stepwise progression from basic to complex information with minimal learner engagement in the experience. Many of the assumptions of behaviorist models are built on the classic work of Thorndike (1913), Pavlov (1927), Skinner (1953), and Wolpe and Lazarus (1966), as well as some of Bruner's earliest writings (1966).

Cognitive Theories

As more scientists focused on teaching and learning, behaviorist theories and their assumptions evolved from teacher focused to learner focused. Theorists such as Piaget (1954), Lewin (1951), Gagne (1974), Bloom (1956), and Johnson, Johnson, and Stanne (2000) examined cognition and the ways that learners process information. By the mid-20th century, a new method of teaching and learning, known as *constructivism,* appeared in the literature (Bruner, 1966). This method of teaching and learning proposes that learners construct new ideas based on previous knowledge and experiences. Today many cognitive and behavioral psychologists support this view, which asserts that learners engage or become active in the learning process instead of passively receiving information. In this view, learners actively seek information, problem solve, collaborate with others, and apply information to realistic problems. Most cognitive and learning experts believe that active learning is superior to passive learning.

Change Theories

The more common teaching-learning methods used by nurses while teaching patients require strategies that empower the patient to exercise healthy behaviors that do not conflict with the patient's value system. The themes of patient empowerment and patient value systems are based on change models and concepts such as Rosenstock's health belief model (1974), Bandura's concept of self-efficacy (1977), Rotter's locus of control (1990), Festinger's cognitive dissonance theory (1957), and stages of readiness described by Prochaska and DiClemente (1982). Change theories are also very useful when exploring the implementation of change in the health care environment. E. M. Rogers' diffusion of innovations theory (2003) is one example of a theory that has been used to address the evolutionary changes in health care related to Informatics and Health Information Technology (HIT).

Humanistic Theories

In humanistic theory, learning is self-motivated, self-directed, and self-evaluated. The teacher provides information and support to help learners increase their cognitive and affective functioning. Humanistic theories are the oldest classic theories and include andragogy or adult-centered learning (Knowles, 1984), hierarchy of needs (Maslow, 1970), self-directed learning (C. Rogers, 1969), reality theory of self-awareness learning (Glasser, 1965), perceptual-existential theory or self-determined learning (Combs, 1965), situated learning (Lave & Wenger, 1991), and values clarification learning (Dewey, 1938).

Teachers who use humanistic theories will encourage learners to set their own goals and work toward them. For example, a nurse might ask a client with diabetes, "When do you think you'll be ready to give your own insulin injection? What activities or steps would help you get ready to do this?"

Chances are that as a nurse you have or will use a combination of the preceding theories in teaching and learning, depending on the type of instruction, the learner, and the desired outcome. Regardless of the theoretical approach of the teaching-learning process, all effective instruction is based on fundamental principles that include matching the instruction with the type of learning that is required and developing a sense of mutuality and trust between teacher and learner.

TEACHING AND LEARNING PRINCIPLES

Teaching and learning can be formal or informal in nature. *Formal learning* is planned instruction with objectives or goals that match the intended learned skills or concepts with the most effective method of delivery. According to the classic cone of experience, a learning theory by Edgar Dale (1969), learners remember:

- 10% of what they read
- 20% of what they hear
- 30% of what they see
- 50% of what they see and hear
- 60% of what they write
- 70% of what they discuss
- 80% of what they experience
- 95% of what they teach

Although reading and listening to information may be the most ineffective method of learning, it is often the most appropriate or feasible method, especially if the information or content is abstract in nature and requires few or no motor skills. On the other hand, content that requires motor skills are best learned by actively engaging in the learning such as experiential learning, simulations, or role-play (Dale, 1969). Regardless of the level of learning required, the more an individual engages in the content, the more likely the person is to learn the material. Learners, whether they are patients, family care givers, or colleagues, often learn best by teaching the information to someone else. Table 10-1 provides examples of types and levels of learning and matching strategies based on Dale's cone of experience theory.

Informal ways of learning are also effective. *Informal learning* results from interactions with others through networking, coaching, and mentoring. Learning that occurs in groups or from interactions with others, known as *collaborative* or *cooperative learning,* engages the learner in the information (Johnson et al., 2000; Walker & Elberson, 2005). Furthermore, learners who participate in their own learning are able to attach purposeful meaning to the content based on previous experiences. Perhaps this is one reason why the most successful learning often takes place in groups, such as weight loss groups, grief support groups, and parenting groups, in which individuals help one another and the teacher is seen more as a guide, coach, or a facilitator.

Self-directed learning is another form of informal learning and often seen in the adult learner who seeks out information on topics of interest. This type of learning could be related to their profession, personal interests, or a combination of both. For instance, the nurse who plays the piano may seek information on how music is used in the care of stroke patients. Self-directed learning may result from *incidental learning,* which consists of learning from mistakes, assumptions, beliefs, attributions, and internalized meanings. Incidental learning is often a byproduct of another activity and motivates the learner to purposefully seek out more information to broaden the understanding of the concept or phenomenon. With more and more learners engaged in online learning, hybrid learning, and *massive open online courses* (MOOCs), emphasis is placed on ways to enhance self-directed learning. Massive open online courses offer an alternative to the traditional tuition-based course for learners interested in a self-paced, Internet-based, learning experience that is heavily focused on community and less on instructor engagement. Although self-directed learning may be incidental, it also can be purposeful when combined with tutorials, access to resources, and guided lessons. Supplemental resources that are developed with various learning styles in mind (e.g., videos, podcasts, concept maps) encourage the learner to use what is known and "comfortable," but also to try other methods he or she has not previously considered. These methods are useful for both the nurse who wants to increase his or her understanding of a topic, and the nurse who wishes to provide education to a client.

TABLE 10-1   Teaching and Learning Based on Dale's Cone of Experience Theory (1969)

INFORMATION/SKILL	LEVEL OF LEARNING	TEACHING-LEARNING STRATEGY
Insulin injections	Concrete motor skill	Simulation, demonstration
Heart-healthy diet	Cognitive skill	Audiovisual or media, pictures, or audio only
Medical vocabulary terms	Abstract information	Text, reference materials

Transfer of Knowledge

The key to successful learning is determining how important the information is to the learner's ability to function effectively in his or her daily life and world. What is the motivation for learning? The more the learning environment resembles the actual environment, the more likely learning will be applied (Knowles, 1980). Focusing on behavior rather than knowledge, setting realistic expectations, and establishing rewards can enhance learning transfer. Behavior, however, is not changed by knowledge alone. To influence behavior, a learner must not only have knowledge of the desired behavior, but also believe that he or she is able to perform or adopt the new information (self-efficacy) and must value or desire (attitude) the behavior (Bandura, 1977). Factors that inhibit transfer of learning include, but are not limited to, readiness to learn, anxiety level, environmental factors, stress levels, complexity of the content or tasks, ability to learn, and emotional readiness (Bastable, 2006).

Mutuality and Trust

The most successful teaching-learning experiences involve a process in which an interpersonal relationship of shared mutuality and trust is established between the teacher and the learner. This relationship might be teacher to student nurse, nurse to nurse, or nurse to client. In such a relationship, the teacher is viewed as the knowledge and information expert, and the learner is seen not only as the individual in need of information and support, but also as the expert on how the information is best suited to his or her life. The emphasis is on the learner actively engaging, discovering, and taking responsibility for new ways of acting and problem solving. Mutuality and trust is prevalent in nurse and patient relationships because the nurse is often considered the expert on health matters and the patient is the information seeker.

CHARACTERISTICS OF EFFECTIVE TEACHERS

Most of us teach the way we were taught, imitating the behaviors of the best teachers we have known and minimizing behaviors of those teachers we did not like. To be an effective teacher, however, requires that we develop a sound educational theory and research base, learn the specifics of the teacher-learner roles, find new ways of interrelating, and continually explore

new teaching methods that we might use in our various roles (as a nurse, teacher, or peer). In addition, we must be able to critique our own performance and be willing to accept constructive criticism from others.

Many lessons can be learned from classroom teachers, but sometimes learning that occurs in a classroom involves nothing more than obtaining information on a topic. It is also important to note that the traditional classroom setting is no longer the "norm." Many learners interact in online learning environments that include formal learning (college courses), interactive chat rooms, wikis, blogs, and listservs. Nurses engaged in teaching often require more advanced teaching and learning skills because patients may need to obtain and understand information, with guidance in using the new knowledge to change their health behaviors. Nurses must be prepared to guide the learner toward credible resources. Sometimes nurses practice paternalism—that is, they overextend their power of authority over the patient. This method is ineffective; instead, nurses should practice a shared decision-making model, such as nurse coaching.

Nurse coaching is a rapidly evolving concept that is being embraced in many areas of the nursing profession. It can be applicable to the nurse–client relationship as well as the roles of nurse educator, nurse preceptor, and nurse mentor. Nurse coaching is a client-centered approach to teaching and learning that focuses on effective communication skills, observation skills, the ability to provide quality feedback, leadership, trust-building, problem identification and solving, decision making, conflict management, and goal setting. The goal of coaching is to assist the client (e.g., patient, student nurse, new graduate, nurse leader) in recognizing his or her own goals, experiences, prior knowledge, strengths, and limitations in the development of a plan to achieve the desired outcome(s). Donner and Wheeler (2009), in partnership with The International Council of Nurses (ICN) and the Honor Society of Nursing, Sigma Theta Tau International (STTI), have developed a coaching workbook to teach nurses the principles and skills of coaching (http://www.nursingsociety.org/Education/ProfessionalDevelopment/Documents/Coaching%20and%20Mentoring%20Workbook_STTI.pdf).

Regardless of the type of learning required, all teaching should be tailored to the learner's age, educational level, culture, and native language. This is a challenge for nurses who must teach complex medical processes to the lay public; however, numerous websites provide information and learning materials for various populations. For example, EthnoMed (http://ethnomed.org/ethnomed) is a site dedicated to providing material and information for culturally diverse populations. In addition, the National Network of Libraries of Medicine (http://nnlm.gov/outreach/consumer/multi.html) houses patient information in more than 12 different languages. With all educational material, but especially web-based information, nurses must ensure accuracy and reliability of the information obtained.

Health Literacy is an important concept when creating and sharing educational materials. Health literacy is defined as "the degree to which individuals have the capacity to obtain, process, and understand basic health information and services needed to make appropriate health decisions" (National Research Council, 2004). Health literacy is not simply the ability to read. It requires a complex group of reading, listening, analytical, and decision-making skills, and the ability to apply these skills to health situations. For example, it includes the ability to understand instructions on prescription drug bottles, appointment slips, medical education brochures, doctor's directions, and consent forms, and the ability to negotiate complex health care systems. The National Network of Libraries of Medicine website provides helpful information on health literacy (http://nnlm.gov/outreach/consumer/hlthlit.html). Health literacy is also addressed in Chapter 13 of this book.

CHARACTERISTICS OF EFFECTIVE LEARNERS

The process of learning often requires engaging in a relationship with a teacher, a nurse, or another person with knowledge. At other times, learners manage their own learning (self-directed learning), which requires both self-direction and motivation for the learner and creative engagement efforts by the teacher. No matter the format, learners must be motivated or accountable for retrieving or receiving information to gain the desired or required knowledge.

Learners are motivated for different reasons. For some, knowledge is necessary to remain healthy, whereas other learners may seek knowledge for professional opportunities or for enjoyment. The motivation for learning can be powerful and should be harnessed to enhance learning. For example, a man who needs to learn how to use an inhaler is generally quite motivated because without it he has trouble breathing. On the other hand, some learners are less interested in learning if they perceive that gaining knowledge or changing behavior is less important than some other factor. For example, a 46-year-old woman has learned that as a result of being overweight, along with other factors, she has developed hypertension. As part of her treatment regimen, she has been prescribed hypertensive medications and instructed to lose 20 pounds. Unless she perceives that her weight is a true cause of the hypertension, she is not likely to change her eating and exercise behaviors—especially if she experiences positive results with the hypertensive medication alone.

Learners must understand their own motivating factors for seeking knowledge and use those factors to enhance learning. Furthermore, learning is enhanced when learners understand their own ways of learning, what works best, and how they might engage in activities to promote the best learning outcomes.

Learning Styles and Preferences

All individuals have experienced some form of teaching and learning; therefore it is likely that most learners can identify their own best method for learning. Each learner has a unique way of processing information, and the various delivery methods can either enhance or distract from the learning that takes place. For this reason, teachers must be aware of the various learning styles so that appropriate strategies can be used to promote learning. The classifications of learning styles are dependent on the type of learning inventory that one completes and the source that is used to determine the learning style. Many scientists have examined learning styles, which has led to numerous classifications. Nonetheless, three domains of learning have come to be considered essential: visual, auditory, and tactile/kinesthetic. These three domains may be combined and then aligned with styles of learning based on individual preferences. You can determine your own learning style by taking a free online learning style survey at http://metamath.com/lsweb/dvclearn.htm or http://www.vark-learn.com/english/index.asp. Learning strategies for individual styles are also provided on these websites.

Working with individuals with various learning styles or assuming responsibility for your own learning will lead to more successful outcomes if you consider the following basic principles in relation to learning styles (Bastable, 2006):

1. Knowledge of the style of the teacher and the style of the learner offers clues about the way one learns, and learning activities can be adjusted accordingly.
2. Nurses functioning in the role of teacher should refrain from teaching exclusively by their own learning style. Full ranges of techniques are often necessary to deliver content, even when teaching to individuals with similar learning styles.
3. Teachers should help learners (even patients) to identify their own style of learning so that the best learning approach can be identified.
4. All learners should have the opportunity to learn through techniques that are best suited to their learning style. For example, individuals who are visual learners prefer videos, movies, or simulations.
5. All learners should be encouraged to explore their various learning preferences to seek out strategies that are most conducive to their learning.
6. Those functioning as teachers must have a "toolbox" full of resources, strategies, and techniques rather than relying on one source for delivering content. Often, learners will need remediation or review, which requires several different sources.

Technology Influences on Teaching and Learning

Learners, whether students enrolled in formal coursework or everyday information seekers (e.g., health consumers), have access to information that until about 15 years ago was available only to a select few. With the advent of the Internet, finding information is no longer the problem. Instead, paring down volumes of information and ensuring that the information is accurate and reliable is the challenge. Before the Internet, information was available through print, video, or word of mouth. Obtaining accurate information involved in-depth research, numerous phone calls, or interviews with reliable sources. In essence, experts served as the clearinghouses of information. If, for example, a patient needed information about his or her newly diagnosed disease, the physician or nurse gave information verbally, by phone, or by printed brochures available only at a health care facility. Internet-empowered information seekers are leading a revolution of informed consumers, including health care consumers. Armed with unprecedented access to health-related information via the Internet, today's health care consumer is demanding more involvement in his or her own care, as well as access to more choices about how health care is organized, delivered, and reimbursed. This development alone influences the teaching-learning methods that nurses must adopt while accessing information and teaching patients or other nurses (see Chapter 13).

Internet-Supported Teaching and Learning

Access to information via the Internet has become one of the most significant defining characteristics of the present *Information Age,* in which computers network with one another. The Pew Research Center's Pew Internet & American Life Project (http://pewinternet.org) "provides information on the issues, attitudes and trends shaping America and the world." The Project produces reports exploring the impact of the Internet on families, communities, work and home, daily life, education, health care, and civic and political life. According to their May 2013 survey, 85% of U.S. adults use the Internet and 72% of Internet users said they looked online for health information in the past year (September 2012 survey). According to the Pew researchers, the most commonly researched topics are specific diseases or conditions, treatments or procedures, and physicians or other health care providers (Pew Research Internet Project, 2013).

This increase in Internet use owes, in part, to more readily available access to computers, smartphones, and other mobile devices, and the Internet in general, the ever-increasing amount of information that can be obtained quickly, and the development of more online multimedia technologies. Teaching styles that use a variety of methods and tools (e.g., mobile technology, video, interactive tutorials, virtual learning environments) can enhance learning and attend to a variety of learning styles.

Because individuals rely on the Internet for information ranging from personal health to financial investments, it is crucial for learners to evaluate these resources. Currently standards do not exist to ensure accuracy of online information. Essentially anyone can publish anything on the Internet. Unlike traditional print resources, web resources rarely use editors or content experts. Multiple tools and criteria are available for evaluating websites, but there are key elements to guide learners in evaluating information on the Internet (Box 10-1).

BOX 10-1 **Evaluating Information on the Internet**

Credibility

- Who is the owner/sponsor of the site? Is it a not-for-profit organization? (Look at the domain or site sponsor located after the "dot" in the address. For example: .edu = education, .gov = government, .org = organization, .com = commercial, .mil = military.)
- Is it current? When was it last updated?
- Is there an editorial process?

Content

- Is it accurate?
- Is it complete?
- Is it free from spelling and grammar errors?
- Is it a reliable source?
- Is it free from opinion or bias?
- Is there a disclaimer?
- Does the author of the website have the education, expertise, or experience to be a trustworthy source?
- Is there a privacy statement?

Disclosure

- What is the purpose of the site?

Links

- Are the links appropriate to the content being described?
- Are all links functional?
- Are all links to credible sources?

Design

- Is it readable and appealing?
- Is it easy to navigate, and does it have a search function?

Interactivity

- Is there a mechanism for feedback or comments?
- Are there listservs?
- Is there a contact source?

Caveats

- Are there advertisements?
- Is there commercial funding?

Health on the Net (HON) is a foundation that guides Internet users to reliable and trustworthy sources of health information. Health on the Net is considered the gold standard for evaluating health-related web-based information. A website that displays the official HON seal has applied for and met HON criteria. Health on the Net has also developed a toolbar that automatically verifies the accreditation status of health-related websites (this toolbar can be downloaded at www.hon.ch). The National Library of Medicine also provides numerous resources to assist the consumer in identifying credible websites (http://www.nlm.nih.gov/medlineplus/evaluatinghealthinformation.html).

Teachers and learners can find a wealth of peer-reviewed learning resources in the online repository Multimedia Education Resource for Online Learning and Teaching (MERLOT) at http://www.merlot.org. Membership is free with multiple benefits and resources for members.

Online Learning

By far most individuals use the Internet as a self-directed learning tool to access information; however, the Internet is capable of supporting other teaching-learning methods. For example, the Internet connects networked computers so that the scope of learning extends beyond the physical walls of a learning institution or facility. Higher education has evolved greatly in the past few years owing in part to the advances in technology, which have contributed to an increased number of students seeking online options. Nursing education has been affected by these events as well. As nurses engage in online learning, they increase their own awareness of the opportunities and resources available for the education of clients and colleagues.

Online learning includes both synchronous and asynchronous learning. Video conferencing, for example, connects individuals who are not physically located in the same place. This method of connecting individuals in real time by video streaming is known as *synchronous learning*. Alternatively, *asynchronous learning* allows individuals to share information or ideas in delayed time. Examples of asynchronous learning are e-mail correspondence, electronic bulletin boards, listservs, blogs, or information posted on websites. Both forms of learning have advantages and disadvantages. Overall, asynchronous learning does not promote live discussion, but it may be advantageous to learners who need additional time for processing information. It may also improve writing skills because all responses are text-based.

Of course, it has been well documented that the greatest advantage of asynchronous learning is the scheduling flexibility for learners (Billings & Halstead, 2009). Because this form of learning does not take place in real time, a learner can choose to engage in the learning at a time that is convenient and fits his or her busy schedule.

Synchronous learning, on the other hand, engages the learner in the teaching-learning process at the same moment with the teacher and/or other learners. This method promotes collaborative or cooperative learning because information is processed with a group of learners. This real-time dialogue may be necessary for some learners or for comprehension of some forms of information. However, synchronous learning requires the use of robust and advanced technology by both the teacher and the learner. At a minimum, the learner and teacher must have broad bandwidth Internet access to support videos, audio, videostreaming, chat rooms, webcasts, or other synchronous methods.

Instructional Technologies

The Internet dramatically changed the ways information is obtained, but technology itself also influences teaching and learning. To offer effective teaching, whether with patients or colleagues, nurses need to seek technology-rich and interactive learning environments that engage the learner. In fact, the generation of children and young adults who have been exposed to technology their entire lives, commonly known as *Millennials* (those born between 1981 and 2000), are described as technologically savvy, creative, innovative, preferring real-time communication, multitaskers, self-inventive, like to be entertained, get bored easily, and desire instant responses and access to information (Hansen & Erdley, 2009; Hoover, 2009; Thielfoldt & Scheef, 2004; Trueman & Miles, 2011). These individuals often learn best in environments that are rich in multimedia, moving and navigating freely through their experience (Mayer, 2001).

The Pre-Millennial generations, those who remember a world without personal computers (PCs), typically process information in a sequential order similar to a book, but engage in the learning more readily when the information is interactive or presented in multiple media (multimedia). Technologies that support multimedia have changed how learners access information and how they interact with information, other learners, and the teacher. For example, collaborative learning (learning in teams, pairs, or small groups) to problem solve (situated learning) is no longer limited to individuals who are physically located in the same room. With advances in mobile technology, networked notebooks/laptops, or with a PC, groups can connect from around the world to learn and problem solve together. Smartphone use has greatly increased in the past few years, contributing to the large numbers of individuals seeking health information online. According to the Pew Resource Center's May 2013 survey, 91% of American adults have a cell phone, and 56% of American adults have a smartphone. Additionally, 31% of cell phone owners, and 52% of smartphone owners, have used their phone to find health/medical information. The findings from the survey also revealed that 19% of smartphone owners have used an app to track or manage their health (Pew Research Internet Project, 2013).

Smartphones are also being increasingly used in the academic and classroom settings for real-time access to up-to-date information, as audience response systems, and creative collaboration. The rapidly growing world of mobile applications (apps) has become a major topic in the world of health care, with applications being developed for just about every condition and population. The EDUCAUSE Center for Applied Research (ECAR) is investigating the ways that mobile technologies, such as hand-held technology, enhance learners' educational experiences. Overall, the research suggests that mobile technology shows promise as a teaching-learning tool and will likely penetrate most formal education settings in the future (Wentzel, Lammeren, Molendijk, Bruin, & Wagtendonk, 2005). Kaminski's PATCH (Pretest for Attitudes Toward Computers and Healthcare) Assessment Tool is useful for teachers and learners to assess their own feelings about the use of computers and technology in the education and practice environments. The assessment tool and personal plan of action to develop your own desired level of computer literacy are free and available at this website: http://nursing-informatics.com/niassess/plan.html.

Most recently, the Internet supports collaborative teaching-learning groups through IP telephony or voice-over-IP (VoIP). This technology allows individuals to talk to one another online. This method of collaboration is cost effective because there are several free applications to support VoIP and there are no additional costs to establish the voice connection (Federal Communication Commission, 2009). Clearly the advantage of VoIP is to connect learners who,

BOX 10-2   Educational Technology Web Resources

- Campus Technology online magazine (www.campus technology.com)
- Carnegie Foundation: Education Nurses: A Call for Radical Transformation (http://www.carnegiefoundation.org/newsroom/press-releases/educating-nurses-call-radical-transformation)
- Educational Technology and Mobile Learning (http://www.ttsechnology.com/)
- Edudemic: Connecting Education and Technology (http://www.edudemic.com/)
- Innovative Educator Blogspot (http://theinnovativeeducator.blogspot.com/)
- Institute of Medicine Report: The Future of Nursing: Leading Change, Advancing Health (http://www.iom.edu/Reports/2010/The-future-of-nursing-leading-change-advancing-health.aspx)
- Office of Educational Technology (http://www.ed.gov/edblogs/technology/)
- Quality and Safety Education for Nurses (QSEN) Institute (www.qsen.org)
- Technology: Key to Transforming Nursing Education (Robert Wood Johnson Blog) (http://www.rwjf.org/en/blogs/human-capital-blog/2011/10/technology-key-to-transforming-nursing-education.html)

before networking capabilities, would have been difficult (if not impossible) to connect without extensive time commitments, travel, and expenses. Each member of the learning group brings unique experiences and perspectives to the situated learning environment, which promotes constructivist approaches to learning. Of course, there are associated disadvantages, including the technical support needed to connect learners via networked computers, the learning curve associated with using collaborative technologies, and the change in the way learners must communicate so that the technology does not interfere with their learning (pauses, delays in audio transmission, frequent disconnections).

Other more extensive web tools, known as Web 2.0 and Web 3.0 tools, are available for learners and teachers. With technology advancements and increased access to web-based programs and applications, some fascinating tools have emerged, many of which were never intended to be learning tools. Box 10-2 lists a few of the educational technology resources available. Social networking, or tools designed to connect people, have evolved and become mainstream for Millennial learners. These tools serve not only to connect

individuals, but also to share information and promote collaboration. For example, Facebook and Twitter connect friends, friends of friends, and those with common interests. These tools support photo and video sharing, live chat sessions, links, and notes. Other similar social networking and collaborative tools allow teachers and learners to share documents, files, and contact information and to set up live meetings using chat features or video applications. Nurses and other professionals may use these applications to connect with like-minded individuals or those with similar expertise. One such tool, LinkedIn, allows professionals to connect and share friends, resources, and contact information. Moodle, a free open-source collaborative tool, also supports networking but is slightly different because it is secure and not available to the public, which means that only individuals who are invited to the site may participate in networking. This application is most commonly used to support classrooms because it can be a secure site and it organizes and manages content. Other tools, most known for social networking, also provide multiple opportunities for the digital learning environment. Pinterest, Instagram, YouTube, Vimeo, and Vine all offer exciting and innovative free resources for creative educational expression.

Blogs, wikis, and services such as Twitter also connect people with common interests; all three allow document and image sharing, posting, and journaling. A blog or a "tweet" can be used to update learners about ongoing activities and store information for easy retrieval. These tools are often used to supplement professional conferences for those persons unable to attend but interested in learning more about the conference presentations and proceedings. The use of hashtags on Twitter allows learners to follow a specific topic of interest (e.g., disaster recovery in Haiti) without having to identify or follow an individual's account.

Wikis offer several benefits for both teachers and learners. A wiki is a collaborative site in which members can create and edit content. Wikispaces (www.wikispaces.com) is one free wiki site created for teachers with multiple options and formats available. Wikis are useful tools for both face-to-face and online learning environments to support group collaboration, faculty–student engagement, creativity, and formative assessment. Additionally, wikis are generally easy to navigate and a good way to introduce digital media to those without a lot of experience with technology.

BOX 10-3 Digital Media and Software Resources for Teaching and Learning

- Animoto: free and easy video producing software (www.animoto.com)
- Audacity: Free, open-source software for recording and editing sounds (http://audacity.sourceforge.net/)
- Camtasia/Jing: screen capture and screencasting tool (www.techsmith.com)
- Coursera: MOOC platform (https://www.coursera.org/)
- Doodle: event scheduling tool (www.doodle.com)
- Dropbox: cloud-based file/data storage system (www.dropbox.com)
- Evernote: free productivity tool (www.evernote.com)
- Explain Everything App: design, screencasting, and interactive whiteboard tool (www.explaineverything.com)
- Facebook: social networking site (www.facebook.com)
- Feedly: RSS reader/aggregator (www.feedly.com)
- GoAnimate: simple animated video production software (www.goanimate.com)
- Google Drive/Docs: free web-based word processing, presentation, spreadsheets, collaboration, forms, data storage, and communication (https://drive.google.com/)
- Google Plus/Hangouts: video meetings, chats, online office hours (www.plus.google.com)
- Instagram: photo and video sharing site (www.instagram.com)
- iSpring: e-learning tool for creating courses, quizzes, and narrated presentations (http://www.ispringsolutions.com/)
- Pinterest: content sharing service (www.pinterest.com)
- Polleverywhere: learner/audience response system (www.polleverywhere.com)
- Prezi: presentation creating and sharing software, nonlinear (www.prezi.com)
- ProProfs Quiz Maker: online quiz/test creator (http://www.proprofs.com/quiz-school/)
- SurveyMonkey: online survey tool (www.surveymonkey.com)
- Today's Meet: private backchannel, real-time audience connection (https://todaysmeet.com)
- Trello: personal and collaborative productivity tool (www.trello.com)
- Twitter: online social networking and microblogging service (www.twitter.com)
- VoiceThread: cloud-based storytelling application (http://audacity.sourceforge.net/)
- Wikispaces: free educational wiki (www.wikispaces.com)
- Wix: free website builder (www.wix.com)
- Wordle: word cloud generator (www.wordle.net)
- Wordpress: free website builder, blogging site (www.wordpress.com)
- YouTube: video hosting and sharing site (www.youtube.com)

Social bookmarking is another type of Web 2.0 tool that allows individuals with similar interests to share their bookmarks or favorite websites. Because the Internet lacks a clear organized structure, it is often difficult to find information or to retrace previous search steps. Bookmark sharing increases one's capacity to locate specific information. Bookmarks are shared when individuals post their bookmarks to a public server, rather than on their personal Internet browser. Individuals who subscribe to the same social bookmarking service then have access to one another's bookmarks. Many bookmarking services, some free, are available: SocialMarking (http://socialmarking.com), AddThis (http://addthis.com), and Delicious (http://delicious.com).

Video, film, audio equipment, software applications, interactive whiteboards, projection systems, and PCs are other forms of technology used frequently to promote learning. Box 10-3 lists several of the popular digital media and software resources used in teaching and learning. Each technology is best suited for a particular form of learning and should be matched to the desired outcome(s).

Technology offers many benefits to the teacher and learner to enhance education efforts, but we must know our goals, objectives, and learner characteristics before choosing a technological tool. In many cases multiple forms of technology (multimedia) are used to support teaching and learning and are effective when matched with the appropriate level of learning. Caution, however, should be used when selecting the delivery method for instruction because selecting the wrong medium can distract the learner, making the instruction ineffective.

CREATING EFFECTIVE TEACHING-LEARNING PLANS

The effectiveness of a teaching-learning plan is limited to the teacher's knowledge and skill on the topic to be taught, as well as the teacher's knowledge about learning, teaching, and evaluation. In professional practice you may design a teaching-learning plan for a student, new graduate, a group of experienced nurses, a patient, a group of patients, or a community group. Each of these requires consideration of the specific needs of the population as well as the methods used to share information and assess the learning. Nurses, therefore, must have some basic knowledge about teaching and learning, and not solely rely on the methods they experienced as learners. Developing a teaching-learning plan is similar to the nursing process and includes assessing the learner, developing learner objectives, selecting teaching-learning strategies, implementing the teaching plan, and evaluating outcomes.

Assessing the Learner

There are some key elements that should be explored when assessing the learner's needs. These include (1) knowledge level, (2) developmental characteristics (e.g., age, reading ability), (3) preferred learning style, (4) motivation or readiness to learn, (5) anxiety level, (6) health values, and (7) health status. Many of these factors have already been discussed in this chapter. It is, however, necessary to gather information about these factors through questioning or interviewing. Susan Bastable, a well-known patient education expert, suggests that interviewing (or any form of communication with a patient) can be enhanced by beginning with short phrases (2006). This technique can apply to any type of learner, whether a patient, a student, or a peer. These short phrases are icebreaker questions such as, "How was the traffic coming in today?" This strategy not only helps to develop rapport with the patient, but also allows the nurse to assess the general well-being of the patient, such as discomfort or irritability. During the initial stages of the interviewing, teachers (nurses) should give patients a sense of what is about to occur, thereby developing trust and setting the stage for the educational experience. This map of what is to occur may be an outline of the material or simply a spoken phrase informing the patient of the information that will be reviewed.

Assessing Special Groups

Learners who are from an unfamiliar culture or who are challenged in some way often have complex and unique learning needs. Assessing the special characteristics of these learners will aid in identifying learning needs and choosing teaching strategies that are appropriate and effective.

Cultural Considerations. Nurses who are teaching to diverse populations must be sensitive to cultural traditions, taboos, and values that facilitate or interfere with the teaching-learning process. For example, in the Asian population it is important to "save face," and these learners may not indicate a lack of understanding or may be uncomfortable answering questions, especially those concerning bodily and sexual functioning. Because Africans respect authority figures, they may be reluctant to ask questions if the questions seem to challenge the teacher.

When a learner from an unfamiliar culture is being assessed, a systematic appraisal of his or her beliefs and values is essential. If the learner is a patient, then the nurse must gather information about the patient's cultural preferences and health care practices. Barriers to communication and preferred methods of learning must also be identified, because both may be culturally based. Several free web-based programs are available to assist in translating documents into different languages (e.g., http://babelfish.com). Such tools are useful as a beginning step in translating teaching materials. However, all documents translated in this manner should be checked by a native speaker to ensure cultural congruency.

Challenged Populations. It is critical for the teacher to carefully assess the learner's reading level and ability to understand the written word when printed materials are used for teaching. This assessment must respect the learner's dignity, because many people are embarrassed by their reading difficulties. For instance, a statement about forgetting one's reading glasses may indicate illiteracy. In this case, nurses should offer to read the content to the learner and attempt to find materials that illustrate the information. When developing or selecting reading materials, the nurse must ensure that the reading level is appropriate for the target audience. For printed materials, the reading level can be determined by most word processing programs. Websites that evaluate readability and grade level of content are also available (http://www.readability-score.com). As a general rule of thumb, experts recommend that all materials prepared for adults be written at a sixth-grade level (Badarudeen & Sabharwal, 2008).

Individuals who are visually or hearing impaired may require adapted educational materials. Reading materials in large print or audiotapes can be used with visually impaired learners, and sign language or closed-captioned videos can be used with those who are hearing impaired. Advances in technology offer many opportunities for visually impaired learners. Adaptive reading devices can translate websites so that the information these learners receive is as similar as possible to that accessed by learners who are not visually impaired. For those with language barriers, an interpreter may be needed. Individuals who have impaired mobility may require adaptations in the teaching plan to accommodate their level of functioning.

Developing Learner Objectives

It is sometimes difficult for new teachers to develop concise and measurable learner objectives. With an increased emphasis on outcomes in both the educational and practice settings, it is imperative that the teacher understands the need for objectives that are matched to the assessments and desired outcomes. The purpose of learner objectives are (1) to communicate what the leaner is to know and do, (2) to guide the selection and use of teaching materials, and (3) to evaluate whether the learner actually learned what the teacher tried to teach. For example, "Today we will watch a video of patients giving themselves insulin injections (media), tomorrow we will practice preparing an insulin injection together (demonstration and return demonstration), and the next day you will have the opportunity to give your own insulin injection (evaluation)."

Bloom divided learning objectives into two categories: cognitive (Bloom, 1956) and affective (Krathwohl, Bloom, & Masia, 1964). *Cognitive objectives* are concerned with the learner's mastery of different levels of cognition along a continuum from simple to complex. Bloom's taxonomy was revised in the mid-nineties to be more reflective of the desire for measureable objectives by changing the six cognitive levels to overt verbs: (1) Remembering (formerly knowledge), (2) Understanding (formerly comprehension), (3) Applying (formerly application), (4) Analyzing (formerly analysis), (5) Evaluating (formerly evaluation), and (6) Creating (formerly synthesis). There are many good resources available to assist with the development of measureable objectives, including the website devoted to instructional design by Northern Illinois University (http://www.niu.edu/facdev/programs/handouts/blooms.shtml), Old Dominion University (http://ww2.odu.edu/educ/roverbau/Bloom/blooms_taxonomy.htm), and a comprehensive and interactive website by Iowa State University (http://www.celt.iastate.edu/teaching/RevisedBlooms1.html). Northern Illinois University's

resources include a revised Bloom's digital taxonomy map. Kathy Schrock's Guide to Everything (http://www.schrockguide.net/bloomin-apps.html) includes many technology-based resources for utilizing the revised Bloom's taxonomy, including smartphone and Web2.0 applications (apps).

Following are examples of cognitive objectives:
- Lists correct signs and symptoms of health problem (remembering)
- Summarizes the relationship between exercise and weight loss (understanding)
- Implements 30 minutes of exercise three times weekly (applying)
- Calculates amount of hidden fat in restaurant offerings before ordering (analyzing)
- Monitors weight loss progression as compared to diet and exercise habits (evaluating)
- Creates low-fat, low-calorie versions of favorite family recipes (creating)

Affective objectives describe changes in the learner's interests, attitudes, appreciations, values, and emotional sets or biases. Levels of affective objectives include (1) receiving, (2) responding, (3) valuing, (4) organizing a value system, and (5) characterizing a value complex. Following are examples of affective objectives:
- Accepts that present weight is unhealthy (receiving)
- Shows willingness to comply with health belief of increased exercise to decrease weight (responding)
- Desires to attain optimal weight (valuing)
- Forms judgment about the responsibility of the individual for maintaining optimal weight (conceptualization of a value)
- Revises health beliefs about weight, diet, and exercise as new information becomes available (value complex)

Much more has been written about cognitive objectives than about affective objectives in the general educational and nursing literature. This may owe, in part, to the complexities of influencing affective domains of knowing. Present changes in society, the global economy, and health care seem to indicate the need to pay as much, if not more, attention to the affective domain of learning.

The *psychomotor domain of learning* requires learners to perform motor skills, which is accomplished through practice to master the skills with precision, accuracy, and complete execution of the task. Psychomotor skills are most commonly associated with lab or clinical learning. Psychomotor skills are best learned by observing the skills of a more experienced person, imitating the behaviors in a controlled environment through practice, and adapting the skills to other situations.

The following are examples of psychomotor objectives:

- Demonstrates proper techniques for specified physical activity (demonstration)
- Illustrates documentation of physical activity in log sheet (application)
- Prepares a meal following the recommended healthy eating guidelines (synthesis)

A lesser-known taxonomy, *SOLO (Structure of Observed Learning Outcomes)* taxonomy, first described by John Biggs (http://www.johnbiggs.com.au/academic/solo-taxonomy/) and Kevin Collis, is a complexity-based classification system used to assess a learner's work based on quality and not just the identification of specific tasks. The SOLO taxonomy represents five levels of increasing complexity in a learner's understanding of a concept: (1) Prestructural, (2) Unistructural, (3) Multistructural, (4) Relational, and (5) Extended Abstract. James Atherton's website (http://www.learningandteaching.info/learning/solo.htm) provides easy-to-understand visual representations of the five levels of complexity.

Selecting Teaching-Learning Strategies

Primary steps in effective teaching and learning are setting the climate and selecting appropriate strategies. Some obvious ways to facilitate a climate conducive to learning include attention to room size, temperature, noise level, seating arrangements, lighting, and availability of supplies and technological resources. The degree of formality that sets the tone of the teaching-learning experience is also important. For example, teaching about dietary and activity recommendations to patients recovering from stroke may involve a more formal presentation. In contrast, a class for new parents on how to bathe a baby may be more informal and relaxed.

Cognitive capacity, psychosocial development, and physical maturation and abilities of the learner are important considerations when one is choosing a teaching strategy (Billings & Halstead, 2009). Selection of appropriate strategies is also influenced by cultural and environmental factors.

Questioning Techniques. Teacher questioning that enhances critical thinking has a positive impact on meeting learner needs. Two aspects of the teacher's questioning technique are important: phrasing the questions and probing the responses. Clearly phrased questions are stated simply, using words that are easily understood; they focus on the content and emphasize specific thinking skills. For example, "When you had your last asthma attack, were you near someone who was smoking?" or "How do you plan to increase your physical activity without jeopardizing your cardiac status?"

After a learner has responded, the teacher should follow up with probing questions to clarify exactly what the patient means (e.g., seeking a more exact description of pain intensity). Probing strategies include asking questions that increase awareness of potential motivations, refocusing the conversation when it begins to wander from the topic at hand, and inquiring about emotional reactions to the situation.

Lecture. In many situations a lecture format of teaching is used; this format is most appropriate when the learner needs basic knowledge on a topic before more advanced forms of learning can occur (Billings & Halstead, 2009). The lecture may be supplemented by written materials or more interactive learning techniques (Novotny & Griffin, 2006). For example, an experienced nurse who is mentoring a new registered nurse (RN) might inquire (use questioning techniques) about the mentee's knowledge about blood gas analysis. If the new RN has minimal knowledge about blood gas analysis and interpretation, it will be necessary to review the basic information about oxygen and carbon dioxide before practicing blood gas analysis and interpretation. This teaching would most likely be presented in a lecture format (either synchronous or asynchronous) because the information is fundamental to understanding how to analyze blood gas results. The learning could be enhanced for a tactile, or hands-on, learner if the lesson also included a demonstration of collecting a blood sample along with a return demonstration.

Demonstration. Frequently a learning situation involves a demonstration in which a teacher shows an individual or group how to perform a particular task. Demonstrations may be presented in a live format or recorded for learners to view on their own time. If prerecorded, it is important that the learner has the opportunity to ask questions in a public forum or via private discussion with the teacher. Live sessions may also be recorded for repeated offerings as review or for those who may miss the live demonstration.

To facilitate a live demonstration, prepare the materials before the audience gathers and analyze the steps ahead of time. Additional tips include:

1. Start the session on time.
2. Arrange the groups around you so that all can see.
3. Explain ahead of time what will happen and what to expect.
4. Demonstrate slowly and deliberately.
5. Explain each step.
6. Allow time for questions after each step.
7. Use humor to keep people alert.
8. End with a final summary and more questions.
9. Have the learners return the demonstration.

Group Discussions. A group discussion is a purposeful conversation and deliberation on a topic of mutual interest conducted under the guidance of the leader. Discussion enables participants to express opinions and to learn about topics of mutual interest. This technique provides maximum opportunity for the acceptance of personal responsibility for learning and sharing experiences and opinions with others. Focus groups are types of group discussions that are often used in research and to obtain information from the patient-consumer point of view. As with other teaching-learning methods, discussion groups may be synchronous (in a "live" environment) or asynchronous (e.g., blogs or wikis).

Role-Playing and Case Studies. Case studies, or fictitious data regarding a situation, often guide role-playing activities. This technique requires that selected members of a learning group spontaneously act out specific roles. Role-playing is used to bring participants into the closer experience of feeling and reacting to a problem. It promotes understanding of one's own and others' feelings and viewpoints. Types of role-playing include the following:

1. Drama: Helps participants gain insight into other people or situations (plot, characters, and scenes are developed previously)
2. Exercise: Larger, more complex, and prolonged version of role-playing in which groups are interacting
3. Psychodrama: Directed primarily at the therapeutic treatment of individuals
4. Simulation games: Learners act out their understanding and insight in handling "live" problems or "critical incidents" using gaming techniques

Choice of media can also enhance teaching and learning and may help determine the strategy selected for learning. Questions to ask in choosing and using media, as well as their individual differences and special considerations, are summarized in Table 10-2.

Evaluating the Teaching-Learning Experience

Evaluation consists of determining the worth of something. This process includes obtaining information for use in judging the worth of a program, product, procedure, or objective, or the potential utility of alternative approaches designed to attain specified objectives. In planning, designing, implementing, and validating teaching-learning experiences, knowledge of the theories, and methods of evaluation is extremely important.

Three evaluation methods can be used concurrently in teaching and learning: formative, summative, and peer evaluation. *Formative evaluation* takes place while the teaching-learning experience is in progress. Its purpose is to identify needed changes in material, content, or teaching style so as to better meet overall program learning objectives (Billings & Halstead, 2009). *Summative evaluation* occurs near the end of a teaching-learning episode and may focus on learner satisfaction, the level of learner performance, the incidence of occurrences related to the subject area (e.g., fewer episodes of hyperglycemia secondary to testing blood glucose levels more frequently), improved self-care skills documented through a home visit, or satisfaction with a lifestyle change (e.g., change in diet or exercise documented through a follow-up phone call). Information from summative evaluations is used to judge the value of the present teaching-learning experience as compared with alternative methods of experiences.

Although learners are certainly important evaluators of teacher effectiveness, teachers should also be evaluated by peers, particularly if they are novices and are expected to grow and develop. *Peer evaluation* conducted by a colleague or an outside observer offers a different perspective on the effectiveness of the entire teaching-learning episode. An evaluation of this type requires an experienced teacher who can evaluate against more sophisticated criteria, such as selection and organization of content, use of the literature, evidence of learning needs assessment, ability to ask or answer difficult questions, and quality of teaching style.

Despite efforts to plan effective teaching and learning, learners may not learn or gain the desired

TABLE 10-2   Choosing and Using Teaching-Learning Materials

MEDIA	ADVANTAGES	CONSIDERATIONS
Audio	Useful for individuals and groups; involves auditory sense Useful for both face-to-face and online learning Economical, easy to prepare Can be used independently	Assess hearing with individuals, room size with groups Requires knowledge of chosen software applications and compatibility with course management system (if applicable)
Books/pamphlets/ printed materials	Useful for individuals; involves visual sense Easy to use Allows learner to self-pace Easy to reference	Assess reading ability and level of material Cost; must obtain permission to copy Texts go out of date rapidly
Software applications (computer, smart-phones, iPads, tablets, etc.)	Allows self-pacing, multisensory involvement Sequential programs; can be used by all learner levels	Requires added time to learn use Expensive equipment Professional programming required
Internet websites	Appeals to visual and auditory learners if sites use multimedia to present material Interactive, multisensory Hyperlinks to additional resources Can support video, sounds, images, animation, and text	Limited to only users with Internet access Computer monitors not designed for paragraph reading; therefore limits information to list format Requires more development time
Films/videos	Suitable for groups; involves sight, hearing Can stimulate emotions, build attitudes May be available from a public library Useful for compression of time and space Ability to self-produce with new technologies available on smartphones and mobile devices	Does not permit self-pacing Difficult to produce Expensive to buy; allow time for order Requires special equipment and/or knowledge of video producing/sharing software
Flipcharts/ chalkboards	Suitable for groups; involves sight Allows step-by-step sequence of material Inexpensive	Bulky to transport Teacher's back to audience while writing Not reusable
Models/real objects	Useful for individuals/small groups Multisensory involvement Permits demonstration and practice	May not be easy to obtain Can be costly Models often easily damaged
Posters/overheads	Useful for individuals/small groups; involves sight Easy to produce, inexpensive May be reused, easy to store	Requires viewing space and/or equipment Avoid crowding; consider color, size, and space For best appearance, have professionally developed
Slides/electronic slides	Suitable for large groups Inexpensive, easy to produce and duplicate Easy to add or subtract material	Requires expensive equipment to develop and to project slides once developed

outcome. According to Bastable (2006), barriers to learning may include any of the following: (1) lack of time to learn, (2) stress related to the need for learning or the circumstance that requires learning, (3) negative influences from the teaching-learning experience, (4) personal characteristics of the learner, (5) inappropriate level or amount of required learning, (6) lack of support, (7) denial that learning needs exist, and (8) the inconvenience and complexity of the information to be learned. In cases in which barriers exist, it is helpful to identify the factors that impede learning and determine what methods of teaching will improve learning based on the barriers. This may require repeated efforts with a variety of methods. Engaging other family members, support individuals, or caretakers in the teaching-learning experience is appropriate and may be absolutely necessary in some cases.

FUTURE TRENDS IN TEACHING AND LEARNING

Technology is changing the way we teach and learn. Future teaching and learning experiences will focus on information management, problem solving, decision making rather than memorization, and interdisciplinary collaboration with teachers and learners through global access. Nurses and patients have access to devices that fit in the palms of their hands. These devices are not only promoting quick and easy access to information, but also influencing the way health is managed. For example, applications are available on hand-held devices that allow patients with asthma or diabetes to store daily health logs and send the information via the Internet to their health care providers. These logs also can be accessed online on any computer for those who do not own hand-held technology. Such technology allows teachers and students to connect with one another for sharing information, teaching, and learning; therefore teaching methods in the future will center on more experiential learning, such as interactive online simulations. Technologies that are currently available via hand-held devices are also available through cellular phones that connect to the Internet using VoIP. This technology has endless potential because cellular phone technology is the fastest-growing market in the world.

At present, some teaching and learning occurs in virtual environments, whereby users become characters (known as *avatars*) acting in simulated settings such as emergency departments or operating rooms to learn skills and techniques. One of the most common virtual environments used in education is Second Life (learn more by visiting http://secondlife.com/whatis). Beyond learning, technology is influencing the way we provide care. Advances in telehealth and telemedicine have greatly improved access to care and provide services that have been difficult to obtain, especially in remote areas. Telehealth is discussed in more detail in Chapter 19.

This ongoing explosion of knowledge and emergence of major scientific developments mean that nurses must become continuous lifelong learners who recognize the importance of how to think critically, how to accept the need to relearn, and how to deal with change. Teaching and learning remain essential aspects of the professional nurse's role. To effectively implement the teaching or learning role, the nurse must possess or acquire a thorough understanding of the teaching-learning process. Furthermore, nurses must take into account variations in a learner's health status, risk factors, cultural considerations, and myriad other factors to develop effective teaching-learning experiences. The need to adapt teaching and learning to new practice environments and the ever-changing health values of the nation will continue to challenge the nursing profession.

SUMMARY

Driven by advancements in technology, communication, and nursing education transformation, teaching and learning in the nursing profession has evolved in recent years. Selected teaching-learning theories and principles that characterize both effective teaching and effective learning were discussed. Technological influences related to internet-supported teaching and learning, online learning, and instructional technologies were addressed. Specific skill sets for creating an effective teaching-learning plan such as assessment of learners, groups, or populations; cultural considerations; development of learning objectives; selection of teaching-learning strategies; and evaluation of the teaching-learning experience were explored from both the perspectives of the teacher and that of the learner. Finally, future trends on the near horizon were introduced.

SALIENT POINTS

- Behaviorist theories are based on the premise that learning occurs through a stimulus-response sequence, followed by consistent feedback.

- Cognitive theories propose that learning is related to an internal change in perception that is influenced by both internal and external variables.

- Change theories are based on strategies that empower patients to exercise healthy behaviors or health-managing behaviors that are not in conflict with the patient's value system.
- Humanistic theories state that learning is self-initiated and should promote the development of insight, judgment, values, and self-concept.
- Learners have different preferred styles of learning (ways in which they perform best). Awareness of the various learning styles influences the choice of teaching-learning strategies and can enhance learning.
- The Internet is dramatically changing the teaching-learning process because teachers and learners now have access to information that, just decades ago, was available only to a select few.
- Advancing technology is changing the way teachers deliver information and the way individuals learn information.

- The teaching-learning process parallels the steps of the nursing process—assessment, planning, implementation, and evaluation.
- Assessment of the learner is multifaceted and includes demographic, psychosocial, cultural, physical, behavioral, and cognitive factors.
- Planning the teaching-learning experience focuses on developing measureable learner objectives and selecting appropriate teaching-learning strategies.
- For successful implementation of the teaching plan, the environment must be conducive to learning.
- Evaluation of the teaching-learning experience includes the level of achievement of learner objectives and the effectiveness of the teacher.
- Among the future trends in teaching and learning are a reliance on information retrieval and management, the development of critical thinking and problem-solving skills, and a focus on experiential learning for the continuous lifelong learner.

CRITICAL REFLECTION EXERCISES

1. Using one of the resources suggested, determine your own learning style. Ask a colleague to do the same. Compare and contrast your results. What types of learning activities do you find most effective and enjoyable? Using these results, design two learning activities (one for you and one for your colleague) to teach a nursing skill (e.g., abdominal assessment).

2. Evaluate the effectiveness of the teaching-learning process in your own area of clinical practice. What are the typical activities of the teacher and the expected outcomes of the learner? What evaluation methods are used to determine whether learning objectives are achieved? What changes would you make in the teaching-learning process to improve its effectiveness?

3. Select a clinical teaching topic of your choice (e.g., diabetes management for a newly diagnosed 16-year-old male athlete). Using the revised Bloom's taxonomy, develop learner objectives advancing from the simple (Remembering) to complex (Creating). What teaching strategies would you use for these objectives? How would you assess the outcomes?

4. Choose a disease in a specific population (e.g., asthma in children). Search the Internet for resources. Evaluate two websites based on the evaluation criteria. Do the sites meet the criteria in Box 10-1? Explain.

5. Select a disease in a specific population (e.g., postpartum depression in teen mothers). Search the Internet for tools and resources that help patients understand and manage their conditions (e.g., websites, blogs, mobile apps, journals). How do the credible sources differ from the noncredible? How can you teach the learner to identify a credible site? How can these tools be used?

6. Analyze teaching materials (e.g., care plans, pamphlets, audiovisuals) in use at your facility. Are technology-based materials noted? How are they evaluated? Are the materials free from educational, gender, or cultural bias? Select two of these materials and describe the changes that need to be made to make them culturally acceptable and to include Internet and mobile technology resources.

REFERENCES

Atherton, J. S. (2013). *Learning and teaching; About the site.* [Online: UK]. Retrieved February 26, 2014 from htt p://www.learningandteaching.info/ learning/about.htm. Read more: About the site http://www.learning andteaching.info/learning/about.ht m#ixzz2uRNkXGIv. Under Creative Commons License: Attribution Non-Commercial No Derivatives.

Badarudeen, S., & Sabharwal, S. (2008). Readability of patient education materials from the American Academy of Orthopaedic Surgeons and Pediatric Orthopaedic Society of North American websites. *The Journal of Bone and Joint Surgery, 90,* 199–204.

Bandura, A. (1977). Self-efficacy: Toward a unifying theory of behavioral change. *Psychology Review, 84,* 191–215.

Bastable, S. B. (2006). *Essentials of patient education.* Sudbury, MA: Jones & Bartlett.

Billings, D. M., & Halstead, J. A. (2009). *Teaching in nursing: A guide for faculty* (3rd ed.). St. Louis: Saunders.

Bloom, B. (1956). *Taxonomy of educational objectives: Handbook I. Cognitive domain.* New York: Davis McKay.

Bruner, J. (1966). *Toward a theory of instruction.* Cambridge, MA: Harvard University.

Combs, A. (1965). *The professional education of teachers.* Boston, MA: Allyn & Bacon.

Dale, E. (1969). *Audiovisual methods in teaching* (3rd ed.). New York: Holt-Dryden.

Dewey, J. (1938). *Experience and education.* New York: Macmillan.

Donner, G., & Wheeler, M. (2009). *Coaching in nursing: An introduction.* Retrieved from http://www.nursingso ciety.org/Education/ProfessionalDeve lopment/Documents/Coaching% 20and%20Mentoring%20Workbook _STTI.pdf.

Federal Communication Commission. (2009). *Voice over internet protocol.*Retrieved March 28, 2009, from http:// www.fcc.gov/voip.

Festinger, L. (1957). *A theory of cognitive dissonance* (1st ed.). Stanford, CA: Stanford University Press.

Gagne, R. (1974). *Essentials of learning for instruction.* Hinsdale IL: Dryden.

Glasser, W. (1965). *Reality therapy.* New York: Harper & Row.

Hansen, M., & Erdley, S. (2009). You-Tube and other Web 2.0 applications for nursing education. *Online Journal of Nursing Informatics, 13*(3). Retrieved from http://ojni.org/13_3/ Hansen_Erdley.pdf.

Hoover, E. (2009). The millennial muddle. Retrieved from The Chronicle of Higher Education website. http://chronicle.com/article/The-Millenial-Muddle-How/48772/.

Internet and World Stats. (2009). *Internet usage statistics: The big picture.* Retrieved March 26, 2009, from http://www.internetworldstats.com/ stats.htm.

Johnson, D. W., Johnson, R. T., & Stanne, M. B. (2000). *Cooperative learning methods: A meta-analysis.* Retrieved April 18, 2005, from http://www.co-operation.org/pages/cl-methods.html .

Knowles, M. (1980). *The modern practice of adult education: From pedagogy to andragogy.* Chicago: Follett.

Knowles, M. (1984). *The adult learner: A neglected species* (3rd ed.). Houston: Gulf.

Krathwohl, D. R., Bloom, B. S., & Masia, B. B. (1964). *Taxonomy of educational objectives: Handbook II. Affective domain.* New York: David McKay.

Lave, J., & Wenger, L. (1991). *Situated learning: Legitimate peripheral participation.* Cambridge, UK: Cambridge University Press.

Learning. (n.d.). *Merriam-Webster. com.* Retrieved March 1, 2014, from http://www.merriam-webster.com/dictionary/learning

Lewin, K. (1951). *Field theory in social science.* New York: Harper & Row.

Maslow, A. (1970). *Motivation and personality.* New York: Harper & Row.

Mayer, R. E. (2001). *Multimedia learning.* New York: Cambridge University Press.

National Research Council. (2004). *Health literacy: A prescription to end confusion.* Washington, DC: The National Academies Press.

Novotny, J. M., & Griffin, M. T. (2006). *A nuts and bolts approach to teaching nursing* (3rd ed.). New York: Springer.

Pavlov, I. (1927). *Conditioned reflexes.* (G. V. Anrep, Trans.). London: Oxford University Press.

Pew Research Internet Project. (2013). *Health fact sheet.* Retrieved from http://www.pewinternet.org/fact-sheets/health-fact-sheet/.

Pew Research Internet Project. (2013). *Mobile technology fact sheet.* Retrieved from http://www.pewinternet.org/fact-sheets/mobile-technology-fact-sheet/.

Piaget, J. (1954). *The language and thought of the child* (3rd ed.). London: Routledge & Kegan Paul.

Prochaska, J. O., & DiClemente, C. C. (1982). Transtheoretical therapy toward a more integrative model of change. *Psychotherapy: Theory, Research, and Practice, 19*(3), 276–287.

Rogers, C. (1969). *Freedom to learn.* Columbus, OH: Merrill.

Rogers, E. M. (2003). *Diffusion of innovations* (5th ed.). New York: Free Press.

Rosenstock, I. (1974). Historical origins of the health belief model. *Health Education Monographs, 2*(4), 324–473.

Rotter, J. B. (1990). Internal versus external control of reinforcement: A case history of a variable. *American Psychologist, 45*(4), 489–493.

Skinner, B. (1953). *Science and human behavior.* New York: Macmillan.

teaching. (n.d.). *Merriam-Webster. com. Retrieved* March 1, 2014, from http://www.merriam-webster.com/thesaurus/teaching

Thielfoldt, D., & Scheef, D. (2004). *Generation X and the millenials: What you need to know about mentoring the new generations.* Retrieved from American Bar Association website http://apps. americanbar.org/lpm/lpt/articles/ mgt08044.html.

Thorndike, E. (1913). *The psychology of learning.* New York: Teachers College Press.

Trueman, M. S., & Miles, D. G. (2011). Twitter in the classroom: Twenty-first century flash cards. *Nurse Educator, 36*(5), 183–186.

Walker, P. H., & Elberson, K. L. (2005). Collaboration leadership in a global technological environment. *Online Journal of Issues in Nursing.* Retrieved June 10, 2010, from http://www.nursi ngworld.org/MainMenuCategories/A NAMarketplace/ANAPeriodicals/OJI N/TableofContents/Volume102005/ No1Jan05/tpc26_516012.aspx.

Wentzel, P., Lammeren, R. V., Molendijk, M., Bruin, S. D., & Wagtendonk, A. (2005). *Using mobile technology to enhance students' educational experiences.* Boulder, CO: Educause.

Wolpe, J., & Lazarus, A. (1966). *Behavior theory techniques: A guide to the treatment of neurosis.* Oxford, UK: Pergamon Press.

CHAPTER 11

Legal Aspects of Nursing Practice

*Nayna C. Philipsen, PhD, JD, RN, CFE, FACCE and
Patricia C. McMullen, PhD, JD, CRNP, FAANP*

(e) http://evolve.elsevier.com/Friberg/bridge/

OBJECTIVES

At the completion of this chapter, the reader will be able to:

- Describe the constitutional and administrative law principles foundational to nursing practice.
- Analyze contract law and its effect on the nurse's employment relationships.
- Differentiate torts of relevance to nursing practice.
- Discuss strategies the nurse can use to reduce legal exposure.

PROFILE IN PRACTICE

Elizabeth Frey, JD, RN
Dugan, Babij & Tolley, LLC, Baltimore, Maryland

As a nurse attorney in Baltimore, Maryland, I handle medical malpractice cases on behalf of the plaintiff (the patient or injured party). I thoroughly enjoy handling these cases for three primary reasons.

First, my goals as a practicing nurse were and are the same as my present goals. They are to be a patient advocate and to improve the quality of patient care. I believe that I am able to reach these goals as a lawyer practicing in the area of plaintiff medical malpractice.

Second, I believe the patient who has been injured as the result of medical negligence is the underdog, if you will, and I prefer to represent those who are less fortunate. The patient generally does not have the same level of resources that physicians, hospitals, and insurance companies have, such as money, influence, and advanced education. Other factors that place the plaintiff at a comparative disadvantage in these cases include tort reform and the difficulty and cost involved in finding a qualified physician who is willing to review records and be an expert witness (which usually means testifying against a fellow physician). And, of course, the plaintiff has the burden of proof.

Third, I believe plaintiff medical malpractice is one of the best areas of law in which to use a nursing background. Most of my time is spent investigating cases

before the filing of a lawsuit and then, after the suit is filed, performing discovery, in which a nursing background is invaluable. As with any case, you must know and understand the facts and applicable law. To obtain the facts in a medical malpractice case, it is necessary to acquire the client's medical records, review them, and know and understand the client's condition, as well as the care and treatment he or she received. When the client contacts you because of an unfavorable outcome, you need to determine whether that negative outcome is a risk or consequence that occurred in the absence of negligence or whether it was the result of medical negligence. To do this you must research the medical literature and determine what kind of medical experts are needed to render the necessary opinions. Then you must contact and retain the required experts. Where I have found my nursing background most helpful is in discussing cases with expert witnesses and in deposing physicians and other health care providers. You must have a strong knowledge and understanding of health care to handle such cases, and my nursing background has been invaluable in this regard. In fact, almost every medical malpractice law firm (plaintiff and defense) I am familiar with has at least one nurse attorney on staff.

INTRODUCTION

Nurses practice within a framework of legal principles on a daily basis. Legal concepts, expectations, and consequences surround all health care professionals in the United States. An informed and safe nurse must be aware of the effect these legal aspects have on nursing practice to reduce exposure to adverse legal consequences.

Law is the sum total of human-made rules designed to help people maintain order in their society and settle their problems in a nondestructive manner. *Statutory law* is established through the legislative process and expands each time Congress or state legislatures pass new legislation. *Common law* is established by previous court decisions and expands each time a judge makes a legal ruling in a case.

The function of law is to create and interpret relationships. *Public law* defines and interprets relationships between individuals and the government. The major categories of public law are constitutional law, administrative law, and criminal law. *Private law* defines and interprets the relationship between individuals. Private law includes contract law and tort law.

These areas of law have an effect on the practice of nursing. Constitutional law defines the clients' and nurses' constitutional rights and remedies. Administrative law includes the licensing and regulation of nursing practice, as well as areas such as collective bargaining. Criminal law usually involves the nurse as a witness. However, it can also involve the nurse as a defendant who is accused of a criminal offense. Contract law identifies the common types of employer–employee relationships and determines the risks and protections inherent in each type of relationship. Tort law is concerned with the reparation of wrongs or injuries inflicted by one person on another. It defines the legal liability for the practice of nursing and identifies the elements essential for each tort. This chapter describes the interaction between law and nursing in three major areas: administrative law, employment law, and civil (or tort) law.

ADMINISTRATIVE LAW IN NURSING

All states have a "police power" to enact legislation to protect the health, safety, and welfare of their citizens. The power of the state to license nurses and other health care professionals originates in the U.S. Constitution

(*Dent v. West Virginia*, 1889). The 10th Amendment allows the states to enact legislation that is not preempted or prohibited by federal law. Each state constitution has a health and welfare clause empowering it to pass such legislation.

Boards of Nursing (boards) are state agencies legislatively created by the state nurse practice acts (NPAs). Like other government agencies, the boards develop regulations that give the public "notice" of how laws passed by the legislature will be implemented in their agency. The boards also enforce their regulations.

Nurses are licensed under state NPAs. The NPAs establish entry requirements into the profession, set definitions of nursing practice, and establish guidelines for professional discipline when a nurse fails to obey state laws or becomes incompetent. For most nurses, licensing is their only direct contact with the board. However, many find themselves tangentially involved with the board through some level of conflict about the definition of nursing. Fewer nurses have direct contact with the board's disciplinary unit.

Licensure

Licensure is an exercise of the state's police power that the state legislature uses to protect the health, safety, and welfare of its citizens. Through state licensure statutes, the state controls entry into the profession, the discipline of licensees who fail to comply with minimal standards, and the nursing activities of unlicensed practitioners ("nurse imposters"). Boards are composed largely of the professionals whom they regulate. Nurses themselves, typically with some consumer representation and input, implement the standards because their specialized knowledge best qualifies them to evaluate and oversee nursing practice.

All the states, the District of Columbia, and the U.S. territories have laws and regulations controlling nursing licensure and practice. National guidelines serve as useful references for nurses in proposing and implementing state laws. The American Nurses Association, the American Association of Colleges of Nursing, the National Organization of Nurse Practitioner Faculties, and other professional groups develop definitions and standards of nursing education, practice, and ethics that are often incorporated into state NPAs. These NPAs are implemented through a state agency called the *health professions board*, *nursing board*, or a similar title. Rules and regulations promulgated by the board give meaning to the NPA.

The most visible function of NPAs is the control over entry of new members into the nursing profession. Nursing and other professions have been scrutinized for entry requirements that may contain bias, discriminate against minorities, or discourage diversity (*Turner v. State Board of Nursing*, 2012). Entry requirements typically include completion of an approved nursing education program, satisfactory performance on a standardized licensure examination, competency in spoken English, and strong moral character. Laws regulating nursing practice vary from state to state, with each state placing its individual requirements on the profession. All state NPAs, however, intends are designed to ensure the health and safety of the patients receiving care by nurses. Licensing is supposed to protect the public from incompetence and abuse. Does a blanket license, covering practice over a broad range of specialties, accomplish that purpose? Do re-credentialing tests scrutinize actual competence? Other licensure questions facing the nursing profession include the following: Is licensure too restrictive in its limits on entry into the profession? Do the tests and criteria used actually identify the individuals who are safe and competent nurses, or do they shut out good nurses who are different from a homogenized stereotype? Do licensure requirements protect the public, or do they protect nursing professionals by eliminating competition? Should national licensure for nurses be established so that nurses could easily practice across state boundaries?

Although a national nursing license is not currently available, an interstate mutual recognition model of nurse licensure, also known as the *Nurse Multi-State Licensure Compact* (or "the Compact"), was approved by the National Council of State Boards of Nursing (NCSBN) in 1998. To participate in the Compact, each state legislature must enact the model Compact. The first state to pass the Compact into law was Maryland in 1999. As of February 2015 24 states had passed the nurse licensure Compact (NCSBN, 2015). The Compact allows a nurse who holds a license in the state of legal residency (the state used as residence on the federal tax return) to practice in other states that have enacted the Compact. The Compact for nursing works like the compact law of a century earlier, which enabled states to recognize automobile licenses so drivers could cross state lines (Philipsen & Haynes, 2007). The nursing licensure Compact is the result of technological advances, including the Internet and the increasing ease of transportation and communication in health care. The goal of the Compact is to ensure public protection and enhance access to safe and competent nursing care for patients who are across state lines from their nurse. These patients may be receiving services through telenursing, by a traveling nurse, or by a nurse who regularly drives across a state line to get to work. Nurses must have licenses in all of the non-Compact states where they practice. Because the nurse who is practicing on a Compact license is subject to each state's laws, the Compact nurse must be familiar with and comply with the NPA for each state in which he or she works.

Because state laws governing advanced practice registered nurses (APRNs) vary more significantly than those governing entry into nursing, a model setting standards for multistate certification took longer to develop. In September 2008 the NCSBN endorsed a new Consensus Model for APRN Regulation: Licensure, Accreditation, Certification, and Education. However, until states pass model legislation agreeing to recognize one another's advanced practice regulations, APRNs must continue to obtain APRN certification (a procedure that is in addition to, and separate from, RN licensure) in each state where they are practicing.

Control over Practice

The power to control entry into the profession and the power to take disciplinary action on the license of practitioners were developed to assure the public of safe, qualified practitioners. An indirect result of those powers is that the boards have some ability to exert control on the nursing market. Licensure grants a privileged place in the occupational hierarchy, but it is a position challenged both by the public and by other professionals who fear the surrender of power. Nurses also control the quality and standards of nursing care in the state through the disciplinary process of nurses in the NPAs. Thus as in many other professions, NPAs leave public consumers of nursing care dependent to a large degree on members of the profession to control access to nursing services and to maintain the quality of nursing care. The result is that nurses have the duty to advocate for patients, at the bedside and before the licensing board, for high-quality care from competent licensed practitioners. The ability of nurses to meet this great responsibility is sometimes challenged by members of the public who fear competing professional incentives. Some have also argued this is too much power to give any profession because professionals may be reluctant to discipline their own colleagues.

This power is also challenged by other professionals, from physicians to wound care specialists and lay midwives, who are afraid nursing's scope of practice will compete with their own professional and financial incentives. Nurse practice acts (NPAs) permit nurses to function under a broad definition of nursing while restricting the practice of non-nursing personnel who might otherwise deliver many services provided by nurses.

Enforcement of the prohibition against the unauthorized practice of nursing is exemplified by the practice of lay midwifery. Some states define midwifery as an advanced practice area within nursing and prohibit the practice of midwifery by non-nurses. Practicing lay midwives are not registered by the board of nursing and may be served with cease-and-desist orders. Boards may also request criminal charges for misrepresentation against lay midwives with the local office of the state's attorney (*Clemons et al. v. The Wellpoint Co., Inc.,* 2013; *People of the State of Illinois v. Jihan,* 1989). Some boards have administrative fining powers for unlicensed practitioners, which they can impose on lay midwives. These powers are invoked regardless of client satisfaction and often in spite of public protest. Boards argue that a threat to the public safety and welfare is inherent whenever unlicensed practice occurs, regardless of the specific situation. Similar policies and procedures have prevented nursing from taking over functions that have been absorbed into medical specialties. The jurisdiction of the nursing board may overlap with other professions that perform some of the same functions as nursing. For example, the expanded role of the nurse has resulted in clashes with physicians at the regulatory level (*Sermchief v. Gonzalez,* 1983). Although nursing boards have moved to limit the practice of unlicensed lay midwives, medical boards and organizations have moved to limit the practice of several types of advanced practice nurses (*California Society of Anesthesiologists, et al. v. Brown et al.,* 2012).

The preceding arguments illustrate the restrictive nature of licensing by limiting entry and practice. Is licensing too restrictive, or is licensing too permissive by granting "blanket" licenses? Does licensure today permit nurses to practice beyond their actual competence? No individual nurse can competently perform all the services nurses are licensed to deliver. Although most nurses practice only in a limited field

(e.g., surgery, obstetrics, oncology), a nursing license permits a nurse to practice in all areas of nursing. In addition, after initial licensure, many states require little or no demonstration of continuing competency to practice. However, initial credentials do not guarantee competency in the indefinite future. For this reason, some states and health care agencies are requiring mandatory continuing education or advanced certification as an indicator of ongoing competency (Philipsen, Lamm, & Reier, 2007).

Delegation in Nursing Practice

Most state NPAs authorize registered nurses to delegate, or assign, certain nursing care tasks to a non-nurse, although the nursing process itself cannot be delegated. Some nurses, knowing they are accountable for the care they delegate to their nursing assistants and other nursing extenders, are fearful of delegation. However, nurses who delegate reasonably and responsibly do not need to fear the task of delegating. Safe delegation requires that the nurse understands the requirements for delegation, such as assessing the task, selecting a nursing assistant/delegatee who is both competent and allowed by law to perform the task, explaining the importance of the task, and evaluating and giving feedback after the delegated task is complete. The 2006 Joint Statement on Delegation by the NCSBN and the ANA (NCSBN & ANA, 2006) is available online (www.ncsbn.org/Joint_statement.pdf).

Disciplinary and Administrative Procedures

A board of nursing usually has both regulatory and adjudicatory power. The regulatory power authorizes the board to develop rules and regulations for nursing licensure, nursing education, and nursing practice. The adjudicatory power authorizes the board to investigate, hear, and decide the outcomes of complaints that involve violations of the act and of the rules and regulations promulgated by the board. As mandated by the NPA, the board must ensure that a licensed nurse continues to practice within the standard of care, behaves professionally and ethically, and obeys all relevant state laws. The NPA contains or incorporates a number of grounds to achieve this. The disciplinary action is on the license of the nurse, and that license may be suspended or revoked by the board.

It is important to understand the responsibility of state boards is to protect the current and future safety of the public. Their delegated powers are to protect the public from unfit nurses, not to punish bad nurses. Boards can only limit or deny a nursing license. They cannot incarcerate a nurse, and they cannot require a nurse to compensate a patient for damages, financial or otherwise. Most board actions cannot be used in a lawsuit against a nurse. If an injured patient does seek monetary damages, he or she must file a civil lawsuit against the nurse. If an individual thinks a nurse has acted criminally, that person must contact the office of the state attorney.

A professional license is property protected by the U.S. Constitution. This means it cannot be limited or taken away without due process. Each state has an Administrative Procedure Act that guides the procedures within state agencies to guarantee this due process right. Each state agency has its own regulations that describe how the agency implements the law. These regulations can vary greatly from state to state and even among professional boards within a state. A board of nursing in one state may hear all arguments concerning nursing issues. The board in a neighboring state may delegate this action to an administrative law judge or a hearing officer. Within a state, a board of nursing may hear its own cases, whereas another professional board in the same state may have its cases heard by an outside hearing officer.

Due process requires the right to be heard, and it requires notice. A licensed nurse has a duty to be aware of the state's NPA. The NPA is considered notice to nurses in that state about the grounds for which they may lose their license to practice. Further notice comes when a nurse receives a charging document. This paper advises the nurse that the board has probable cause to believe the nurse is violating the NPA. It has to be specific enough to give the nurse notice about what any defense could be and about the time and place of the hearing.

Due process further requires that a nurse be afforded the right to appeal any decision made by the board that seems improper. This appeal is usually to the state civil courts. Appeal is typically limited to procedural issues, such as whether the board had a right to hear the case or whether the board gave the nurse proper due process rights.

Although all NPAs have commonalities, each state has its own unique legislation. The nurse who moves from one state to another or practices in multiple states through the Compact should obtain a copy of each state's NPA. The differences in state NPAs can be significant. For example, one state may impose no legal duty on a nurse to report the incompetence of a physician. In the next state, the nurse may find that failure to report such a physician can result in the loss of the nurse's license. The nurse needs to be familiar with the requirements of the local NPA for licensure, the boundaries and definitions of practice, the areas for discipline on practice, and the procedures in place to protect the nurse in case the board challenges the license.

The Americans with Disabilities Act

In 1990 the federal government enacted the Americans with Disabilities Act (ADA). The ADA (U.S. Department of Justice, 1990) prohibits discrimination based on disability in employment. It also prohibits disability-related discrimination by state and local governments, by private companies, and by commercial facilities. This is a federal law and, like the constitutional right to due process, it applies to all state boards. Updated information about ADA requirements can be found online (www.ada.gov). The entire text of the ADA is also available online (www.ada.gov/pubs/ada.htm).

Formerly the boards could interact with disabled nurses without regard or accommodation for their disability. Now disabled nurses, such as those with a drug dependence who are compliant with treatment, those with a physical impairment, and those with a mental illness, are granted special confidentiality, as long as it is consistent with patient safety. This is intended to encourage nurses to seek treatment and self-report, to report other nurses who need treatment, and to ensure the disabled are not the object of discrimination. Some boards have responded to this mandate by creating their own internal resources to comply with the ADA, such as a rehabilitation committee. Others have made arrangements with external groups, such as rehabilitation services that are provided privately or by a professional organization. A nurse in treatment for a protected disability does not have a public record connected with that disability.

The ADA also requires the professional boards to make any special arrangements to facilitate access to practice by nurses. Examples are special communication services for the sensory impaired and reasonable accommodations at the entrance to the site for licensure examinations or disciplinary hearings.

NURSING AND EMPLOYMENT LAW

Most nurses work as employees rather than as employers or independent contractors. Nurse employees deal daily with the tension of being professionally independent and responsible for their actions in practice, while simultaneously being constrained by the standards and requirements of their employer. At some time, every nurse will be faced with making a decision about accepting a work assignment. Similarly, the nurse is likely to be faced with decisions about delegation of nursing functions to unlicensed assistive personnel. How can nurses' voices be heard and valued in creating work environments that promote the delivery of high-quality care? What avenues of redress do nurses have if they experience employee/management problems, such as hospital downsizing or cross-training of nonprofessionals to carry out nursing functions under their supervision? How can nurses tell whether they are employees or part of management for bargaining purposes?

Contract Law

Nurses who are employed work under some form of contract. A contract is a promissory agreement between two or more parties that creates (or modifies or destroys) a legal relationship (Bix, 2012). A contract can be in writing, or it can be in spoken language with specific terms, in which case it is called an *express contract*. A contract also can be based solely on the conduct of the parties. These contracts are referred to as *implied contracts.*

An enforceable contract must first be for the performance of legal goods or services. A nurse cannot contract to practice medicine. Second, the parties must have legal capability to make the contract. For example, they must all have the mental ability to understand their actions and must be old enough to make a legal agreement. Third, all parties at the time of the contract must agree to do something, and they must agree on what that something is. Finally, there must be "consideration" (i.e., some kind of trade in which each party gets something from the contract). In a typical nurse employment situation, the employer receives nursing services, and the employee receives financial reimbursement.

All states have a "statute of frauds" that limits the enforcement of some contracts not written. These vary and are usually not significant to a nurse employee situation. However, a nurse who wants to prove the specific terms of a contract will obviously have difficulty with an oral contract.

Of more significance is the state "parole evidence rule." This rule provides that if oral agreements are made that differ from the written contract, the courts will not allow them to add to or change the written contract. Overcoming a written contract can be difficult for nurses, although it can be done—for example, by showing fraud or duress by the employer. When a nurse agrees to an employment position, he or she should be familiar with the employment contract, should obtain it in writing, and should not rely on oral agreements not part of the written contract. What about the role of the contract when the nurse is being terminated from employment or wants to leave employment? A contract can be legally terminated when it has been completely performed, its terms have been met, both parties agree to a change, it becomes impossible (e.g., through the death of a party or the destruction of the subject matter), or both parties agree to annul the contract. A contract can also be terminated by a breach, which means one of the parties fails to meet the terms of the agreement. When that happens, the other party can sue in civil court for any damages. For instance, an employee could sue for lost wages, and an employer could sue for lost profits. The Fair Labor Standards Act (FLSA) sets standards for overtime pay, minimum wage, family and medical leave, child labor, and workers' compensation. The U.S. Department of Labor provides a detailed description of the provisions of the FLSA online (www.dol.gov/compliance/laws/comp-flsa.htm). A nurse employee in a private setting could also file a grievance with the National Labor Relations Board (NLRB). Of utmost importance for nurses to understand is that most employment contracts are not individual contracts but are "at will." The following section clarifies this concept.

Employment at Will

Employment at will means the employee has the right to quit employment at any time for any reason, or "at will." The employer has the parallel right to terminate the employee at any time for any reason, also at will. The law of employment at will considers the employee and employer to have equal power, an assumption nurse employees know does not reflect employee–employer realities. For this reason, it is a harsh legal doctrine. An example is an employee who is terminated for reasons that are against the public good, such as for joining a union or serving on a jury. Courts have found ways to restrict this doctrine, but they are limited to public policy, implied contract, and good faith. Employees terminated against an implied contract are those who can show this contract included hospital procedural manuals and personnel handbooks, employer's conduct or policy, or (rarely) oral promises. An informed nurse employee must be familiar with such manuals and handbooks, document any oral promises, and get them in writing as soon as possible. What else can nurses do to enhance their protection as employees?

Labor Law

Collective bargaining by nurses is a relatively recent activity. In 1974 Congress extended coverage of the National Labor Relations Act (NLRA) to apply to workers in certain health care organizations. By the early 1990s, approximately 18% of registered nurses were represented by unions (AFL-CIO Department of Professional Employees, 2014). This means they had formed a collective bargaining unit and could bargain with the employer as a group, in good faith, to make an agreement regarding similar interests in wages, hours, and working conditions. Collective bargaining agreements contain grievance procedures guaranteed to all employees. Furthermore, they usually contain a clause protecting the nurse employee from discharge except for "good cause." Nurses who work in a unionized facility cannot bargain individually with the employer. The employer must bargain with the union, which must represent all employees, whether or not they join the union (McMullen & Philipsen, 1994). Nurse employees can enforce employment agreements under the NLRA, enacted on July 5, 1935 (29 U.S.C. 141-178). The provisions of the NLRA are enforced through the National Labor Relations Board (NLRB) and various federal courts. The NLRB is a federal agency charged with implementing the NLRA, in much the same way the nursing board implements the NPA. Because the NLRA is federal law, its protections apply in all states.

Only nurses who are employees can participate in collective bargaining with the union. The NLRA also has a special provision allowing "professionals" to bargain collectively. In the past, many nurses who supervised health care workers, such as nursing assistants, were able to participate in collective bargaining under the professional exemption. Some nurse supervisors, however, were, and still are, excluded from collective bargaining participation and protection. In May 1994, the Supreme Court narrowed the NLRA coverage of professional nurses. In a split decision, the court found that nurses who supervised others in a nursing home were part of management because such activities were "in the interest of the employer" (*NLRB v. Health Care and Retirement Corporation of America*, 1994). Of note, subsequent NLRB cases have determined many types of nurses do not fall into the supervisory category and are eligible to participate in collective bargaining. In the case of *Providence Alaska Medical Center v. Alaska Nurses' Association and the American Nurses Association* (1996), affirmed on appeal to the federal court, the NLRB determined that charge nurses, neurological outpatient rehabilitation nurses, and on-call home health leaders were not supervisors under Section 2 (11) of the NLRA because they did not exercise "independent judgment in directing employees" and were therefore able to engage in collective bargaining. In *NLRB v. Kentucky River Community* (2001) the Supreme Court concluded that charge nurses are supervisors, and not employees, under the NLRA. As a result every nurse has to ask whether supervision of other employees might be interpreted as "management," thereby depriving the nurse of the right to collective bargaining and its protections.

Compliance Programs

Nurses are often employees of health care organizations, which have to comply with multiple state and federal laws and programs. A compliance office is responsible for developing and implementing related policies and procedures. The purpose of the compliance program is to promote conformity to legal requirements within the institution by identifying potential concerns and correcting and preventing the recurrence of any identified problems. Compliance programs should include a confidential disclosure program, such as a toll-free telephone line, that allows employees to report suspected violations of federal or state health care program requirements or of the company's policies and procedures to the compliance officer. Nurses should be able to make these reports anonymously and be protected from retaliation or any other adverse action for making a report in good faith. Nurses should become familiar with their employer's written standards of conduct and compliance program. Nurse employees typically receive annual training that covers health care compliance policies, procedures, and related legal requirements.

Government Employees

The NLRA applies only to privately employed nurses. Federal employees, such as nurses who work for the Veterans Administration, are covered under the Civil Service Reform Act of 1978. The employment rights of state employees are governed by each state's public employee statutes.

TORT LAW IN NURSING

Another area of the legal system of particular importance to nurses is that of tort law. Torts are private or civil wrongs, in contrast to crimes, which are wrongs committed against the state (Goldberg, Sebok, & Zipursky, 2012; Schwartz, Kelly, & Partlett, 2010). The plaintiff, or person filing the lawsuit, files a tort action to recover damages for personal injury or property damage occurring from negligent conduct or unintentional misconduct (Schwartz et al., 2010). Unintentional torts are those in which persons incur harm or injury as a consequence of an unintended, wrongful act by another person. Negligence and the related legal concept of malpractice are examples of unintentional torts (Goldberg et al., 2012; Schwartz et al., 2010). Several types of torts are often encountered in legal actions against nurses. These include negligence, assault, battery, false imprisonment, lack of informed consent, and breach of confidentiality. A brief discussion of each of these types of torts follows. Case examples of various torts are included in Box 11-1.

Negligence and Malpractice

Negligence occurs when a person fails to act in a reasonable manner under a given set of circumstances (Schwartz et al., 2010). For example, if a person drinks excessively at a party, drives down the highway, and injures another motorist, the injured motorist could file a tort suit for negligence. Driving a car under the influence of alcohol or drugs is not typically considered reasonable conduct. Consequently, in addition to possible criminal action by the state where the accident happened, a negligence lawsuit probably also would result.

Unreasonable conduct by a nurse or other professional is a specific type of negligence, one referred to as *malpractice*. The nurse has the legal duty to provide the patient with a reasonable standard of care. This is usually described as "what the reasonably prudent nurse would do under the same or similar circumstances." In malpractice cases, the issue is whether the conduct of the nurse is below the standard established by law for the protection of others or whether the care given by the nurse involves an unreasonable risk for causing damage to another (Goldberg et al., 2012; Schwartz et al., 2010). The courts, based on long-established legal precedent, usually place the responsibility of establishing that the nurse acted wrongly on the injured patient. The nurse is initially assumed to be innocent of the malpractice charge. Consequently, the plaintiff patient has the responsibility of proving that the nurse's conduct was unreasonable. In some cases the nurse is able to resolve the patient's charges out of court through an alternative dispute resolution strategy (Philipsen, 2008). To successfully negotiate a settlement or defend in court, the nurse responds to a patient complainant/plaintiff, who must provide evidence related to four elements:

1. *Duty.* A duty is a legal obligation toward the patient (Schwartz et al., 2010; Scott, 1998). A nurse's signature in the patient's medical record may be enough to prove that the nurse had a duty to the patient. For purposes of establishing the element of duty in a malpractice case against a nurse, the question is, "Did the nurse have a legal obligation toward this patient?"

2. *Breach of duty.* This element of negligence and malpractice considers whether the nurse's conduct violated the duty to the patient (Schwartz et al., 2010). To determine whether a breach of duty occurred, the plaintiff must show that the nurse's conduct did not comply with reasonable *standards of care* rendered by an average, like-specialty provider under similar circumstances (Schwartz et al., 2010). A number of methods are used to determine whether the nurse's care was reasonable. Expert witness testimony, nursing texts, professional journals, standards developed by professional organizations, institutional procedures and protocols, and equipment guidelines developed by manufacturers can all be used to decide whether the nurse's care complied with reasonable care (Aiken & Catalano, 1994; Glannon, 2010; Guido, 2013; Schwartz et al., 2010; Sharpe, 1999). Use of careful documentation techniques, such as those specified in the documentation guidelines, will help the nurse

BOX 11-1   Charting Basics

Documentation is always vital for nurses. Knowledge of a few basic rules can help nurses protect themselves in the event of a lawsuit. These rules can also help communicate the quality of nursing care that is delivered. Helpful tips include the following:

- Never alter or falsify a record. You will lose all your credibility if it is discovered that you altered or falsified a record.
- If you make a written error, draw one line through it and explain why (e.g., wrong chart). Never use correction fluid or a sticker over an error. You want others to clearly see what you have changed so that you maintain your credibility and your client goals.
- Know and adhere to your agency's policies and guidelines. Policies and guidelines help convey what the expectations are in your facility. They are frequently evaluated in lawsuits to determine whether what the nurse did or did not do complies with reasonable standards of care. Consequently the policies and guidelines need to delineate what the reasonable expectations are. But they should not be so stringent that they cannot reasonably be accomplished.
- Document in clear and chronological order. If you need to go back, chart a "late note." If a lengthy delay in charting occurs, explain why. Keeping orderly records is important. Remember always to date and time all notations. Nurses often leave blank spaces in the chart so that others can come back and make additions. However, blank spaces leave room for a sanitized record. Avoid gaps in charting. No one expects you to prolong a code to make a timely nursing entry. If you code a patient at 0900 and your adrenaline finally becomes manageable at 1100, make a late entry note. This will make sense to attorneys, judges, and other health team members.

- Record accurate and complete information. If an abnormality occurs, chart your appropriate actions. Complete information is data that another member of the health care team would need to care for that particular patient reasonably. If you fill your charting with irrelevant details, other providers will have a hard time locating the important facts. Part of your nursing role is to separate the critical information from the filler.
- If you identify a patient's abnormality, chart your appropriate nursing actions. Remember to record the physician's response to your concerns. An unsatisfactory response (or no response) from a physician warrants a call to your nursing superior.
- State objective, factual information. Avoid conclusive statements such as "well," "good," "fine," and "normal."
- Sign your legal name and title. Always make your charting legible. A plaintiff's attorney can use illegible charting to his or her advantage.
- Keep records in a safe and confidential manner. Institutions and professionals are charged with the responsibility of maintaining a patient's privacy.
- Unusual circumstances warrant an incident report, but do not refer to the incident report in your notes. Incident reports are designed to improve the quality of care rendered in an institution. They are not designed to communicate the needs of a particular patient. Generally, incident reports are not discoverable during a lawsuit. Courts want to promote quality care in institutions. However, if you refer to the incident report in your patient's chart, a little-known legal doctrine, incorporation by reference, may be applied. Under this doctrine, the incident report becomes part of the patient's record and not just the institution's quality assurance program and is consequently discoverable.

Modified from McMullen, P., & Philipsen, N. (1993a). Charting basics 101. *Nursing Connections, 6*(3), 62-64.

to establish that the care delivered was reasonable (Box 11-2).

3. *Causation.* This element addresses two issues: whether the nurse's action or inaction caused the patient's injury and whether the patient's injury was foreseeable (Aiken & Catalano, 1994; Glannon, 2010; Guido, 2013; Schwartz et al., 2010). To determine whether the nurse's action or inaction caused the injury to the patient, lawyers frequently use the "but for" test (Schwartz et al., 2010), which asks, "But for the acts or inaction of the nurse, would the injury to the patient still have occurred?" The second part of the causation element looks at whether the nurse could have reasonably anticipated that his or her conduct might lead to patient harm (Aiken & Catalano, 1994; Guido, 2013).

4. *Damages.* For a patient to recover damages from a nurse in a malpractice suit, he or she must have suffered some type of damage (i.e., injury, harm). For example, if the nurse gave the patient the wrong medication but the patient did not experience any adverse effects, the damage element would be missing and the malpractice suit would be unsuccessful.

Assault and Battery

The common law has long recognized the right to be free from offensive touching or even the threat of offensive touching. An assault is a deliberate act in which one person threatens to harm another person without his or her consent and has the ability to carry out the threat (Schwartz et al., 2010). A battery is a nonconsensual touching, even if the touching may be of benefit

---

BOX 11-2   Giving Oral Testimony

- Bring your own attorney with you to review any records, for depositions or trials, to answer interrogatories, or for other legal requests if you are a party to a lawsuit.
- Never go to a deposition or a trial after working an off-shift, when you may be mentally exhausted.
- Thoroughly prepare for your testimony.
- Bring a recent, thoroughly updated copy of your resume or curriculum vitae with you to the deposition or trial.
- During your testimony, always tell the truth.
- Dress professionally for your trial or deposition.
- If you are asked a question that is lengthy or convoluted, ask that it be restated and then rephrase it in your own words.
- Do not testify regarding the medical standard of care.
- If you become fatigued during your testimony, ask for a brief break.
- Try to remain calm throughout the testimony.
- If asked whether a source is "authoritative" or a "classic," almost always answer "no."
- Maintain eye contact during testimony.
- Do not waive your signature.

Modified from McMullen, P., & Pepper, J. (1992). Surviving the legal hot seat. *Nursing Connections, 5*(2), 33-36.

---

to the patient (Schwartz et al., 2010). For example, a lawsuit for assault could result when a nurse threatens to medicate a competent person against his or her will. Battery would occur when the nurse actually administers the medication to the unwilling patient.

In some circumstances, such as restraint situations, the law allows providers to touch patients without their consent. However, special circumstances and procedural safeguards must be adhered to so as to excuse the battery. Initially, courts look at whether the battery was needed to protect the patient, health care team members, or the property of others (e.g., a patient threatens to set a fire in an emergency department). Next, courts examine whether restraining the patient was the least intrusive method to control the patient. For example, could the patient have been placed in a quiet room rather than being placed in a restraint? Finally, courts typically inquire whether the health care team regularly reassessed the need to continue using the restraint. If the health care team can demonstrate that it has complied with these requirements and with institutional procedure, nonconsensual touching will be excused. Consequently, nurses need to be sure they provide detailed documentation to indicate that (1) the patient

was a threat to self, others, or the property of others; (2) the restraint was the least intrusive means to control the patient; (3) regular reassessment of the need to continue the restraint occurred; and (4) the restraint was discontinued as soon as possible. Many hospitals and clinical facilities have specific procedures and protocols dealing with the application of restraints. Every nurse needs to be familiar with applicable agency policies.

Informed Consent

Informed consent lawsuits focus on whether the patient was given enough information before a treatment to make an informed, intelligent decision, including the decision to refuse treatment. The legal mandate for informed consent in the United States is unambiguous and overwhelming. It is based on the 14th Amendment constitutional right to privacy and self-determination and the liberty interest, on the 1st Amendment constitutional Free Exercise Clause, and on state and federal legislation, as well as on common law. Informed consent requires that the patient receive adequate information concerning the nature of the proposed treatment and its purposes, the material risks and benefits of the proposed treatment and of doing nothing (based on best evidence and including discomfort), and the choice to refuse or accept. In other words, did the patient get enough information so that he or she was the ultimate decision maker regarding whether to pursue or abandon the proposed treatment?

Courts have made strong statements supporting informed consent. The right to informed consent was articulated in a landmark 1914 New York Court of Appeals case in which the court stated that, "Every human being of adult years and sound mind has a right to determine what shall be done with his own body" (*Schloendorff v. Society of New York Hospital*). In 1997 a Massachusetts court stated, "Basic to the informed consent doctrine is that a physician has a legal, ethical and moral duty to respect patient autonomy" (*Feeley v. Baer*, 1997). Consent may be express or implied. Express consent is given in spoken or written direct words. Implied consent is consent inferred from the patient's conduct. Even if the patient does not sign a consent form expressly consenting to a proposed treatment or procedure, courts sometimes find that the patient gave implied consent to the treatment or procedure by coming to the health care facility and submitting to the treatment or procedure. For example, coming to an emergency department implies the patient is seeking emergency treatment. An early case found that holding out an arm to receive a vaccination implies consent to the vaccination (*O'Brien v. Cunard S.S. Co.*, 1891). In most circumstances, express written consent is the standard.

The patient may accept or refuse any treatment, even lifesaving procedures. Nearly all states today treat the failure to provide the necessary information so a patient can make an informed decision regarding the risks and benefits of care as negligence under the informed consent doctrine. In other states the plaintiff files a battery action alleging that the failure to give adequate treatment information constituted nonconsensual touching. The right to informed consent and informed refusal was affirmed at the federal level by the Patient Self-Determination Act of 1991.

Recognized exceptions exist to the doctrine of informed consent. If a patient was admitted to an emergency department with a severe, hemorrhaging abdominal injury that required the immediate removal of his spleen, this would be within the *emergency exception* to the mandate to provide the usual explanation of the splenectomy procedure and obtain informed decisions about care from the patient. Some courts have allowed a provider to avoid full disclosure to a patient if disclosure of information might lead to further harm to the patient. This exception is known as *therapeutic privilege*. For example, if the provider thought a psychiatric patient's knowledge of terminal cancer would lead the patient to commit suicide, the provider might exert therapeutic privilege and not reveal the cancer to the patient.

Regardless of the situation, the caregiver does not have authority to stand in the place of the patient to provide informed consent for the treatment he or she is providing (Philipsen, 2000). Consent must be obtained from the patient or the patient's legal representative. In any exception, the practitioner must seek the best possible substitute for informed consent by the patient. In emergencies, implied consent permits the caregiver to save a life but does not waive the patient's right to informed consent as expeditiously as practical. Patients who are unconscious, incompetent, or minors are unable to provide their own informed consent. The caregiver must locate the person with (1) the patient's power of attorney for health care, (2) the next of kin designated by state law, or (3) the court-appointed guardian who

has the power to make decisions for the patient, in that order. Parents are generally responsible for making the health care decisions for their minor children, unless the parents are not acting in the child's best interest. The caregiver must inform the patient, the patient's guardian, or the patient's *surrogate for health care decisions* of the patient's care options and must obtain consent for treatment. A true exception is court-ordered care; for example, drug treatment or psychiatric care ordered during sentencing by a criminal court. When in doubt, the nurse should consult with the facility's attorney.

Typically responsibility for the consent procedure rests in the hands of the practitioner who will be performing the treatment, frequently a physician, and the nurse serves as a witness. When the nurse signs the witness portion of the consent form, he or she is attesting that the signature on the consent form is the patient's. If the nurse witnesses the physician giving the pertinent information regarding the treatment or procedure, the nurse may want to write "consent procedure witnessed" below his or her signature. If a lawsuit later develops concerning whether the provider gave the patient information concerning the procedure or treatment, the "consent procedure witnessed" statement can furnish powerful evidence that the patient did receive adequate information. Today's advanced practice nurses often perform procedures and treatments that require consent, such as suturing, obstetrical care, and administration of medications. In these circumstances, the APRN is the practitioner who must ensure the patient has enough information to make an informed decision regarding a proposed treatment.

False Imprisonment

False imprisonment occurs when a person is unlawfully confined within a fixed area. The confined person must be aware of the confinement or harmed as a result of the confinement. To prevail in a false imprisonment action, the patient must prove that he or she was physically restrained or restrained by threat or intimidation and that he or she did not consent to the restraint (Schwartz et al., 2010). False imprisonment suits may involve situations in which a patient was kept in a mental health facility against his or her will and without a judicial order, or a restraint device was applied to a patient against his or her will.

The laws on false imprisonment vary from state to state. Most states allow some degree of patient confinement if the patient poses a serious threat of harm to self, others, or the property of others. In deciding whether a valid confinement occurred judges and juries often look at the reasonableness of the decision to confine the patient, how long the patient was confined, whether the need for the confinement was regularly reassessed, and whether the least restrictive methods for detention of the patient were used.

Breach of Confidentiality

Confidentiality is the duty of health care providers to protect the secrecy of a patient's information, no matter how it is obtained (McMullen & Philipsen, 1993b). Until recently patients had few legal remedies when the privacy of their medical records was breached. Today, state and federal laws provide patients with legal remedies to compensate them for confidentiality breaches.

One such law is the Health Insurance Portability and Accountability Act (HIPAA), which was enacted by Congress in 1996 (PL 104-191; 42 U.S.C. §§1320d et seq.), along with the regulations issued under HIPAA governing the privacy of personal health information (the Privacy Rule, at 45 C.F.R. §§160 and 164) and the security of such information (the Security Rule at 45 C.F.R. §164.302 et seq.), which set a minimum standard governing uses and disclosure of this information. This legislation also protects individuals from losing their health insurance when leaving or changing jobs (portability), and it increases the government's authority over health care fraud and abuse (accountability). The HIPAA established that although the health care practitioner who created a health record owns that record, the information that it contains belongs to the patient. The HIPAA Privacy Rule prohibits the release of identifiable personal health information in any form without the patient's permission. Penalties for failure to comply with the Privacy Rule involve a substantial fine and/or prison term for those who use individual health information for commercial or personal gain or to inflict harm. The Security Rule provides two standards to ensure the authenticity of electronic patient records: The Integrity Standard and the Person or Entity Authentication Standard (45 C.F.R. §§164.31). As the electronic medical record becomes commonplace and new patient privacy issues surface, nurses should expect that additional regulations will be promulgated under HIPAA.

Several cases demonstrate why valid concerns exist about medical record confidentiality. In *Doe v. Roe* (1993), a flight attendant asked her treating physician not to reveal her HIV status to her insurer or her employer. The physician verbally promised not to reveal her HIV status. Several months later, the flight attendant found that her entire chart, complete with HIV information, had been forwarded to her employer. The attendant recovered damages against the physician for breach of confidentiality and for breaching his expressed oral promise not to disclose her HIV status. Breach of confidentiality lawsuits have also resulted when psychiatric, drug, and alcohol treatment information was released. In a more recent case, a patient, John Doe, presented to a clinic to be treated for a sexually transmitted disease. One of the nurses at the clinic was related to Mr. Doe's girlfriend. The nurse sent the girlfriend several text messages notifying her that Mr. Doe was being treated for a sexually transmitted infection. The nurse was fired from her position for revealing confidential patient information (*Doe v. Guthrie Clinic, Ltd.,* et al., 2012).

A strict level of confidentiality typically exists for patients receiving drug or alcohol abuse treatment. Providers are usually prohibited from even disclosing information on whether a certain person is a patient. In addition, the state where a nurse is practicing may have laws that identify who has authority to control access to medical records of patients who are incapacitated, incompetent, minors, or deceased. Information concerning special situations is available through the office of the state's attorney general and through the employer's legal counsel. Issues related to privacy and confidentiality are also addressed in Chapter 12 on ethics.

Disaster Nursing

Nurses who respond to disaster are typically volunteer nurses, working either through a recognized nonprofit organization such as the American Red Cross or through a government agency. As long as the volunteer nurse acts in good faith and within their scope of practice, he or she is protected from tort actions. Special provisions in most NPAs permit practice across state borders for emergencies. The Good Samaritan Acts, which were designed to encourage individuals to volunteer to help in emergencies, also protect volunteer nurses. In addition, special tort laws protect nurses who may be working as disaster volunteers under the coordination of a state or federal government agency, in the same way employees of that agency are protected (Howie, Howie, & McMullen, 2012).

CRIMINALIZATION OF UNINTENTIONAL ERROR

In rare cases officials of the local criminal courts have charged health care providers criminally for patient deaths that resulted from unintentional error. This is an extreme example of a common response to error: to punish the individual who made the error. Errors are seldom due to one individual failure, and that reaction is unlikely to make the system safer. In addition, one element of a crime is that it must include the *intent to do wrong*. Carelessness is not a crime, unless the individual was so reckless as to show intentional disregard for others, as in the case of drunk driving or waving a loaded handgun. All nurses make mistakes, but mistakes do not create criminal intent, regardless of patient outcome. Criminalization of health care providers in the past decade has been initiated by complaints related to medication errors, patient abandonment, and disaster care.

When bad outcomes in health care are criminalized, they are likely to receive public attention. In 1998 workers at the Faith Clinic in Libya were sentenced to death when the government blamed them for spreading AIDS to the children they were treating for AIDS. They were freed after negotiations with the European Union in 2007 (Garrett, 2006; U.S. Department of State, 2008). In 1996 three nurses at Centura St. Anthony Hospital North outside Denver, Colorado, were charged with administering the wrong dose of a medication to an infant, who died. Two of the nurses pled guilty in a plea bargain, but the nurse who refused to plead guilty was acquitted by a jury (Plum, 1997). In December 2008 in San Luis Obispo, California, Dr. Hootan C. Roozrokh was acquitted after being charged criminally with speeding the death of an organ donor (Superior Court of California County of San Luis Obispo, 2008). Perhaps the case with the greatest amount of publicity in recent times involved the Hurricane Katrina tragedy. With no food, water, oxygen, or basic medical supplies, in sweltering heat, and with outside help late in arriving, nurses and doctors at Memorial Medical Center in New Orleans, themselves victims of the disaster, were unable to save all of their patients. The Louisiana attorney general charged one physician and two nurses with euthanasia (*Louisiana v. Anna M. Pou, Lori L. Budo, and Cheri A. Landry*, 2006; Night, 2007). Eventually charges were dropped against the nurses in return for their testimony, and in July 2007 a grand jury refused to indict the physician. In another high-profile case, nurses recruited to the United States from the Philippines were charged in New York's Suffolk County Court with abandoning their patients when they resigned from their job because of abuse by their recruiter. Details are available online from the Philippine Nurses Association of New York (www.pnanewyork.org/articles/sentosa.html).

These cases discourage the recruitment of nurses and other caregivers, discourage the reporting of errors, discourage participation in lifesaving organ donation, and discourage caregivers from volunteering in disaster. In response, authoritative bodies have begun to emphasize the need to stop blaming the individual for bad outcomes in health care systems. The Joint Commission (TJC) sets standards for health care organizations and issues accreditation to institutions that meet those standards. In 2006 TJC stated solutions must make health care systems safer and prevent mistakes from reaching patients instead of focusing on individuals. The Institute of Medicine, in their 2004 report, *To Err Is Human: Building a Safer Health System*, stated:

> The focus must shift from blaming individuals for past errors to a focus on preventing future errors by designing safety into the system ... when an error occurs, blaming an individual does little to make the system safer and prevent someone else from committing the same error. Health care is a decade or more behind other high-risk industries in its attention to ensuring basic safety. (p. 5)

The Committee for Disaster Medicine Reform (www.cdmr.org) is an organization formed in response to the criminal charges following Hurricane Katrina. It promotes legislation and takes other measures to protect health care professionals from "unwarranted criminal allegations and wrongly placed lawsuits" (www.cdmr.org/intro.html). Nurses and other health care professionals must work together to enforce a policy against the criminalization of error. Belonging to an authoritative professional organization, such as the ANA, is one act every nurse can take to effectively advocate for nursing and for patients.

SUMMARY

A basic understanding of the impact of legal principles on nursing practice is essential to safe and effective performance as a nurse. An understanding of the role of the state board of nursing in the control and regulation of nursing practice is also important. A thorough knowledge of employment rights and responsibilities when nurses enter into employment contracts can make nurses better negotiators. Knowledge of tort law is crucial to understand the duties and liabilities in our system and to serve as both a professional and patient care advocate.

SALIENT POINTS

- The power of the state to license nurses is derived from the U.S. Constitution.
- Licensing of health professionals is intended to protect the health, safety, and welfare of the public.
- Nurse practice acts (NPAs) define the practice of nursing, identify the scope of nursing practice, set the requirements for licensure, and provide guidelines for licensure disciplinary action.
- A nurse who is charged with a violation of a state's NPA has a right to due process in the investigation and hearing of the charge.
- The Americans with Disabilities Act grants special confidentiality to nurses who are in treatment for protected disabilities.
- Nurses work under a contract, which is an express or implied agreement with an employer that creates a legal relationship.
- A collective bargaining agreement establishes a contractual relationship between the union and the employer.
- Torts are private civil wrongs against individuals, in contrast to crimes, which are wrongs against the state.
- Negligence occurs when a person fails to act in a reasonable manner.

- Malpractice occurs when the conduct of a nurse or other professional practices below the established standard.
- Assault is a threat to touch or harm another person.
- Battery is nonconsensual touching, even if the touching is beneficial to the patient.
- The principle of informed consent requires that the patient be given enough information before treatment to make an informed, intelligent decision about whether to pursue or abandon treatment.
- False imprisonment occurs when a person is unlawfully confined within a fixed area.
- Information about a patient belongs to the patient; the health care provider is duty bound to keep information about a patient confidential and generally cannot share it unless the patient gives permission.
- Disaster nurses who act in good faith and within their scope of practice are protected from tort claims.
- The criminalization of nursing errors is rare and a violation of public policy.
- One way that nurses can advocate for changes in health care policy or law is to join an authoritative professional organization such as the American Nurses Association.

CRITICAL REFLECTION EXERCISES

1. Review your state NPA and delineate the definition and scope of nursing practice. Evaluate its relevance for today's health care environment.
2. Discuss the administrative and disciplinary functions of state boards of nursing.
3. How does the right of due process protect the nurse? How does it protect the public?
4. What must a plaintiff prove to recover damages in the following situation?

An IV was left in place for 5 days, although the hospital policy specified 2 days. As a result, the patient sustained a thrombosis and inflammation at the site.

5. Discuss the concepts of employment law as they relate to your employment situation.
6. Apply knowledge of tort law to formulate risk reduction strategies that could protect the nurse against legal action.

WEBSITE RESOURCES

American Nurses Association: http://nursingworld.org/. The professional organization for registered nurses is a resource for standards for practice and safety, policy, and advocacy.

National Council of State Boards of Nursing: https://www.ncsbn.org/index.htm. The nonprofit organization where state boards come together, share goals and concerns, and develop policy statements and model laws, as well as the national nursing licensure examination (NCLEX).

National Institutes of Health, Institute of Medicine. *To err is human: Building a safer health system*: www.nap.edu/books/0309068371/html. This report by the Institute of Medicine estimates that as many as 98,000 people in the United States die each year as a result of medical errors. The report examined primarily hospital-based errors. Common errors and suggested solutions are addressed.

National Labor Relations Board: www.nlrb.gov. Facts about the NLRB, labor law, weekly summaries, press releases, rules and regulations, and decisions are all available on this free government website. Information is available in Spanish and English.

Nurses Service Organization: http://www.nso.com. This free website provides the Risk Advisor Newsletter, a nursing malpractice case of the month, and valuable information on malpractice/liability questions. Malpractice insurance information is also available.

U.S. Department of Health and Human Services: http://www.hhs.gov/regulations/. The HHS website includes links to statutes related to nursing and health care such as HIPAA and HITECH, as well as regulations and links to rules and comments for all HHS Divisions, including the Agency for Healthcare Research and Quality (AHRQ), the Centers for Disease Control and Prevention (CDC). The Centers for Medicare and Medicaid Services (CMS), and the Health Resources and Services Administration (HRSA).

U.S. Department of Justice. Americans with Disabilities Act: http://www.usdoj.gov/crt/ada/adahoml.htm. The ADA website gives valuable information on the history of the ADA, provisions of the Act, enforcement considerations, settlement information, technical assistance, new or proposed regulations, and ADA mediation information.

VersusLaw: www.versuslaw.com. VersusLaw is a legal search engine. Cases from all states and the federal government are available. There is a modest fee to use the site.

REFERENCES

AFL-CIO Department of Professional Employees. (2014). Nursing: A profile of the profession. Fact sheet. Available online at http://dpeaflcio.org/programs-publications/issue-fact-sheets/nursing-a-profile-of-the-profession/

Aiken, T. D., & Catalano, J. T. (1994). *Legal, ethical and political issues in nursing*. Philadelphia: Davis.

Bix, B. H. (2012). *Contract law: Rules, theory & context*. New York: Cambridge University Press.

California Society of Anesthesiologists et al. v. Brown et al., 204 Cal App 4th 390; 138 CalRptr. 3rd 745, 2012 Cal. App. Lexis 308 (2012).

Clemons et al. v. The Wellpoint Co., Inc. 2013 U.S. Dist. Lexis 35899, 35 I.E.R. Cas (BNA), 536, U.S. Dist. N.Y. 2013.

Committee for Disaster Medicine Reform. Retrieved March 8, 2010, from http://www.cdmr.org/intro.html

Dent v. West Virginia, 129 U.S. 114, 9 S. Ct. 231, 32 L. Ed. 623 (1889).

Doe V. Guthrie Clinic Ltd. et al., 710 F.ed 492 (NY 2012).

Doe v. Roe, No. 0369 N.Y. App. Div., 4th Jud. Dept. (May 28, 1993).

Feeley v. Baer, 424 Mass. 875, 876, 679 NE2d 180, 181 (1997).

Garrett, L. A. (2006). *Six imprisoned health care workers in Libya are pawns in a far larger strategic game, with enormous repercussions*. Council on Foreign Relations. Retrieved December 6, 2013, from http://www.cfr.org/publication/11821/six_imprisoned_health_care_workers_in_libya_are_pawns_in_a_far_larger_strategic_game_with_enormous_repercussions.html?breadcrumb=%2Fregion%2F146%2Flibya

Glannon, J. W. (2010). *The law of torts* (4th ed.). New York: Wolters Kluwer.

Goldberg, J. C. P., Sebok, A. J., & Zipursky, B. C. (2012). *Tort law: Responsibilities and redress* (3rd ed.). New York: Wolters Kluwer.

Guido, G. W. (2013). *Legal and ethical issues in nursing* (6th ed.). Upper Saddle River, NJ: Prentice Hall.

Howie, W. O., Howie, B. A., & McMullen, P. C. (2012). To assist or not assist: Good Samaritan considerations for nurse practitioners. *Journal for Nurse Practitioners*, 81(9), 688–692.

Institute of Medicine. (2004). *To err is human: Building a safer health system*. Washington, DC: Institute of Medicine.

McMullen, P., & Pepper, J. (1992). Surviving the legal hot seat. *Nursing Connections*, 5(2), 33–36.

McMullen, P., & Philipsen, N. (1993a). Charting basics 101. *Nursing Connections*, 6(3), 62–64.

McMullen, P., & Philipsen, N. (1993b). Medical records: Promoting patient confidentiality. *Nursing Connections*, 6(4), 48–50.

McMullen, P., & Philipsen, N. D. C. (1994). The end of collective bargaining for nurses? NLRB v. Health Care and Retirement Corp. *Nursing Policy Forum*, 1(1), 34–39.

Mills v. Moriarty, 302 A.D 2d 436, 754 N.Y.S.2d 901; N.Y. App. Div. LEXIS 1312, (2003).

National Council of State Boards of Nursing and American Nurses Association. *Joint Statement on Delegation.* (2006). Retrieved December 6, 2013, from https://www.ncsbn.org/Delegation_joint_statement_NCSBN-ANA.pdf

National Council of State Boards of Nursing and American Nurses Association. (2008). *Consensus model for APRN regulation: Licensure, certification, education & regulation.* Retrieved December 6, 2013, from https://www.ncsbn.org/7_23_08_Consensue_APRN_Final.pdf

National Council of State Boards of Nursing. (2015). *Nurse licensure compact.* Retrieved from https://www.ncsbn.org/nlc.htm

Night, S. S. (2007). *Hurricane force winds destroy more than physical structures.* Retrieved December 6, 2013, from http://punctiliopartners.com/Development/Articles/(SN)%20Pou%20New%20Orleans.pdf

NLRB v. Health Care and Retirement Corporation of America, 511 U.S. 571, 114 S. Ct. 1778, 128 L.Ed. 586, 62 U.S.L.W. 4371, 146 L.R.R.M. (B.N.A.) 31, 18 Lab.Cas. 11,090 (May 3, 1994).

NLRB v. Kentucky River Community, 121 S.Ct. 1861 (2001).

O'Brien v. Cunard S.S. Co., 28 N.E. 266 (Mass. 1891).

People of the State of Illinois v. Jihan, 537 N.E.2d 751m 127 Ill.2d 379, 130 Ill. Dec. 422 (1989).

Philipsen, N. (2000). In the patient's best interest: Informed consent or protection from the truth? *The Journal of Perinatal Education*, 9(3), 243.

Philipsen, N. (2008). Resolving conflict: A primer for nurse practitioners on alternatives to litigation. *The Journal for Nurse Practitioners*, 4(10), 766–772.

Philipsen, N., & Haynes, D. (2007). The multistate licensure compact: Making nurses mobile. *The Journal for Nurse Practitioners*, 3(1), 36–40. Retrieved December 6, 2013, from http://www.medscape.com/viewarticle/551037

Philipsen, N., Lamm, N., & Reier, S. (2007). Continuing competency for nursing licensure. *The Journal for Nurse Practitioners*, 3(1), 41–45.

Plum, S. D. (1997). Nurses indicted: Three nurses may face prison in a case that bodes ill for the profession. *Nursing 97*, 27(7), 32–35. Retrieved December 6, 2013, from http://journals.lww.com/nursing/Citation/1997/07000/Nurses_indicted__Three_Denver_nurses_may_face.18.aspx

Providence Alaska Medical Center v. Alaska Nurses' Association and the American Nurses Association, 121 F.3d 548(1997), 320 NLRB No. 49 (January 3, 1996).

Schloendorff v. Society of New York Hospital, 211 N.Y. 125, 105 N.E. 92 (1914).

Schwartz, V. E., Kelly, K., & Partlett, D. F. (2010). *Prosser, Wade, and Schwartz's torts: Cases and materials* (12th ed.). St. Paul, MN: Foundation Press.

Scott, R. W. (1998). *Health care malpractice: A primer on legal issues for professions.* New York: McGraw-Hill.

Sermchief v. Gonzalez, 660 S.W.2d 683 Mo. (1983).

Sharpe, C. C. (1999). *Nursing malpractice.* Westport, CT: Auburn House/Greenwood.

State of Louisiana v. Anna M. Pou, Lori L. Budo, and Cheri A. Landry. (2006). Retrieved March 1, 2009, from http://news.findlaw.com/nytimes/docs/katrina/lapoui706wrnt.html

Superior Court of California County of San Luis Obispo. (2008). *The People of the State of California v. Hootan Roozrokh*, Defendant. Case No. F405885. Retrieved December 6, 2013, from http://www.cacj.org/documents/2009_Syllabus/Fall_Docs/Defendants-MPA-in-Support-of-Motion-to-Compel-Discovery-12-11-07.pdf

Turner v. State Board of Nursing, 2012. U.S. Dist. LEXIS 58255 (April 24, 2012 Decided).

U.S. Department of Justice. (1990). Americans with Disabilities Act of 1990. (ADA). Retrieved December 6, 2013, from http://www.ada.gov/pubs/ada.htm.

U.S. Department of State. (2008). *Country reports on human rights practices.* Retrieved December 6, 2013, from http://www.state.gov/g/drl/rls/hrrpt/2007/100601.htm

Ethical Dimensions of Nursing and Health Care

Elizabeth G. Epstein, PhD, RN and Frances Rieth Ward, PhD, RN, MBE

(e) http://evolve.elsevier.com/Friberg/bridge/

OBJECTIVES

At the completion of this chapter, the reader will be able to:

- Identify resources and strategies to address practice problems.
- Define key terms in ethics language.
- Describe the nursing role in ethically challenging situations, including the use of an ethical framework.

- Define moral distress and moral residue and how they commonly arise in nursing.
- Identify the nursing contribution to ethics on four professional levels: patient, unit, organization, and national/global.

PROFILE IN PRACTICE

Frances Rieth Ward, PhD, RN, MBE

After nursing school, I began working in pediatric nursing (primarily neonatal intensive care). Although ethical issues abound in any practice site, I began having more and more questions regarding ethical issues that I witnessed daily, and wanted some guidance. I went back to school for master degrees in nursing and bioethics, and pursued a PhD in nursing, with my dissertation focused on decision making about clinical research in neonates. Although the questioning continues, I gained valuable insight into examining ethical issues on more than a surface level, in discovering appropriate resources, and in becoming more comfortable with issues dealing with ethics and in helping others to do similarly. I am presently involved with an academic health science center, teaching clinical and research ethics to nursing and medical students, generating policy with a local hospital ethics committee, and ensuring research safeguards as a member of the Institutional Review Board (IRB).

Elizabeth G. Epstein, PhD, RN

I had little knowledge of clinical ethics as a new nurse, and even less knowledge about my role as a nurse in ethically challenging situations. As a neonatal intensive care nurse, I encountered many situations that left me with a feeling of unease, but the idea of using my clinical expertise or my insights to contribute to solutions never occurred to me. I only knew I hurt about these situations, many of which I can remember vividly to this day.

I remember clearly the moment I realized that ethics would be my career. I was a doctoral student at the University of Virginia and my interest at the time was the neonatal intensive care unit (NICU) nurse's role in neonatal development. Ethics was the farthest thing from my mind. In one class, a guest lecturer, Dr. Ann Hamric, spoke about her career as a nurse and how her encounters with morally troubling cases led her to pursue a career in ethics. That was the moment I changed my research focus and the trajectory of my career. Dr. Hamric became (and still is) my mentor. She and I have spent hours together talking about the importance of nursing in ethical conundrums and about how to address the moral distress that scars health care providers of all professions.

I now know that nurses must bring their expertise and knowledge to ethically challenging situations. I also know that nurses can influence the environment in which they practice and, in doing so, create a practice environment that promotes collaboration and high-quality patient care. I consider myself extraordinarily lucky to have an opportunity to study these aspects of nursing and health care through my research, to teach them to bright and engaged students, and to practice them as a member of the Ethics Consult Service and the Moral Distress Consult Service at the University of Virginia.

INTRODUCTION

We are sometimes asked why nurses must learn about ethics. In the questioner's words, "Aren't nurses 'by definition' ethical? What should we expect to learn?" Gallup surveys repeatedly find that the American public believes nurses to be the most honest and ethical of all professions (Gallup, 2013). Are those who are truly ethical attracted to the nursing profession and thus imbue the discipline with innate morality? Why should nurses and nursing students waste their time appraising ethics theories or reasoning if we are "already there"?

A nurse may mean well, be a caring individual, and a highly skilled clinician, but this does not prepare the nurse for the complex and ethically challenging clinical situations that occur every day in health care. Moreover, the ethical issues nurses face are not only at the patient level, but are often at the organizational level as well and involve interactions among families, nursing colleagues, medical colleagues, and administrators. Health care professionals must learn about ethics—not to help them be ethical people but to help them understand and contribute to ethically challenging clinical situations that arise, and to recognize the ethical aspects of their profession with every patient encounter. Good intentions are not sufficient to frame and analyze complex situations. The literature notes that nurses are often reluctant to participate in discussions regarding ethical decisions because of their own presumed knowledge deficits (Grady et al., 2008; Laabs, 2012; Ulrich et al., 2007). However, the nursing role is critical in identifying ethically justifiable solutions to clinical problems and to ethical issues at the organizational level. This is why it is important for nurses to learn about ethics.

Given that the writings about health care ethics are vast both in number and scope, what is important—indeed, essential—for the nurse practicing at the bedside to know and understand? We believe that nurses must have a foundational understanding of the language of ethics, of applied frameworks for ethical reasoning, and of resources to facilitate learning. This chapter is intended to build the student's knowledge base with regard to ethics in general and nursing ethics more specifically. We discuss the nurse's role in ethically challenging clinical and organizational situations and provide resources for further learning.

TO BEGIN: WHAT IS ETHICS?

Ethics is a form of philosophy derived from the Greek word *ethos*, which is roughly interpreted as character. In a broad sense ethics is an attempt to establish a foundation for determining good and bad conduct. When referring to an individual's behavior, it has become common practice to use the term *morals* instead of *ethics*. *Normative* ethics describes the accepted ways of conducting ourselves and asks the question, "What should I do?" For example, suppose a nurse made a medication error that resulted in no harm to a patient. Should he or she tell the patient about the mistake? If the nurse were to draw on normative ethics in this situation, he would arrive at the answer to tell the truth. Telling the truth is accepted ethical practice. Normative ethics attempts to provide standards for determining what is morally right or wrong. Conversely, *descriptive* ethics describes the actual practices that occur. The questions, "How are problems solved?" and "How do people behave?" are addressed with this type of ethics (Vaughn, 2013). In a recent study of nurse and physician experiences with infant death in the NICU (Epstein, 2008), an expected (normative ethic) finding was that decisions to withdraw aggressive treatment from terminally ill infants would be based largely, if not solely, on the best interests of the infant. In reality, however, end-of-life decision making is much more nuanced and involves the relationship between the parent and the staff, the comfort of the staff with end-of-life discussion, and the best interests of the family as well as the infant. This is descriptive ethics—the ethical reasoning that occurs in actual fact.

Therefore although normative ethics might describe how we *ought* to behave, descriptive ethics describes how we *do* behave. How does a health care team determine what *should* be done? This is the practice of *applied* ethics—the use of ethical frameworks to identify ethically justifiable solutions to thorny clinical issues. A judicious appreciation of applied ethics depends on conceptual precision (Paul & Elder, 2013). Is it ethics or is it religion? Is it ethics or is it law? Nuanced deliberation may well come to a direct halt if a participant claims that a proposed action is unethical. For example, consider the case of Bradley and Mary. Bradley and Mary are adult siblings whose mother is critically ill and has little hope of recovery. They are in a heated discussion about whether or not to withdraw aggressive treatment (mechanical ventilation) and Bradley states, "Mary, withdrawal is a sin! How can you suggest such a thing? This goes against my religious beliefs and it's unethical." Consider religious pronouncements regarding sin related to feeding tube withdrawal in the case of Terry Schiavo (e.g., Roig-Franzia, 2005). Given that the decisions in this case became framed around discussions of "quality of life" vs. "sanctity of life," it is unsurprising that public commentary developed religious overtones. Sin is a religious construct. Other religious traditions may delineate the construct differently, but each of the religious traditions expects their own view to be regarded as a universal ethical construct. This perspective fails to appreciate that sin and many other concepts (e.g., miracle, salvation) are theological concepts with varied interpretations and do not constitute an ethical perspective (Paul & Elder, 2013). The practice of applied ethics would not take the pronouncement of religious beliefs as a trump card that inhibits further discussion. Instead, applied ethics might allow for redirection of the discussion to ethically grounded concepts (e.g., mother's preferences, risks, harms, benefits, quality of life) and away from a topic as sensitive and unresolvable as religion.

Ethics and the law may be similarly confused. What would be the reason for ethical deliberation if any dilemma could be reduced to whether or not it was against the law? Confusion may exist because ethics and the law share many features. Both use a similar language. Both try to regulate individual actions and both present behavioral standards from which individuals and society may learn. Law and ethics do have distinct differences. The law defines the floor of acceptable behaviors, and punishments for infractions are often public. Goals of ethics, on the other hand, are aspirational—the ceiling of acceptable behavior; ethical sanctions are often private in nature. In historical observations of health care, law and ethics seldom reach a decision at the same time. Situations in which law has followed ethics' pronouncements include tort law evolution and practice guidelines. Conversely, the law weighed in on issues dealing with informed consent, standards of care, and health care provider duties (e.g., Gostin, 2002) before the literature on ethics related to these concepts was established. Ethics has an active presence in case law (court rulings that may be cited as precedent): The NJ Supreme Court established a patient's right to refuse treatment (McFadden, 1995) and influenced the requirement of access to mechanisms for resolution of ethics disputes at accredited health care institutions; the U.S. Supreme Court impelled the emphasis of advance directives and health care proxies (Lewin, 1990) and determined that there is no constitutional right to die, thus opening the door for state regulation of physician assisted suicide.

Given that applied ethics is the practice of using ethical frameworks to solve dilemmas and that it is a separate process from consideration of religious beliefs or legal aspects, the next question is "What is an ethical dilemma?" Beauchamp and Childress (2013) define ethical or moral dilemmas as those "circumstances in which oral obligations demand or appear to demand that a person adopt each of two (or more) alternative but incompatible actions, such that the person cannot perform all the required actions" (p. 11). In a particular situation, a person could take action A or action B but not both, and neither A nor B alone is entirely satisfactory. The first step in applied ethics is to identify the actions that are justifiable. This is where the law and religion may need to be considered. For example, suppose an 18-year-old patient comes to the clinic concerned that she may be pregnant. A pregnancy test confirms that she is indeed pregnant. An ethical analysis of the situation may conclude that an abortion is an ethically justifiable solution. However, if the patient herself is against abortion on religious grounds, the abortion option drops from the list of ethically justifiable solutions. Additionally, if abortion were illegal, it would not be an ethically justifiable solution either. Once ethically justifiable solutions are identified, the next step is attempting to discover which action (A or B) is the better of the two. To help guide reasoning in terms of identifying appropriate actions and determining which is best, engaging ethical theory can be useful.

ETHICAL THEORY

Normative ethics address classifications of ethical theories, including those that are "act-based" (e.g., utilitarianism and deontology) or "agent-based" (e.g., virtue ethics). These theories of morality provide a foundation for understanding what we ought to do in a certain circumstance and a rationale for why the actions identified are morally right or morally wrong. Although there are many ethical theories, three are commonly used in the health care field. Each has significant strengths and, unfortunately, each has significant drawbacks as well. None of the theories will produce all of the morally right (or wrong) actions in every situation. The first theory, virtue ethics, centers on the character of the person acting. Historically, Western nursing and medicine were highly virtue-centric. A "good" doctor or a "good" nurse would know the right action to take. "Good" (in nursing) involved many characteristics, such as obedient, attentive to detail, caring, sturdy, Christian, white. We now know that most of these "goods" are not moral goods and that a good doctor or nurse cannot possibly know the right thing to do based on his or her virtues alone. However, might it help the doctor or nurse to identify right and wrong actions if they are capable of empathy? Of kindness? Of trustworthiness? Many would argue that possessing certain virtues can be helpful in that they are alerted to moral problems in the workplace, that is, they can recognize moral issues because they can feel that something is not quite right. In addition, a highly compassionate nurse may be able to find morally right and wrong actions that an uncaring or hard-hearted nurse may never see. Virtue-based ethics can be helpful, but in terms of being a reliable ethical theory that will provide the guidance that today's clinicians need to resolve complex ethical challenges, it is insufficient.

Theresa Drought (2002) described that being a nurse is to experience the privilege of bearing witness and that witnessing suffering, death, hope, and recovery cannot help but to change how one sees the world and his or her place in it. Although we are born with certain attributes, there are also traits acquired throughout life, whether through experience, one's profession, or one's conscious choosing (Drane, 1994). As nurses, we have undoubtedly been changed by what we have experienced and we exhibit the behaviors of our profession as a result.

The second ethical theory centers on the duties of the person acting. What is one obligated to do? This theory is called deontology and arises largely from Immanuel Kant (1724–1804). This theory begins with the acknowledgment that every person has inherent dignity and worth and that acting ethically means acting in such a way that respects others' (and one's own) dignity and worth. Kant's categorical imperative (the foundational principle upon which all obligations arise) is to act such that you always treat others and yourself as an end and never only as a means

(Degrazia, Mappes, & Brand-Ballard, 2011). For example, Mike is interested in meeting a famous musician. He learns that the musician is going to a big party at a neighbor's house down the street from where you live. This neighbor is not Mike's friend and, although they have lived on the same street for 15 years, the disparate election stickers on their cars have not facilitated substantial conversation between them. Mike could introduce himself to the neighbor and be very friendly in the hopes that the neighbor would offer an invitation to the party. According to the deontological perspective, this would be wrong because Mike would be using his neighbor only as a means of getting what he really wants, which is to try to meet the famous musician.

The strengths of this theory are that it makes intuitive sense to make use of identified duties (do not lie, do not kill, keep your promises) that most who are morally minded value. It also emphasizes our need to reason through problems so as to identify the proper duty and apply it. Rather than relying on personal character (kindness, empathy), this theory calls on us to draw on common rules of conduct. The drawbacks are many, however. When more than one duty is apparent in a given situation, there is no method of prioritizing them to discern which duty to follow. For instance, suppose you had promised your professor that you would help her collect data this afternoon. However, when you called home to check on your infant son, the babysitter informed you that he had a fever and had vomited twice. Your duties here are in conflict—keeping a promise versus attending to one's sick child. How do you know which duty to follow so as to be morally right? Deontology cannot help you. In addition, deontology does not take into consideration the outcomes of acting on duties. Suppose the year is 1943 and you are a German citizen living in Nazi Germany. A family of Jews is hiding in your attic. One day the Nazis come to your door and ask if you are hiding anyone. As a deontologist, you might determine that your duty is to tell the truth. The outcome would be disastrous, however. So, again, deontology provides little guidance in terms of identifying duties we should adhere to so as to resolve moral problems. However, this theory cannot always identify the "right" action to take.

The third ethical theory, utilitarianism, places emphasis on the outcomes of a situation. Mill (1806–1873) and Bentham (1748–1832) suggested that right action is determined by identifying actions that yield the greatest good for the greatest number (Beauchamp & Childress, 2013). If that goal is met, the action is morally right. Many utilitarians accept rules as guidelines and do not discount them entirely. However, unlike a deontologist, a utilitarian could justify lying to the Nazis because the outcome, saving the lives of the Jews in the attic, is far better than allowing them to be discovered.

Utilitarian applications abound in health care. Examples include the Affordable Care Act and vaccination programs. Both seek to achieve the greatest good (health care insurance to most Americans or immunity from disease) for the greatest number of people. Another example would be planning for an epidemic or natural disaster. These plans include triaging such that those who have a chance at survival are given priority over those who are unlikely to survive and whose care would use valuable resources (staff, equipment, time) without the benefit of a good outcome.

Utilitarian thinking is helpful in that it allows attention to be paid to the greater good. On an individual level, utilitarian thinking can be helpful in considering the potential outcomes of several treatment plans—which outcomes are desired? Which are possible? Which of the treatment plans might help the patient achieve his or her desired outcome? Weaknesses of this theory include the potential to downplay the needs of the minority or even harming the minority to achieve the greatest good for the greatest number. An extreme oft-used example would be the following.

Nurse Peters is caring for four patients: (1) Mr. Frederickson, a homeless man with no support system and a belligerent personality who is admitted with serious injuries following a pedestrian accident; (2) Ms. Delaney, a married housewife and mother of two young children who is on the kidney transplant list; (3) Mr. Pfeffercorn, a 78-year-old healthy man who is in need of a corneal transplant; and (4) Mrs. Divers, a 58-year-old woman with liver failure who is on the liver transplant list. A utilitarian could (conceivably) determine that not treating Mr. Frederickson (allowing him to die) would be an appropriate action to take because, in doing so, three lives (Delaney, Pfeffercorn, and Divers) could be saved or improved by harvesting his organs. This action does not sit well, however. It might be justifiable using utilitarian thinking, but we know that something is not quite right about this action.

In summary, there are many ways to think about ethical problems. We could consider the problem in terms of the person who will act and whether that person possesses virtues that would assist in making the right decision. Alternatively, we could consider the actions themselves. Given a certain situation, what are our obligations and duties? What rules shall we live our lives by and how should we apply those rules? Finally, we could consider the outcomes of whatever action we take. Which action will yield the greatest good?

A BRIEF HISTORY OF NURSING ETHICS

Caring for sick, suffering, recovering, and dying patients and their families is inescapably a moral practice. Nurses have been considering the question of "What ought I do now for my patient" for generations. *How* they have considered this question, given the context of their practice, has changed dramatically over the years. However, important lessons are learned from every stage in nursing ethics' history.

In the early years of professional nursing, the nurse's personal behavior and values were the foundation of nursing ethics. A nurse of high moral character was one who would provide ethically grounded care. This was a time when nurses were subservient to doctors, when there were few technological aspects to nursing, and when nursing was extraordinarily "hands on." Thus virtues such as obedience, sincerity, and graciousness (Fowler, 1997) were important. This was also a time when nurses were primarily white women from upper-class families, so virtues like Christian, good posture, and poise (Fowler, 1997) were not so surprising. Nursing schools were charged with providing a "moral training ground" designed to promote development of nurses with strong moral character (Fowler, 1997, p. 24). Although it is easy to brush many of the stated virtues off as irrelevant for today, the nursing profession actually carries forward many lessons learned from this era. Although nursing schools are no longer considered "moral training grounds," much honing of moral character occurs during training. Attending to the ideas of respect for the dignity of persons and for privacy, rules about appearance during clinicals (i.e., no crop tops), and mindfulness about not expressing job dissatisfaction to patients are all grounded in the early virtues of nursing. Conversely, some of the virtues extolled so reverently in the past have remained there. Gone, thankfully, is the misbelief that the white, upper-class, Christian woman is the ideal nurse. We have learned that diversity brings creativity and broadened perspectives, so critical to effective nursing practice.

Nursing ethics developed from these early days as nursing became increasingly viewed as a profession, and as nursing in the context of society and health care shifted. The first code of ethics was written in the 1920s and centered on nursing duties—to self, to patient, and to doctors.

It was not until 1950 that the American Nurses' Association (ANA) adopted a Code of Ethics and by then, significant shifts in the nurse's role had occurred. This and later versions reflected a sense of empowerment and accountability, as military nurses served in the world wars and, especially, in Vietnam and as health care technologies became increasingly complex. The independence, professionalism, and accountability achieved during these difficult times was here to stay. The current (2015) Code of Ethics speaks to the nurse's obligations to patient, self, colleagues, and professional practice. The ANA Code of Ethics for Nursing is available in a view-only PDF for ANA members and non-members at the following link: http://nursingworld.org/MainMenuCategories/ThePracticeofProfessionalNursing/EthicsStandards/CodeofEthics.aspx.

The International Council of Nurses (ICN), a federation of national nurses' associations serving nurses in more than 128 countries, also published a code of ethics in 1953, with its most recent revision appearing in 2012 (ICN, 2012). The ICN Code of Ethics for Nursing can be accessed at: http://www.icn.ch/about-icn/code-of-ethics-for-nurses/.

NURSING ETHICS IN PRACTICE: FOUR LEVELS

The ANA Code of Ethics provides a foundation for understanding nursing ethics today. There are essentially four levels of nursing ethics—the patient, professional, organizational, and national/global level. Each level brings a different perspective of nursing ethics to light, and involves a different way of ethical thinking as well. Here, we review each of the four levels one-by-one, highlighting the important features as well the ethical contribution from nursing.

Historically nurses have not viewed themselves as key players in these types of situations because they are not the medical decision makers, and often nurses and other staff shy away from involvement because they feel they lack the knowledge about ethics that is necessary to analyze the situation and arrive at appropriate solutions. It is critical, however, that today's nurse recognize himself or herself as an important contributor in ethically challenging clinical situations. As so beautifully put by nurse and ethicist, Theresa Drought (2002):

> In all of our work we bear witness to the experience of others. We witness the inexorable wear of disease, the environment and time on the human body. We witness the love that binds humankind: the mother stroking the cheek of her newborn child; the son stroking the cheek of his dying mother; the friend holding a hand during a bout of pain. We witness the wonton senselessness of vice and violence: the victim of a drunken driver; the woman beaten by her husband; the teenage victim of a gang shooting. The moral challenge for us as nurses is to explicate meaning and identify the duties that follow from what we are privileged to witness. (p. 238)

The nurse is in the unique position of being able to see clinical situations from many angles at once. The nurse learns from the patient and family about their past experiences, their deepest fears, their beliefs, and how they interpret the current situation. At the same time the nurse understands the pathophysiological basis of the disease, treatment options, likely outcomes, and the expected clinical trajectory. All of this is important information and can be very helpful in assessing and analyzing an ethical dilemma. To participate in finding solutions, the nurse must know himself or herself to be an ethical practitioner (Taylor, 2011) and must be able to convey relevant and important information in a constructive way.

Carol Taylor (2011) has delineated the features of an ethical practitioner; these include clinical competence, trustworthiness, demonstration of commitment to advancing the patient's best interests, accountability, ability for collaboration and conflict mediation, and the capacity to recognize the ethical aspects of practice, including patient care, technology, resource use, and care delivery. Engaging these features on a daily basis ensures that nurses seek circumstances in which they can contribute to resolution of ethical problems and be accountable for their actions. A key factor is conveying relevant information to other team members. This is critical and does not, surprisingly, require a tremendous amount of ethics knowledge. It does, however, require that nurses be able to identify relevant features of a case. Cases can be at the patient level, the unit level, the organizational level, or the national/global level.

Patient-Level Ethics

Most commonly, we think of ethics as being at the bed-side—encountering a difficult patient situation as it unfolds. To illustrate the potential for nursing input, we provide the following case:

Father Frank Fowler is a 70-year-old Roman Catholic priest. His power of attorney for health care was his long-time colleague and friend, Father Jeremy Lewis. Father Fowler is a patient in the ICU, following surgery for a GI obstruction. He has a history of diverticulitis, coronary artery disease, and hypertension. He has experienced several complications following surgery, including respiratory failure and pseudomonas sepsis. He was intubated and on a ventilator while critically ill. He now has a tracheostomy and remains ventilator dependent. His sepsis is improving dramatically and he is alert and oriented. He cannot speak, but can write and has a good relationship with you, his nurse.

Father Fowler is described by his colleagues, including the nuns from the convent associated with his church, as ornery and difficult, even in the best of circumstances. However, he has devoted friends and, to many congregants, he is a beloved leader.

At one point early on in his admission, Father Fowler refused to cooperate with treatment recommendations. These refusals were believed to be part of an arduous postoperative adjustment. At the time, in fact, Father Fowler agreed that the postoperative course had been difficult and that he was unafraid to die—both of these led him to refuse aggressive treatments. However, after talking with his friend, Father Lewis, he felt better and stronger and expressed a wish to carry on and to "see things through." For the past several weeks, Father Fowler has been ill-tempered and uncooperative, but he has been accepting treatments. This week, he is again unwilling to continue treatment. His condition has improved, though, and there is hope for a good outcome. The critical care and surgical teams acknowledge his right to refuse treatment, but they are a bit perplexed given his current clinical picture.

He has stated to the nurse and to the critical care physician that he wants the ventilator stopped. The physician told him that if the ventilator was stopped, he would die, and Fr. Fowler expressed that he understood this outcome through nodding his head appropriately.

He had seemed to several nurses to be depressed during this hospitalization. When he had become septic and critically ill, the focus was on sustaining his life and antidepressants were never started. Now, Father Fowler is refusing to talk to a psychiatrist or to take antidepressants. He did say, however, that he wanted to continue treatment until Father Lewis could visit. He also wanted to speak with his longtime friend and colleague, Sister Mary Jane. He enjoyed their company and wanted to hear their perspectives.

The critical care physician and surgeon are concerned about his clinical picture and his desire to withdraw the ventilator. This would take a huge emotional toll on the staff and on them to withdraw life-sustaining treatment for a completely lucid person who seemed to be doing so well. They are considering contacting the ethics consult service.

Case adapted from Ford and Dudzinski (2008).

What can Fr. Fowler's nurse contribute in this situation? Most importantly, the nurse can provide information and interpretation. The Four Topics approach to ethical decision making (Jonsen, Siegler, & Winslade, 2006) can be effective for both. The Four Topics approach involves ordering the information that is known about a case in four discrete sections: medical indications, patient preferences, quality of life, and external factors. By separating the relevant facts of the case into these four categories, the nurse is able to identify key issues that require further investigation or that will play a role in the ethical analysis of the case. In Fr. Fowler's case, the quadrant might go as follows:

Medical Indications. This section includes relevant medical data. Fr. Fowler is currently in the ICU following surgery for a GI obstruction. He has a history of diverticulitis, coronary artery disease, and hypertension, and has experienced complications following surgery, including respiratory failure and pseudomonas sepsis. He now has a tracheostomy and is ventilator dependent. His condition is improving. He is alert and can communicate through writing. His health care providers are concerned that he is suffering from depression.

Patient Preferences. This section is intended to provide a clearer picture of how the patient is thinking about his or her treatments, what his or her stated preferences are, and whether there are any directives that could be helpful. Fr. Fowler has stated that he wants the ventilator to be stopped. In the past he has refused treatments, but he changed his mind after speaking with his friends. Now, Fr. Fowler seems sure of himself, although again he would like to speak with his friends before making his final decision. He understands that treatments can be removed or withheld.

Quality of Life. This section provides some idea of the quality of the patient's life before the illness, during the illness, and after the illness. Health care providers often discuss quality of life issues, but they must be careful to acknowledge that they cannot judge another person's quality of life. Only the patient can make this judgment. For example, a young patient who suffers severe spinal injuries in a motor vehicle accident and who is now quadriplegic may, in fact, perceive herself to have a very good quality of life. It might not be the life she had imagined or hoped for, but she (and many others in her situation) may find her life to be entirely worth living. We, as health care providers, have no say in how one perceives the quality of their life. In Fr. Fowler's case, we are unsure of his *past* quality of life, but the evidence is there that he led a parish, has parishioners who cherish him, and has deeply valued friendships. His *current* quality of life might be perceived by him to be poor. What is making his quality of life poor, especially when his condition has improved substantially? What would need to change to help him see his life differently? Might clinical depression be influencing his decision? Finally, what is his *future* quality of life likely to be? The health care team believes that he is likely to have a "good outcome," but what does that mean? What are they expecting his future life to be like, and, more importantly, will that qualify as a "good outcome" for Fr. Fowler?

External Factors. This section includes other factors that are or could be relevant to the case, such as insurance coverage, home safety/conditions, companionship, availability of caregivers, financial issues, and so on. For Fr. Fowler, we know little about his financial issues. We can assume he is covered by Medicare, but do not know his insurance status beyond this. His insurance status will dictate any long-term care decisions that are made. He is unmarried, but has dear friends. Their ability to provide care for Fr. Fowler is unknown.

Having completed the four sections, we can see gaps in our current knowledge about Fr. Fowler and can interpret some of the important factors. A significant gap is our lack of understanding of Fr. Fowler's past, current, and future quality of life. Here, the nurse can play an

important role. He or she can ask Fr. Fowler about what his life was like before his illness, what he enjoyed, what he looked forward to, and what gave him purpose. The nurse could ask about what, in his current state, is so dissatisfying. What kinds of things are burdensome? Why does he want the ventilator stopped when his condition is improving? What is keeping him from talking with a psychiatrist? The nurse could investigate the meaning of a "good outcome." Further clarification of this is certainly necessary. A good outcome could mean anything from a ventilator-dependent patient being discharged to a skilled nursing facility to an independently functioning patient being discharged to home. The goals of care must be clarified and then articulated to Fr. Fowler. Would the expected outcomes be satisfactory, allow him to enjoy his life? Other gaps in the case include whether or not he has an advance directive, what his insurance status is, whether he is concerned about his financial status. The nurse can certainly be helpful in finding this information. So, Fr. Fowler's nurse plays an important role in filling out the picture as it is presented. Once this is done, the work of analysis begins.

Case Analysis. There are myriad ways in which an ethically challenging case can be analyzed. Most familiar to health care providers is the using the principlism theory articulated by Beauchamp and Childress in the 1970s. This approach has since become the foremost used framework for analysis in health care settings. Four principles are applied to cases: respect for autonomy, beneficence, nonmaleficence, and justice. Within each principle are content areas that provide further guidance in applying the principle to the case. Briefly, let us discuss Fr. Fowler's case using the principlist approach and incorporating information gleaned from the Four Topics approach.

Respect for Autonomy. This principle addresses the idea that a person's wishes ought to be respected (assuming they do not overly burden others or violate the law—there are limits). This is true for people who are capable of making autonomous decisions. Such people must have liberty (be free from influencing factors), agency (be able to make decisions), and understanding (have enough information to make decisions) (Beauchamp & Childress, 2013). Factors that influence another's decision may render that person unable to make independent decisions. Others who demand a person act a certain way (i.e., the grandmother of an infant who insists that the mother bottle feed the infant rather than breastfeed) or severe depression can be influencing factors. Not included in this category, generally, are religious beliefs, even very restrictive religious beliefs. For example, a patient who practices as a Jehovah's Witness may request that no blood products be used, even if this means that she may die. This is not to say that this patient's request should not be explored a bit more deeply to ensure that it is truly her belief and not the demands of others influencing her opinion, but if this is truly what the patient believes, her wishes ought to be followed. In Fr. Fowler's case, there is no reason to question his ability to make decisions. He is alert and conversant. If his mental outlook is appropriately investigated during the assessment phase, it may or may not be deemed to be an influencing factor, which speaks to his liberty in terms of decision making. Fr. Fowler appears to have an understanding of the benefits and burdens of continuing treatment, especially if the vague concept of a good outcome has been explored. If Fr. Fowler has liberty, agency, and understanding, he may choose to have aggressive treatments withdrawn.

Also within the principle of respect for autonomy are guidelines for surrogate decision makers and the informed consent process. Suppose that Fr. Fowler was unable to make decisions about his medical treatment. He would require someone to decide for him; this is a person he can designate while he has decision-making capacity, as he did when he chose Fr. Lewis. For those who have not designated someone to make decisions for them, individual states have determined who the surrogate decision makers should be and in what order they would become surrogates. In the Commonwealth of Virginia, for example, surrogate decision makers are prioritized as follows: designated guardian, patient's spouse, adult child, patient's parent, adult sibling, and other relative in descending order of blood relationship (Virginia Statutes Health Care Decisions Act). This means that if a patient has been living with someone for 20 years but is not married, that person may not legally be able to make decisions for the patient. The nurse can play an important role in this by ensuring that patients have designated the person they wish to make decisions for them, should they become unable to do so while in the hospital. In Fr. Fowler's case, it would be important to include Fr. Lewis in discussions about treatment withdrawal (if that was acceptable to Fr. Fowler).

Beneficence. This principle calls on us as health care providers to do good for our patients—to prevent and remove harm. First, it is incumbent upon health care providers to identify the potential harms and benefits of the different options available. In Fr. Fowler's case, withdrawing treatment would lead to his death—certainly a harm, and an irreversible one, but there are worse harms than death for many patients. Death is not necessarily the worst possible outcome. One harm of not withdrawing aggressive treatment may be that Fr. Fowler goes on to have a life-long disability that he would rather not endure. The "rather not endure" aspect of this harm is important because it too is a harm in and of itself. Purposely refusing to follow a capable person's wishes is a called *paternalism*. Sometimes, paternalism is acceptable. Examples include situations in which safety is a primary concern (e.g., insisting that a patient who is in traction following orthopedic surgery use the bedpan rather than following his wish to get up to use the commode) or when a patient asks that the health care provider do something that is not legal (e.g., the patient asks the provider to administer opioids for the purpose of ending his life). Many times, however, overriding a patient's wish is unacceptable. Fr. Fowler may be one such case, but this is not entirely clear. We do not know why Fr. Fowler is asking for discontinuation of aggressive treatment and we do not know what he considers to be harms and benefits of continued treatment versus discontinuation.

Nonmaleficence. This principle also involves harms, similar to beneficence. The difference is that the focus is on not inflicting harm rather than preventing or removing harm. It is not difficult to think of situations in health care where pain or suffering is actually inflicted on patients, such as getting a patient up to walk soon after a surgical procedure. There is little doubt that this is painful. However, *not* doing so leads to much greater harms. These actions matter little in the context of the principle of nonmaleficence. Inflicting *unnecessary* harm is central to this principle. So, in Fr. Fowler's case, would we be inflicting harm if we discontinued treatment? How about if we continued treatment? Again, Fr. Fowler's view of "harms" would be helpful here.

Justice. This final principle speaks to the idea of distribution of goods, particularly scarce goods. It generally applies to communities, societies, or even organizations, rather than individual patients and hence has little relevance in Fr. Fowler's case. The usefulness of this principle comes into play when considering unit, organization, or national/global levels of ethics.

Using the principlist approach, it is clear that Fr. Fowler is a capable decision maker and as such, health care providers ought to abide by his wishes. However, it is much less clear why he wants these treatment modalities to be stopped. What does he consider the harms of the current treatments? Before proceeding with withdrawal per his wishes, a fuller understanding of Fr. Fowler's perceived harms and benefits seems necessary. The nurse could take the lead in investigating this. What if Fr. Fowler writes, "This tracheostomy makes my ability to talk to my friends and congregants impossible; I can't write everything I want to say. If I can't communicate with my congregants, how am I going to do the work I set out for myself to do?" How enlightening! The issue is not that he wants to die or that the treatments are too burdensome, but that he cannot see how he can continue to do the work he loves to do. Is there a different tracheostomy tube he could use that would enable him to speak? Is there hope that he may, with time and therapy, be able to have the tracheostomy tube removed? This new information sets the case on a different path, leads the team and the patient down a different road than the one that they all had been on. The nurse's work of breaking out the important aspects of the case into the four topics helped to identify key features of the case as well as gaps in knowledge. The case analysis targeted those key features and those gaps, and framed them in such a way as the team could understand what information was needed and for what purpose. The team needed Fr. Fowler's perspective on harms and benefits so as to fully understand the case.

Beyond the Principles: Rules for Health Care Providers. In addition to the four principles, several rules apply to health care situations, including *privacy* and *confidentiality*, *veracity*, and *fidelity*. *Privacy* involves not only treating a patient's information as private, but protecting patient's privacy as well. Most nurses are now familiar with the requirements of the Health Insurance and Portability and Accountability Act (USDHHS, 1996) and its stipulations certainly should be followed. More troublesome are the situations that seem quite minor, but are violations of privacy or *confidentiality*— the elevator or hallway discussions about patients, telephone conversations that can be overheard, the presence of patients at the nurses' station where patient information is exchanged. The nurse must be mindful of what is being said in public areas and is obligated to take action when violations of privacy or confidentiality occur.

The principle of *veracity* is defined as the obligation to tell the truth and to not lie or deceive others (Fry & Veatch, 2006). Truthfulness has long been regarded as fundamental to the existence of trust among individuals and has special significance in health care relationships (Fry & Grace, 2007). Over and over again, studies have shown that patients and families want to receive honest information, and that this is what health care teams ought to strive for (Institute of Medicine, 2001).

Fidelity. Fidelity is another rule that speaks to the obligations of persons to others or to organizations. Nurses have multiple simultaneous obligations and often, it is difficult to determine which obligations are strongest. The ANA Code of Ethics (2015) would say that one's obligation to the patient is most important. However, there are many situations in which maintaining a commitment to the patient jeopardizes future relationships with colleagues, and this risk is not insubstantial. Gordon and Hamric (2006) found that nurses' experiences of being in situations where they could choose to call an ethics consult often involved an assessment of risk in terms of relationships to medical colleagues. Some took the risk and others declined to call a consult because the perceived risk was too high. Thus, identifying one's obligations and considering them is not such an easy task. It is not so simple as to put the patient first.

Unit- and Organizational-Level Ethics

Much of what nursing ethics is extends beyond the patient. Daniel Chambliss' sociological study of ethical issues faced by nurses in the hospital setting revealed that the most problematic issues are derived not from individual patients, but from the system itself (1996). Chambliss noted that the repeated situations of poor communication, planning, and follow-through are what challenge the nurse's ability to do the work that needs to be done.

The ethical environment certainly influences perceptions and behavior. Penticuff and Walden (2000) found that nurses were more likely to get involved in resolving ethically challenging cases if they perceived their unit to be supportive of such work. Others studies have shown that nurses who perceive their units to have a better ethical climate (more collegial, administrative support, good avenues of communication) tend to have lower levels of moral distress (Hamric & Blackhall, 2007; Pauly, Varcoe, Storch & Newton, 2009). This is a growing area of research interest and one which the nursing contribution could be substantial and influential because nurses are called on to contribute to the building and maintenance of strongly ethical health care environments (ANA, 2001).

Moral Distress. Moral distress was first defined in the 1980s but has only recently begun to be studied and better understood. First described in nurses, moral distress is now known to affect every type of health care provider, including physicians, respiratory therapists, psychologists, chaplains, social workers, and more (Austin et al., 2005; Hamric & Blackhall, 2007; Hamric, Borchers, & Epstein, 2012; Schwenzer & Wang, 2006; Sporrong et al., 2005). A recent definition of *moral distress* is "the experience of being seriously compromised as a moral agent in practicing in accordance with accepted professional values and standards" (Varcoe, Pauly, Webster, & Storch, 2012). That is, moral distress occurs when one believes they know what the correct ethical action to take is, but is constrained from taking that action (Jameton, 1993). Many providers who experience moral distress note that what is so damaging is that they believe they are forced to do something that is morally wrong.

There are two stages to moral distress: initial moral distress and moral residue. Initial moral distress occurs in the moment, while the problematic situation is taking place. The level of moral distress may rise (crescendo) over time as the situation becomes more entrenched and difficult to resolve (Figure 12-1). Then, once the situation has passed, the level of moral distress drops dramatically, but it never returns to zero (or to the level it was before the problematic situation). This residual moral distress is called *moral residue*. We know this exists because when we ask health care providers who have been in morally distressing situations 5, 10, or 30 years ago what they recall about the situation, they can recount in vivid detail the complexities of the case, where they were and how they felt (frustrated, angry, hurt, trapped). There is currently a concern that over time, repeated exposure to morally distressing situations will lead to burnout or to providers becoming less engaged in the ethical aspects of their work. These are real concerns. Some, but not all, studies of nurses have shown that moral distress levels increase with increasing years in a position (Elpern, Covert, & Kleinpell, 2005; Hamric & Blackhall, 2007). The crescendo effect (see Figure 12-1) is a model that requires more testing but is supported by significant qualitative and quantitative evidence, especially for nurses (Epstein & Hamric, 2009).

Few studies have published strategies to address moral distress. However, one of the most powerful strategies we have found is that naming the problem when it arises can be empowering and can decrease the amount of anxiety. It is not uncommon to hear providers say that they believed themselves to be weak or to be unable to handle the stresses of the job before they understood the concept of moral distress. Knowing one is not alone is a relief to many providers. In addition

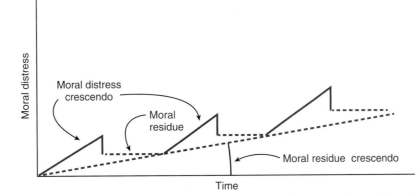

FIGURE 12-1 Crescendo effect (solid lines indicate moral distress, dotted lines indicate moral residue). (Permission received from Epstein, E. G., & Hamric, A. B. (2009). Moral distress, moral residue, and the crescendo effect. *Journal of Clinical Ethics, 20*(4), 330-342.)

to recognizing moral distress in ones' self and others, beginning dialogue within the unit about moral distress is important. Building supportive networks, learning more about moral distress, and working together to identify the sources of moral distress and design strategies to reduce moral distress—all of these are good steps toward being prepared to work in units in which morally distressing situations tend to occur.

Ethics Consult Services/Committees. One prospect for facilitation of ethical reflection and understanding for practicing nurses is consultation with the organization's ethics committee (EC). Daily decisions that nurses make often have ethical components, and mirror both the values of the persons making those decisions and those of the profession of nursing. Articulation of those values may require careful consideration, and may be assisted by those who are expert in the language and nuance of ethical deliberation. The Joint Commission requires hospitals to have structures in place to resolve situational conflict with ethical components; ECs at most hospitals have become the means for doing so.

Mandates for ECs include: education (of members and other employees); consultation and mediation of conflict; generation of policy; and research/ quality improvement to ensure policies are working as envisioned. An EC comprises members of various disciplines and the community. It is this multiplicity of perspectives, experiences, and professional disciplines that facilitate collaboration in creditable ethical decision making and policy development. Nursing is an integral part of these committees, and those who are members should be experienced in clinical practice, expert in communication, and practiced in the art of negotiation. Price (1995) observes that nurses as members of ECs provide a specific perspective that includes a "holistic view" of patients and families, an appreciation of power differentials experienced by families and staff, and a pragmatic understanding of proposed solution implementation for conflicts about ethical issues.

Ideally, members of ECs are consulting and writing policy on issues including guidelines for end of life, informed consent, treatment refusal, professionalism, and resource allocation. Through EC member presentation on ward rounds or grand rounds, awareness may permeate the entire organization; this education allows for sensitization to issues of ethics. EC resources ought to be available to all members of the health care team and to patients and families; organizational mechanisms should allow anyone to ask for case consultation.

Gordon and Hamric (2006) studied nurses' perceptions of "risk, power dynamics, and regret" with requests for ethics consultation. These researchers found that even with those nurses who were aware of ethics committee resources, a majority of them did not know how to request ethics consultation. Nurses in this study expressed reluctance to ask for ethics consultation primarily because of their fears of disrupting collegial relationships with attending physicians and other members of the health care team.

Indeed, the small group of nurses who stated they did feel comfortable making a request for an ethics consultation were the ones who reported supportive colleagues and managers, and trusting relationships with their attending physicians. This notion of ethical climate's relation to constructive working conditions and relationships evokes Walker's (1993) conception of keeping "moral space" open within health care environments. The purpose of this kind of space is to facilitate an "integrated and inclusive process of moral negotiation …" (Walker, 1993, p. 40). Achieving this kind of inclusiveness is difficult with interdisciplinary expectations and conflict. Shannon (1997) explored possible origins for the nature of interdisciplinary ethics conflict, noting that nurturing sensitivity to disciplinary perspectives may help attenuate discord.

National/Global Level

There are numerous resources in health care ethics available to nurses on national and international levels. The ANA, for example, is the professional organization representing the interests of all registered nurses in the United States. Membership in this organization provides access to extensive and print copies of texts relevant to discussions of ethics in nursing. Even without membership, it is possible to read the ANA Code of Ethics for Nurses and the various position papers on ethics and human rights (e.g., assisted suicide, forgoing nutrition, and access to therapeutic marijuana) on the ANA website (www.nursingworld.org). A search of the position statements of the ANA illustrates the distinction in application between law and ethics. Capital punishment and assisted suicide, whereas legal in more than a few states (as of this writing, the death penalty—with lethal injection the primary method used by states—is legal in 32 states, and physician-assisted death is legal in five states), are firmly opposed by the ANA. In contrast, the ANA supports patients' access to therapeutic marijuana while acknowledging that its use is prohibited by many state laws. The ANA cites core values as espoused in the Code of Ethics for Nurses that undergird these position statements. The ANA website also provides extensive dialogue and further resources for ethical issues experienced by nurses.

The ICN, founded in 1899 by nurses in Germany, the United Kingdom, and the United States, is a federation of more than 128 national nurses' associations providing international guidelines for nursing practice and policy worldwide. This organization works with the World Health Organization, and represents nursing at the annual World Health Assembly. The ICN Code of Ethics for Nurses, freely available on their website, http://www.icn.ch/about-icn/code-of-ethics-for-nurses/, emphasizes working collegially with co-workers to advance the health of individual patients, communities, and the natural environment. Policy statements (approved by all member associations) include those on ethical nurse recruitment, health care waste, and elimination of female genital mutilation.

SUMMARY

Nurses in today's health care system need a foundational understanding of ethics in order to practice. The health care system is complex, patient situations are complex, and the nurse's role in both is critical and often not intuitive. Understanding moral philosophy, professional ethics, nursing professional values, and nursing ethics provides a foundation for ethical nursing practice and decision making. When confronted with a challenging situation, it is not necessary for the nurse to be able to analyze the situation and identify ethically appropriate actions. However, it is necessary for the nurse to provide information that may be helpful in the analysis (through consideration of the four topics approach) to participate in the resolution of the case to the extent possible, to be accountable for that participation, and to know when to call the ethics consult service. It is also important that the nurse be aware that although the ethical challenge may be centered on the patient, there are often unit and organizational components at play. These should certainly be considered carefully and seriously and the nurse can play an influential role in that too. And, finally, the ANA Code of Ethics for Nurses calls on us to be active on the national and global levels as well—to speak up, to work for social justice, to advance nursing practice, and to be engaged.

SALIENT POINTS

- Nurses play an important role in identifying and framing ethical problems at the bedside, on the unit, within the organization, within the nation, and on a global scale.
- Frameworks are available to help make sense of clinical, psychosocial, economic, and other contextual details so that they can be thoroughly considered in the process of finding good solutions to ethical problems.
- All health care providers can experience moral distress. Recognizing moral distress in self and others and acting on it may promote a healthy work environment.

CRITICAL REFLECTION EXERCISES

1. Think through the following scenario: Mr. Jones was a 64-year-old dying patient. Nurse Stiles cared for Mr. Jones on many occasions and learned that Mr. Jones had been a musician "back in the day" and that he had once had a close-knit family including two siblings. About 10 years ago there had been an argument and this divided Mr. Jones from his siblings. Since then, he has had very little contact with them. Mr. Jones and Nurse Stiles talk frequently about the old days and about the way he wants his life to end. He has not told either sibling that he is dying and says he "wants to keep it that way." Nurse Stiles has two siblings also, with whom she gets along well. Although Nurse Stiles understands Mr. Jones' wishes,

she feels that if his siblings knew of their brother's situation, they could come and see him and make amends before Mr. Jones dies.

- What actions would be appropriate if you considered only Nurse Stiles' virtues?
- What actions would be appropriate if you considered only Nurse Stiles' duties and obligations?
- What actions would be appropriate if you considered only the potential outcomes of the situation?

2. Consider what resources are available to you if you were to encounter an ethically challenging case at your institution. Discuss with your student peers what the available resources are and how you access them as a professional nurse.

WEBSITE RESOURCES

American Medical Association—*Principles of Medical Ethics*: http://www.ama-assn.org/ama/pub/category/2512.html

American Nurses Association: http://www.nursingworld.org/MainMenuCategories/EthicsStandards This site contains information on general ethics as well as moral distress.

Bioethics.net: http://www.bioethics.net/

American Society for Bioethics and Humanities (ASBH): www.asbh.org

End-of-Life Nursing Education Consortium (ELNEC): http://www.aacn.nche.edu/elnec

End-of-life/Palliative Education Resource Center: http://www.eperc.mcw.edu/EPERC.htm

International Medical Interpreters Association (IMIA) Code of Ethics: http://www.imiaweb.org/code/default.asp

International Council of Nurses (ICN): www.icn.ch

Joint Commission Resources (ethics): http://www.jcrinc.com/Chapter-1-Defining-Main-Components/Developing-and-Implementing-an-Ethical-Infras/Ethics-Framework/

Kennedy Institute of Ethics: http://kennedyinstitute.georgetown.edu/

National Association of Social Work Code of Ethics: http://www.socialworkers.org/pubs/code/code.asp

National Hospice and Palliative Care Organization: http://www.nhpco.org/palliative-care-0

National Human Genome Research Institute: http://www.genome.gov/issues/

National Institute of Health—State of Science Conference Statement on Improving End of Life Care: http://sccmcms.sccm.org/SCCM/Publications/Critical+Connections/References/December+2005/

Nuffield Council on Bioethics: http://www.nuffieldbioethics.org/

Respecting Choices: http://www.respectingchoices.org/index.asp

Society of Critical Care Medicine—Statement on End of Life Decisions: http://sccmcms.sccm.org/SCCM/Professional+Resources/Critical+Care+Ethics/EndOfLifeCare.htm

The Hastings Center: http://www.thehastingscenter.org/

US National Library of Medicine Bioethics Information Resources: http://www.nlm.nih.gov/bsd/bioethics.html

JOURNAL RESOURCES

American Journal of Bioethics
Cambridge Quarterly Journal of Ethics
Hastings Center Report

HEC Forum
Journal of Clinical Ethics
Journal of Medical Ethics

Journal of Medicine and Philosophy
Kennedy Institute of Ethics Journal
Nursing Ethics

REFERENCES

ANA. (2015). *Code of ethics for nurses.* Retrieved from http://nursingworld.org/MainMenu Categories/EthicsStandards/CodeofEthicsforNurses/Code-of-Ethics.pdf

Austin, W. M., Rankel, M., & Kagan, L. (2005). To stay or to go, to speak or to stay silent, to act or not to act: Moral distress as experienced by psychologists. *Ethics and Behavior, 15*(3), 197–212.

Beauchamp, T., & Childress, J. (2013). *Principles of biomedical ethics* (7th ed.). New York: Oxford University Press.

Chambliss, D. (1996). *Beyond caring: Hospitals, nurses, and the social organization of ethics.* Chicago: University of Chicago Press.

Degrazia, D., Mappes, T. A., & Brand-Ballard, J. (2011). *Biomedical ethics* (7th ed.). New York: McGraw Hill.

Drane, J. (1994). Character and the moral life: A virtue approach to biomedical ethics. In E. DuBose, R. Hamel, & L. O'Connell (Eds.), *A matter of principles? Ferment in U.S. bioethics* (pp. 321–331). Valley Forge, PA: Trinity Press International.

Drought, T. (2002). The privilege of bearing witness. *Nursing Ethics, 9,* 238–239.

Elpern, E. H., Covert, B., & Kleinpell, R. (2005). Moral distress of staff nurses in a medical intensive care unit. *American Journal of Critical Care, 14,* 523–530.

Epstein, E. G. (2008). End-of-life experiences of nurses and physicians in the newborn intensive care unit. *Journal of Perinatology, 28,* 771–778.

Epstein, E. G., & Hamric, A. B. (2009). Moral distress, moral residue, and the crescendo effect. *Journal of Clinical Ethics, 20*(4), 330–342.

Ford, P. J., & Dudzinski, D. M. (2008). *Complex ethics consultations: Cases that haunt us.* Cambridge, UK: Cambridge University Press.

Fowler, M. (1997). Nursing's ethics. In A. J. Davis, M. A. Aroskar, J. Liaschenko, & T. S. Drought (Eds.), *Ethical dilemmas and nursing practice* (4th ed.). Stamford, CT: Appleton & Lange.

Fry, S. T., & Grace, P. J. (2007). Ethical dimensions of nursing and health care. In J. L. Creasia, & B. J. Parker (Eds.), *Conceptual foundations: The bridge to professional nursing practice* (4th ed) (pp. 273–299). St. Louis: Mosby.

Fry, S. T., & Veatch, R. M. (2006). *Case studies in nursing ethics* (3rd ed.). Sudbury, MA: Jones & Bartlett.

Gallup (2013). http://www.gallup. com/poll/1654/honesty-ethics-professions.aspx

Gordon, E. J., & Hamric, A. B. (2006). The courage to stand up: the cultural politics of nurses' access to ethics consultation. *Journal of Clinical Ethics, 17,* 231–254.

Gostin, L. O. (2002). *Tarasoff v. Regents of California.* In *Public health law and ethics: A reader.* Accessed February 2014, from http://www.publichealthla w.net/Reader/docs/Tarasoff.pdf

Grady, C., Danis, M., Soeken, K., O'Donnell, P., Taylor, C., Farrar, A., & Ulrich, C. (2008). Does ethics education influence the moral action of practicing nurses and social workers? *American Journal of Bioethics, 8*(4), 4–11.

Hamric, A. B., & Blackhall, L. (2007). Nurse-physician perspectives on the care of dying patients in intensive care units: Collaboration, moral distress, and ethical climate. *Critical Care Medicine, 35,* 422–429.

Hamric, A. B., Borchers, C. T., & Epstein, E. G. (2012). Development and testing of an instrument to measure moral distress in healthcare professionals. *AJOB Primary Research, 3*(2), 1–9.

Institute of Medicine. (2001). *Crossing the quality chasm: A new health system for the 21st century.* Washington, DC: National Academy Press.

International Council of Nurses (2012). *ICN Code of ethics for nurses.* Retrieved from http://www.icn.ch/about-icn/code-of-ethics-for-nurses/

Jameton, A. (1993). Dilemmas of moral distress: Moral responsibility and nursing practice. *AWHONNS Clinical Issues in Perinatal & Womens Health Nursing, 4*(4), 542–551.

Jonsen, A., Siegler, M., & Winslade, W. (2006). *Clinical ethics: A practical approach to ethical decisions in clinical medicine.* 6 ed. New York: McGraw-Hill.

Kaiser Family Foundation. (2013). *Key facts about the uninsured populations.* Retrieved from http://kff.org/uninsured/fact-sheet/key-facts-about-the-uninsured-population/

Laabs, C. A. (2012). Confidence and knowledge regarding ethics among advanced practice nurses. *Nursing Education Perspectives, 33*(1), 10–14.

Lewin, T. (1990). Nancy Cruzan dies, outlived by a debate over the right to die. *NY Times, December, 27* 1990. Accessed February 2014, from http://www.nytimes.com/1990/12/27- /us/nancy-cruzan-dies-outlived-by-a-debate-over-the-right-to-die.html

McFadden, R. D. (1995). Karen Ann Quinlan, 31, dies. *NY Times, June 12, 1995.* Accessed February 2014, from http://www.nytimes.com/1985/06/12/ nyregion/karen-ann-quinlan-31-dies-focus-of-76-right-to-die-case.html

Paul, R., & Elder, L. (2013). *Ethical reasoning.* Dillon Beach, CA: Foundation for Critical Thinking.

Pauly, B., Varcoe, C., Storch, J., & Newton, L. (2009). Registered nurses' perceptions of moral distress and ethical climate. *Nursing Ethics, 16*(5), 561–573.

Penticuff, J., & Walden, M. (2000). Influence of practice environment and nurse characteristics on perinatal nurses' responses to ethical dilemmas. *Nursing Research, 49,* 64–72.

Price, D. (1995). An ethical perspective: Ethics committees and nurses. *Journal of Nursing Law,* 57–64.

Roig-Franzia, M. (2005). Schiavo case goes to federal judge. *Washington Post, March 22, 2005.* Accessed February 2014, from http://www.washingtonpost.com/ wp-dyn/articles/A53153- 2005Mar21.html

Schwenzer, S. K., & Wang, L. (2006). Assessing moral distress in respiratory care practitioners. *Critical Care Medicine, 34*(2), 2967–2973.

Shannon, S. (1997). The roots of interdisciplinary conflict around ethical issues. *Critical Care Nursing Clinics of North America, 9,* 13–28.

Sporrong, S. K., et al. (2005). We are white coats whirling around: Moral distress in Swedish pharmacies. *Pharmacy World and Science, 27,* 223–239.

Taylor, C. (1995). Rethinking nursing's basic competencies. *Journal of Nursing Care Quality, 9,* 1–9.

Taylor, C. (2011). *Fundamentals of nursing: The art and science of nursing care* (7th ed). Philadelphia: Wolters Kluwer Health/Lippincott Williams & Wilkins.

Ulrich, C., O'Donnell, P., Taylor, C., Farrar, A., Danis, M., & Grady, C. (2007). Ethical climate, ethics stress, and the job satisfaction of nurses and social workers in the United States. *Social Science and Medicine, 65*(8), 1708–1719.

US Department of Health and Human Services (USDHHS). (1996). *Health information privacy.* Accessed January 2014, from http://www.hhs.gov/ocr/privacy/

Varcoe, C., Pauly, B., Webster, G., & Storch, J. (2012). Moral distress: Tensions as springboards for action. *HEC Forum, 24,* 51–62.

Vaughn, L. (2013). *Bioethics: Principles, issues, and cases* (2nd ed.). Oxford, UK: Oxford University Press.

Virginia Statutes Health Care Decisions Act §54.1-2981-§54.1 2993. Accessed February 2, 2014 from http://www.nrc-pad.org/images/stori es/PDFs/virginia_adstatute.pdf

Walker, M. U. (1993). Keeping moral space open: New images of ethics consulting. *Hastings Center Report, 23,* 33–40.

Information Management

Kelly K. Near, MLS, MSN, RN, WHNP-BC

ℯ http://evolve.elsevier.com/Friberg/bridge/

OBJECTIVES

At the completion of this chapter, the reader will be able to:

- Compare the definitions of informatics, information management, and information literacy.
- Describe the qualities of an "information literate" person.
- Recognize the need for standardized languages for information retrieval in electronic systems.
- Understand the differences between keyword searching and searching using a controlled vocabulary in a citation database.

- Recognize the importance of citation management.
- Describe and give examples of the advantages of evidence-based practice to patient care.
- Explain the process of developing an answerable clinical question for improved information retrieval.
- Understand the expanding use of personal health records and describe some concerns that consumers may have with them.

👤 PROFILE IN PRACTICE

Kelly K. Near, MLS, MSN, RN, WHNP-BC
Hospital and Community Services Librarian, University of Virginia, Charlottesville, Virginia

I've been in nursing in some form or fashion for a long time. Initially, after I received my ADN degree I worked in different settings—hospitals, nursing homes, home health, critical care, medical, and gynecology surgery departments. I liked nursing but not really nursing "tasks" or procedures. What I liked best was getting to know my patients and talking to them about their lives and their experiences. For a while, I toyed with the idea of going into counseling psychology and received a bachelor's degree in Human Services but decided I would have to complete a doctorate degree and hundreds of hours of internship before I could practice. For a single parent, that was a little too time-intense. Since I have long been interested in the politics and provision of women's reproductive health, this led me to my women's health nurse practitioner (NP) certification. Working in well-women's health was much more my style, and in the beginning of my NP practice I had lots of autonomy. I felt I could spend an adequate time on patient education. Workplace efficiency, insurance requirements, and economic pressures ultimately decreased the amount of time I had with patients and the job satisfaction, so I looked for other career options. I've always loved reading and quiet contemplation offered by libraries so I decided to pursue a master's degree in library science. The transfer of information and the many factors that can impact communication are areas rich with expanding knowledge and research, and librarians remain important players in the implementation of innovative findings in these fields. Interest in the provision of health care information led me to my current job as the Hospital and Community Services Librarian at the Claude Moore Health Sciences Library at the University of Virginia. My background helped me understand the information needs of students, practicing nurses, and patients. I'm very glad that I'm now in a position to assist clinicians and consumers in finding and using reliable health care information.

INTRODUCTION

Information from all disciplines is expanding rapidly. In health care, the flood of electronic data may be compromising provider's abilities to find and use the best information. For clinicians, the "danger of missing key information while drowning in data is real" (Flood, Gasiewicz, & Delpier, 2010, p. 101). Internet search engines, like Google, return millions of hits per search term. Databases such as MEDLINE, the bibliographic database from the National Library of Medicine, contain millions of references from health sciences journals and health care records systems are generating giant data sets that are being used to develop targeted treatments based on an individual's genetic makeup. It is now possible for even an inexpensive personal computer to have terabytes of data storage. The global Internet data traffic is expected to reach 7.7 zettabytes per year by 2017 (Cisco, 2013). For nurses the skills and resources needed to filter and process this abundant information have become essential to improving patient care.

Recognizing that health care providers need to be equipped with basic computer skills, information literacy, and an understanding of informatics and information management, the Technology Informatics Guiding Education Reform (TIGER) initiative was formed in 2006. This summit brought together over 70 stakeholders who, after extensive evaluation of the state of informatics research, education, and practice, developed the TIGER Nursing Informatics Competencies Model. This Model contains three parts: Basic Computer Competencies, Information Literacy, and Information Management (The TIGER Initiative, 2008). The TIGER Initiative, along with the National League for Nursing 2008 position statement, and the best practices from the American Association of Colleges of Nursing (2008), strongly urges the nursing profession to develop informatics competencies in order to deliver safer and more efficient care through the use of information technology. This chapter will describe the skills and concepts nurses need to know in order to manage information in the technology-based health care world.

INFORMATION MANAGEMENT

Health informatics includes the study of systems and information technology in health care but "its focus is information management, not computers" (Sewell & Thede, 2013, p. 4). *Information management* is a process consisting of collecting data, processing data, and communicating that data as information or knowledge (The TIGER Initiative, 2008). Nurses have always managed patient data and are central to the communication of the information needed for ongoing patient care. Nurses must organize and develop medication records, orders, and care plans, whether that information is found in a written chart or an electronic medical record. The evolving information landscape, however, requires students and nurses to develop a renewed interest in best practices and processes and a desire to use computerized resources to answer the many questions that arise in nursing education, practice, and research.

INFORMATION LITERACY

Information literacy is the set of skills needed to find, retrieve, analyze, and use information (Association of College and Research Libraries, 2000). It incorporates informatics and information management processes. According to the Association of College and Research Libraries (ACRL), the *information literate person* is able to determine the extent of information needed and access the needed information effectively and efficiently. The ACRL has developed information literacy competency standards and the Institute of Medicine (IOM) has also endorsed competencies that include the ability to search for and evaluate sources of evidence. After 2 years of research the ACRL has recently completed information literacy standards for nurses. The standards require nurses to have the "ability to identify an information need; find and evaluate information; assess information; use information ethically; and to use information for the purpose of best practice" (ACRL, 2013, para. 3).

In spite of the importance of information management for nurses and the need to teach information literacy skills in nursing education, a review by Flood, Gasiewicz, and Detpier (2010) found very few specific examples of integrating information literacy into nursing curricula. Another review found that "nursing education programs are not uniformly helping graduates acquire the information management skills needed to function competently in our information overloaded profession" (Hunter, McGonigle, & Hebda, 2013, p. 112). To improve these nursing skills, it is helpful to establish connections with a library, especially a medical library, because they are important sources of instruction for nurses and faculty learning about the ever more complex world of information management.

Basic Information Literacy Skills

Effectively searching an online library catalog might seem to be a skill that all nurses have acquired, yet some may never have used this type of resource for scholarly writing. These online catalogs usually contain records of print or e-books and online or print journal titles owned by the institution. Most will list other resources such as bibliographic or citation databases, institutional repositories of dissertations and theses, and other unique resources. Students searching for scholarly journal literature will find that the best source for organized information on a topic is a citation database because, unlike an Internet search, content in a database has been evaluated for authority and accuracy. A *citation* in a bibliographic database is a record that contains details about a publication. MEDLINE, from the National library of Medicine, is a biomedical journal article citation database. It contains information about the article, such as the title, the authors' names, the journal name and volume, and often an abstract of the article. The citation record may link to the full text of an article if it is freely available or if the institution owns a subscription to the online version of the journal. It is essential that nurses be able to retrieve an article from a citation database. Once an article is found, nurses should be able to evaluate the reliability, validity, accuracy, authority, timeliness, and point of view or bias of the article (Association of College and Research Libraries, 2000). Not all literature is of high quality, even if published in a journal, and the ability to evaluate an article is an important component of information literacy. Obtaining the skills to appropriately find and use scholarly information will enhance the nurse's ability to implement evidence-based practice (EBP) and conduct research in the future.

Information Retrieval

To be useful, information must be logically categorized and easily retrievable. Libraries have traditionally collected and cataloged nursing and medical information in books and databases, but now information can be stored in multiple places and retrieval has become an exercise in critical thinking. Where to go to find the correct source to answer a question is a complex task. A student's need to access information for an academic assignment in a baccalaureate nursing program will differ from that of an RN on a hospital unit required to find and evaluate the evidence available for recommending a change in practice. Whether the information is accessed from the electronic medical record on a bedside computer, the student's laptop, tablet computer, or mobile phone, the nurse must assess the reliability of the resource retrieved and effectively search through its content for the appropriate data, document, or website.

Standardization of Health Care Information

The Health Information Technology for Economic and Clinical Health (HITECH) Act from the American Recovery and Reinvestment Act of 2009 (U.S. Department of Health and Human Services, 2009) calls on health care providers to adopt, implement, and effectively utilize health information technology that allows for the electronic exchange and use of information in compliance with standards. That systems must be able to exchange information across platforms is also implicit in the definition of the *electronic health record* as an "interoperable health care record that can contain data from many electronic medical records and also personal health records (PHRs)" (Sewell & Thede, 2013, p. 231). It is essential that the standardization of nursing data occurs in order to facilitate the documentation and retrieval of this critical information across varied electronic systems.

Nursing Languages. Nurses have collected information since Florence Nightingale began conducting her research in 1882, yet Sewell and Thede (2013) comment on the "invisibility of nursing" wherein, historically, nursing's contributions to patient care have not been adequately described or documented and nursing's value has not been easily measured. Before the 1970s, nursing data and narrative notes were often purged and destroyed (p. 281). Today, there are many groups working to standardize nursing terminologies in order to make the value of nursing care explicit and comparable in electronic systems. Nurses understand that the terms *decubitus ulcer* and *bed sore* are the same, but various information systems might not classify them in the same way. A common language allows for quality improvement based on data that is retrievable and equivalent to that of other hospitals and health care providers. The North American Nursing Diagnosis

Association began a data standardization process by developing the first set of nursing diagnoses in 1982. The Nursing Minimum Data Set (NMDS) was developed in 1984 and recognized by the American Nurses Association (ANA) in 1999. The purpose of the NMDS was to establish comparability of nursing data across clinical populations, settings, geographic areas, and time; to describe the nursing care of clients and their families in a variety of settings; and to stimulate nursing research (Werley, Devine, Zorn, Ryan, & Westra, 1991). Other examples of nursing terminologies are the Fifth Edition Clinical Care Classification (formerly known as Home Health Care Classification), International Classification for Nursing Practice, Nursing Intervention Classification, Nursing Outcome Classification, Omaha System (used primarily in community and public health settings), and Perioperative Nursing Data Set. Currently there are 12 terminologies recognized by the American Nurses Association as standards that apply to nursing (American Nurses Association, 2012a). All of these terminologies have been added to the Unified Medical Language System (UMLS) designed by the US National Library of Medicine. Two components of UMLS include the Metathesaurus and the Semantic Network determined by semantic types and their relations. The Metathesaurus currently contains more than two million concepts submitted from more than 130 source vocabularies (U.S. National Library of Medicine, 2013). Kim, Coenen, and Hardiker (2012) studied existing overlapping concepts across the nursing terminology systems in the UMLS that could compromise the interoperability of nursing data. Their investigation demonstrated that improvements were needed in the representation of nursing domain knowledge in the UMLS. Stakeholders must continue their efforts to improve cross-mapping of nursing terminologies in order to support the applicability of any nursing problem lists derived from these interdisciplinary vocabularies. The ability to find and retrieve standardized nursing information from electronic medical records and other resources is essential in order to continue to make "visible" the importance of nursing practice to health care outcomes.

Controlled Vocabularies in Journal Article Databases. Nursing students are often required to search in electronic databases to find articles as references for academic papers. The *Merriam-Webster Online Dictionary* defines *database* as "a usually large collection of data organized especially for rapid search and retrieval (as by a computer)" (2014). The Cumulative Index to Nursing and Allied Health Record (CINAHL; EBSCO Information Services, 2013), is a database that provides the most comprehensive coverage of nursing literature. It indexes the contents of more than 3000 journals going back to 1981 and also includes records of nursing dissertations, book chapters, and some conference proceedings. The CINAHL is only available through a specific vendor and it requires a paid subscription through a school or other institution. The institution's subscription type will allow varied levels of access to the full text of the CINAHL's contents. This database can be searched using keywords but it also contains a "common language" or *controlled vocabulary* of Subject Headings. These terms follow the structure of Medical Subject Terms (MeSH), the controlled vocabulary used in MEDLINE. PubMed, the freely available version of MEDLINE (www.pubmed.gov), contains 22 million citations from MEDLINE, life science journals, and online books. PubMed does not include the full text of journal articles but it does link to articles contained in PubMed Central, a free full text database of medical and scientific literature. The MEDLINE database is also available from various vendors, and these vendors can add features that benefit searchers. Ovid MEDLINE (www.ovid.com) enhances searching by suggesting appropriate terms based on the user's keyword queries and displays searches so that they can be easily combined. The CINAHL also aids students and nurses by connecting natural language terms used by a searcher to an index of preferred subject terms. This is called *mapping*. If a student inputs the term *bed sores* into the search box in CINAHL, the keyword is mapped to the preferred Subject Heading *pressure ulcer*. The same mapping would take place if other synonyms were used in the initial search such as *decubitus ulcers* or even if alternative spellings and singular rather than plural terms were used, as when inputting the term *bedsore* instead of *bed sores*. Scope Notes that define the subject term are also included in CINAHL and MEDLINE. Both of these databases are set up with a hierarchical structure that allows searchers to narrow or expand their search. Expanding a search is known as *exploding* a term. Exploding the subject term *pressure ulcer* in CINAHL would result in a search that also contains citations related to specific types of pressure ulcers such as *heel ulcer* and

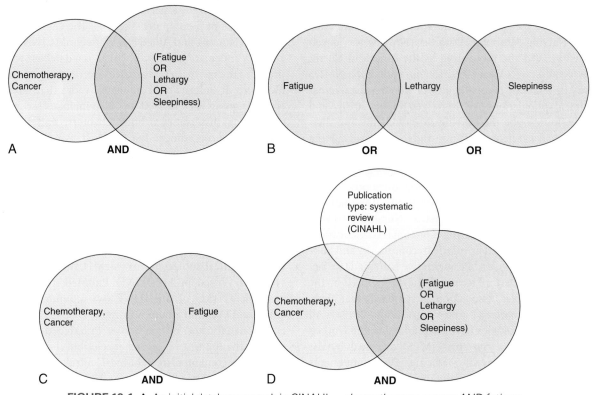

FIGURE 13-1 A, An initial database search in CINAHL—*chemotherapy, cancer AND fatigue*— retrieves articles with both terms present in the citation. **B,** An expanded search uses *OR* to string synonyms together. *Fatigue OR lethargy OR sleepiness* broadens the search to include articles with any of the terms in the citation. **C,** A search on *chemotherapy, cancer AND (fatigue OR lethargy OR sleepiness)* retrieves results with chemotherapy, cancer AND any of the synonyms that are connected by OR. **D,** The search results may be further reduced by other categorical limits, such as "publication type: systematic review," in CINAHL.

deep tissue injury. A broader term to use would be *skin ulcer.* To explode the term *skin ulcer* would result in citations about all types of skin ulcers, not just pressure ulcers. In MeSH and CINAHL, subheadings are available to limit a search even more precisely. When searching for articles about pressure ulcers, nurses may choose to limit their retrieval by using one or more of 40 narrower subheadings, ranging from "complications" to "prevention and control." There is also an ability to limit retrieval in CINAHL and MEDLINE to only those articles in which the topic is the major subject of an article by choosing the "Focus" feature in CINAHL and Ovid MEDLINE, or the Restrict to MeSH Major Topic choice in PubMed's MeSH Database (Figure 13-1).

Combining and Limiting Searches. In most databases, searches can be combined using an advanced search feature that uses connecting terms called *Boolean operators.* Two Boolean operators are AND and OR. Figure 13-2 shows how a search for *skin ulcer AND diabetes mellitus, Type 2* will decrease the amount of citations retrieved because the articles have to include both terms, but searching for *skin ulcer OR diabetes mellitus, Type 2* will increase the amount because the search will result in all the articles that are about either one of these terms or both. Often using the OR Boolean operator can result in a large amount of irrelevant citations and hours of frustration for searchers. However, most databases include helpful ways to filter results using various limits to

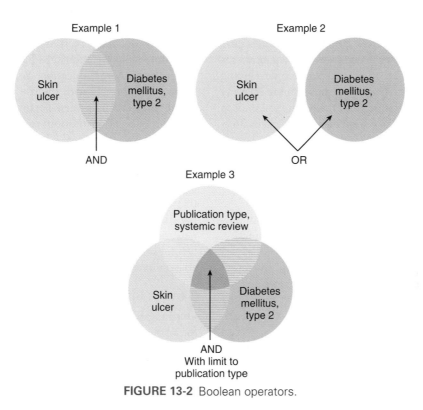

FIGURE 13-2 Boolean operators.

the articles retrieved. In MEDLINE and CINAHL, searches can be limited to article type and publication years among other filters. For example, searchers may specify that their results only include publication types such as systematic reviews or randomized controlled trials, or they may want to limit to research articles in CINAHL. For students, another valuable limit in CINAHL is a filter for only those journals that are peer-reviewed. This helps the searcher know that the articles retrieved are from scholarly sources and therefore, more authoritative.

Even though CINAHL and MEDLINE are the major databases needed for searching the medical and nursing literature, there are numerous other databases such as PsycINFO (www.apa.org/psycinfo/), Academic Search Complete (www.ebscohost.com/academic/academic-search-complete), and ERIC (http://eric.ed.gov/) that can be helpful for nurses, especially now that there is an increasing focus on interdisciplinary research in health care.

Using keywords for searching in a database or search engine is often the simplest way to find journal citations depending on the information need. Students might have an assignment to complete an academic paper on a topic such as burnout among nurses and the assignment requires a defined number of journal articles. Adequate citations that fit these criteria may potentially be retrieved by using a search engine and students often prefer to use familiar sources for searching to complete assignments, turning to resources such as Google Scholar (http://scholar.google.com/), or Wikipedia (http://www.wikipedia.org/). Because contents of many databases are indexed by search engines, this strategy can be appropriate for assignments that don't require that the instructor be able to replicate the student's search or for an extensive literature search for evidence-based projects. Although nurses may be successful in gathering articles through search engine keyword queries, they should be encouraged to develop skills to search databases using controlled vocabularies when available, as this allows others to evaluate the inclusiveness and breadth of the search by recreating it. Comprehensive searching is difficult even for the most knowledgeable searcher but most databases have online help sections and tutorials to help the novice searcher. If the search does require a comprehensive literature search or a search for evidence-based information, it is helpful to consult with a librarian for help developing appropriate search strategies. It is important to save any search terms that were used and the results so as not to have to recreate the search from memory at a later time. Most databases have a "save search" option so search results can be saved temporarily or permanently, or results can be e-mailed or saved in a file.

Mobile Computing Resources

Information retrieval through mobile devices is now an integral part of nursing education and practice. Handheld computers, tablets, and smart phones are increasingly becoming a part of nursing education and bedside care. Nurses use these devices to talk directly with other clinicians, or use text-messaging or e-mail (Broussard & Broussard, 2013). Some institutions allow access to the electronic medical record and the Internet through wireless devices and they may be used in education to provide podcasts, instructional videos, evidence-based guidelines, and reference materials. Although there is no clear evidence that these devices have a positive impact on clinical outcomes (Divall, Camosso-Stefinovic, & Baker, 2013), rapidly providing nurses with the best evidence in order to make a decision at the point of care is an important goal for time-pressed clinicians. A common use of these devices is for retrieving drug information at the point of care. A popular free drug information resource for nurses is Epocrates Rx (http://www.epocrates.com/). Along with quick access to information, this resource allows users to include local formularies in search results. Other drug information resources include *mobile* Micromedex 2.0, and Lexicomp's Nursing Lexi-Drugs database. These and hundreds of other medical "apps" are available either for free or often for a low cost for Apple iOS (iPad, iPhone, iPod Touch) and Android powered devices. Despite the many advantages of mobile devices in the workplace and in education, there are concerns when implementing these new technologies such as "cost, frequent releases of new products, accessibility, interference, disease transmission, and confidentiality" (Phillippi & Wyatt, 2011, p. 451). With rapid development of medical apps, it can be difficult to assess their quality. Wu et al. (2011) also found that though clinicians perceived an increase in efficiency from the use of smart phones, nurses in their study noted a perceived decrease in the quality of interprofessional relationships because of overreliance on electronic communication. Younger students may be very comfortable with the use of these devices for social connections in their personal lives but because of these concerns, institutions must develop the appropriate infrastructure for the implementation of mobile devices in practice and clear policies for their use. The ANA in 2011 published *Principles for Social Networking and the Nurse: Guidance for the Registered Nurse* that can be used as general guide for nurses and nursing students for maintaining professional standards in new media environments. Medical librarians are also a helpful source for finding the highest quality and reliable online resources.

Citation Management

Once a searcher has found a number of relevant citations for a paper or project from a database search, whether the search was done from a desktop computer or smartphone, keeping these expanding collections stored in files on a computer is no longer adequate (Glassman & Sorensen, 2012). Information literate nurses must now understand the use of citation management software. Sometimes referred to as *bibliographic* or *reference management software*, these programs allow users to store, organize, output, and share their bibliographic citations online as well as on a local device (Childress, 2011). Most allow users to gather references automatically from article databases and format papers and citations instantly in a variety of styles, such as American Psychological Association (APA). Users can generate bibliographies and save references in a personal database that they may then share with others. Glassman and Sorensen (2012) note that, traditionally, citation management software has been developed for desktop and laptop computers, but now there is new focus on the use of these tools on mobile devices for easier "sharing, collaborating and social bookmarking" (p. 223). Some common citation management tools in academic libraries are EndNote, Mendeley, RefWorks, and Zotero. EndNote and RefWorks are commercial products, whereas Zotero (http://www.zotero.org) and Mendeley (http://www.mendeley.com/) are freely available online. Mendeley, Zotero, and RefWorks also include mobile citation management apps. Most mobile reference management tools are available for iOS (i.e., iPad, iPhone, iPod Touch) and Android devices. Once again, it is important to collaborate with a librarian for help with answering questions about basic features of these products, such as how to import citations from particular library databases, how to use word processors to input citations during the writing process, and how to generate a bibliography in a preferred output style.

EVIDENCE-BASED PRACTICE

Evidence-based practice (EBP) has been called the "key to delivering the highest quality of health care and ensuring the best patient outcomes" (Melnyk & Fineout-Overholt, 2011, p. 3). In *Johns Hopkins Nursing Evidence-Based Practice Model and Guidelines*, EBP is defined as a "problem-solving approach to clinical decision making within a health-care organization that integrates the best available scientific evidence with the best available experiential (patient and practitioner) evidence" (Newhouse et al., 2007, p. 3). Learning the steps for retrieving, analyzing, and using best evidence tests the information literacy skills of any clinician, but Melnyk and Fineout-Overholt (2011) note that if clinicians are able to find and use information about best practices and if patients are confident that their providers use the best evidence in their care, outcomes are better for all. Research has clearly established that there are numerous advantages to basing nursing practice on evidence. Evidence-based practice results in improvements in the quality of patient care, better patient outcomes, decreased health care costs, and enhanced work satisfaction for nurses (Brockopp, Moe, Corley, & Schreiber, 2013; Melnyk, Fineout-Overholt, Stillwell, & Williamson, 2009, 2010; Poe, White, Sigma Theta Tau International & Johns Hopkins University, 2010). In addition, EBP is a part of the new standards for Magnet Recognition, the measure awarded by the American Nurses Credentialing Center as a means of recognizing hospitals that offer excellent nursing care (Drenkard, 2013). The new standards contain a renewed focus on outcomes and stress more relevant data collection. The Institute of Medicine also encourages nurses to lead and manage collaborative efforts with physicians and other members of the health care team and to conduct research and to redesign and improve practice environments and health systems (Institute of Medicine (US) Committee on the Robert Wood Johnson Foundation Initiative on the Future of Nursing, 2011). However, even with these institutional calls to incorporate EBP into all nursing

care, barriers to implementing these practices are still present. Challenges to implementing EBP include lack of time, resources, and organizational support (Shaffer et al., 2013). The EBP process has been comprehensively described by many authors (Melnyk and Fineout-Overholt, 2011; Poe et al., 2010; Rosswurm & Larrabee, 1999; Sackett, 2000; Titler et al., 2001) and models have been developed to help clinicians understand the components and implementation of EBP. The Johns Hopkins Nursing Evidence-Based Practice Process involves three major components called PET: Practice Question, Evidence, and Translation (Newhouse et al., 2007), whereas Melnyk et al. (2010) list these seven steps of EBP:

Step Zero: Cultivate a spirit of inquiry.
Step 1: Ask clinical questions in PICOT format.
Step 2: Search for the best evidence.
Step 3: Critically appraise the evidence.
Step 4: Integrate the evidence with clinical expertise and patient preferences and values.
Step 5: Evaluate the outcomes of the practice decisions or changes based on evidence.
Step 6: Disseminate EBP results.

The steps of EBP often begin with the formulation of an answerable clinical question yet as Levin and Feldman (2013) found, clarifying that question can still be a challenge for clinicians. Learning to articulate a clearly defined question is a skill that should be practiced as it will aid in the selection of the best resource to consult for an answer. When choosing a resource to search, it is important to know if the information needed is a background question or a foreground question (Noble, 2001). Background questions are those that look for general knowledge or summary information about a disease, a problem, or a population. An example of a background question would be, "What is the pathophysiology of pressure ulcers?" These types of questions may be best answered by a textbook, an online textbook such as UpToDate (http://www.uptodate.com/) or possibly even a review article. Foreground questions ask for specific knowledge to inform clinical decisions and these types of questions tend to be more complex than background questions (Fineout-Overholt & Johnston, 2005). Quite often, foreground questions investigate comparisons. A foreground question might be, "Are there special beds or mattresses that are more effective than standard hospital beds for preventing pressure ulcers in nursing home populations?" Foreground questions are best answered by searching scholarly journal databases such as MEDLINE or CINAHL or specific evidence-based collections such as the Cochrane Database of Systematic Reviews (http://www.cochrane.org/).

Framing the Clinical Question

Framing and focusing a question in a structured way helps the nurse search for and retrieve relevant answers. The Cochrane Collaboration recommends that the clinical question should specify the types of population (participants), types of interventions (and comparisons), and the types of outcomes that are of interest. The acronym PICO (Participants, Interventions, Comparisons and Outcomes) helps to serve as a reminder of these (Higgins & Green, 2011). Other formulations use the PICOT template (Population, Intervention, Comparison or Control, Outcomes, and Time). The T in this format stands for "time frame." This component is included when it is important to know the time it takes for the intervention to achieve the outcome or when a population has been followed for a particular length of time. (Huang, Lin, & Demner-Fushman, 2006; Melnyk & Fineout-Overholt, 2011) An example of using the PICO format with the question of whether there are special types of mattresses that help prevent pressure ulcer formation in nursing home residents would be organized like this:

Population—Nursing home residents
Intervention—Special mattresses
Comparison—Standard mattresses
Outcome—Prevention of pressure ulcers

A library specialist is important to include in any group searching for evidence to initiate or change a clinical practice because formulating a well-developed question and conducting a comprehensive search using controlled vocabulary can be challenging.

Levels of Evidence

After a literature search for evidence has been completed, the next step for the clinician is to review the citations by scanning the abstract or retrieving and reading the full text of articles to determine which articles best answer the clinical question. The searcher must then assess the level of the evidence each article represents. Organizations such as the Cochrane Collaboration and JBI, the Joanna Briggs Institute

(http://joannabriggs.org/) develop systematic reviews and meta-analyses considered to be the "gold standard" of health care evidence. A systematic review finds all the existing primary research on a topic that meets certain criteria and this is assessed using stringent guidelines to establish whether or not there is conclusive evidence about a specific treatment or test (The Cochrane Collaboration, 2014). Cochrane only selects randomized controlled trials (RCTs) to combine for their systematic reviews or meta-analyses because randomized controlled trials are considered to have the most rigorous study design. Randomly assigning subjects in an experiment is like flipping a coin as to who receives an intervention or not. This minimizes the bias inherent in other types of studies. Meta-analysis is the statistical combination of results from two or more separate studies (Higgins & Green, 2011) and this can represent an even higher level of evidence because the combined numbers of participants increases the certainty of the results. Qualitative studies represent a lower level of evidence because this type of research is not generalizable as is quantitative research like RCTs. Many organizations and authors have developed various frameworks for establishing their own levels of evidence. Levels range from 1 through 8 in Melnyk and Fineout-Overholt's scale, 1-3 in DynaMed (https://dynamed.ebscohost.com/content/LOE), or 1-5 at the Oxford Centre for Evidence Based Medicine (CEBM, 2013) (http://www.cebm.net/?o=1025). Usually the lowest level of evidence on a scale is considered to be case studies or narrative opinions of experts, although some put animal studies at the bottom (Figure 13-3).

After completing a comprehensive database search, research evidence for a decision may be lacking, so it is important in the decision-making process to examine and evaluate other types of available evidence. Other sources of evidence may come from clinical guidelines and recommendations from national and local professional organizations (Newhouse et al., 2007). A good source for clinical guidelines is the National Guidelines Clearinghouse (http://www.guideline.gov/) developed by the Agency for Healthcare Research and Quality (AHRQ), that is freely available online. It is important to remember that not all clinical guidelines can be considered evidence based. It is necessary to read the guideline to determine how the guideline was classified as well as which ranking scale was used for its recommendations.

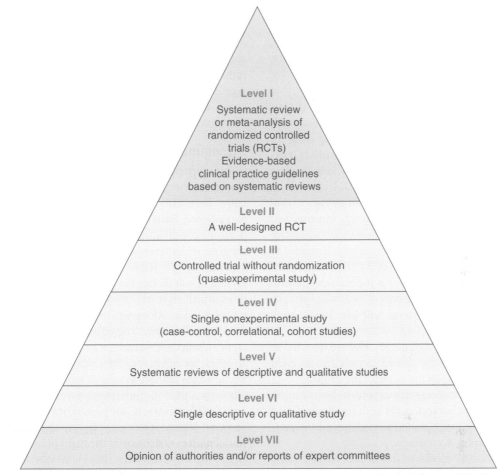

FIGURE 13-3 Levels of evidence pyramid. (From Lobiondo-Woods, G., & Haber, J. (2010). *Nursing research* (7th ed.). St Louis: Mosby.)

Critical Appraisal

Establishing the evidence level of an article is important but this is only part of critically appraising the quality of a study. Critical appraisal requires specific skills. Time is needed to establish if a study provides valid and reliable evidence that can be applied to the clinician's and the patient's specific circumstances. To assist busy clinicians, new consolidated resources are being developed that can be quickly accessed at the point of care. These resources, for example, DynaMed, Essential Evidence Plus (http://www.essentialevidenceplus.com/), Mosby's Nursing Consult (http://www.nursingconsult.com/nursing/index), and the Joanna Briggs Institute, Evidence Summaries, contain pre-filtered evidence-based information in which all content has already been evaluated and given a strength of evidence or strength of recommendation rating. Most of these resources are also available for mobile devices.

One way for nurses to learn more about critical appraisal of research studies is to institute a journal club. Journal clubs usually meet face-to-face to discuss a particular article of interest to a group. Berger, Hardin, and Topp (2011) note that journal clubs both educate nurses and improve clinical practice by helping them to learn how to translate research into improved patient care. Nurses learn to analyze the quality of studies and become more familiar with the process of critical appraisal in a supportive setting. Nurses may be too busy to meet face-to-face, however, so the authors suggest forming a virtual journal club using a blog format that allows text-based interactions between participants.

Other publishers may have online journal clubs as one of their evidence-based tools available to users. Such online journal clubs often guide the user through an appraisal of different types of literature for their quality.

Implementing Evidence-Based Practice

Once evidence has been gathered and appraised, clinical judgment is required before implementation is considered. Describing the process of implementing evidence into clinical practice has been comprehensively outlined by Melynk and Fineout-Overholt, Sackett, Poe and others (Melnyk & Fineout-Overholt, 2011; Poe et al., 2010; Sackett, 2000). Expert support and guidance from administration and experienced research mentors will always be necessary in order to promote the collaborative effort and find the time in a busy unit schedule needed to complete an EBP project. Shaffer et al (2013) have developed a set of recommendations for the bedside nurse to consider when implementing an evidence-based project:

- Realize that the EBP process will take longer than anticipated.
- Identify and involve staff nurses who are invested in the project. The group should include five to eight nurses, depending on the scope of the project.
- Involve clinical and research experts to help identify the scope of the project, assist with the process, and establish a realistic timeline to understand the concept and to plan accordingly.
- Identify an EBP model to follow that all can easily understand and use.
- Set goals and a timeline. Be prepared to modify the timeline as needed.
- Communicate the plan not only to each member of the team but also to the nurse manager and all appropriate staff members responsible for project implementation.
- Remember the following three key words: time, patience, and perseverance (pp. 359-360).

Keeping Current with New Evidence

Results of new studies are published every day; so many databases such as CINAHL and MEDLINE allow users to save their searches so that they can be updated as new information appears. In these databases, searches may be saved as alerts and users then receive an e-mail or an RSS feed with any new citations that match the search strategy. Nurses may also sign up for journal table-of-contents services either through a database or directly through the publisher's website. Many journals are published for specialty areas such as critical care or perianesthesia nursing, so receiving information about the current contents of a specific journal can help nurses keep up on the latest topics in their field. Online services such as Medscape (http://www.medscape.com/) deliver free journal articles and news to users based on a personalized registration profile.

Dissemination

It is important to the nursing profession that information from new research and programs be widely disseminated. There are various venues for presenting content to an audience. Poster sessions are presentations of information by individuals or representatives of teams at a congress or conference with an academic or professional focus. Poster guidelines are determined by the specific event and will dictate the size, orientation, or other features identified by the event sponsors such as deadlines for submission. Along with poster presentations, nurses are often called upon to give individual or panel presentations about their research at a meeting or asked to write an article for publication in a scholarly journal. In order to encourage authors to submit information about their scholarly activities, conference providers will often send out a "call for abstracts" for posters or presentations. The *Merriam-Webster Online Dictionary* defines *abstract* as a brief written statement of the main points or facts in a longer report, speech, etc. (2014). Weinert (2010) notes that the importance of the abstract is often overlooked and a well-crafted abstract is essential for having nursing research and writing noticed and accepted. Faculty and clinical mentors must be readily available for new nurse authors learning the article submission process. One method of providing this type of support is described by Hoke and Papa (2014) who developed a three-part workshop that included a process of peer review to provide authors with guidance and encouragement for the development of successful abstracts.

CONSUMER HEALTH INFORMATION

Personal Health Records

The Healthcare Information and Management Systems Society (HIMSS) defines *personal health records* (PHRs) as electronic records "used by patients to manage their relevant health information and to promote health maintenance and chronic disease management. PHRs are interactive, common data sets of electronic health information (EHRs) and e-health tools" (HIMSS, 2013, para 1). In a 2012 position statement, the ANA supported the development of PHRs but stressed that the PHR should be secure and "only available to the consumer or their designated health care providers" (American Nurses Association, 2012b, para. 1).Personal health records can be part of The Medicare and Medicaid Electronic Health Record (EHR) Incentive Programs that provide financial incentives for the *meaningful use* of certified EHR technology to improve patient care. To receive an EHR incentive payment, providers have to show that they are "meaningfully using" their EHRs by meeting thresholds for a number of objectives. The meaningful use objectives are grouped into five patient-driven domains that relate to health outcomes policy priorities:

- Improve Quality, Safety, Efficiency
- Engage Patients and Families
- Improve Care Coordination
- Improve Public and Population Health
- Ensure Privacy and Security for Personal Health Information (HealthIT.gov, n.d.).

The "Blue Button" is a technology that allows consumers to download their personal health information online and U.S. military veterans have had access to their online records since 2010. The Veterans Administration (VA) was first to display the Blue Button symbol on its patient portal but now many other health care providers and plans are using this technology. Leadership of the initiative to promote this technology is now being overseen by the Office of the National Coordinator for Health Information Technology. Technology is being developed that will allow consumers to better share their Blue Buttoned-information with others they trust and plug them into new apps and tools. "With more than half of Americans using smart phones today and an abundance of popular health apps and tools such as digital pedometers, glucose monitors, and sleep sensors, consumers are becoming an undeniable part of the equation for better health and health care through health information technology" (Ricciardi, 2013, para. 8).

Health Literacy

It is hoped that the information accessible through a PHR will help health care consumers in making informed health decisions although concerns need to be addressed around the issue of the literacy level of its users. The Patient Protection and Affordable Care Act of 2010, Title V, defines *health literacy* as the degree to which an individual has the capacity to obtain, communicate, process, and understand basic health information and services to make appropriate health decisions. Concerns regarding health literacy were described in 2004 by the IOM who convened the Committee on Health Literacy to write *Health Literacy: A Prescription to End Confusion*. In the description of the book, the National Academies Press notes that in order to "maintain their own health and the health of their families and communities, consumers rely heavily on the health information that is available to them. This information is at the core of the partnerships that patients and their families forge with today's complex modern health systems." The authors note that many Americans cannot understand the information given to them by health care personnel (Nielsen-Bohlman et al., 2004). The National Assessment of Adult Literacy (NAAL) has found that over a third of U.S. adults would have trouble with common health tasks, such as following directions on a prescription drug label or adhering to a childhood immunization schedule using a standard chart (U.S. Department of Education, 2006). Berkman et al. (2011), in their review, found that low health literacy was consistently associated with decreased ability to understand health messages, less ability to understand labels and take medication appropriately, lower receipt of screening mammograms and flu vaccinations, more hospitalizations, greater use of emergency care, and, among elderly people, worse overall health status and higher mortality rates.

Nurses have a duty to recognize the diverse information needs of their patients and use tested strategies to assist them. Koh et al. (2012) found that certain procedures help patients deal with complicated and confusing forms and instructions:

- Simplifying and making written materials easier to understand using things like simple pictograms when educating about medications.
- Improving providers communication skills by having providers receive feedback on their education methods with low literacy patients.
- Improving patients' self-management skills by developing self-care, picture-based educational materials, and using scheduled telephone follow-up to reinforce adherence to necessary medication regimens and instructions (pp. 2-3).

Patient education information is provided by hundreds of different vendors. Some of these commercial vendors such as Micromedex CareNotes (Micromedex.com) and Krames StayWell (kramesstaywell.com) can be integrated into the electronic medical record. Many commercial products provide information at a targeted reading level—usually fifth to eighth grade, and often provide their patient information in multiple languages.

Consumer Health Information Resources on the Internet

In 2013 Fox found that 72% of U.S. patients searched for online health information. Most used search engines such as Google or Bing to begin their search. Though patients persistently use the Internet for information, they still turn for help from health care providers for serious health concerns or questions (Fox & Duggan, 2013) This raises an opportunity for nurses not only to provide tailored education to patients seeking information at the point of care, but to educate patients on how to access quality information when searching on their own. The National Library of Medicine's consumer health database, MedlinePlus (http://medlineplus.gov) is considered to be one of the most reliable sources of advertisement-free health information on the Internet. MedlinePlus contains information on over 900 health topics in English and Spanish, plus videos, tutorials, and other multimedia content. It has easy-to-read information as well as links to information in multiple languages. This is a resource that should be recommended to patients and consumers as a place to start a search for health care information. There are also thousands of other competing health information sources found on the Internet. Many of these are commercial sites such as WebMD, which permit advertisements on their pages, while many are provided by organizations such as the American Academy of Family Physicians (familydoctor.org) or the American Cancer Society (www.cancer.org/). The information seeker needs, at a minimum, to be aware of the authority of the authors of such sites and the currency of the information, and users need to be able to verify the information they find at a site by finding similar information from other sources. Many consumers like to use the Internet to find others who share a particular medical condition. Websites such as PatientsLikeMe (www.patientslikeme.com/) allow patients to connect with others online to discuss concerns about symptoms and medical treatments. These sites promote open sharing but there is always a need to understand the level of privacy afforded by the site before disclosing personal health information.

▌ SUMMARY

Health care resources and processes are rapidly evolving. Nurses must learn the most effective ways to manage the information generated by new electronic systems in order to provide quality care. Although sometimes challenging in practice, students as well as bedside nurses need well-developed information retrieval skills to ensure that they are finding the best available evidence. Nurses should also take an active part in synthesizing and critically appraising information in order to implement best practices in their settings. Health care consumers are now seeking health information at expanding rates and nurses can offer essential guidance in helping these consumers find quality resources that are appropriate to their level of health literacy.

▌ SALIENT POINTS

- Nurses must position themselves to manage the expanding amount of information being generated in academic and health care settings.
- Information literacy requires the development of skills to find, analyze, and use electronic information.
- Information can be retrieved from multiple formats, including the Internet, bibliographic databases, electronic medical record, and personal health records.
- Mobile resources will continue to play a large part in data entry and point-of-care retrieval.
- Nursing stakeholders must continue to improve the cross-mapping of nursing terminologies in larger electronic records systems to ensure the interoperability and inclusion of critical nursing data.
- Learning effective strategies for finding reliable information will become increasingly important as

the majority of health care institutions broaden their focus on the provision of evidence-based care.

- Collaboration with a librarian, especially a medical librarian, is important when developing a comprehensive literature search for medical or nursing information.
- Evidence-based practice requires time for skill development and support from administrators in order for bedside nurses to be successful in its implementation.

- Personal health records are improving consumer's access to personal medical information although privacy concerns should continue to be addressed.
- Research has shown that limited health literacy leads to poorer health care outcomes so nurses have an obligation to make sure that the information they provide is understandable and sensitive to the patient's unique needs.

CRITICAL REFLECTION EXERCISES

1. Find the website of an academic medical library such as the Hardin Library of the Health Sciences (www.lib.uiowa.edu/hardin/) or the Duke Medical Center Library (https://mclibrary.duke.edu/) and determine if they provide subject guides for nursing or evidence-based practice.
2. Conduct a search for a topic (e.g., pressure ulcer) that can be mapped to a Subject Heading in CINAHL. Compare the results to a keyword search for the same topic in a search engine such as Google or Bing.

3. Develop a clinical question in the PICOT format and consider how you would begin to search for the answer to this question in a database such as MEDLINE or CINAHL.
4. Search MedlinePlus.gov for the topic "asthma." Find and review an interactive tutorial on this topic and determine how you might use this resource for patient care.

WEBSITE RESOURCES

Academic Search Complete (www.ebscohost.com/academic/academic-search-complete)

American Academy of Family Physicians (http://familydoctor.org)

American Cancer Society (www.cancer.org/)

Cochrane Database of Systematic Reviews (http://www.cochrane.org/)

DynaMed (https://dynamed.ebscohost.com/content/LOE)

Epocrates Rx (http://www.epocrates.com/).

ERIC (http://eric.ed.gov/)

Essential Evidence Plus (http://www.essentialevidenceplus.com/)

Google Scholar (http://scholar.google.com/)

Joanna Briggs Institute (http://joannabriggs.org/)

Krames StayWell (http://kramesstaywell.com)

MedlinePlus (http://medlineplus.gov)

Medscape (http://www.medscape.com)

Mendeley (http://www.mendeley.com/)

Micromedex CareNotes (http://Micromedex.com)

Mosby's Nursing Consult (http://www.nursingconsult.com/nursing/index)

National Guidelines Clearinghouse (http://www.guideline.gov/)

Ovid MEDLINE (www.ovid.com)

Oxford Centre for Evidence Based Medicine (http://www.cebm.net/?o=1025)

PatientsLikeMe (www.patientslikeme.com/)

PsycINFO (www.apa.org/psycinfo/)

PubMed (www.pubmed.gov)

UpToDate (http://www.uptodate.com/)

Wikipedia (http://www.wikipedia.org/).

Zotero (http://www.zotero.org)

REFERENCES

abstract. (2014). In *Merriam-Webster Online Dictionary*. Retrieved from http://www.merriam-webster.com/dictionary/abstract

ACRL Association of College and Research Libraries. (2013). *Information literacy competency standards for nursing*. Retrieved from http://www.ala.org/acrl/standards/nursing

American Association of Colleges of Nursing. (2008). *The essentials of baccalaureate education for professional nursing practice*. Retrieved from http://www.aacn.nche.edu/education-resources/BaccEssentials08.pdf

American Nurses Association. (2012a). *ANA recognized terminologies that support nursing practice*. Retrieved from http://www.nursingworld.org/npii/terminologies.htm

American Nurses Association. (2012b). *Electronic personal health record*. Retrieved from http://www.nursingworld.org/electronicphr

Association of College and Research Libraries. (2000). *Information literacy competency standards for higher education*. Retrieved from http://www.ala.org/acrl/sites/ala.org.acrl/files/content/standards/standards.pdf

Berger, J., Hardin, H.,K., & Topp, R. (2011). Implementing a virtual journal club in a clinical nursing setting. *Journal for Nurses in Staff Development, 27*(3), 116–120.

Berkman, N. D., Sheridan, S. L., Donahue, K. E., Halpern, D. J., & Crotty, K. (2011). Low health literacy and health outcomes: An updated systematic review. *Annals of Internal Medicine, 155*(2), 97–107.

Brockopp, D. Y., Moe, K., Corley, D., & Schreiber, J. (2013). The Baptist Health Lexington evidence-based practice model. *Journal of Nursing Administration, 43*(4), 187–193.

Broussard, B., & Broussard, A. (2013). Using electronic communication safely in health care settings. *Nursing for Women's Health, 17*(1), 59–62.

CEBM Centre for Evidence Based Medicine. (2013). *Oxford Centre for evidence based medicine—levels of evidence.* Retrieved from http://www.cebm.net/index.aspx?o=1025

Childress, D. (2011). Citation tools in academic libraries: Best practices for reference and instruction. *Reference & User Services Quarterly, 51*(2), 143–152.

Cisco. (2013). *Cisco global cloud index: Forecast and methodology, 2012–2017.* Retrieved from http://www.cisco.com/en/US/solutions/collateral/ns341/ns525/ns537/ns705/ns1175/Cloud_Index_White_Paper.html

The Cochrane Collaboration. (2014). *Cochrane reviews.* Retrieved from http://www.cochrane.org/cochrane-reviews

database. (2014). In *Merriam-Webster Online Dictionary.* Retrieved from http://www.merriam-webster.com/dictionary/database.

Divall, P., Camosso-Stefinovic, J., & Baker, R. (2013). The use of personal digital assistants in clinical decision making by health care professionals: A systematic review. *Health Informatics Journal, 19*(1), 16–28.

Drenkard, K. (2013). Change is good. *Journal of Nursing Administration, 43*(10), 489–490.

EBSCO Information Services. (2013). *CINAHL | cumulative index to nursing and allied health.* Retrieved from http://www.ebscohost.com/nursing/products/cinahl-databases/the-cinahl-database

Fineout-Overholt, E., & Johnston, L. (2005). Teaching EBP: Asking searchable, answerable clinical questions. *Worldviews on Evidence-Based Nursing, 2*(3), 157–160.

Flood, L. S., Gasiewicz, N., & Delpier, T. (2010). Integrating information literacy across a BSN curriculum. *Journal of Nursing Education, 49*(2), 101–104.

Fox, S., & Duggan, M. (2013). *Health online 2013.* Retrieved from http://www.pewinternet.org/2013/01/15/health-online-2013/

Glassman, N.,R., & Sorensen, K. (2012). Citation management. *Journal of Electronic Resources in Medical Libraries, 9*(3), 223–231.

HealthIT.gov. (n.d.). *EHR incentives & certification: Meaningful use definition & objectives.* Retrieved from http://www.healthit.gov//providers-professionals/meaningful-use-definition-objectives/

Higgins, J., & Green, S. E. (March 2011). *Cochrane handbook for systematic reviews of interventions version 5.1.0. the Cochrane collaboration.* Retrieved from www.cochrane-handbook.org

HIMSS. (2013). *Personal health records (PHRs) and patient portals | patient engagement | HIMSS resource library.* Retrieved from http://www.himss.org/resourcelibrary/TopicList.aspx?MetaDataID=1498&navItemNumber=13562

Hoke, L. M., & Papa, A. M. (2014). Increasing the odds, using peer review promotes successful abstract submission. *Clinical Nurse Specialist CNS, 28*(1), 46–55.

Huang, X., Lin, J., & Demner-Fushman, D. (2006). Evaluation of PICO as a knowledge representation for clinical questions. *AMIA...Annual Symposium Proceedings / AMIA Symposium. AMIA Symposium,* 359–363.

Hunter, K., McGonigle, D., & Hebda, T. (2013). The integration of informatics content in baccalaureate and graduate nursing education. *Nurse Educator, 38*(3), 110–116.

Institute of Medicine (US). Committee on the Robert Wood Johnson Foundation Initiative on the Future of Nursing. (2011). *The future of nursing: Leading change, advancing health.* Washington, DC: National Academies Press.

Kim, T. Y., Coenen, A., & Hardiker, N. (2012). Semantic mappings and locality of nursing diagnostic concepts in UMLS. *Journal of Biomedical Informatics, 45*(1), 93–100 doi:http://dx.doi.org/10.1016/j.jbi.2011.09.002.

Koh, H. K., Berwick, D. M., Clancy, C. M., Baur, C., Brach, C., Harris, L. M., et al. (2012). New federal policy initiatives to boost health literacy can help the nation move beyond the cycle of costly 'crisis care'. *Health Affairs (Project Hope), 31*(2), 434–443.

Levin, R. F., & Feldman, H. R. (2013). *Teaching evidence-based practice in nursing* (2nd ed.). New York: Springer.

Melnyk, B. M., Fineout-Overholt, E., Stillwell, S. B., & Williamson, K. M. (2009). Evidence-based practice: Step by step. Igniting a spirit of inquiry: An essential foundation for evidence-based practice: How nurses can build the knowledge and skills they need to implement ERP. *American Journal of Nursing, 109*(11), 49–52.

Melnyk, B. M., Fineout-Overholt, E., Stillwell, S. B., & Williamson, K. M. (2010). Evidence-based practice: Step by step: The seven steps of evidence-based practice. *The American Journal of Nursing, 110*(1), 51–53.

Melnyk, B. M., & Fineout-Overholt, E. (2011). *Evidence-based practice in nursing & healthcare: A guide to best practice* (2nd ed.). Philadelphia: Wolters Kluwer/Lippincott Williams & Wilkins.

Newhouse, R. P., Dearholt, S. L., Poe, S., Pugh, L. C., White, K. M., Sigma Theta Tau International, et al. (2007). *Johns Hopkins nursing evidence-based practice model and guidelines.* Indianapolis, IN: Sigma Theta Tau International Honor Society of Nursing.

Nielsen-Bohlman, L., Panzer, A. M., Kindig, D. A., Institute of Medicine (U.S.) & Committee on Health Literacy. (2004). *Health literacy a prescription to end confusion.* Retrieved from http://site.ebrary.com/id/10062734.

Noble, J. (2001). *Textbook of primary care medicine* (3rd ed.). St Louis: Mosby.

Phillippi, J. C., & Wyatt, T. H. (2011). Smartphones in nursing education. *CIN: Computers, Informatics, Nursing, 29*(8), 449–454.

Poe, S., White, K. M., Sigma Theta Tau International, & Johns Hopkins University. (2010). *Johns Hopkins nursing evidence-based practice.* Indianapolis, IN: Sigma Theta Tau International.

Ricciardi, L. (2013). *The blue button movement: Kicking off national health IT week with consumer engagement.* Retrieved from http://www.healthit.gov/buzz-blog/electronic-health-and-medical-records/blue-button-movement-kicking-national-health-week-consumer-engagement/

Rosswurm, M. A., & Larrabee, J. H. (1999). A model for change to evidence-based practice. *Image: The Journal of Nursing Scholarship, 31*(4), 317–322.

Sackett, D. L. (2000). *Evidence-based medicine: How to practice and teach EBM* (2nd ed.). Edinburgh: Churchill Livingstone.

Sewell, J. P., & Thede, L. Q. (2013). *Informatics and nursing: Opportunities and challenges* (4th ed.). Philadelphia: Wolters Kluwer Health/Lippincott Williams & Wilkins.

Shaffer, S. T., Zarnowsky, C. D., Green, R., et al. (2013). Strategies from bedside nurse perspectives in conducting evidence-based practice projects to improve care. *Nursing Clinics of North America, 48*(2), 353–361.

The TIGER Initiative. (2008). *The TIGER initiative informatics competencies for every practicing nurse: Recommendations from the TIGER collaborative.* Retrieved from http://www.thetigerinitiative.org/docs/TigerReport_InformaticsCompetencies.pdf.

Titler, M. G., Kleiber, C., Steelman, V. J., Rakel, B. A., Budreau, G., Everett, C., et al. (2001). The Iowa model of evidence-based practice to promote quality care. *Critical Care Nursing Clinics of North America, 13*(4), 497–509.

U.S. Department of Education. (2006). *The health literacy of America's adults: Results from the 2003 national assessment of adult literacy.* Retrieved from http://nces.ed.gov/pubs2006/2006483.pdf

U.S Department of Health and Human Services. (2009). Health information technology for economic and clinical health (HITECH) Act, title XIII of division A and title IV of division B of the American recovery and reinvestment act of 2009 (ARRA). Retrieved from http://www.healthit.gov/sites/default/files/hitech_act_excerpt_from_arra_with_index.pdf

U.S. National Library of Medicine. (2013). *Unified Medical Language System (UMLS).* Retrieved from http://www.nlm.nih.gov/research/umls/knowledge_sources/metathesaurus/

Weinert, C. (2010). Are all abstracts created equal? *Applied Nursing Research, 23*(2), 106–109.

Werley, H. H., Devine, E. C., Zorn, C. R., Ryan, P., & Westra, B. L. (1991). The nursing minimum data set: Abstraction tool for standardized, comparable, essential data. *American Journal of Public Health, 81*(4), 421–426.

Wu, R., Rossos, P., Quan, S., Reeves, S., Lo, V., Wong, B., et al. (2011). An evaluation of the use of smartphones to communicate between clinicians: A mixed-methods study. *Journal of Medical Internet Research, 13*(3), e59.

Diversity in Health and Illness

Ishan C. Williams, PhD and Cathy L. Campbell, PhD, RN, ANP-BC

OBJECTIVES

At the completion of this chapter, the reader will be able to:

- Describe nursing care strategies that may be used to provide care to a diverse patient population.
- Describe methods used to become culturally competent.
- Identify societal factors affecting the delivery of culturally responsive nursing care in the United States.
- Identify barriers to and resources for minority access to care in the United States.

- Describe the differences in the concepts of race, culture, and ethnicity.
- Discuss strategies to approach diverse populations in the provision of culturally relevant care.
- Discuss how strategies to approach diverse populations can improve the outcomes for patients, families, communities, and health care organizations.

👤 PROFILE IN PRACTICE

INTERPROFESSIONAL COLLABORATION IN LIMPOPO PROVINCE, SOUTH AFRICA
Cathy L. Campbell, PhD, ANP-BC
University of Virginia, School of Nursing, Rural and Global Research Center
Marianne Baernholdt, PhD, MPH, RN
University of Virginia, School of Nursing, Rural and Global Research Center
University of Virginia, Department of Public Health Sciences
Rebecca Dillingham, MD, MPH
University of Virginia, School of Medicine
University of Virginia, Center for Global Health
Violet M. Mabunda, Bsc
Department of Health, Vhembe District, Thohoyondou, Limpopo province, South Africa
Mary Malaleke, PhD, RN
University of Venda, Department of Advanced Nursing Science, Thohoyondou, Limpopo Province, South Africa
James Plews-Ogan, MD
University of Virginia, School of Medicine
Margaret Plews-Ogan, MD
University of Virginia, School of Medicine
Lizzy Netshikweta, PhD
University of Venda, Department of Advanced Nursing Science, Thohoyondou, Limpopo Province, South Africa

Limpopo province is the northernmost province in South Africa. It shares a border with Mozambique and Zimbabwe. With a population of 5,227,200, the residents of this rural province are challenged by poverty, limited access to clean water, health care, and the impact of the HIV/AIDS virus (Coovadia et al., 2009). Limpopo province is divided into five health districts, and the Vhembe district is the northernmost district (Vhembe District Municipality, 2013). The University of Virginia (UVA) in Charlottesville has a 10-year partnership with the University of Venda (UNIVEN) and two rural villages working on the Water and Health in Limpopo Project (WHIL). The UNIVEN is unique in terms of geographic location. It is the only university in the country close to three bordering countries, namely, Botswana, Mozambique, and Zimbabwe.

Building on the foundation of the UNIVEN-UVA relationship in 2012, an additional partner was added, the Limpopo's Department of Health (DOH) in the Vhembe District in 2012, the first time such tripartite collaboration had occurred. The Vhembe Health District developed a list of five priority areas in which they sought collaboration with the UVA and UNIVEN. The priorities included mental health, environmental and occupational health services, health promotion, maternal child and women's health, and malaria (Vhembe Health District, 2013).

The Vhembe health district wanted to focus health promotion as it related to the education of community health workers (CHWs) on the chronic illnesses of diabetes mellitus and hypertension. Limpopo's DOH relies heavily on community workers for many health care services. The patient-to-nurse ratio for all of South Africa is 417:1, whereas in Limpopo the ratio is 536:1 (South African Nursing Council [SANC], 2012). Capitalizing on this unique interprofessional partnership between the UVA and UNIVEN, an interdisciplinary team was created to design and implement a 2-day training on diabetes mellitus and hypertension for CHWs in two rural health centers in the Limpopo province. A variety of teaching methods were used, such as hands-on skills demonstration and practice, story boarding (participants visually depict their baseline knowledge or experience with a topic), role-play, experiential learning activities, small group work, and clinical narratives to teach knowledge and skills related to diabetes mellitus and hypertension management. Each participant also was given a fact sheet to be used as a resource guide in his or her clinical work once the training was completed.

All of the partners involved anticipated that there would be challenges to implementing this project, as there are with any cross-cultural endeavor. The first challenge was to decide the language in which the training should be conducted. The DOH, Vhembe District, requested that the training be done in English, because it was a language common to all of the participants. However, during the first day of training, it was clear that the plan needed to be modified. The UNIVEN faculty and staff present at the workshop partnered with UVA students and faculty so that each group of participants had an interpreter available for all of the activities. Each day of training ended with a role-play in which the participants demonstrated the knowledge and skills they learned during the session. The participants performed the role-play in their native language along with assistance from the faculty or student interpreter. This change allowed for freer expression and ultimately a richer experience for the participants.

The linguistic challenge also was apparent when we reviewed the evaluations. The participants completed a two-page survey. The first page contained a questionnaire that was completed with a series of check marks using the 5-item Likert-type scale (strongly agree-agree-neutral-disagree-strongly disagree). The second page had space for a narrative or free form comments. When the evaluations were reviewed, the first page was completed correctly or as expected; however, the narrative comments on the second page were written in the native language of the participant. As a result, an interpreter will continue to support the project to translate the comments from this training and for future work so as to expand the curriculum to include other health conditions.

A second challenge was to identify strategies to incorporate dietary topics in the training, given the cultural, social, and economic implications of diet and nutrition. To address this, the UVA students undertook novel approaches and collaborated with DOH colleagues. One approach included a field trip to local grocery stores and markets to discover the food that was available in the larger city where UNIVEN is located and that was close to where the research team lived. Another approach reviewed circulars (inserts from local grocery stores). Based on this research, laminated cards were developed with common foods, including the nutritional value that was used in the workshop. At tea time, samples of lower-fat foods or protein alternatives such as fruit or peanut butter sandwiches were provided. Initially, the participants provided feedback that the peanut butter sandwiches at tea were not well received. However, things turned around at lunch. Our DOH colleagues provided a mixture of local foods with an emphasis on locally grown vegetables, lean meat, and an edible caterpillar protein source, maponi (mapone) worms. The participants were more appreciative of the lunch menu because it reflected more culturally appropriate choices.

Sixty CHWs completed the training. Across all trainings, 94% of participants felt better able to help their patients as a result of the training, 93% noted that they could use the information they learned in their daily work, and 76% reported that what they learned would change their practice. As an outcome of the workshop, a training manual for hypertension and diabetes mellitus management is now available for use across the Limpopo District.

In summary, the historical tripartite collaboration UNIVEN, DOH, and UVA was essential to the success of the CHW trainings. The UNIVEN faculty students provided critical interpretation of the language and culture and the DOH staff helped to incorporate traditional foods into our training. The close linkage to the DOH, the community partner for UNIVEN and UVA, made it likely that knowledge, skills, and resources from the trainings could be applied in clinical practice. In the future, research studies can evaluate the effects on health outcomes at an individual or community level based on these changes to clinical practice.

INTRODUCTION

America is more of "mixed salad" than a "melting pot" and is composed of diverse groups of individuals. Yet the nursing profession in the United States does not reflect the diversity of the population it serves. This is a significant challenge for the nursing profession and for the 83.2% of non-Hispanic white nurses (American Association of Colleges of Nursing [AACN], 2013). The nursing profession needs to address recruitment of a diverse workforce and the preparation of professional nurses who are competent to deliver culturally responsive care. Professional nurses must develop the knowledge, skills, and values to provide culturally sensitive care. Professional nursing is uniquely positioned to address health care disparities within the health care delivery system. This chapter explores the relationship between diversity and health and offers frameworks for exploring culture and care. Specific nursing-related barriers, strategies, and resources are identified for developing cultural competency in health care delivery.

Diversity and Health

We live in a pluralistic society, and it is becoming more evident that cultural differences, if not acknowledged, will increasingly serve to isolate and alienate us from one another. It is not enough to simply educate people about cultural differences; one must also confront these competing standards of truth. Given that health care professionals learn from their culture the "art" of being healthy or ill, it is imperative for health professionals to treat each patient with respect to his or her own cultural background. *Culture* can be defined in multiple ways. In general, most definitions encompass socially inherited and shared beliefs, practices, habits, customs, language, and rituals. It shapes how people view their world and how they function within that world. It can transcend generations. The one unifying theme in defining culture is that it is *learned*. Much of what we believe, think, and act is attributable to culture. Hence one's culture can profoundly determine what is perceived as health versus illness. There are also numerous definitions for diversity. Many people define *diversity* simply as racial or ethnic differences. This chapter considers diversity more broadly to encompass differences that may be rooted not only in culture, but also in age, health status, gender, sexual orientation, racial or ethnic identity, geographical location, or other aspects of

sociocultural description and socioeconomic position (Kennedy, Fisher, Fontaine, & Martin-Holland, 2008). Given the importance of culture in how we define ourselves and our environment, each person must be treated with respect and his or her cultural sensitivity must be valued.

How nurses incorporate the patient's cultural diversity in their general plans of care can mean the difference between success and failure (Stanfield & Brown, 2013). Cultural issues are crucial to all clinical care and management of illness because culture shapes health-related beliefs, values, and behaviors. Thus, providing culturally responsive care requires that the nurse, when confronted with culturally diverse patients, is attuned to the cultural cues while balancing sensitivity, knowledge, and skills to accommodate social, cultural, biological, psychosocial, and spiritual needs of the client respectfully (Kulbok, Mitchell, Glick, & Greiner, 2012). When clinicians are focused only on the signs and symptoms of a disease and do not reflect on and explore the physical, social, cultural, and symbolic environments of the people who are seeking care, there is a distortion of reality and a strong possibility that the needs of patients and their caregivers will not be met (Campinha-Bacote, 2002; Leininger, 1991; Stanfield & Brown, 2013).

The importance of being sensitive to cultural diversity cannot be overemphasized. The ability to build on strengths, and understand and respect diverse cultures results in interventions that can lead to healthy practices and behaviors. Health and illness can be perceived in a variety of ways. Acknowledging the significance of culture in people's problems as well as solutions is essential. Numerous expectations exist regarding appropriate treatment and care. Cultural values and social norms greatly affect the interaction and outcomes for both nurses and patients (Box 14-1).

As the United States continues to increase in diversity, nurses will be providing care for patients from many different backgrounds. It would be unrealistic for nurses to know the cultural traits of every diverse group (Engebretson, Mahoney, & Carlson, 2008). Instead, nurses must appreciate cultural diversity and demonstrate due respect and appropriate caring behaviors.

Many theoretical frameworks provide contextual bases for understanding and providing culturally *and* linguistically appropriate care. Leininger's 1991 theoretical framework for transcultural nursing emphasizes

BOX 14-1   Case Study: Visiting

When Ellen began her clinical rotation on a large American-Indian (Lakota) reservation, her thinking revolved around what she could teach the community workers. She spent days traveling many miles with various community health representatives (CHRs). These were American-Indian men and women who had approximately 1 month of training (sometimes in addition to other training and student experiences). They then assumed roles as providers, visiting homes of other tribe members, doing routine and basic care, and acting as liaisons between the American-Indian population and the biomedical system. Slowly, Ellen realized how Lakota culture shaped the CHRs' and other residents' perceptions of health, illness, and their expectations for treatment and care. As the weeks went on and Ellen learned to be open to new ways of knowing and doing things, her interpretations changed, as her following journal entries indicate:

Week 1: "The CHRs don't really do anything. They just go and drink coffee and sit down and visit."

Week 2: "I think they just visit because they don't know what else to do. They even talk about themselves and their kids' problems. And they are all quiet a lot. Sometimes, they hardly talk about the patient's problem."

Week 3: "You know, something happens when the CHRs visit, but I don't know what it is. I don't see how their visiting works, but I see that people appreciate it."

Week 4: "The patients do what the CHRs want them to do. Something goes on, but I don't get it; they never actually tell the patients what to do."

Week 5: "I still don't see how the visiting works when the CHRs don't do much instruction. They do other things—wash the quadriplegic man's long hair, dress decubitus ulcers, weigh babies—but mostly they visit. Somehow it works."

Week 6: "I've got it. Visiting is what the CHRs do. That is what is important and how they intervene. It is because of the visiting that the patients respond, not because of what the CHRs do when they visit."

the commonalities and differences among worldviews of diverse health systems (Figure 14-1). This depiction of the many interrelated dimensions of culture and care is useful for exploring important meanings and patterns of care. She focused on comparative culture care examined through a holistic and multidimensional lens (Leininger, 2002). The purpose of the theory is to provide culturally congruent, safe, and meaningful care to clients from different or similar cultures. Furthermore, it posits that worldview as well as cultural and social structures influence care outcomes related to culturally congruent care; generic emic (folk) practices (an

attempt to understand the viewpoint of the people themselves) and professional etic nursing practices (according to the principles, methods, and interests of the observer) influence outcomes; and the three modes for transcultural care actions and decisions (culture preservation and/or maintenance; cultural care accommodation and/or negotiation; and cultural care repatterning and/or restructuring) provide culturally congruent care (Leininger, 2002). Further discussion of Leininger's framework occurs in Chapter 5.

Another model for examining cultural competence in nursing care is the Campinha-Bacote Model of Cultural Competence (Campinha-Bacote, 2002). In this model, nurses continuously work toward cultural competence by addressing five constructs: cultural awareness, cultural knowledge, cultural skill, cultural encounters, and cultural desire. The final—and perhaps the most important—concept in the model is cultural desire or wanting to become culturally competent (Campinha-Bacote, 2002, www.transculturalcare.net).

The Campinha-Bacote Model of Cultural Competence is an interactional dynamic model of cultural competence that requires achievement of all five identified constructs. The process of cultural awareness occurs when the nurse is able to examine his or her own values, biases, and stereotypes. It also requires the nurse to examine the potential cultural biases (racism) that may exist within the health care setting. The process of cultural knowledge occurs when nurses educate themselves about the worldviews of other cultures and ethnic groups. This cultural knowledge may include learning how disease processes and management may vary depending on the cultural group. Cultural skill occurs when the nurse can conduct a relevant cultural assessment. Hence, it is achieved when cultural data are used to develop and implement a culturally relevant treatment plan. Cultural encounters encourage the nurse to engage directly with patients from different ethnic and cultural backgrounds to modify existing beliefs about a cultural group and prevent potential stereotyping. Finally, cultural desire addresses the motivation of the health care provider to acquire new knowledge about different cultures. This last construct is based solely on the nurse's intrinsic need to acquire new cultural knowledge and cannot be driven by external regulations or requirements (Kulbok et al., 2012).

Similar to the Campinha-Bacote model, the U.S. Health Resources Services Administration attempted to

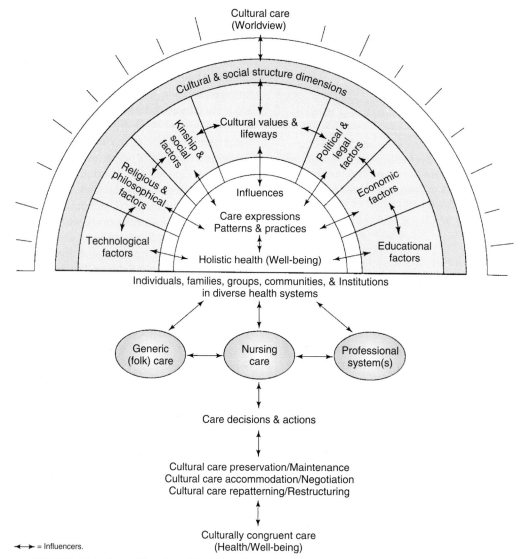

FIGURE 14-1 A modification of Leininger's model of transcultural nursing. (Modified from Leininger, M. M. [1991]. *Culture care diversity and universality: A theory of nursing.* New York: National League for Nursing; with permission of the National League for Nursing, New York, NY.)

identify the critical domains of cultural competence for health care providers and organizations with enhanced national Culturally and Linguistically Appropriate Services (CLAS) in Health and Health Care Standards (United States Department of Health and Human Services [USDHHS], 2013, available at minorityhealth. hhs.gov). The CLAS standards are comprised of eight domains: governance, leadership, workforce, communication, language assistance, engagement, continuous improvement, and accountability. By addressing all eight domains, health care providers and organizations can achieve cultural competence.

VALUES THAT SHAPE HEALTH CARE AND NURSING

The discipline of nursing reflects the values and norms of a society; in the United States, these values and norms are predominantly Eurocentric, middle class, Christian, and androcentric in view. In general the American culture tends to value personal freedom and independence (Ulrich et al., 2010) as well as individual achievement over the common good (Beauchamp & Childress, 2009; Shaw & Degazon, 2008). For example, the concept of a single autonomous decision maker that is the hallmark of a Eurocentric worldview does not accurately capture the involvement of family members and other significant people in health care decision making (Stanfield & Brown, 2013). The notion that everyone be treated exactly the same is idealized and unrealistic. Traditionally, health care providers are presumed to know more about their patients' needs than do the patients themselves. This concept, known as *paternalism*, is discussed further in Chapter 12. Although there is a growing movement to listen and incorporate patients' goals and beliefs in their care, this continues to be a challenge when patients' beliefs differ greatly from those of the providers of health care.

NURSING'S CHALLENGE

Nursing is in a strategic position to provide care to diverse groups with diverse expectations, problems, and goals. Not surprisingly, nurses manage patients who are generally underserved. Today's nurses attend to both population-based and individual patterns and needs (Farrell, McCabe, & Jevit, 2013). Many nurses realize that respectful encounters with topics such as race, ethnicity, religion, politics, gender, sexual orientation, and belief systems outside biomedicine are essential to providing effective nursing care (Stanfield & Brown, 2013). However, some nurses still practice with the inherent belief that patients who disagree with them are wrong. Others acknowledge the diversity they encounter but are overwhelmed by its complexity. Despite these perceived difficulties, the integration of patients' beliefs and values can result in effective nursing care (Farrell et al., 2013).

The paucity of nurses prepared in nursing school to manage diversity effectively is daunting. A commitment to diversity is a value in many schools of nursing; however, faculty members may lack the skills and resources to incorporate diversity into their syllabi, teaching strategies, and course evaluation (Kennedy et al., 2008). Moreover, the lack of diversity among nursing faculty and students in nursing schools further compounds this issue. The Sullivan Commission

(2004) report on diversity in the health care workforce underscored the scarcity of minority faculty and students in nursing. A report by the American Association of Colleges of Nursing (AACN), Enrollment and Graduations in Baccalaureate and Graduate Programs in Nursing 2010–2011 (AACN, 2013) provides descriptive information about minority nursing students and faculty. Students from minority backgrounds represented 26.8% of students in entry-level baccalaureate programs, a 0.8% increase from the 2008 data, 26.1% of master's students, and 22.3% of students in research-focused doctoral programs. In terms of gender breakdown, men accounted for 11.4% in 2013. Although a 3% increase in minority students enrolling in baccalaureate nursing education is promising, the future still looks bleak for minority faculty. The majority of faculty members in schools of nursing are not minorities either. In fact it is estimated that only 12.3% of full-time nursing school faculty come from minority backgrounds, and only 5.4% are male (AACN, 2013). Without representation from diverse ethnic, racial, and gender perspectives, the potential for disseminating alternate views on providing culturally responsive care diminishes. For the first time the lack of diversity in the educational experience of health care professionals and in the workforce has been linked to issues of quality and patient safety. Patient safety is explored in more detail in Chapter 20. The scarcity of diverse perspectives in race, ethnicity, culture, and language in health care settings increases the possibility for discordance during health care visits. Racial and language discordance can have an impact on patient and family health care literacy and negatively affect the safe, timely, and effective use of medications and other treatments (Stanfield & Brown, 2013).

Members of diverse groups are increasingly acknowledged to have rights to their own distinct lifestyles, values, and norms (Stanfield & Brown, 2013). In nursing the ability to communicate and work interculturally and to understand culture-based care and caring practices is viewed as essential to providing high-quality, effective care (Kulbok et al., 2012). Our education must reflect the diversity of the individuals and communities we serve.

DECREASING BIASES

The concepts of race and ethnicity are commonly thought to be dominant elements of culture. However, culture, as defined in the preceding, is much broader than this, and each concept has a different meaning. No one definition can encompass the meaning of race. The most widely used methods for defining races are those based on skin color, facial features, ancestry, and national origin. Many social scientists argue that most racial definitions are imprecise, arbitrary, derived from custom, and vary among cultures. Hence, defining human beings on the basis of race is related more to sociopolitical constructs than to science. The U.S. Office of Management and Budget (1997) responded to criticism and revised its standards for classifying federal data on race and ethnicity. The new standards set five categories for data on race, including (1) American Indian or Alaska Native, (2) Asian, (3) Black or African American, (4) Native Hawaiian or other Pacific Islander, and (5) White. A separate designation for data on ethnicity includes two categories: (1) Hispanic or Latino and (2) not Hispanic or Latino. Racial and ethnic categories set forth in the standards should not be interpreted as being primarily biological or genetic in reference. Race and ethnicity may be thought of in terms of social and cultural characteristics as well as ancestry. Often people fail to consider other factors that influence culture and determine how people think and behave—for instance, age, educational level, income level, geographical residence, length of residency in the United States, and specific health care beliefs about time, personal space, and eye contact, to name just a few.

Ethnicity is usually defined as membership of a person in a particular cultural group. Ethnic groups usually have a sense of shared common origins, distinct history, or collective cultural individuality (Spector, 2004). Thus, people may be in the same ethnic group, yet have different nationalities. Ethnicity appears to be a more viable mechanism than race for examining similarities and differences. However, in the United States, race still influences everyday social experience; it is one major issue that today's nurses must confront to manage diversity effectively.

More than 3000 different cultural groups exist in the world. Regardless of their ability to interact with 20 or 200 patients, nurses must be sensitive to recognize and confront their own biases that may hinder their ability to provide quality care (Kulbok et al., 2012). A *bias* can be defined as influence in a particular, typically unfair direction (prejudice). To manage diversity effectively, nurses must be sensitive to both differences and similarities, knowledgeable about expected patterns of behavior, and skillful at integrating their sensitivity and knowledge into appropriate assessment and interventions. Information about acceptable patterns of behavior and their interpretation always should be tested against an individual's perception of a specific situation. Not verifying one's own perception with that of the individual may lead to biases and stereotyping.

Nurses should identify their own personal prejudices and biases because these biases may distort the level of care that is provided. Self-awareness or cultural awareness is the first step toward becoming culturally competent (Leininger, 2002; Purnell & Paulanka, 2003). Biases can be so intrinsic that the nurse is unaware of them. Research studies have found that health care providers can unknowingly bias the care provided to patients on the basis of race or gender (Campesino, 2008; Cully, 2006; Kirk et al., 2005). With open communication and changing prejudgments of a person's cultural beliefs and customs, intrinsic biases can be mitigated. Figure 14-2 illustrates the positive and negative consequences to biases.

"COLOR BLIND" AND OTHER OXYMORONS

The U.S. Census and Healthy People 2020 (HP 2020) provide valuable information about how populations have changed over time. Rarely have these organizations focused on the cultural values, beliefs, and practices or preferences of a particular subgroup.

As a result there is limited evidence to understand one's behavior around health care issues. However, we can learn how the health of our nation is changing by examining the trends over time.

Between 2000 and 2010, life expectancy has increased and infant mortality has decreased for all racial/ethnic groups (National Center for Health Statistics, 2012). Overall the trends in health status have steadily been improving. Recent studies have shown that racial and ethnic minorities continue to experience a lower quality of health services and they are less likely to receive routine medical procedures (Haider et al., 2013; Hasnain-Wynia, et al., 2007; McClelland et al., 2013). Additionally, racial and ethnic minorities have higher rates of morbidity and mortality than nonminorities (National Center for Health Statistics, 2012). These disparities continue to exist even after controlling

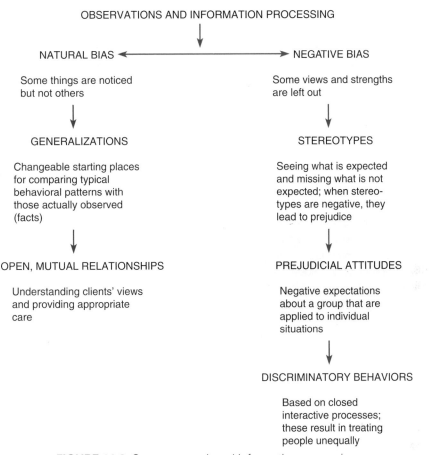

OBSERVATIONS AND INFORMATION PROCESSING

NATURAL BIAS ← → NEGATIVE BIAS

Some things are noticed but not others

Some views and strengths are left out

GENERALIZATIONS

STEREOTYPES

Changeable starting places for comparing typical behavioral patterns with those actually observed (facts)

Seeing what is expected and missing what is not expected; when stereotypes are negative, they lead to prejudice

OPEN, MUTUAL RELATIONSHIPS

PREJUDICIAL ATTITUDES

Understanding clients' views and providing appropriate care

Negative expectations about a group that are applied to individual situations

DISCRIMINATORY BEHAVIORS

Based on closed interactive processes; these result in treating people unequally

FIGURE 14-2 Open versus closed information processing.

for gender, condition, age, and socioeconomic status. In 2013, the National Healthcare Disparities Report (NHDR), produced by the Agency for Healthcare Research and Quality (AHRQ, 2013) on behalf of the U.S. Department of Health and Human Services (USDHHS), reported that although health care quality is improving, access to health care is getting worse, and the disparities are not changing.

Recent evidence shows that African Americans have the most severe burden of human immunodeficiency virus (HIV) of all racial/ethnic groups in the United States. They account for a higher proportion of HIV infections at all stages of disease from new infections to deaths. For example, the estimated rate of new HIV infections for black women (38.1/100,000 population) was 20 times as high as the rate for white women, and almost five times as high as that of Latinas (Centers for Disease Control [CDC], 2013). American Indians (AI)

and Alaska Native (AN) mothers were twice as likely to lack prenatal care and experienced high infant mortality at a rate 1.7 times higher than non-Hispanic white mothers (CDC, 2013). Moreover, the AI and AN infant mortality rate from sudden infant death syndrome (SIDS) is higher than any population group (CDC, 2013).

Clearly, access to health care varies greatly for African Americans, Hispanics, and other racial/ethnic minorities compared with whites, as well as for poor communities compared with more higher-income populations (Hanchate et al., 2012; Rosenbaum, 2011; Safford et al., 2012). These disparities may be partly attributed to higher rates of unemployment and jobs without health benefits among minority populations. In 2012, the census bureau estimated that 48 million people in the United States are uninsured (United States Census Bureau, 2013). Having health insurance is consistently associated with access to health care and the quality of care

(Meropol et al., 2009). A large number of studies find race-based differences in the receipt of primary health care and therapeutic procedures for a broad range of conditions and health outcomes (Brooks-Carthon, Jarrin, Sloane, & Kutney-Lee 2013), even after adjustments in insurance status and severity of disease (Ibrahim & Franklin, 2013; Pathman, Fowler-Brown, & Corbie-Smith, 2006). Regarding the effectiveness of local and national initiatives to reduce surgical procedural differences between African-American and white older adults, over a 10-year period (1992–2001) racial disparities continue to exist (Jha, Fisher, Li, Orav, & Epstein, 2005). In fact, access to five surgical procedures significantly differed between African-American and white older adults. Differentiated care still exists within the American health care system.

One easy but ineffective method for avoiding the difficult work of addressing racial issues is to be "color blind." Pretending that everyone in society is equal and that issues of disparate access are in the past perpetuates societal patterns of differential treatment based on race, culture, and so forth (Campbell, 2007; Hassouneh, 2006). This approach to health care simply denies that variations in life experiences exist. For example, the disparities that exist between African Americans and whites in their use of hospice services at the present time have been linked to the different social realities for these populations during the period when hospice was first introduced in the United States (Carrion, Park, & Lee, 2012). The hospice movement had its genesis in the late 1960s and early 1970s as an alternative to hospital-based care for people with life-limiting illness. At this same time, African Americans were not looking for an alternative to hospital-based end-of-life care; they were seeking equal access to the services available to whites in their communities. For them, the hospice alternative was perceived as second-rate care—a myth that persists today in many minority communities (Campbell, 2007; Taxis, 2006). This is an example of how patients can become resentful when their unique experiences are ignored. Many aspects of racism and other biases can be institutionalized such that individuals fail to recognize that these societal structures have created an environment for disparities to exist. This failure to consider the unique experiences of minorities further perpetuates and condones the behavior (Hassouneh, 2006). Acknowledging and challenging the currently existing biases within oneself and health care institutions are first steps in eliminating disparities. Simply

increasing one's knowledge about different cultural groups of people does not necessarily negate biased attitudes that may be internalized, nor does increasing one's knowledge about the cultural beliefs and practices mean that the health professional will be able to effectively interact with someone from another cultural group (Campesino, 2008).

Diversification of America

The United States has become increasingly diverse in the last century. According to the U.S. Census Bureau (2011) in 2010 there were 50.5 million Hispanics in the United States (16% of the total population), a 43% increase from the year 2000. The non-Hispanic population grew relatively slower over the same decade, only a 5% increase. Ninety-seven percent of all respondents to the 2010 census reported only one race (229.7 million). The largest group reported the white alone (223.6 million or 72%) followed by the black or African American alone population (38.9 million/13%). The next largest minority group identified their race as Asian alone (14.7 million/5%). The Asian population grew faster than any other race group between 2000 and 2010. American Indian and Alaska Native alone represented 2.9 million respondents (0.9%), whereas the smallest major race group was Native Hawaiian and other Pacific Islander alone (0.5 million/0.2%).

The U.S. Census Bureau (2011) predicts that within the next 90 years non-Hispanic whites will account for 40% of the U.S. population. Simply stated, in less than a century, racial and ethnic minorities will become the majority in the United States. In 2011, five states and the District of Columbia were found to be "majority-minority." Majority-minority states are those where more than 50% of the population is made up of people other than single-race non-Hispanic whites. Hawaii led the nation with a population that was 77% minority in 2010, followed by California (60%) and New Mexico (60%). About 55% of Texas' population was minority in 2010 and the District of Columbia's population was 65% majority-minority, which was lower than reported in 2000. Next in line, although not majority-minority states but significant proportions of the population were minority, were Nevada, Maryland, Arizona, Florida, and Georgia, each with a minority population approached 50%. Nevada had the highest proportion minority (46%).

As the racial and ethnic diversity of the U.S. population continues to increase, so does the need for health care professionals to acquire knowledge about such populations to provide culturally responsive care. Although some people may find these projections threatening and others may find them hopeful, nursing at times seems to be stuck between "fight and flight" in managing such realities. Demanding conformity to a single set of norms is no longer acceptable. Social variation continues despite a homogenized culture that permeates every household with standardized fast food and consumer expectations. As a society, the United States is moving toward a truer democracy and nursing must adapt to this reality.

INDIVIDUAL VERSUS GROUP IDENTITY

The delivery of nursing care is usually individualized to the patient. However, for many cultures the nurse must be more cognizant of the influence of the patient's family. In fact, in some cultures nursing care decisions are not considered solely the wishes of the patient (the American way) but must take into consideration the wishes and decisions of all family members. In many Asian and African cultures, decisions are made by groups or by heads of groups. Although care may be individualized for each patient, nurses must become comfortable with managing patients in the collective terms of their families. Also, nurses must recognize that the process of acculturation differs for everyone. That

is, acculturation may occur at different rates among families of the same cultural background, as well as among members of the same family. In fact, each community, whether grouped by culture, ethnicity, religion, sexual orientation, or another self-identified category, will have its own variations within the group (Agar, 2006; Engebretson et al., 2008), including treatment preferences or health-related behaviors. Ignoring these issues will perpetuate the problems of stereotyping and prejudice, which can lead to misdiagnosis and culturally incompetent care.

CARE BARRIERS AND RESOURCES

Although the diversity within the American population should be celebrated, this factor can pose barriers to health care delivery because of issues related to language, economics, and potential distrust of health providers (Box 14-2). For example, many older African Americans have a general distrust of health care providers, an opinion rooted, at least partly, in the Tuskegee syphilis study in which 399 poor African-American sharecroppers in Macon County, Alabama, were denied treatment for syphilis and deceived by physicians of the U.S. Public Health Service from 1932 to 1972 (Brandon, Isaac, & La Veist, 2005). One goal of the Tuskegee syphilis study was to chronicle the natural evolution of syphilis in the African-American community to see

---

BOX 14-2 Case Study: Barriers to Care

Joy, a community health nurse (CHN), prepared to visit an older American-Indian man, Mr. Murphy, who had been hospitalized with bronchitis, and an elderly American-Indian woman, Mrs. Bird, who was characterized as "noncompliant" with her dialysis treatment and who consumed alcohol. Joy had numerous other clients who could use home visits, but in the rural area in which they lived, homes were miles apart and difficult to locate, roads were often treacherous, and few people had phones for verifying availability. Each attempted visit involved the time of a translator as well as the CHN.

When Joy and the translator arrived at the home of Mrs. Bird, she was away having a healing ceremony. Joy interpreted this as a good sign; perhaps she would return to dialysis after the ceremony. "What else can I do?" Joy asked herself. "I can't leave her a note; she does not read English." Next, Joy and the translator moved on to the small home of Mr. Murphy. They asked whether he was taking his medicine, and he showed them several bottles of pills, still full. They ask whether he had eaten breakfast. He described bacon and eggs.

But the unwashed dishes in the sink lacked evidence, and the wood stove that served both to heat the tiny dwelling and for cooking was not warm. "One order of Meals on Wheels coming up," quipped Joy to the translator when they returned to the car, "at least when they can get back there. But the pills? Mr. Murphy knows I want him to take them. He says he has them for when he needs them. I will try to visit him more often and have others check on him, but I must respect his choices."

1. If you had been that visiting nurse, how would you have responded to each of the clients? In your response, make sure that you demonstrate your understanding of the culture.
2. How could the knowledge of cultural practices have been used to help patients be successful with their treatment plan?
3. How might it have been possible to incorporate traditional healing or folk remedies with mainstream Western medicine when developing a treatment plan for Mr. Murphy and Mrs. Bird?

whether it differed from the same disease process in the white community. Hence these poor, uneducated African-American men were told they were being treated for "bad blood." However, government officials went to extraordinary measures to block the men from receiving treatment for their syphilis. Many argue that the distrust engendered by this study is a significant factor in the low participation of African Americans in clinical trials, organ donation efforts, and routine preventive care.

As discussed earlier, nurses need to be prepared to attend to the various culturally and linguistically diverse populations' preferences and needs to access the health care services they need. In particular, often there is a need for greater access to interpreters and culturally appropriate communication and education. If not addressed, patients may feel that they have experienced racism or discrimination. As a result, patients may not participate fully in their health care plans or in the decision-making process with health care providers. Addressing these barriers and ensuring that health care organizations invest in culturally tailored programs that are in line with the needs of diverse communities, the United States can achieve better health care.

Resources

The increasing racial and ethnic diversity of the U.S. population makes it essential that nurses acquire knowledge and develop a skill set to provide care that is culturally responsive. The Office of Minority Health (U.S. Department of Health and Human Services [USDHHS], 2007) has developed several excellent resources for health care providers, including a three-module training series on cultural competence called Culturally Competent Nursing Modules. Introduced in 2007, the training program consists of an introduction followed by the three modules. Modules can be studied separately or as a group, and nurses can earn up to 9 hours of continuing education credit. The content is based on the National Standards for CLAS. The modules are self-directed, interactive, and web based. A DVD version is available so that the content can be used in a group setting. Case studies and reflective exercises provide an opportunity for nurses to explore issues of diversity in the health care setting, such as honoring religious beliefs and practices, incorporating alternative and complementary treatments into the plan of care, and creating a health care environment that is truly inclusive (USDHHS, 2007).

Another resource sponsored by the Office of Minority Health is the Think Cultural Health website (USDHHS, 2009). The site (www.thinkcultural health.hhs.gov) offers the latest resources and tools to promote cultural competence in health care and includes free online courses accredited for continuing education credit as well as additional resources to help providers and organizations promote respectful, culturally congruent, high-quality care to an increasingly diverse patient population. Additional content includes online courses such as "A Physician's Practical Guide to Culturally Competent Care" and "Culturally Competent Nursing Care," as well as interactive tools such as the "Health Care Language Services Implementation Guide" (USDHHS, 2009). Another recent and free online course on effective communication, developed by the U.S. Department of Health and Human Services, Health Resources and Services Administration (HRSA, 2013) has been provided to improve not only health care communication overall, but specifically improve communication with a focus on medically underserved patients (i.e., those who are low income, uninsured, and/or whose English proficiency is low; http://www.hrsa.gov/culturalcompetence/index.html).

Nurses are in a unique position because they often function as the gatekeepers between the patient and the health care system. Thus, they facilitate flow of information from patients to health care providers while maintaining the dignity of the patient. Nurses must have a good knowledge of the health behaviors and beliefs of a diverse group of patients. This knowledge can be acquired from a variety of methods (e.g., listening to patients and families, reading books, accessing computer-based programs). Hassouneh (2006) cautions nursing students, practicing nurses, and nursing faculty about relying solely on a "cookbook" approach to learning culturally responsive care. Cultural assessment is a dynamic process that begins with willingness of the student to explore not only the person's culture, but also their own biases that might prevent a full exploration. The placement of unique value on holism positions nurses to understand, respect, and protect the individual differences within the patient populations served.

Cultural Assessment Strategies

Cultural assessment has two aspects: the desire to acquire knowledge of a different culture and the strategies for acquiring knowledge of that different culture. The desire to acquire knowledge of a new culture is an intrinsic process. No one can force the nurse to acquire this knowledge. To assist with the continuous appraisal of cultural competence, the acronym ASKED, based on the Campinha-Bacote Model of Cultural Competence (Campinha-Bacote, 2002), was developed to assist health care providers in understanding several key concepts that influence the health care process. Some of these areas include recognizing one's own biases and prejudices, conveying skills in a sensitive manner to all, familiarizing oneself with diverse worldviews about health care, and seeking out opportunities to learn from someone who is different from oneself. Addressing these key areas of cultural competence is critical for one's journey to becoming culturally competent. This is an excellent model to examine desire for cultural knowledge acquisition.

Once the desire for obtaining cultural knowledge is present, developing a framework of strategies to acquire the knowledge is important. Categories of strategies for a basic cultural assessment are presented in Box 14-3. These strategies are helpful in identifying general lifestyles and health patterns that may help in nursing care planning and interventions. Nurses should never assume that particular beliefs, practices, or supports do or do not exist. Expected patterns always must be contrasted with actual, individual situations. Finally it is important to recognize that the process of becoming culturally competent and being sensitive to others' cultural beliefs occurs along a continuum. Nurses will be at different points on the continuum—and each individual nurse may be at a different point of the continuum with each minority group served.

Linking Diversity to Outcomes for Patients/Families and the Organization

Over the last 20 years, health care organizations have developed diversity initiatives to seek employees "who looked like people in the community they serve." Health Care Organizations recruited people of color as employees, created diversity committees, community advisory boards, and created events to demonstrate a commitment to diversity. Although diversity initiatives to date have been started with the best intentions,

---

BOX 14-3   Approaches Recommended for All Cultural Groups

- Provide a feeling of acceptance.
- Establish open communication.
- Present yourself with confidence. Introduce yourself. Shake hands if it is appropriate.
- Strive to gain your client's trust, but don't be resentful if you don't get it.
- Understand what members of the cultural or subcultural group consider to be "caring," both attitudinally and behaviorally.
- Understand the perceived relationship between your client and authority.
- Understand your client's desire to please you and his or her motivations to comply or not comply.
- Anticipate diversity. Avoid stereotypes based on sex, age, ethnicity, socioeconomic status, and so forth.
- Do not make assumptions about where people come from. Let them tell you.
- Understand the client's goals and expectations.
- Make your goals realistic.
- Emphasize positive points and strengths of health beliefs and practices.
- Show respect, especially for men, even if you are interested in the women or children. Men are often decision makers about follow-up.

- Be prepared for the fact that children go everywhere with some cultural groups as well as with poorer families, who may have few child care options. Include them.
- Know the traditional, health-related practices common to the group with whom you are working. Do not discredit them unless you know they are harmful.
- Know the folk illnesses and remedies common to the group with whom you are working.
- Try to make the clinic setting comfortable. Consider colors, music, atmosphere, scheduling expectations, pace, tone, seating arrangements, and so forth.
- Whenever possible and appropriate, involve the leaders of the local group. Confidentiality is important, but the leaders know the problems and often can suggest acceptable interventions.
- Respect values, beliefs, rights, and practices. Some may conflict with your own or with your determination to make changes. But every group and individual wants respect above all else.
- Learn to appreciate the richness of diversity as an asset, rather than a hindrance, in your work.

the outcomes have not been measurable or sustainable because the diversity initiatives were not fully integrated into an organization's strategic plan or linked directly to patient/family outcomes such as access to quality care, effective patient/family-provider communication or satisfaction with care provided (Davidson, 2011).

Successful organizations will make the business case for "seeking differences that matter" as a strategy to maintain the health and resilience of the organization so it can meet its mission. Davidson (2011) suggests that Directors of Diversity initiatives should become "Chief Learning Officers" to guide the discovery at all levels of the organization. Rather than focusing on diversity as a nebulous concept, the focus should be on a four-step process described by Davidson: (1) identify strategically relevant differences; (2) develop strategies to learn about the relevant differences; (3) integrate what is salient to the target population into programs and services; and (4) create results from the relevant differences. Once an organization captures relevant differences, services or programs can be integrated in the strategic plan. The outcomes for patients/families and the healthcare organization can be evaluated. The process will ensure that an organization meets the needs of people in its service area and ultimately positively impact the organization's financial viability (Davidson, 2011; National Hospice and Palliative Care Organization [NHPCO], 2007).

SUMMARY

America is composed of a diverse group of individuals; yet 83.2% of nursing professionals are non-Hispanic whites (AACN, 2013). Thus, there is a great need for nurses to engage in learning experiences that create new ways of examining culture and diversity. Many note that the United States is not so much a "melting pot" as a "tossed salad." If this is true, nurses must strive to understand the similarities and dissimilarities among the patient populations served. Remaining cognizant of personal intrinsic biases and those that permeate throughout the health system is vital.

Because nurses serve as gatekeepers to the health care system, they are in a unique position to help bridge the gap in the disparities that exist for diverse patients. As nurses acquire cultural competencies, they in turn will help break the barriers that divide in the health care system.

Dr. Josepha Campinha-Bacote (2006) spoke to the progress toward cultural competence in nursing education: "I contend that nursing is on a progressive course toward successfully answering the question, 'How do we effectively teach cultural competence in nursing education?' We must realize that it is a journey that reflects an ongoing transformational process" (p. 244).

SALIENT POINTS

- Cultural views of individuals and groups influence perception of health and health care.
- Diversity management uses affirmation and encouragement to move toward development of the client's full potential.
- Open and honest communication can facilitate nurse-client relationships to provide a better understanding of clients' perspectives of health and illness.
- Health care professionals and institutions may possess intrinsic biases against differing cultures; thus nurses must remain hypervigilant to identify and correct those biases.
- Culturally congruent care incorporates those cultural characteristics (e.g., religion, social relations, education, language) deemed important by the client.

- Cultural assessment in nursing involves systematic appraisal of beliefs, values, and practices of the client.
- Nurses must remain mindful not to make automatic assumptions about patients based on their cultural affiliation.
- Nurses must remain motivated to learn about different cultures to provide culturally relevant care.
- Nurses will either learn to manage diversity or be managed by it.
- Nurses can lead health care organizations in the exploration of "what differences matter?" to the communities we serve.

CRITICAL REFLECTION EXERCISES

1. Discuss strategies nurses could implement to promote culturally sensitive care.

2. Discuss current barriers within health care institutions that hinder culturally appropriate care.

3. How could a nurse develop the requisite balance of cultural sensitivity, knowledge, and skills needed to manage diverse clients effectively?

4. In your experience, what strategies work well for practice of culturally acceptable nursing assessment, communication, and intervention?

REFERENCES

Agar, M. (2006). Culture: Can you take it anywhere? *International Journal of Qualitative Methods, 5*(2). Retrieved on January 30, 2009, from https://ejournals.library.ualberta.ca/index.php/IJQM/article/view/4384/3513.

Agency for Healthcare Research and Quality. (July 2013). National Healthcare Quality & Disparities Reports. Rockville, MD. Retrieved on December 3, 2013, from http://www.ahrq.gov/research/findings/nhqrdr/index.html.

American Association of Colleges of Nursing (AACN). (2013). *Fact Sheet: Enhancing diversity in the nursing work force*. Retrieved on November 16, 2013, from http://www.aacn.nche.edu/Media/FactSheets/diversity.htm.

Beauchamp, T., & Childress, J. (2009). *Principles of biomedical ethics* (6th ed.). New York: Oxford.

Brandon, D. T., Isaac, L. A., & La Veist, T. A. (2005). The legacy of Tuskegee and trust in medical care: Is Tuskegee responsible for race differences in mistrust of medical care? *Journal of the National Medical Association, 97*, 951–956.

Brooks-Carthon, M., Jarrin, O., Sloane, D., & Kutney-Lee, A. (2013). Variations in postoperative complications according to race, ethnicity, and sex in older adults. *Journal of the American Geriatrics Society, 61*(9), 1499–1507.

Campbell, C. (2007). Respect for persons: Engaging African-Americans in end-of-life research. *Journal of Hospice and Palliative Care Nursing, 9*(2), 74–78.

Campesino, M. (2008). Beyond transculturalism: Critiques of cultural education in nursing. *Journal of Nursing Education, 47*(7), 298–304.

Campinha-Bacote, J. (2002). A culturally competent model of care. Retrieved on May 28, 2014, from http://www.transculturalcare.net.

Campinha-Bacote, J. (2006). Cultural competence in nursing curricula: How are we doing 20 years later? *Journal of Nursing Education, 45*(7), 243–244.

Carrion, I. V., Park, N. S., & Lee, B. S. (2012). Hospice use among African Americans, Asians, Hispanics, and Whites: Implications for practice. *American Journal of Hospice & Palliative Medicine, 29*(2), 116–121.

Centers for Disease Control, National Center for Health Statistics. (2012). *Health, United States, 2012: With special feature on emergency care*. Hyattsville, MD. Retrieved on December 3, 2013, from http://www.cdc.gov/nchs/data/hus/hus12.pdf.

Centers for Disease Control. (2013). *HIV among African-Americans (February 2013)*. Retrieved on December 3, 2013, from http://www.cdc.gov/hiv/statistics.

Centers for Disease Control (CDC). (2013). *Health disparities affecting minorities: American Indians and Alaska Natives*.

Coovadia, H., Jewkes, R., Barron, P., Sanders, D., & McIntyre, D. (2009). The health and health system of South Africa: Historical roots of current public health challenges. *The Lancet, 374*, 817–834.

Cully, L. (2006). Transcending transculturalism? Race, ethnicity and health care. *Nursing Inquiry, 13*, 144–153.

Davidson, M. (2011). *The end of diversity as we know it*. San Francisco: Berrett-Koehler.

Engebretson, J., Mahoney, J., & Carlson, E. (2008). Cultural competence in the era of evidence-based practice. *Journal of Professional Nursing, 24*(3), 172–178.

Farrell, B., McCabe, M. S., & Jevit, L. (2013). The Institute of Medicine report on high quality cancer care: Implications for oncology nursing. *Oncology Nursing Forum, 40*(6), 603–609.

Haider, A. H., Hashmi, Z. G., Zafar, S. N., Hui, X., Schneider, E. B., Efron, D. T., et al. (2013). Minority trauma patients tend to cluster at trauma centers with worse-than-expected mortality: Can this phenomenon help explain racial disparities in trauma outcomes? *Annals of Surgery, 258*(4), 572–579.

Hanchate, A., Lasser, K. E., Kapoor, A., Rosen, J., McCormick, D., D'Amore, M., & Kressin, N. R. (2012). Massachusetts Reform and Disparities in Inpatient Care Utilization. *Medical Care, 50*(7), 569–577.

Hasnain-Wynia, R., Baker, D. W., Nerenz, D., Feinglass, J., Beal, A. C., Landrum, M. B., et al. (2007). Disparities in health care are driven by where minorities seek care: Examination of the hospital quality alliance measures. *Archives of Internal Medicine, 167*, 1233–1239.

Hassouneh, D. (2006). Anti-racist pedagogy: Challenges faced by faculty of color in predominantly white schools of Nursing. *Journal of Nursing Education, 45*(7), 255–262.

Ibrahim, S. A., & Franklin, P. D. (2013). Race and elective joint replacement: Where a disparity meets patient preference. *American Journal of Public Health, 103*(4), 583–584.

Jha, A. K., Fisher, E. S., Li, Z., Orav, J. E., & Epstein, A. M. (2005). Racial trends in the use of major procedures among the elderly. *New England Journal of Medicine, 353,* 683–691.

Kennedy, H. P., Fisher, L., Fontaine, D., & Martin-Holland, J. (2008). Evaluating diversity in nursing education. *Journal of Transcultural Nursing, 19*(4), 363–370.

Kirk, J. K., Bell, R. A., Bertoni, A. G., Arcury, T. A., Quandt, S. A., & Goff, D. C. (2005). A qualitative review of studies of diabetes preventive care among minority patients in the United States, 1993–2003. *American Journal of Managed Care, 11,* 349–360.

Kulbok, P. A., Mitchell, E. M., Glick, D., & Greiner, D. (2012). International experiences in nursing education. *International Journal of Nursing Education Scholarship, 9*(1), 1–21.

Leininger, M. (2002). Culture care theory: A major contribution to advance transcultural nursing knowledge and practices. *Journal of Transcultural Nursing, 13,* 189–192.

Leininger, M. M. (1991). The theory of culture care diversity and universality. In M. M. Leininger (Ed.), *Culture and diversity and universality: A theory of nursing (NLN Publication No. 15-2402)* (pp. 5–68). New York: National League of Nursing.

McClelland, R. L., Jorgensen, N. W., Post, W. S., Szklo, M., Kronmal, R. A., et al. (2013). Methods for estimation of disparities in medication use in an observational cohort study: Results from the multi-ethnic study of stherosclerosis. *Pharmacoepidemiology & Drug Safety, 22*(5), 533–541.

Meropol, N. J., Schrag, D., Smith, T. J., Mulvey, T. M., Langdon, R. M., Jr, & Blum, D. (2009). American Society of Clinical Oncology guidance statement: The cost of cancer care. *Journal of Clinical Oncology, 27*(23), 3868–3874. doi http://dx.doi.org/10.1200/JCO.2009.23.1183.

National Hospice and Palliative Care Organization. (2007). *Inclusion access toolbox.* Alexandria, VA: Author.

Office of Management and Budget. (1997). *Revisions to the standards for the classification of federal data on race and ethnicity.* Retrieved on December 3, 2013, from http://www.whitehouse.gov/omb/fedreg/1997standards.html.

Pathman, D. E., Fowler-Brown, A., & Corbie-Smith, G. (2006). Differences in access to outpatient medical care for Black and White adults in the rural south. *Medical Care, 44*(5), 429–438.

Purnell, L. D., & Paulanka, B. J. (2003). *Transcultural health care: A culturally competent approach.* Philadelphia: Davis.

Rosenbaum, S. (2011). The patient protection and affordable care act: Implications for public health policy and practice. *Public Health Reports, 126*(1), 130–135.

Safford, M., Brown, T. M., Muntner, P. M., Durant, R. W., Glasser, S., Halanych, J. H., et al. (2012). Association of race and sex with risk of incident acute coronary heart disease events. *JAMA, 308*(17), 1768–1774.

Shaw, H. K., & Degazon, C. (2008). Integrating the core professional values of nursing: A profession, not just a career. *Journal of Cultural Diversity, 15*(1), 44–50.

South African Nursing Council (SANC). (2013). *South African Nursing Council Geographic Distribution 2012.* Retrieved on December 3, 2013, from http//www.sanc.co.za.

Spector, R. E. (2004). *Cultural diversity in health and illness* (6th ed.). Upper Saddle River, NJ: Pearson/Prentice-Hall.

Stanfield, D., & Browne, A. J. (2013). The relevance of indigenous knowledge for nursing curriculum. *International Journal of Nursing Education Scholarship, 10*(1), 1–19.

The Sullivan Commission. (2004). *Missing persons: Minorities in the health professions.* Retrieved on December 3, 2013, from http://www.aacn.nche.edu/Media/pdf/SullivanReport.pdf.

Taxis, J. C. (2006). Attitudes, values, and questions of African Americans regarding participation in hospice programs. *The Journal of Hospice and Palliative Care Nursing, 8*(2), 77–85.

Ulrich, C. M., Taylor, C., Soeken, K., O'Donnell, P., Farrar, A., Danis, M., & Grady, C. (2010). Everyday ethics: Ethical issues and stress in nursing practice. *Journal of Advanced Nursing, 66*(11), 2510–2519.

U.S. Census Bureau. (2011). U.S. Department of Commerce. *Overview of Race and Hispanic Origin: 2010.* Retrieved on December 4, 2013, from www.census.gov/population/www/socdemo/race/race.html.

U.S. Census Bureau. (2013). U.S. Department of Commerce. *Income, poverty, and health insurance coverage in the United States, 2012.* Retrieved on February 13, 2014, from www.census.gov/newsroom/releases/archives/income_wealth/ch12-165.html.

U.S. Department of Health and Human Services, Health Resources and Services Administration. (2013). *Health literacy free online course.* Retrieved from http://www.hrsa.gov/culturalcompetence/index.html.

U.S. Department of Health and Human Services, Office of Minority Health. (2007). *Culturally competent nursing modules.* Retrieved from https://www.thinkculturalhealth.hhs.gov/CCNM.

U.S. Department of Health and Human Services, Office of Minority Health. (2009). *Think cultural health.* Retrieved from http://www.thinkculturalhealth.hhs.gov.

Vhembe District, Department of Health. (2013). *Vhembe district wish list for 2013 technical assistance in partnership with University of Venda and University of Virginia* [Unpublished].

Vhembe District Municipality. (2013). *Location.* Retrieved from http://www.vhembe.gov.za/index.php?page=location.

PART III

Themes in Professional Nursing Practice

15 | CHAPTER

Health and Health Promotion

Sandra P. Thomas, PhD, RN, FAAN

(e) http://evolve.elsevier.com/Friberg/bridge/

OBJECTIVES

At the completion of this chapter, the reader will be able to:

- Compare several definitions and models of health.
- Compare several models of health behavior.
- Describe psychological, behavioral, and environmental factors related to wellness.
- Apply the stages of change model to a selected health behavior.

- Apply the health belief model (HBM) to a selected health behavior.
- Describe the use of evidence-based interventions to promote behavior change.
- Describe the goals of *Healthy People 2020*.
- Compare several types of community-level health promotion programs.

PROFILE IN PRACTICE

Leslie El-Sayad, MSN, RN, FNP

Nurse Practitioner, Morgan County Medical Center, Wartburg, Tennessee

During more than 20 years in primary care in rural eastern Tennessee, I have tried to avoid burnout and becoming jaded concerning my patients' motivations or lack thereof. But questions flit across my mind, unbidden, when patients make decisions that adversely affect their health. I think to myself, "Isn't it as plain as the nose on her face what she should do? Haven't I discussed that with her enough times?" Two principles have helped remind me to respect the patient's viewpoint on health.

First, no one sets out deliberately to make a wrong decision. This idea is based on one of nursing theorist Ernestine Wiedenbach's beliefs about the individual: Whatever the individual does represents his or her best judgment at the moment of doing it. Given their immediate circumstances (and rural poor populations are more affected by immediate circumstances than those with more available options), past experiences, knowledge base, physical and mental state, and social or economic pressures at the time a decision is made, patients will make the best decisions they are capable of making.

Therefore there is no looking back or chastising—only going forward with new knowledge. We cannot presume to know what is best for another person.

Second, symptoms by themselves may have no meaning to a person unless they have a significant effect on his or her life. A person may have no wish to change anything. Long lectures about the benefits of better health habits are demeaning and will not be helpful. A person may walk around with large tumors, constant dyspepsia, extreme dyspnea, or gnarled and painful joints, but an ingrown toenail will bring him to the provider because he could not wear his boots. Risk factors do not have a one-to-one relationship to disease. They are risk factors, not guarantees of poor outcomes. Despite scientifically based predictions, patients will not buy into your suggested preventative measures if they see no gain. It is difficult to promote health, but it is my job. Keeping the above principles in mind saves my sanity and helps me respect my patients' abilities on behalf of their health.

INTRODUCTION

Ricky Jones is a 45-year-old long-distance truck driver who once used amphetamines heavily to help him stay awake while driving. He presently weighs 205 pounds (height 5 feet 8 inches, medium frame [BMI 31.2]) and expresses disgust with his weight and lack of physical fitness. After his annual physical examination, the nurse practitioner collaboratively sets initial goals of increasing Ricky's level of exercise and achieving a 10-pound weight loss. As Ricky departs he wryly expresses a wish that amphetamines were still readily available so that he could diet more easily.

Many Americans share Ricky's longing for an easy way to lose weight or become fit. Millions of dollars are spent on books, tapes, pills, and exercise machines. But the outcomes Ricky seeks are not easy to achieve. Changing health behavior is difficult. Nurses, such as the family nurse practitioner profiled, know how difficult it is to motivate well people to undertake behaviors that lessen the likelihood of future illness. Some health professionals have a mistaken notion that the mere provision of didactic information will bring about health-promoting actions. But studies show that although individuals are often aware of the risks associated with behaviors such as alcohol use and smoking, they modify their thinking about these risks rather than taking the more difficult route of changing the behaviors (Leffingwell, Neumann, Leedy, & Babitzke, 2007). Information is the solution only when ignorance is the problem. Health care providers need a more sophisticated understanding of the principles of behavior change to help their patients make health-promoting decisions. This chapter explores a variety of evidence-based interventions to change health behavior.

CONCEPT OF HEALTH

Before discussing specific health behaviors, it is important to define *health*, a concept that remains something of an enigma. Is health a state, a process, or a goal? To the average layperson it is *illness* that compels attention, a departure from taken-for-granted smooth functioning. Likewise, traditional medical and nursing curricula have prepared health professionals to care for the acutely ill. Many textbooks still place greater emphasis on morbidity and mortality than on health promotion.

In contemporary nursing literature many authors assert that nursing has a mandate to promote holistic health. What does this mean? Unfortunately, some people think that *holistic* means "new age" or "alternative," something outside traditional beliefs or practices. Because the term is frequently misused, it may be useful to trace its origin. The word *holism* was first used in a 1926 book by Jan Smuts (p. 99), the first prime minister of South Africa and a lifelong student of biological evolution. Smuts rejected the mechanistic explanation of the world that was pervasive in his time. He saw physical matter and the mind as inseparable, and he believed that holism, a dynamic striving toward integration, was the ultimate principle of the universe. Not until the late 1950s and 1960s did these ideas begin to infiltrate the American health care delivery system. In medicine Halbert Dunn began to speak of "high level wellness," the ultimate integration of body, mind, and spirit as an interdependent whole (1959, 1971). In nursing Martha Rogers (1970) wrote about unitary human beings who are not reducible to parts or symptoms. She also emphasized the indivisible whole of person and environment.

Concurrent with the gradually shifting perspective of health professionals, a consumer wellness movement burgeoned that was linked to the other human liberation movements of the 1960s and 1970s such as the civil rights and women's movements. Public dissatisfaction with paternalistic medical treatment and mystifying medical terms, along with a better educated, more affluent populace, contributed to a thirst for information about holistic therapies and self-care. Americans became preoccupied with self-care clinics, self-help groups, and the tantalizing potential of peak wellness and self-actualization. Education of the public for self-care became an important element of federal government policies and public health initiatives, such as the Healthy People initiative, first begun in 1979 and reformulated each succeeding decade. Motivated by escalating costs of care for sick workers, corporations began to demand that employees assume more responsibility for their health and provided them with incentives such as exercise rooms, walking trails, and healthier meal options in the employee cafeteria. Although strong public interest in health-related information is encouraging, one of the nurse's most important tasks today is helping people decipher the bewildering mélange of pseudoscience and conflicting advice disseminated via the Internet.

EVOLVING CONCEPTIONS OF HEALTH

Nursing interventions to promote health are guided by ideas about human beings and the meaning of the concept of health. Smith (1983) traced evolving conceptions of health across the centuries, categorizing them into four models (Table 15-1).

Clinical Model

Listed first is the narrowest view of health, the clinical model, perhaps more readily recognizable to nurses as the "medical model." Health is simply the absence of disease or disability in this model. On examination of the physiochemical system of the patient, the health care provider would declare "health" if no signs of any incipient illnesses were detected. Unfortunately, this narrow conceptualization of health is still dominant in many health care settings.

Role Performance Model

The role performance model depicts health as the ability to fulfill one's customary social roles. Thus if a young mother is able to adequately carry out her childcare activities, she would be deemed healthy. If she cannot perform these activities, she would be considered ill. The problem with this view of health is the distressful and stultifying nature of many people's occupational or familial roles. Can individuals trapped in unsatisfying jobs or marriages achieve optimal health? What is the health impact of juggling multiple roles or experiencing

role conflict? What if performance in one role (worker, for example) so dominates one's existence that performance in another role (parent) is compromised?

Adaptive Model

Based largely on the ideas of Dubos (1965), the adaptive model emphasizes the ability to adapt flexibly to ever-changing environments and challenges. Continuous readjustment to life's stressful demands is necessary. Healthy people are resilient and hardy. Disease is viewed as a failure of adaptation. Although the adaptive model achieved popularity in nursing, as exemplified in the work of theorists such as Callista Roy (2009), there is a still broader conceptualization of health.

Eudaemonistic Model

Drawn from the Greek philosophers and from the humanistic psychologist Abraham Maslow (1961), the eudaemonistic model depicts health as the complete development of the individual's potential, an exuberant well-being. Clearly this model emphasizes the human capacity for growth. Within nursing, theorist Margaret Newman (2000) has proposed that health is expanding consciousness.

For this chapter a broad concept of health was selected, consistent with the broader view exemplified in Smith's adaptive and eudaemonistic models and Dunn's description of high-level wellness. Adopting a broader view of health has several implications for nursing practice. For one thing, separating mind, body, and spirit becomes impossible. Moreover, the patient's embeddedness in family, friendships, culture, and the environment cannot be ignored. Also, the patient's own power for healing is recognized. The role of the nurse is that of *facilitator* of the patient's own innate capabilities for healing and growth. Skilled counseling is as important as technical competence.

HEALTH PROMOTION AND DISEASE PREVENTION

The terms *health promotion* and *disease prevention*, although often used synonymously, actually have different meanings. Flowing logically from adaptive or eudaemonistic views of health, health promotion refers to activities that protect good health and take people beyond their present level of wellness. By achieving lean and fit bodies and well-managed stress levels, individuals

TABLE 15-1	**Models of Health**
MODEL	**CONCEPTION OF HEALTH**
Clinical	Elimination of disease as identified through medical science
Role performance	Ability to perform social, occupational, and other roles
Adaptive	Ability to engage in effective interaction with environment
Eudaemonistic	Self-actualization of individual; optimal well-being

Modified from Smith, J. (1983). *The idea of health: Implications for the nursing profession.* New York: Teachers College Press.

have a greater likelihood of achieving a high quality of life and reaching the goal of self-actualization. In contrast, disease prevention efforts are derived from the clinical model of health. Emphasis is frequently placed on avoidance, deprivation, or restraint. Behaviors are undertaken to prevent specific diseases. Mortality statistics demonstrate the importance of lifestyle modifications to prevent premature death. The chief causes of death in the United States are strongly related to unhealthy behaviors such as smoking and overeating (Box 15-1).

MODIFICATION OF HEALTH ATTITUDES AND BEHAVIORS

Convincing empirical evidence shows that healthy lifestyles can significantly reduce the mortality rate from cardiovascular diseases, cancer, obesity, diabetes, and human immunodeficiency virus/acquired immunodeficiency syndrome (HIV/AIDS). Therefore the modification of health attitudes and behavior is one of the most important responsibilities of every nurse. As shown in Figure 15-1, a comprehensive model of wellness includes interacting factors such as psychological characteristics, health-promoting behaviors, and aspects of the environments in which people live and work. Both attitudes and behaviors are modifiable by health care providers, as well as some (but not all) aspects of environments.

BOX 15-1 The 15 Leading Causes of Death in the United States, 2010

1. Heart disease
2. Malignant neoplasms
3. Chronic lower respiratory diseases
4. Cerebrovascular diseases
5. Accidents
6. Alzheimer's disease
7. Diabetes mellitus
8. Nephritis, nephrosis
9. Influenza and pneumonia
10. Suicide
11. Septicemia
12. Chronic liver disease and cirrhosis
13. Essential hypertension and hypertensive renal disease
14. Parkinson's disease
15. Pneumonitis

Murphy, S. L., Xu, J., & Kochanek, M. (2013). Deaths: Final data for 2010. National Vital Statistics Reports, 61(4). Hyattsville, MD: National Center for Health Statistics.

The sections that follow examine a number of these modifiable factors. Although a comprehensive wellness model includes organismic variables (e.g., genetic predispositions) and demographic characteristics (e.g., age, income, gender), these are not amenable to modification by health care providers. We instead emphasize the factors that can be affected by nurses.

Psychological Attitudes and Characteristics Associated with Wellness

Self-Concept. Many theorists consider a healthy self-concept (and closely related concepts such as self-acceptance or self-esteem) essential for wellness. Persons who feel better about themselves are more inclined to enact self-care behaviors that promote good health. Abundant data demonstrate that self-destructive habits such as drug abuse are linked to lower self-worth. Although experiences with parents, teachers, and peers all contribute to initial development of self-concept, later life experiences offer opportunities to alter it. A client's negative evaluation of the self can be altered in an ongoing, supportive relationship with a nurse. For example, the nurse can guide the client to recall strengths, such as persistence in confronting life stressors.

Locus of Control. Locus of control is a construct from Rotter's (1954) social learning theory. According to this theory, as individuals are exposed to reinforcements (rewards) for their behavior, they develop beliefs about their ability to control desired outcomes or rewards. Eventually most people have a stable, general expectancy that reinforcements are contingent on their own behavior (termed *internal locus of control*) or an expectancy that rewards are received on a purely random basis or dispensed by powerful others (called *external locus of control*). What does locus of control have to do with wellness? Logically, individuals who have an internal locus of control are more likely to engage in positive health behaviors. They believe that the reinforcement (good health) is directly related to their own actions, not controlled by powerful others (e.g., doctors) or by the vicissitudes of fate. Although questionnaires are available to measure locus of control, a nurse can easily assess it by asking questions such as the following: "What do you think caused you to have this heart attack? Who do you think knows best what you really need? Do you normally follow instructions pretty well, or do you prefer to work things out your own way?" Nursing interventions can be tailored accordingly. If the person has an internal locus

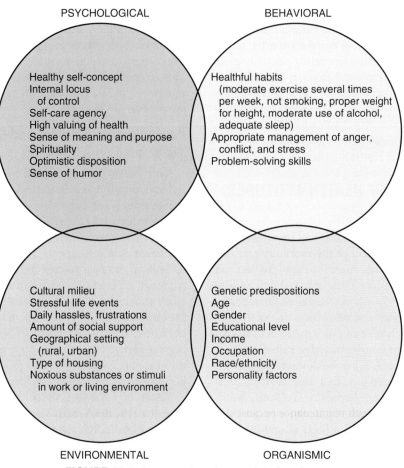

PSYCHOLOGICAL

Healthy self-concept
Internal locus
    of control
Self-care agency
High valuing of health
Sense of meaning and purpose
Spirituality
Optimistic disposition
Sense of humor

BEHAVIORAL

Healthful habits
    (moderate exercise several times
    per week, not smoking, proper weight
    for height, moderate use of alcohol,
    adequate sleep)
Appropriate management of anger,
    conflict, and stress
Problem-solving skills

Cultural milieu
Stressful life events
Daily hassles, frustrations
Amount of social support
Geographical setting
    (rural, urban)
Type of housing
Noxious substances or stimuli
    in work or living environment

Genetic predispositions
Age
Gender
Educational level
Income
Occupation
Race/ethnicity
Personality factors

ENVIRONMENTAL   ORGANISMIC

FIGURE 15-1 A comprehensive model of wellness.

of control, a nurse should allow a high degree of client participation in goal setting and selection of reinforcers. If the person has an external locus of control, providing plenty of concrete guidance and support is important. For example, if the goal is weight loss, suggesting involvement in a program with regular group meetings such as Weight Watchers may be beneficial.

Self-Care Agency/Self-Efficacy. *Self-care agency,* a term coined by nurse theorist Dorothea Orem (2001), refers to the ability to care for oneself, for which the person must have knowledge, skills, understanding, and willingness. In working with a client, assessment of all these factors is necessary. A parallel concept from social cognitive theory called *self-efficacy* (Bandura, 1997) has generated a sizable body of health psychology and nursing literature. According to Bandura's theory, when people perceive that they have efficacy to accomplish a specific behavior (e.g.,

breast self-examination), they are predisposed to undertake the behavior. Studies have established links between self-efficacy and exercise, weight management, smoking cessation, chronic disease management, and medication adherence (Anderson & Anderson, 2003; McAuley, Doerksen, Morris, Motl, Hu, & Wojcicki, et al., 2008; Wingo, Desmond, & Brantley, et al., 2013). This empirical evidence suggests that a nurse's first step in working with many clients is to enhance their belief in personal capability. Research shows that self-efficacy is modifiable through strategies such as anticipatory guidance and persuasive motivational messages (Bandura, 1997).

Values. Values are elements that show how a person has decided to use his or her life. Values serve as a basis for decisions and choices. The nurse must assess whether the client's values promote a healthy lifestyle. How important is health to an individual compared with other life values such as pleasure, excitement, or social recognition? Jackson, Tucker, and Herman (2007) found that individuals who place a higher value on health also display greater involvement in a health-promoting lifestyle. Of course, some people declare that they highly value health, but their behaviors contradict this declaration. A value system may contain conflicting values. For example, highly valuing achievement and financial prosperity may result in overwork and neglect of health. Assisting a client to clarify conflicting values can be a useful intervention. Review previous chapter on ethics for details.

Sense of Purpose. Having a sense of meaning and purpose for one's life may be an important factor in individuals' responsiveness to health providers' instructions. Purpose in life includes having goals for the future and a sense of directedness. Exploring whether clients aim to follow a particular career trajectory, pursue an enjoyable hobby or avocation, or see their children and grandchildren grow and mature is often helpful. Greater purpose in life was associated with lower risk of mortality in a 5-year study of older persons, even when their chronic medical conditions were taken into account (Boyle, Barnes, Buchman, & Bennett, 2009). When assessing a client, it can be thought-provoking to ask about aims to make a difference or leave a legacy. Persons with clear goals may devote more effort to health maintenance because most goals cannot be achieved without good health.

Spirituality. Health researchers and clinicians are increasingly recognizing that spirituality is an integral component of holistic health and wellness. Spirituality is not synonymous with involvement in organized religion, but the sense of connection with a divine wisdom or higher power often motivates practices such as meditation, prayer, and attendance at religious services. Studies have examined the relationship of spirituality and/or religious practice with disease conditions (e.g., heart disease, cancer, mental illness) as well as health risk behaviors (e.g., smoking, excessive drinking, using illicit drugs) (Hart, 2008). Clients may be motivated to take health-promoting actions by a belief that the body is a temple for the spirit.

Optimism. An optimistic disposition has been shown to be important to health in studies conducted for more than two decades. Optimism is a stable personality characteristic with important implications for the manner in which people regulate their actions, particularly actions relevant to health. Optimism includes tendencies to expect the best, look on the bright side, and anticipate good things in the future. It is important

to note that the presence of optimism is not dependent on a person's particular locus of control; expectations of favorable outcomes could be derived from perceptions of being lucky or blessed (external locus of control) or from convictions of personal control (internal locus of control). Higher levels of optimism have been associated with positive health outcomes such as completion of an alcohol treatment program and faster recovery after coronary bypass surgery, bone marrow transplant, and traumatic injury (Carver & Scheier, 2002). An optimistic outlook can be cultivated if it does not come naturally.

Sense of Humor. Although a sense of humor is a socially appealing trait, it also conveys health benefits. The physical effects of mirth have been compared with the effects of exercise. For example, laughing 100 times expends the same number of calories as 10 minutes on a rowing machine (Godfrey, 2004). The efficiency of the respiratory system increases, and the cardiovascular and muscular systems relax. Humor and laughter have been linked to higher levels of endorphins and immunoglobulin A and lower levels of cortisol (Godfrey, 2004). Laughter is an excellent way to dispel stress and tension as well.

Health Behaviors Associated with Wellness

Behaviors associated with wellness are listed in Figure 15-1. The first research about health behaviors was done in the 1950s by social psychologists who sought to explain the public's perplexingly low response to screening programs that were free or low in cost (Hochbaum, 1958). From this work, the Health Belief Model (HBM) was developed by Becker et al. (1977). According to the HBM, an individual's perceptions of his or her susceptibility to a disease (and the severity of that disease), the perceived benefits of taking action, and cues to action (from media, health professionals, or family) contribute to the likelihood of taking preventive actions—provided that barriers are not too great (Becker, Haefner, & Kasl, et al., 1977).

In the 1980s nurse researcher Nola Pender presented a model with similarities to the HBM but with greater emphasis on health-promoting behaviors. Individual characteristics and prior behavior are theorized to affect perceptions of self-efficacy, benefits and barriers to action, and a factor called *activity-related affect*, which refers to the feelings about the behavior in question. For example, is exercise fun or unpleasant? All these factors, as well as interpersonal and situational variables, can influence commitment to a plan of action. Additionally, competing demands such as work or family care responsibilities are taken into account in the prediction of health-promoting behavior, the outcome variable of the model. Based on years of research that tested Pender's Health Promotion Model, the model was revised, deleting constructs with insufficient predictive power (Figure 15-2). According to a synopsis of 38 studies, the

best predictors of health-promoting behavior are perceived self-efficacy, perceived barriers, and prior behavior (Pender, Murdaugh, & Parsons, 2002).

With the exception of Pender's model, most health behavior models fail to acknowledge the powerful role of *affect*. Lawton, Conner, and McEachan (2009) found that affect (the enjoyment of the activity) was a better

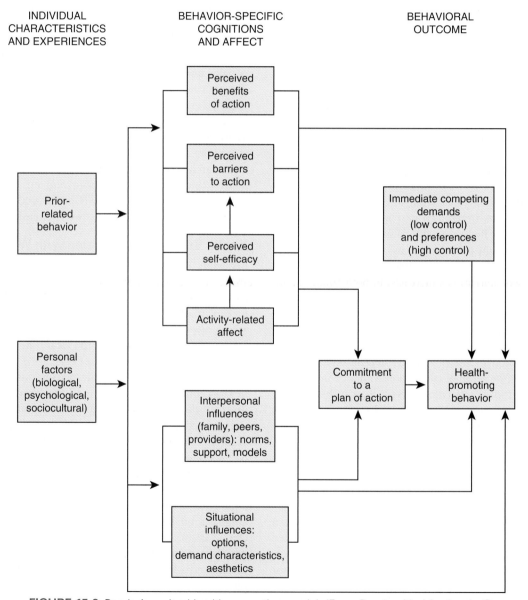

FIGURE 15-2 Pender's revised health promotion model. (From Pender, N., Murdaugh, C. L., & Parsons, M. A. [2002]. *Health promotion in nursing practice* [4th ed.]. Upper Saddle River, NJ: Prentice-Hall.)

predictor than cognitive attitude (harm or benefit of the activity) for four risky behaviors (e.g., excessive drinking) and five health-promoting behaviors (e.g., eating fruits and vegetables). The researchers concluded that "many of the behaviors that most threaten our health and safety may not be reasoned or planned but depend, at least to some extent, on whether they make us feel happy or sad, relaxed or tense" (Lawton et al., 2009, pp. 63–64).

Health Habits. More than 40 years ago, longitudinal studies established that good health habits, such as regular exercise, are correlated with better health status and longevity (Belloc & Breslow, 1972; Breslow & Enstrom, 1980). Given that the benefits of healthful habits are well established, the average American's lack of adherence to the recommended lifestyle regimen is discouraging. We focus here on exercise, diet, tobacco use, sleep, and emotion management.

Exercise. Analysis of a massive database, including the findings of studies involving over 300,000 people, showed that exercise is as effective as prescriptive medications for prevention of diabetes and secondary prevention of heart disease, and *more* effective than prescriptive medications during stroke rehabilitation (Naci & Ionnidis, 2013). Yet, only one in five U.S. adults meets government guidelines for physical activity (CDCP, 2013). Sedentarism has increased in both children and adults with the escalation of hours spent using computers, television, and hand-held electronic devices for entertainment as well as business purposes (Ricciardi, 2005). The prevalence of inactivity rises with age, and women are more likely than men to be inactive at all ages (CDCP, 2013). Like the Hispanic women studied by Im's research team (2010), many women place their families first and are unwilling to set aside time for their own physical activity. Even when an exercise program is started, the usual rate of dropout is 50% in the first few months (Wilbur, Vassalo, & Chandler, et al., 2005). Many people have an aversion to exercise, mentally associating it with competitive sports or regimented calisthenics. Even as health club membership climbs—at least among the more affluent—too many Americans pay someone else to wash the car, use riding mowers to mow the lawn, and treat their treadmills as clothes racks.

Nurses need to spread the word that gym membership and expensive equipment are not necessary for regular physical workouts. Long-term adherence to an exercise program is more likely when the regimen is home based rather than dependent on participation in a group class at a gym (King, Kiernan, & Oman, et al., 1997). If finances preclude purchasing a set of weights, soup cans and other household items can be substituted. Although fear of crime inhibits outdoor exercise, especially among women and older adults (Roman & Chalfin, 2008), nearly everyone can find some safe place to walk (shopping malls are a good alternative for those who live in unsafe neighborhoods). Studies show that walking provides almost all the benefits of more vigorous activity, requires no equipment or fees, and can be done alone or with a companion (Norman & Mills, 2004). Gardening, dancing, and biking are pleasurable activities that are also beneficial to the heart and muscle tone. A person raking leaves burns 288 calories per hour—while also enjoying fresh air and fall colors. Many residents of cities suffer from "nature deficit disorder" and should set aside time to walk or bicycle in parks and nature trails (Walsh, 2011). Clients may be more motivated to exercise when informed of immediate benefits, such as increased energy and improved mood. With the release of natural endorphins, exercise can lift spirits for hours afterward.

Because so many clients are completely sedentary, professionals must remember to begin with realistic and achievable goals, such as 5 to 10 minutes of walking. In an experiment with healthy young college women, aimed at enhancing their exercise self-efficacy, some women dropped out of the study at the time of the pretest because they perceived that a "step test" was frightening and aversive. They were afraid that the subsequent exercise sessions (step aerobics, dancing, and kickboxing) would be far too difficult for them to perform (D'Alonzo, Stevenson, & Davis, 2004). If such apprehensions are present in healthy young women, consider how they could be magnified in older adults. Effective exercise interventions must be tailored carefully. On a positive note, emphasize to clients that as little as 10 minutes a day of moderate exercise can reduce risk for disease and improve quality of life (Listfield, 2009).

Healthy Eating. The United States is in the midst of an alarming obesity epidemic, in which more than one third of adults are obese (Koh, 2010). Not only is obesity (a body mass index greater than 30) rapidly rising, but so is morbid obesity (defined as a BMI greater than 40). By 2030, the global burden of obesity will be staggering: 2.16 billion adults are predicted to be overweight and 1.12 billion obese (Kelly, Yang, Chen, Reynolds, & He, 2008). Childhood obesity has reached unparalleled proportions. The prevalence of obesity in school-age children has quadrupled since the 1970s (Estabrooks, Fisher, & Hayman, 2008). It is clear that the "happy meals" children consume today will have unhappy consequences for their health tomorrow. Some obese children already have the arteries of 45-year-old adults. Among the consequences of the rapidly rising incidence of obesity in the United States is the increased number of adults with hypertension (67 million now compared with 50 million in 1994) (CDCP, 2014). Millions more are prehypertensive, prompting the government to recommend the low-fat, low-salt, low-sweets DASH (Dietary Approaches to Stop Hypertension) diet. The plant-based Mediterranean diet also exerts beneficial effects on blood pressure, especially when supplemented with nuts and extra virgin olive oil (Toledo, Hu, & Estruch, et al., 2013).

Despite widespread media promotion of the USDA's Food Guide Pyramid (MyPyramid) and the Mediterranean diet, Americans consume nowhere near the recommended daily servings of fruits and vegetables. Current intake of flour, grains, and beans is only two thirds of what society consumed in 1910. Each person, on average, consumes 150 pounds of sweeteners (mostly sugar and corn syrup) per year, 25 pounds more than in 1984. Americans drink twice as much carbonated soda as milk. And society still consumes too much fat (U.S. Department of Agriculture, 2008). Falling consumption of fish is another problem, resulting in inadequate intake of omega-3 fatty acids, which could reduce heart attack risk (Campos, Baylin, & Willett, 2008) and improve mood and mental health (Hallahan & Garland, 2005). Because MyPyramid's colorful graphic image contains no text, critics have urged the USDA to provide consumers with more specific guidance. When counseling clients about dietary modifications, nurses may find the *Dietary Guidelines for Americans 2010* more useful. Key recommendations include: (1) consuming half of all grains as whole grains; (2) increasing intake of fat-free or low-fat dairy products; (3) using oils to replace solid fats; (4) replacing high-solid-fat protein foods with lower-solid-fat foods; (5) increasing intake of fruits, vegetables, and seafood; and (6) choosing foods that provide greater amounts of fiber, calcium, potassium, and Vitamin D (U.S. Department of Agriculture, 2010). A simple and easy tool ties in all of these better choices, entitled Choose My Plate. Ten great tips are incorporated into portion size and recommendations. More information can be found at chooseMyPlate.gov (http://www.choosemyplate.gov/).

Food is laden with emotional, social, and cultural significance, complicating attempts at dietary modification. For many clients, foods high in salt may be "soul food" and rich sweets may be "comfort food." Hispanic individuals who cook with lard may think food prepared with other types of fat is unappealing. Immigrants from South Asia view butter and milk as nurturing and are reluctant to reduce these ingredients when preparing their traditional dishes (Patel, Phillips-Caesar, & Boutin-Foster, 2012). Therefore targeting interventions to children while their eating habits are still developing makes good sense. When she learned that one third of school-age children in her state were overweight or obese, the Texas agriculture commissioner (a mother of three) banned junk food from school cafeterias (Booth-Thomas, 2004). Grain bars, nuts, and baked chips replaced candy in the school vending machines. Fresh produce, yogurt, and low-sugar drinks became available to the students. Many nurses have become involved in similar efforts to combat childhood obesity in their own communities.

Complicating nurses' efforts to combat the obesity epidemic is their own predilection to be overweight or obese; more than half of nurses weigh too much (Miller, Alpert, & Cross, 2008). Research shows that laypersons have less confidence in nurses' ability to provide health education when nurses themselves are overweight (Hicks et al., 2008).

Tobacco Use. Smoking is the leading cause of preventable death across the globe (Koh, 2010). In the United States, public smoking has been discouraged by bans in offices, restaurants, and airports. Many Americans have kicked the habit. But smoking prevalence remains high among lower-income groups, and it is rising among girls and women, with a concomitant increase in female lung cancer. Another disturbing trend is water pipe (hookah) smoking, which is becoming popular among college students because of the pleasant flavorings (e.g., apple, coffee) and sweeteners added to the tobacco (Primack, Sidani, Agarwal, Shadel, Donny, & Eissenberg, 2008). Some youngsters have their first smoke in middle school or earlier. These youngsters do not know they are exposed to more than 4000 chemicals each time they light up, including arsenic and radioactive compounds such as polonium. Some of them have the mistaken belief that cigars, water pipes, or chewing tobacco are healthy alternatives to cigarettes. Small cigars flavored like fruit or candy are smoked by 1 in 30 middle and high school students; by the senior year of high school, 1 in 12 acknowledge doing so (King et al., 2014). The statistics on youth tobacco use are deeply disturbing given the addictive potential of nicotine. Adolescent tobacco use is a powerful predictor of adult tobacco use.

Electronic cigarettes are the newest avenue to nicotine addiction, erroneously viewed as much less dangerous than regular cigarettes. Promoted heavily in advertisements featuring glamorous celebrities, electronic cigarette sales have rapidly escalated. By 2017 sales in the United States are predicted to reach $10 billion (Gray, 2013) The long-term consequences of this form of nicotine use are unknown.

Studies have shown that nurse-delivered smoking cessation counseling is effective even when relatively brief; only a few minutes are necessary for a nurse to ask about smoking status, assess a client's desire to quit, and provide evidence-based advice about tactics (Bialous & Sarna, 2004). Approximately 76% of smokers say they want to quit, but they lack specific plans to do so (Herzog & Blagg, 2007). There are many barriers to quitting: withdrawal symptoms, missing the companionship of cigarettes, less control of stress and moods, fear of weight gain, and lack of encouragement from family and friends. Some of the barriers can be dispelled by clear, strong, and personalized advice from clinicians: "Continuing to smoke makes your asthma worse" or "Quitting smoking may reduce the number of ear infections your child has" (Fiore, Jaen, Baker, Bailey, Bennett, & Benowitz, et al., 2008, p. 163). Some parents are surprised to learn that their children are still exposed to the toxins in tobacco smoke even if the parent smokes only while the children are sleeping. "Third-hand smoke" lingers in the home, contaminating surfaces where children crawl and play (Third-Hand Smoke: Another Reason to Quit Smoking, 2008).

Motivating a client to stop smoking is always a challenge. James Prochaska and his research team have studied the stages of change in addictive behaviors (Prochaska, DiClemente, & Norcross, 1992). In working with a client, the Prochaska model is helpful in assessing the client's stage. The Prochaska model is applied to smoking cessation in Table 15-2. Health professionals can promote client movement to subsequent stages by interventions that raise consciousness. For example, a middle-age man in a high-stress job may be startled to learn that smoking does *not*

TABLE 15-2 Prochaska's Transtheoretical Model of Change Applied to Smoking Cessation

Stage 1: Precontemplation	Smokers do not see their smoking as a problem and do not intend to stop within the next 6 months.
Stage 2: Contemplation	Smokers see their smoking as a problem and think about quitting but are not ready to change.
Stage 3: Preparation	Smokers intend to take action in the next month; some have made small changes, such as cutting down on the number smoked or delaying the first smoke of the day.
Stage 4: Action	Smokers adopt a goal of smoking cessation and make an attempt to quit, involving overt behavior change and environmental modification.
Stage 5: Maintenance	Smokers work to prevent relapse and maintain abstinence.

Modified from Prochaska, J. O., DiClemente, C. C., & Norcross, J. C. (1992). In search of how people change: Applications to addictive behaviors. *American Psychologist, 47,* 1102–1114.

improve mood on stressful days; smoking actually worsens mood (Aronson, Almeida, Stawski, Klein, & Kozlowski, 2008). An adolescent girl who uses smoking for weight control may consider cessation when she learns of its negative effects on the skin. Interventions to promote smoking cessation can be guided by the HBM, as shown in Table 15-3. Unless contraindicated, nicotine replacement therapy combats withdrawal symptoms such as irritability and craving. If clients are depressed or have a history of depression, education regarding mood management enhances the likelihood of successful cessation (van der Meer, Willemsen, Smit, & Cuijpers, 2013). Research by Judith Prochaska's team showed that exercise during smoking cessation not only improves mood but also increases the probability of staying smoke-free (Prochaska, Hall, Humfleet, Munoz, Reus, & Gorecki, et al., 2008). During cessation, smokers must break the associations between smoking and familiar environments (e.g., the living room couch) that stimulate craving (Stambor, 2006), so alterations in the environment and daily routines are recommended. Lapses in abstinence are common, and

TABLE 15-3 Application of the Health Belief Model in Interventions to Promote Smoking Cessation

FACTOR	INTERVENTIONS
Perceived susceptibility	Teach about morbidity and mortality statistics of smokers versus nonsmokers.
Perceived severity	Illustrate what happens to lungs and other organs when smoking; show pictures of diseased lungs and wrinkled skin.
Perceived barriers	Identify barriers unique to the individual and counsel regarding common fears about weight gain, greater stress, and irritability.
Perceived benefits	Identify benefits, such as more pleasant breath and body odor; increased energy; decreased cough; improved circulation; enhanced ability to taste; and reduced risk of heart disease and stroke and cancers of the mouth, throat, esophagus, lungs, bladder, and cervix.
Cues to action	Use telephone calls and postcard reminders. Provide pamphlets about cessation strategies. Organize support groups and buddy systems.

clients must be encouraged to resume the strategies that initially helped them to quit. Successful quitters usually make several tries.

Sleep. Sleep does not receive sufficient attention from health care providers, but it is essential to physical and mental health. It affects resistance to infection, ability to concentrate, productivity, and mood. Research shows that a good night's sleep improves thinking and memory (Gorman, 2004). Unfortunately, millions of Americans are sleep deprived; 25% of adults report insufficient sleep at least half the nights of each month (Centers for Disease Control and Prevention, 2009). The odds of sleeping less than 6 hours per night have significantly increased over the past 30 years (Knutson, Van Cauter, & Rathouz, et al., 2010). Even children are sleeping less than experts recommend. For example, preschoolers should sleep 11 to 13 hours, but a survey showed an average of only 10.4 hours; school-age children should sleep 10 to 11 hours but average only 9.5 hours (National Sleep Foundation, 2004). Many parents are unaware of the recommended amount of sleep for their children. Nurses' health promotion efforts must include education about sleep hygiene and sleep disorders.

Emotion Management. Appropriate management of emotions (particularly anger and hostility) is essential to wellness but does not receive sufficient attention in health promotion programming. Mismanaged anger and hostility are linked to coronary artery calcification, increased cardiovascular reactivity, elevated lipid levels, metabolic syndrome, lower pulmonary function, poorer general health, and early death (Chida & Steptoe, 2009; Goldbacher & Matthews, 2007; Harburg, Kaciroti, Gleiberman, Julius, & Schork, Holt-Lunstad, Smith, & Uchino, 2008; McCloskey, Kleabir, & Berman, et al., 2010: Mostofsky, Maclure, & Tofler, et al., 2013). Research by immunologists showed that intensely hostile interactions, such as arguments with a spouse, lower one's immunocompetence (Kiecolt-Glaser, McGuire, Robles, & Glaser, et al., 2002).

Although anger is a normal human emotion, it is pathogenic when it is too frequent, too intense, too prolonged, or managed ineffectively. Habitual suppression is just as problematic as the tendency to have explosive outbursts because suppression of emotion requires great effort and often results in rumination for hours about the incident (Thomas, 2007). Anger also contributes to disease by causing increased consumption of food, cigarettes, alcohol, and other mood-altering drugs.

The health-promoting way of managing anger is to wait until the initial physiological arousal abates, then discuss the anger-provoking incident with the provocateur or a confidant and, finally, take constructive action to resolve the problem. Persons who regularly discuss their anger in this way have lower blood pressure and better health (Thomas, 1997). When resentment about an old grievance has become chronic, it should be released by forgiving the offender. If the offender is deceased or far away, forgiveness can still be accomplished through reflective journaling or a healing ritual. Extensive research by psychologist James Pennebaker (1990; Pennebaker & Chung, 2011) demonstrates the healing power of expressing emotions through confiding in others or writing about painful events. Health promotion efforts by nurses should include instruction about healthy emotional disclosure and anger management. Guidelines for teaching anger management to community groups may be found in Thomas (2001). Interventions should be tailored with regard to age, gender, culture, and customary expression style (whether volatile or suppressive) (Thomas, 2006, 2007).

Problem Solving. Problem-solving skills must be taught to clients who do not know systematic strategies and techniques for enacting healthful habits or making changes in health behavior. For example, recovering alcoholics need to learn ways to slowly sip on nonalcoholic beverages at a party; dieters must practice polite refusal of foods at a family gathering. Middle school students may benefit from role playing a scenario in which they refuse illicit drugs at a party. Individuals who lack assertiveness may need to rehearse firm insistence that sex partners use condoms. Assertiveness can also empower underserved groups to request needed community services or assistance from other members of the health care team. When giving exercise or diet prescriptions to clients, health care providers should ask what problems or barriers they envision; this will point the way to the skills that need to be taught. Research shows that family members, friends, and coworkers often engage in undermining nutrition and exercise decisions, by giving tempting foods, encouraging skipped workouts, and making negative comments (Mackert, Stanforth, & Garcia, 2011). The possibility of undermining should always be explored with clients when behavior changes are undertaken, and counseling should be offered about ways of resisting it. Some clients benefit from problem-solving activities in groups, such as groups conducted with dieters (Hollis, Gullion, Stevens, Brantley, Appel, Ard, & et al., 2008).

EVIDENCE-BASED INTERVENTIONS TO PROMOTE BEHAVIOR CHANGE

Health professionals often use threats of future disease when urging behavior change. However, when people are frightened, they use denial to convince themselves that the threatening event (e.g., HIV/AIDS, cancer) is not likely to happen to them. Such threats of distant adverse outcomes are not as likely to be as successful as approaches that confer immediate benefits and rewards or reduce denial. Motivational enhancement counseling is more effective in producing lifestyle change. Components of the motivational counseling approach are provider empathy, a spirit of collaboration with the client, avoidance of lecturing or arguing, and support of client self-efficacy (Riegel, Dickson, Hoke, McMahon, Reis, & Sayers, et al., 2006). Nurses should remember that many

laypersons hold unfavorable views of the medical establishment and are skeptical about medical practitioners' advice because of prior negative experiences (Hughner & Kleine, 2008). Reluctance to discuss issues such as obesity is common among Hispanics, African Americans, and many other groups (Guarnero, 2013). Therefore establishing a collaborative relationship with clients is the first priority (Thomas & Pollio, 2002). Then readiness to change can be assessed. Surprising readiness to change may be evident when the nurse simply asks screening questions during routine primary care visits, such as "Do you drink more than you should?" For example, a high percentage (75%) of outpatients who screened positive for alcohol misuse indicated readiness to change (Williams, Kivlahan, Saitz, Merrill, Achtmeyer, & McCormick, et al., 2006). When promoting behavior change, be aware that "approach goals" (e.g., increasing consumption of fruits and vegetables) are easier for clients to work on than "avoidance goals" (e.g., decreasing snacks or sweets) (Sullivan & Rothman, 2008).

A health risk appraisal (HRA) is a tool that can be used to provide clients with an estimate of biological age versus chronological age, an assessment of risk factors that may lead to health problems, and specific recommendations for behavioral changes that may lengthen their lives. A variety of computerized HRA instruments are available, as well as paper-and-pencil versions of the tests. Some health risk appraisal tools are limited in scope, focusing only on a specific area, such as risk for coronary heart disease. Others assess broad areas, including the environment, education, stress, family history, and health behavior. These surveys are often administered during health fairs at community centers and shopping malls. An HRA instrument is best used in conjunction with laboratory tests (e.g., cholesterol, triglycerides) and the on-site measurement of some variables by professionals (e.g., blood pressure, triceps skin-fold thickness). Nurses should bear in mind that the accuracy of HRA mortality predictions has been called into question, so focusing on the client's life expectancy is not recommended. Individuals who are given the results of their risk assessment along with a supportive educational process benefit more than persons who simply receive the test results.

The selection of incremental, achievable goals is also essential because clients can be overwhelmed by the prospect of drastic changes such as sweeping dietary modifications. One research team asked overweight adults to make only one small change in food choice and one small change in physical activity per week; significant improvements in waist circumference, intra-abdominal fat, and weight resulted (Lutes, Winett, Barger, Wojcik, Herbert, & Nickols-Richardson, et al., 2008).

A nurse could begin by asking an overweight client about desire to lose weight; if the answer is yes, nurse and client formulate two or three areas to begin work on (e.g., choosing a high-fiber cereal instead of a Danish pastry for breakfast). Such an approach is far more likely to result in compliance than stringent calorie restriction. Clients should be taught that slow weight loss is preferable to rapid loss from fad diets, which can produce ketosis, gout, and other adverse consequences. Even small changes may increase quality of life. For example, older adults (ages 70 to 82) who simply expended energy in routine daily activities, such as household chores and climbing stairs, had a 32% lower risk of mortality over the 6 years of a longitudinal study by Manini, Everhart, Patel, Schoeller, Colbert, & Visser, et al. (2006). Achieving an extra decade of life may be a significant motivator of healthful habits for some individuals. According to longitudinal studies of more than 360,000 patients, people who did not smoke and maintained low cholesterol levels (200 mg/dL or below) and blood pressure (120/80 mm Hg or less) can live up to 9.5 years longer than those less careful about their health (Stamler, Stamler, Neaton, Wentworth, Daviglus, & Garside, et al., 1999). Death from cardiovascular disease, as well as from all other causes, was substantially reduced among adults with this desirable risk profile.

In contrast to interventions that target a single deleterious behavior, success was achieved by one team of researchers who delivered a multiple-behavior intervention to college students. PowerPoint slides were used to enhance the verbal messages. Despite the brevity of the behavioral counseling (25 minutes), significant improvements were found in sleep and health-related quality of life, along with reduced alcohol and marijuana use (Werch, Moore, Bian, DiClemente, Ames, & Weiler, et al., 2008).

When health care providers write prescriptions for exercise or diet, adherence improves (Dobson, 2008). Another strategy with proven effectiveness is contracting. The purpose of writing a contract is to arrange a favorable, positively reinforcing experience when the client performs the desirable health behavior. Elements of a good contract are depicted in Box 15-2. A sample contract for

---

BOX 15-2   Elements of a Good Contract for Behavior Change

- The behavior must be carefully selected and explicitly described.
- The behavior must be measurable (e.g., number of cigarettes smoked, minutes of exercise).
- A data collection plan must be developed (e.g., calendar, log, chart, graph, diary).
- Client and nurse agree on the goals (short-term and long-term) and time frame.
- Client and nurse agree on the reinforcers (extrinsic and intrinsic).
- Reinforcers are specified for step-by-step approximations of the desired behavior.
- Client and nurse sign the written contract and both keep a copy.
- Client and nurse evaluate effectiveness of the plan.
- The plan is revised as needed.

---

weight loss appears in Figure 15-3. Keeping a log or diary also contributes to successful behavior change, especially when attempting to lose weight. In a 2008 study by Hollis and colleagues, food diary keepers lost twice as much weight as those who did not keep food diaries.

An impediment to the use of written prescriptions and contracts is the low functional literacy of Americans. Literacy levels are lower among minorities, the poor, older adults, and those with less education. If giving written materials to clients, use simple, everyday vocabulary. Ascertain clients' comprehension of the behavior change instructions and invite questions before they leave the clinical area. This strategy is known as the *teach-back method*.

ENVIRONMENTAL FACTORS THAT AFFECT WELLNESS

Nurses must look beyond individual capabilities in the quest to help clients become healthier. The range of health-promoting choices available to individuals may be drastically limited by societal forces, structures, and policies. As depicted in Figure 15-1, numerous environmental factors affect wellness.

Culture

The cultural milieu in which a person develops and resides has a profound influence. In successful health promotion initiatives, the help of cultural insiders is solicited so that professionals can be aware of cultural

Desired outcome:	Weight loss of 10 lb
Long-term goal:	To lose 2½ lb per week for 4 weeks
Short-term goals:	1. Maintain 1200 calorie/day diet. 2. Increase water consumption to eight glasses per day. 3. Avoid skipping meals. 4. Ride exercise machine: 　Week 1: 15 minutes 3 times per week 　Week 2: 20 minutes 3 times per week 　Week 3: 25 minutes 3 times per week 　Week 4: 30 minutes 3 times per week 5. Weigh self on Monday mornings. Record weight on flow sheet.
Intrinsic rewards:	Increased self-esteem and confidence Clothes fit better Improved physical fitness and appearance
Extrinsic rewards:	Upon successful completion of each day's regimen, a 20-minute bubble bath At end of each week, movie with a friend At end of contract, purchase of a new outfit

Signature of nurse _____ Signature of client _____ Date _____

FIGURE 15-3 Example of a health behavior change contract.

norms and traditions before interventions are developed. Customs, laws, novels, films, television, and other cultural forces shape ideas about health and how to achieve it. Culture determines whether an individual thinks healthful body movement should take the form of tai chi or jogging, or whether aging should involve accepting wrinkles or having face lifts. Culture can also convey conflicting messages. Paradoxically, Americans are saturated with media images of toned, sleek bodies, while fast-food restaurants beckon at every intersection. A visitor from another planet, confronted with our highly health-conscious but overweight, sedentary population, might conclude that most Americans have a death wish.

Environmental Influences

Nurses' attention to environmental hazards was heightened when the American Nurses Association adopted the Precautionary Principle in 2004. Thousands of new chemicals have been introduced in recent years, but research regarding their effects on human beings is often lacking. Many products commonly used in agriculture, industry, and the home are proving to be harmful. If adverse health effects are suspected, the Precautionary Principle mandates that nurses take precautionary measures even if cause–effect relationships have not been scientifically demonstrated. Nurses are also urged to include an environmental exposure history in routine health assessments (Buchanan, 2005). Clients should be queried about exposures where they live, play, and work.

Many people are exposed to noxious substances or stimuli in the workplace. Asbestos, mercury, radiation, and toxic chemicals such as pesticides are just a few of the hazards workers may encounter. Social and psychological hazards must be considered as well. Racial or sexual discrimination on the job may present a health risk equivalent to (or even greater than) environmental factors such as excessive workplace noise. Queries about a client's place of residence may reveal proximity to polluting industries or hazardous waste sites. Many Americans reside in substandard housing in neighborhoods in which crime and violence are commonplace. Some lack the security provided by a close-knit community of solicitous neighbors. They may have limited coping resources to withstand the daily bombardment of stressful events and hassles.

Stress

What happens when the environment bombards individuals with stressors? Researchers now know that stress is not simply a physiological reaction to environmental stimuli, as conceptualized by Selye (1956), but is instead a psychological appraisal that the environmental demands exceed one's coping resources (Lazarus, 1991). Early stress research focused on major life events such as foreclosure of a mortgage, bereavement, divorce, or job loss, demonstrating that an accumulation of such events could be detrimental to health (Holmes & Rahe, 1967). These major life events are undoubtedly disruptive, but minor daily hassles such as traffic jams, rude salespersons, and tax frustration are disruptive as well (Kanner, Coyne, Schaefer, & Lazarus, 1981). Stress is often associated with gender roles, with males reacting more strongly to masculine-role stressors (work, financial) and females reacting more to stresses within their relationships and caregiving roles (Davis, Burleson, & Kruszewski, 2011).

Allostasis (the continual adjustment of our bodies to stressors) can slide into health-damaging *allostatic load* when stress lasts too long or the body's response is too strong (McEwen & Lasley, 2003). Chronic stress increases vulnerability to diseases, such as cardiovascular disease (Shivpuri, Gallo, Crouse, & Allison, 2012), and accelerates the aging process by shortening the life span of cells (Epel, Blackburn, Lin, Dhabhar, Adler, & Morrow, et al., 2004). Research on a nationally representative sample showed that the risk of premature death was increased in individuals who reported high stress (Keller, Litzelman, Wisk, et al., 2012).

Stress can undermine enactment of health-promoting behavior. For example, during times of high stress people tend to exercise less. Fortunately, stress management modalities, ranging from meditation to yoga to breathing techniques, are widely available. However, health care providers must, once again, keep the environmental context in mind. Individuals in highly stressful environments may choose health-damaging behaviors to help them cope. Low income women report that they smoke to relieve the stresses of poverty and to belong in their social circle; smoking is one of the few coping strategies available to them (Stewart, Greaves, & Kushner, et al., 2011). Millions of American (15% of our population) live in poverty, at or below the federal poverty level (Abramsky, 2013). People living in poverty are not likely to perceive that they can master stress. In fact, when poverty is chronic and resources scant, individuals are likely to have pervasive feelings of powerlessness and a fatalistic outlook about the future (Kaplan, Madden, & Mijanovich, et al., 2013).

Social Support

Loving relationships with significant others may buffer or moderate stress. Connectedness to others is a central element in health throughout life. Considerable empirical evidence shows that social support produces improved resistance to disease, influences recovery from a health crisis such as myocardial infarction, and predicts longevity (Lett, Blumenthal, Babyak, Catellier, Carney, & Berkman, et al., 2007). How does social support result in improved health? Both emotional and instrumental types of support have been identified (Finfgeld-Connett, 2005). Support from relatives and friends can include concrete material help (e.g., money, provision of health information and advice) as well as affirmation of self-worth and encouragement to maintain good self-care practices. Extrafamilial support groups and health professionals can also play a vital role in encouraging exercise, smoking cessation, dieting, and other health-promoting actions. The value of a dieting or jogging "buddy" is well known. Stigmatized and marginalized client populations, such as the homeless, may lack a supportive network. Mobilizing social support can be an essential nursing intervention in such cases.

NATIONAL HEALTH PROMOTION GOALS

Nurses' health promotion efforts must be supported and guided by an adequate understanding of U.S. public policy. The Healthy People documents published in 1979, 1990, 2000, and 2010 by the U.S. Public Health Service (USPHS), Department of Health and Human Services, have focused on both individual and societal influences on health. These widely disseminated publications have drawn attention to health disparities among Americans and provided guidance to state and local planners of public health programs. Health promotion and disease prevention objectives are precisely stated and measurable. The precisely delineated objectives in the Healthy People documents have enabled measurement of the nation's progress. While progress has been made in increasing Americans' life expectancy,

TABLE 15-4   **Selected Examples of National Health Promotion Objectives as Identified in *Healthy People 2020***

FOCUS AREA	GOAL	OBJECTIVE	TARGET
Health Communication and Health Information Technology	Use health communication strategies and health IT to improve population health outcomes, health care quality, and health equity.	HC/HIT 2.2 Increase the proportion of persons who report that their health care providers always explained things so they could understand them.	66% of persons will report that their health care providers always explained things so they could understand them.
Nutrition and Weight Status	Promote health and reduce chronic disease risk through the consumption of healthful diets and achievement and maintenance of healthy body weights.	NWS 10.2 Reduce the proportion of children aged 6 to 11 years who are considered obese.	15.7% of children aged 6 to 11 years will be considered obese.
Tobacco Use	Reduce illness, disability, and death related to tobacco use and secondhand smoke exposure.	TU 3.4 Reduce the initiation of the use of cigars by children and adolescents aged 12 to 17 years.	2.8% of children and adolescents will initiate the use of cigars.

too many people spend their final years burdened by multiple chronic diseases that impair their quality of life. Healthy People 2020 contains four overarching goals: promoting quality of life, healthy development, and healthy behaviors across the lifespan, and creating social and physical environments that promote health (USPHS, 2010). Selected objectives from Healthy People 2020 are shown in Table 15-4.

COMMUNITY HEALTH PROMOTION

Health professionals are collaborating increasingly with community leaders to design interventions such as youth activity programs, nutrition classes, school-based clinics, and health screenings. Among the indicators of a community's health are communication patterns, ability to take organized action, level of social functioning (work and school attendance), proportion of individuals at the poverty level, crime rates, and traditional morbidity and mortality statistics. One type of community intervention has focused on improving the cardiovascular health status of entire communities. Examples include the Stanford Five City Project, the Pawtucket Heart Health Program, and the Minnesota Heart Health Program (National Heart, Lung, and Blood Institute, 1990). These programs attempt to reduce risk factors such as obesity, hypertension, smoking, sedentary lifestyles, and serum cholesterol levels. Community members become involved in media campaigns. Distinct

programs are set up for different groups within the community. Points of contact with community residents include churches, stores, schools, and work sites. Many of these programs have been successful in reducing cholesterol levels, tobacco use, and weight gain and in lowering blood pressure and coronary heart disease risks in general. Competition between "teams" is encouraged in the popular Lighten Up weight loss programs, such as Lighten Up Iowa and Lighten Up Wisconsin. Interstate competition also takes place (Norman & Mills, 2004).

A second type of community program is the Healthy Cities initiatives, first developed in Canada and Europe. The first site in the United States, the Indiana Healthy Community Project, was developed by a nurse (Flynn, Rider, & Bailey, 1992). Rather than focusing on a predetermined health problem such as cardiovascular risk, the Healthy Cities initiatives address a broad range of concerns that are identified by community members, such as gang violence and job creation. Coalitions of community groups are formed to develop programming. For individuals who live in rural areas rather than cities, county-based programs involving county extension agents, such as Walk Kansas, have proven successful (Estabrooks, Bradshaw, Dzewaltowski, & Smith-Ray, 2008). Because lack of public transportation and child care presents barriers to participation in health-promoting activities in rural areas, church buses and vans have been recommended (Kruger, Howell, & Haney, et al., 2012).

Interventions at work sites are increasingly common. An example is Seattle's worksite obesity prevention program, delivered at 33 worksites (Barrington, Ceballos, & Bisho, et al., 2012). Participants were encouraged to consume fewer fast food meals, eat more fruits and vegetables, and increase the amount of physical activity. Additionally, stress was measured by the researchers. Consistent with previous studies, higher stress was associated with lower physical activity and less attentiveness to healthy eating.

School-based interventions, especially those involving contemporary media used by youth, are achieving success in smoking prevention and cessation. For example, Canadian researchers created an interactive website called the Smoking Zine (www.smokingzine.org:81/start), which was supplemented by motivational groups in the classroom and 6 months of e-mail messages to the adolescent students. The intervention provided cessation motivation to the smokers who were most resistant to quitting and prevented nonsmokers from taking up the habit (Norman, Maley, Li, & Skinner, 2008).

Interventions at the neighborhood level are also proving efficacious. Researchers in Portland, Oregon conducted a neighborhood walking program aimed at improving quality of life in older adults (Fisher & Li, 2004). Neighbors walked together, led by a researcher-trained leader, three times a week for 6 months. Physical functioning, mental well-being, and life satisfaction were significantly improved in the 56 intervention neighborhoods compared with control neighborhoods in which residents only received informational materials about aging.

Nurses teamed up with community health workers in the "Sister to Sister" project, to assist low-socioeconomic African American women in subsidized housing to quit smoking (Andrews, Felton, Wewers, Waller, & Humbles, 2005). The community workers were residents of the community and former smokers themselves. They shared their own experiences in smoking cessation during individual sessions and group meetings with the study participants. The project achieved a 2-month abstinence rate of 60%, with study participants showing significant increases in self-efficacy. The support of the community health workers was an important component of the intervention.

Canadian researchers are studying the role of the family as an intermediary between community health promotion programs and subsequent desired changes in family members' risk behaviors. In the Quebec Heart Health Demonstration Project, four types of families (balanced, traditional, disconnected, and emotionally strained) were examined. Balanced families (characterized by a balance between focus on interior of the family and presence in the extrafamilial world) scored highest of the four types on valuing of health and were predicted to be more responsive to community health promotion programming (Fisher, Soubhi, Mansi, Paradis, Gauvin, & Potvin, et al., 1998). Yet to be determined are ways to increase responsiveness of the more poorly functioning families.

Within the last decade, increased emphasis is being placed on tailoring preventive interventions to meet the needs of diverse groups that are culturally different from the participants in scientifically rigorous controlled trials. Programs designed to reduce health disparities or combat problems such as substance abuse or teenage pregnancy may be evidence-based, but mismatched for the particular community (Ramanadhan, Crisostomo, Alexander-Molloy et al., 2012). Castro, Barrera, and Martinez (2004, p. 41) quote a Southwestern community leader who asked (in Spanish), "What good is science if it doesn't help us?" Unless programs are adapted for the intended audience, people will "vote with their feet" (Crowley, Greenberg, Feinberg et al., 2012, p.101). Thus willingness to listen to community input when planning health promotion programs is essential.

The greatest challenge of health promotion in the 21st century may be reaching the more vulnerable and disenfranchised members of society and involving them in strategies to enhance and prolong their lives.

SUMMARY

Changing health behavior is difficult even when doing so would lessen the likelihood of future illness. Although individuals are often aware of the risks associated with poor health behaviors, they modify their thinking about these risks rather than changing the behaviors. Information is the solution only when ignorance is the problem.

Understanding the principles of behavior change helps patients make health-promoting decisions. Using a comprehensive model of wellness identifies the behavioral, psychological, environmental, and organismic factors of attitude and behaviors associated with wellness. Pender's health promotion model assists in predicting the likelihood of successful behavior change based on personal factors and prior-related behavior. Health risk appraisals and contracting are useful to fostering health promotion behaviors. Environmental factors also affect wellness. National health promotion goals to guide health policy are defined in the *Healthy People* initiative.

SALIENT POINTS

- Conceptualizing health more broadly than "the absence of disease" has significant implications for nursing practice.
- Health promotion and disease prevention have different foci, in that health promotion activities aim to take people beyond their present level of wellness, whereas disease prevention efforts are undertaken to prevent specific diseases.
- The major causes of death in the United States are related to lifestyle.
- A comprehensive model of wellness includes modifiable attitudinal and behavioral variables as well as environmental factors and nonmodifiable organismic characteristics.

- Pender's Health Promotion Model is useful in guiding health promotion research and practice.
- Prochaska's transtheoretical model can be used to assess client readiness to change health behavior.
- Motivational interventions are more likely to promote health behavior change than threats of future disease or distant adverse outcomes.
- Health care providers should make greater use of written prescriptions, contracting, and other evidence-based interventions.
- Nurses' health promotion efforts should be guided by national health promotion goals, such as those articulated in *Healthy People 2020*.
- Health promotion initiatives must target families and communities as well as individuals.

CRITICAL REFLECTION EXERCISES

1. Interview three people regarding their definition of health. Compare their definitions to the various theories presented in the chapter, and to your own ideas about health.
2. Assess your own health behavior, and then select one behavior that you desire to change. It can be something you want to *increase,* such as aerobic exercise, *decrease,* such as eating junk food, or *stop,* such as smoking. Develop a plan to change the behavior, and then implement the plan for one month. Critically

assess factors that facilitated or hindered achievement of your behavior change.
3. Select one detrimental health behavior, such as excessive drinking. Review the research literature regarding evidence-based interventions to change this behavior. Is it clear which interventions are most effective? Is sufficient information available about changing the behavior in people of diverse ages, ethnicity, sexual orientation, and socioeconomic status? Develop at least three questions for future research.

WEBSITE RESOURCES

American Council on Science and Health: www.acsh.org
For calculating calories in food and calories burned in activities of daily living: www.caloriesperhour.com
Center for the Advancement of Health: www.cfah.org
Center for Tobacco Cessation: www.centerforcessation.org
The Collaborative on Health and the Environment: www.cheforhealth.org

For general tips on smoking cessation: www.ahrq.gov/consumer/index.html#smokingwww.smokingzine.org:81/start
Healthy People 2020: www.HealthyPeople.gov
For models of health behavior change: www.med.usf.edu/~kmbrown/hlth_beh_models.htm
For nurses who smoke: www.tobaccofreenurses.org
Nutrition information: www.nutrition.gov
For physical activity guidelines: www.health.gov/paguidelines

For tips on achieving better sleep: www.sleepfoundation.org
For treatment of obesity: Agency for Healthcare Research and Quality: www.ahrq.gov/clinic/epcsums/obesphsum.pdf
USDA food pyramid: www.mypyramid.gov
USDA/HHS Dietary Guidelines: www.dietaryguidelines.gov
For weight control information: www.win.niddk.nih.gov/index.htm

REFERENCES

Abramsky, S. (October 7, 2013). America's shameful poverty stats. *The Nation*.

Anderson, N. B., & Anderson, P. E. (2003). *Emotional longevity*. New York: Penguin.

Andrews, J. O., Felton, G., Wewers, M. E., Waller, J., & Humbles, P. (2005). Sister to sister: A pilot study to assist African American women in subsidized housing to quit smoking. *Southern Online Journal of Nursing Research, 6*(1), 1–20.

Aronson, K. R., Almeida, D. M., Stawski, R. S., Klein, L. S., & Kozlowski, L. T. (2008). Smoking is associated with worse mood on stressful days: Results from a national diary study. *Annals of Behavioral Medicine, 36*, 259–269.

Bandura, A. (1997). *Self-efficacy: The exercise of control*. New York: W. H. Freeman.

Barrington, W. E., Ceballos, R., & Bishop, S., et al. (2012). Perceived stress, behavior, and body mass index among adults participating in a worksite obesity prevention program, Seattle, 2005-2007. *Preventing Chronic Disease*, October 9, E152.

Becker, M. H., Haefner, D. P., Kasl, S. V., et al. (1977). Selected psychosocial models and correlates of individual health-related behaviors. *Medical Care, 15*(5), 27–46.

Belloc, N. B., & Breslow, L. (1972). Relationship of physical health status and health practices. *Preventive Medicine, 1*, 409–421.

Bialous, S. A., & Sarna, L. (2004). Sparing a few minutes for tobacco cessation. *The American Journal of Nursing, 104*(12), 54–60.

Booth-Thomas, C. (2004). The cafeteria crusader. *Time, 164*(24), 36–37.

Boyle, P. A., Barnes, L. L., Buchman, A. S., & Bennett, D. A. (2009). Purpose in life is associated with mortality among community-dwelling older persons. *Psychosomatic Medicine, 71*, 574–579.

Breslow, L., & Enstrom, J. E. (1980). Persistence of health habits and their relationship to mortality. *Preventive Medicine, 9*, 469–483.

Buchanan, M. (2005). Rebuilding the bridge. *The American Journal of Nursing, 105*(4), 104.

Campos, H., Baylin, A., & Willett, W. C. (2008). Alpha-linolenic acid and risk of nonfatal acute myocardial infarction. *Circulation, 118*, 323–324.

Carver, C. S., & Scheier, M. F. (2002). Optimism. In C. R. Snyder, & S. J. Lopes (Eds.), *The handbook of positive psychology* (pp. 231–243). New York: Oxford University Press.

Castro, F. G., Barrera, M., & Martinez, C. R. (2004). The cultural adaptation of prevention interventions: Resolving tensions between fidelity and fit. *Prevention Science, 5*(1), 41–45.

Centers for Disease Control and Prevention. (2014). High blood pressure facts. Retrieved from www.cdc.gov.

Centers for Disease Control and Prevention, Epidemiology Program Office. (2009). Perceived insufficient rest or sleep among adults: United States, 2008. *Morbidity and Mortality Weekly Report, 42*, 1175–1179.

Centers for Disease Control and Prevention. (2013). Adult participation in aerobic and muscle-strengthening physical activities—United States, 2011. *Morbidity and Mortality Weekly Report, 62*(17), 326–330.

Chida, Y., & Steptoe, A. (2009). The association of anger and hostility with future coronary heart disease: A meta-analytic review of prospective evidence. *Journal of the American College of Cardiology, 53*, 939–946.

Crowley, D. M., Greenberg, M. T., & Feinberg, M. E., et al. (2012). The effect of the PROSPER Partnership Model on cultivating local stakeholder knowledge of evidence-based programs: A five-year longitudinal study of 28 communities. *Prevention Science, 13*, 96–105.

D'Alonzo, K. T., Stevenson, J. S., & Davis, S. E. (2004). Outcomes of a program to enhance exercise self-efficacy and improve fitness in Black and Hispanic college-age women. *Research in Nursing & Health, 27*, 357–369.

Davis, M. C., Burleson, M. H., & Kruszewski, D. M. (2011). Gender: Its relationship to stressor exposure, cognitive appraisal/coping processes, stress responses, and health outcomes. In R. J. Contrada, & A. Baum (Eds.), *The handbook of stress science: Biology, psychology, and health* (pp. 247–261). New York: Springer.

Dobson, R. (2008). Half of patients given exercise prescriptions are more active. *British Medical Journal, 337*, 894–895.

Dubos, R. (1965). *Man adapting*. New Haven, CT: Yale University Press.

Dunn, H. (1959). High level wellness for man and society. *American Journal of Public Health, 49*, 88.

Dunn, H. (1971). *High level wellness*. Arlington, VA: Beatty.

Epel, E. S., Blackburn, E. H., Lin, J., Dhabhar, F. S., Adler, N. E., & Morrow, J. D. (2004). Accelerated telomere shortening in response to life stress. *Proceedings of the National Academy of Sciences, 101*(49), 17312–17315.

Estabrooks, P., Bradshaw, M., Dzewaltowski, D., & Smith-Ray, R. (2008). Determining the impact of Walk Kansas: Applying a team-building approach to community physical activity promotion. *Annals of Behavioral Medicine, 36*, 1–12.

Estabrooks, P., Fisher, E. B., & Hayman, L. L. (2008). What is needed to reverse the trends in childhood obesity? A call to action. *Annals of Behavioral Medicine, 36*, 209–216.

Finfgeld-Connett, D. (2005). Clarification of social support. *Journal of Nursing Scholarship, 37*(1), 4–9.

Fiore, M. C., Jaen, C. R., Baker, T. B., Bailey, W. C., Bennett, G., Benowitz, N. L., et al. (2008). A clinical practice guideline for treating tobacco use and dependence: 2008 update. A U.S. Public Health Service Report. *American Journal of Preventive Medicine, 35*, 158–176.

Fisher, K. J., & Li, F. (2004). A community-based walking trial to improve neighborhood quality of life in older adults: A multilevel analysis. *Annals of Behavioral Medicine, 28*, 186–194.

Fisher, L., Soubhi, H., Mansi, O., Paradis, G., Gauvin, L., & Potvin, L. (1998). Family process in health research: Extending a family typology to a new cultural context. *Health Psychology, 17*, 358–366.

Flynn, B. C., Rider, M. S., & Bailey, W. W. (1992). Developing community leadership in healthy cities: The Indiana model. *Nursing Outlook, 49*(3), 121–126.

Godfrey, J. R. (2004). Toward optimal health: The experts discuss therapeutic humor. *Journal of Women's Health, 13*, 474–479.

Goldbacher, E., & Matthews, K. A. (2007). Are psychological characteristics related to risk of the metabolic syndrome? A review of the literature. *Annals of Behavioral Medicine, 34*, 240–252.

Gorman, C. (2004). Why we sleep. *Time, 164*(25), 46–56.

Gray, E. (September 30, 2013). Electronic cigarettes could save lives—or hook a new generation on nicotine. *Time*, 39–46.

Guarnero, P. A. (2013). Latino young men and health promotion, emerging adulthood and acculturation: A qualitative exploration. *Issues in Mental Health Nursing, 34*, 806–812.

Hallahan, B., & Garland, M. (2005). Essential fatty acids and mental health. *British Journal of Psychiatry, 186*, 275–277.

Harburg, E., Kaciroti, N., Gleiberman, L., Julius, M., & Schork, M. A. (2008). Marital pairanger-coping types may act as an entity to affect mortality: Preliminary findings from a prospective study (Tecumseh, Michigan, 1971-1988). *Journal of Family Communication, 8*(1), 44–61.

Hart, J. (2008). Spirituality and health. *Alternative and Complementary Therapies, 14*, 189–193.

Herzog, T. A., & Blagg, C. O. (2007). Are most precontemplators contemplating smoking cessation? Assessing the validity of the stages of change. *Health Psychology, 26*, 222–231.

Hicks, M., McDermott, L. L., Rouhana, N., Schmidt, M., Seymour, M., & Sullivan, T. (2008). Nurses' body size and public confidence in ability to provide health education. *Journal of Nursng Scholarship, 40*, 349–354.

Hochbaum, G. M. (1958). *Public participation in medical screening programs: A sociopsychological study*. U.S. Public Health Service Publication No. 572. Washington, DC: U.S. Department of Health and Human Services.

Hollis, J. F., Gullion, C. M., Stevens, V. J., Brantley, P. J., Appel, L. J., & Ard, J. D. (2008). Weight loss during the intensive intervention phase of the Weight-Loss Maintenance Trial. *American Journal of Preventive Medicine, 35*, 118–126.

Holmes, T. H., & Rahe, R. H. (1967). The Social Readjustment Rating Scale. *Journal of Psychosomatic Research, 11*, 213–218.

Holt-Lunstad, J., Smith, T. W., & Uchino, B. (2008). Can hostility interfere with the health benefits of giving and receiving social support? The impact of cynical hostility on cardiovascular reactivity during social support interactions among friends. *Annals of Behavioral Medicine, 35*, 319–330.

Hughner, R. S., & Kleine, S. S. (2008). Variations in lay health theories: Implications for consumer health care decision making. *Qualitative Health Research, 18*, 1687–1703.

Im, E. O., Lee. B., & Yoo, K., et al. (20100. "A waste of time": Hispanic women's attitudes toward physical activity. *Women and Health, 50*, 563–579.

Jackson, E. S., Tucker, C. M., & Herman, K. C. (2007). Health value, perceived social support, and health self-efficacy as factors in a health-promoting lifestyle. *Journal of American College Health, 56*(1), 69–74.

Kanner, A., Coyne, J., Schaefer, C., & Lazarus, R. (1981). Comparison of two modes of stress measurement: Daily hassles and uplifts versus major life events. *Journal of Behavioral Medicine, 4*, 1–39.

Kaplan, S., Madden, V., Mijanovich, T., et al. (2013). The perception of stress and its impact on health in poor communities. *Journal of Community Health, 38*, 142–149.

Keller, A., Litzelman, K., Wisk, L., et al. (2012). Does the perception that stress affects health matter? The association with health and mortality. *Health Psychology, 31*, 677–684.

Kelly, T., Yang, W., Chen, C. S., Reynolds, K., & He, J. (2008). Global burden of obesity in 2005 and projections to 2030. *International Journal of Obesity, 32*, 1431–1437.

Kiecolt-Glaser, J., McGuire, L., Robles, T. F., & Glaser, R. (2002). Emotions, morbidity, and mortality: New perspectives from psychoneuroimmunology. *Annual Review of Psychology, 53*, 83–107.

King, A. C., Kiernan, M., & Oman, R., et al. (1997). Can we identify who will adhere to long-term physical activity? Signal detection methodology as a potential aid to clinical decision-making. *Health Psychology, 16*, 380–389.

King, B. A., Tynan, M. A., Dube, S. R., & Arrazola, R. (2014). Flavored-little-cigar and flavored-cigarette use among US middle and high school students. *The Journal of Adolescent Health, 54*(1), 40–46.

Knutson, K. L., Van Cauter, E., & Rathouz, P. J., et al. (2010). Trends in the prevalence of short sleepers in the UDA: 1975-2006. *Sleep, 33*, 37–45.

Koh, H. K. (2010). A 2020 vision for healthy people. *The New England Journal of Medicine, 362*, 1653–1656.

Kruger, T. M., Howell, B. M., & Haney, A. (2012). Perceptions of smoking cessation programs in rural Appalachia. *American Journal of Health Behavior, 36*, 373–384.

Lawton, R., Conner, M., & McEachan, R. (2009). Desire or reason: Predicting health behaviors from affective and cognitive attitudes. *Health Psychology, 28*, 56–65.

Lazarus, R. (1991). *Emotion and adaptation*. New York: Oxford University Press.

Leffingwell, T. R., Neumann, C., Leedy, M. J., & Babitzke, A. C. (2007). Defensively biased responding to risk information among alcohol-using college students. *Addictive Behaviors, 32*, 158–165.

Lett, H. S., Blumenthal, J. A., Babyak, M. A., Catellier, D. J., Carney, R. M., & Berkman, L. F., et al. (207). Social support and prognosis in patients at increased psychosocial risk recovering from myocardial infarction. *Health Psychology, 26*, 418–427.

Listfield, E. (2009, August 9). 10 minutes to better health. *Parade*, 19.

Lutes, L. D., Winett, R. A., Barger, S. D., Wojcik, J. R., Herbert, W. G., & Nickols-Richardson, S. M. (2008). Small changes in nutrition and physical activity promote weight loss and maintenance: 3-month evidence from the ASPIRE randomized trial. *Annals of Behavioral Medicine, 35*, 351–357.

Mackert, M., Stanforth, D., & Garcia, A. A. (2011). Undermining of nutrition and exercise decisions: Experiencing negative social influence. *Public Health Nursing, 28*, 402–410 2011.

Manini, T. M., Everhart, J. E., Patel, K. V., Schoeller, D. A., Colbert, L. H., & Visser, M., et al. (2006). Daily activity energy expenditure and mortality among older adults. *Journal of the American Medical Association, 296*, 171–179.

Maslow, A. (1961) Health as transcendence of environment. *J Humanistic Psychology, 1*, 1–7.

McAuley, E., Doerksen, S., Morris, K., Motl, R., Hu, L., Wojcicki, T., et al. (2008). Pathways from physical activity to quality of life in older women. *Annals of Behavioral Medicine, 36*, 13–20.

McCloskey, M. S., Kleabir, K., & Berman, M. E., et al. (2010). Unhealthy aggression: Intermittent explosive disorder and adverse physical health outcomes. *Health Psychology, 29*, 324–332.

McEwen, B., & Lasley, E. N. (2003). Allostatic load: When protection gives way to damage. *Advances, 19*(1), 28–33.

Miller, S. K., Alpert, P. T., & Cross, C. L. (2008). Overweight and obesity in nurses, advanced practice nurses, and nurse educators. *Journal of the American Academy of Nurse Practitioners, 20*, 259–265.

Mostofsky, E., Maclure, M., Tofler, G., et al. (2013). Relation of outbursts of anger and risk of acute myocardial infarction. *The American Journal of Cardiology, 112*(3), 343–348.

Murphy, S. L., Xu, J., & Kochanek, M. (2013). Deaths: Final data for 2010. *National Vital Statistics Reports, 61*(4). Hyattsville, MD: National Center for Health Statistics.

Naci, H., & Ioannidis, J. (2013). Comparative effectiveness of exercise and drug interventions on mortality outcomes: Metaepidemiological study. *British Medical Journal, 347*, 15577.

National Heart, Lung, and Blood Institute. (1990). *Three community programs change heart health across the nation* [Special edition]. Infomemo. Washington, DC: Author.

National Sleep Foundation. (2004). "Sleep in America" 2004 poll [Online]. Retrieved from http://www.sleepfoundation.org/_content//hottopics/2004SleepPollFinalReport.pdf

Newman, M. (2000). *Health as expanding consciousness* (2nd ed.). Sudbury, MA: Jones & Bartlett.

Norman, C. D., Maley, O., Li, X., & Skinner, H. A. (2008). Using the Internet to assist smoking prevention and cessation in schools: A randomized, controlled trial. *Health Psychology, 27*, 799–810.

Norman, G. J., & Mills, P. J. (2004). Keeping it simple: Encouraging walking as a means to active living. *Annals of Behavioral Medicine, 28*, 149–151.

Orem, D. E. (2001). *Nursing: Concepts of practice* (6th ed.). St Louis: Mosby.

Patel, M., Phillips-Caesar, E., & Boutin-Foster, C. (2012). Barriers to lifestyle behavioral change in migrant South Asian populations. *Journal of Immigrant and Minority Health, 14*, 774–785.

Pender, N., Murdaugh, C. L., & Parsons, M. A. (2002). *Health promotion in nursing practice* (4th ed.). Upper Saddle River, NJ: Prentice-Hall.

Pennebaker, J. W. (1990). *Opening up: The healing power of confiding in others*. New York: Morrow.

Pennebaker, J. W., & Chung, C. K. (2011). Expressive writing and its links to mental and physical health. In H. Friedman (Ed.), *Oxford handbook of health psychology*. New York: Oxford University Press.

Primack, B. A., Sidani, J., Agarwal, A., Shadel, W., Donny, E., & Eissenberg, T. (2008). Prevalence of and associations with waterpipe tobacco smoking among U.S. university students. *Annals of Behavioral Medicine, 36*, 81–86.

Prochaska, J. J., Hall, S. M., Humfleet, G., Munoz, R., Reus, V., & Gorecki, J. (2008). Promoting physical activity for maintaining non-smoking: A randomized controlled trial. *Annals of Behavioral Medicine, 35*, S102.

Prochaska, J. O., DiClemente, C. C., & Norcross, J. C. (1992). In search of how people change: Applications to addictive behaviors. *The American Psychologist, 47*, 1102–1114.

Ramanadhan, S., Crisostomo, J., Alexander-Molloy, J., et al. (2012). Perceptions of evidence-based programs among community-based organizations tackling health disparities: A qualitative study. *Health Education Research, 27*, 717–728.

Ricciardi, R. (2005). Sedentarism: A concept analysis. *Nursing Forum, 40*(3), 79–87.

Riegel, B., Dickson, V. V., Hoke, L., McMahon, J., Reis, B., & Sayers, S. (2006). A motivational counseling approach to improving heart failure self-care: Mechanisms of effectiveness. *Journal of Cardiovascular Nursing, 21*, 232–241.

Rogers, M. (1970). *An introduction to the theoretical basis of nursing*. Philadelphia: Davis.

Roman, C. G., & Chalfin, A. (2008). Fear of walking outdoors: A multilevel ecologic analysis of crime and disorder. *American Journal of Preventive Medicine, 34*, 306–312.

Rotter, J. B. (1954). *Social learning and clinical psychology*. Englewood Cliffs, NJ: Prentice-Hall.

Roy, C. (2009). *The Roy adaptation model* (3rd ed.). Upper Saddle River, NJ: Pearson Education.

Selye, H. (1956). *The stress of life*. New York: McGraw-Hill.

Shivpuri, S., Gallo, L., Crouse, J. R., & Allison, M. A. (2012). The association between chronic stress type and C-reactive protein in the multi-ethnic study of atherosclerosis: Does gender make a difference? *Journal of Behavioral Medicine, 35*, 74–85.

Smith, J. (1983). *The idea of health: Implications for the nursing profession*. New York: Teachers College Press.

Smuts, J. (1926). *Holism and evolution*. New York: Macmillan.

Stambor, Z. (2006). Specific environments alone can trigger smokers' cigarette cravings. *APA Monitor, 37*(3), 15.

Stamler, J., Stamler, R., Neaton, J. D., Wentworth, D., Daviglus, M. L., & Garside, D. (1999). Low risk-factor profile and long-term cardiovascular and non-cardiovascular mortality and life expectancy: Findings for 5 large cohorts of young adult and middle-aged men and women. *Journal of the American Medical Association, 282*, 2012–2018.

Stewart, M. J., Greaves, L., Kushner, K. E., et al. (2011). Where there is smoke, there is stress: Low-income women identify support needs and preferences for smoking reduction. *Health Care for Women International, 32,* 359–383.

Sullivan, H. W., & Rothman, A. J. (2008). When planning is needed: Implementation intentions and attainment of approach versus avoidance health goals. *Health Psychology, 27,* 438–444.

Third-hand smoke: Another reason to quit smoking. (December 31, 2008). *Science Daily.* Retrieved January 15, 2009, from http://www.sciencedaily.com/releases/2008/12/081229105037.htm.

Thomas, S. P. (1997). Angry? Let's talk about it. *Applied Nursing Research, 10*(2), 80–85.

Thomas, S. P. (2001). Teaching healthy anger management. *Perspectives in Psychiatric Care, 37,* 41–48.

Thomas, S. P. (2006). Cultural and gender considerations in the assessment and treatment of anger-related disorders. In E. L. Feindler (Ed.), *Anger-related disorders: A practitioner's guide to comparative treatments.* (pp. 71–95). New York: Springer.

Thomas, S. P. (2007). Trait anger, anger expression, and themes of anger incidents in contemporary undergraduate students. In E. I. Clausen (Ed.), *Psychology of anger* (pp. 23–69). New York: Nova Science.

Thomas, S. P., & Pollio, H. R. (2002). *Listening to patients.* New York: Springer.

Toledo, E., Hu, F., Estruch, R., et al. (2013). Effect of the Mediterranean diet on blood pressure in the PREDIMED trial: Results from a randomized controlled trial. *BMC Medicine, 11,* 207.

U.S. Department of Agriculture. (August, 2008). Diet quality of Americans in 1994-96 and 2001-02 as measured by the Healthy Eating Index-2005. Nutrition Insight 37. Retrieved January 15, 2009, from http://www.cnpp.usda.gov

U.S. Department of Agriculture and US Department of Health and Human Services. (2010). *Dietary guidelines for Americans 2010* (7th ed.). Washington, DC: US Govt. Printing Office.

U.S. Public Health Service. (1979). *Healthy People: The Surgeon General's report on health promotion and disease prevention.* Washington, DC: U.S. Department of Health, Education, & Welfare.

U.S. Public Health Service. (1990). Healthy People 2000. Washington, DC: U.S. Department of Health and Human Services.

U.S. Public Health Service. (2000). Healthy People 2010. Washington, DC: U.S. Department of Health and Human Services. [Online]. Available at http://www.health.gov/healthy people.

U.S. Public Health Service. (2010). Healthy People 2020. Washington, DC: U.S. Department of Health and Human Services. [Online]. Available at www.Health.gov/healthypeople.

van der Meer, R. M., Willemsen, M. C., Smit, F., & Cuijpers, P. (2013). Smoking cessation interventions for smokers with current or past depression. Retrieved from www.thecochranelibrary.com .

Walsh, R. (2011). Lifestyle and mental health. *American Psychologist, 66,* 579–592.

Werch, C. E., Moore, M. J., Bian, H., DiClemente, C., Ames, S. C., Weiler, R. M., et al. (2008). Efficacy of a brief image-based multiple-behavior intervention for college students. *Annals of Behavioral Medicine, 36,* 149–157.

Wilbur, J., Vassalo, A., & Chandler, P., et al. (2005). Midlife women's adherence to home-based walking during maintenance. *Nursing Research, 54,* 33–40.

Williams, E. C., Kivlahan, D. R., Saitz, R., Merrill, J. O., Achtmeyer, C. E., McCormick, K. A., et al. (2006). Readiness to change in primary care patients who screened positive for alcohol misuse. *Annals of Family Medicine, 4,* 213–220.

Wingo, B. C., Desmond, R. A., Brantley, P., et al. (2013). Self-efficacy as a predictor of weight change and behavior change in the PREMIER Trial. *Journal of Nutrition Education and Behavior, 45,* 314–321.

16 CHAPTER

Genetics and Genomics in Professional Nursing

Dale Halsey Lea, MPH, RN, CGC

ⓔ http://evolve.elsevier.com/Friberg/bridge/

OBJECTIVES

After completion of this chapter, the reader will be able to:

- Define genomic health care.
- Discuss the importance of the *Essentials of Genetic and Genomic Nursing: Competencies, Curricula Guidelines, and Outcome Indicators* to nursing practice.
- Discuss the nursing role in family history assessment.
- Describe nursing roles in genetic testing.

- Explain the nursing role in referral of patients and families for specialized genetic and genomic services.
- List two new ways that genetic testing is being used in clinical practice.
- Identify ethical issues of concern with regard to genomic health care.

👤 PROFILE IN PRACTICE

Barbara J. Ganster, RN, BSN
Nurse Case Manager, Breast Care Center, National Naval Medical Center, Bethesda, Maryland

I work in the breast care center at a military treatment facility (MTF). Every week we hold a multidisciplinary clinic in which newly diagnosed breast cancer patients are seen by the team who will be involved in their care and treatment. I complete a family "pedigree" as part of our evaluation, looking for factors that may indicate a need for genetic counseling and possible genetic testing.

I was completing the pedigree on a patient who, for support, had brought along a friend, a survivor of breast cancer who had been diagnosed in her thirties. While I do a pedigree, I provide education and explain why I am asking the questions. As we spoke, I mentioned to the friend that she had probably already had this conversation with her oncologist. She responded that she had not, but she added that since she had undergone bilateral mastectomies, it wasn't an issue for her. As I continued with the pedigree, I noted several times the friend giving nonverbal clues that had me increasingly concerned that there was more going on in her own family tree.

After I completed my patient's pedigree, I asked to speak with the friend. She did not want to take the focus off my patient, but I was able to reassure her that while the patient met with our social worker, I could spend a few minutes with her. Because this woman was not my patient and was not eligible for care at a MTF, I had to balance educational needs and not do actual counseling.

I offered to do a family pedigree, which revealed several more maternal family members with histories of breast cancer and at least one with ovarian cancer. Also, the woman was of Ashkenazi Jewish ancestry. I encouraged her to take the pedigree to her oncologist, whom she was scheduled to see that week for follow-up. I explained that although she had decreased her risk for breast cancer by having bilateral mastectomies, other cancers were also associated with BRCA mutation, ovarian cancer being the most concerning because survival rates are low, there are no good screening measures, and it usually is not detected early. If she was found to have a mutation, genetic counseling would include additional screening and possible risk-reduction measures.

My patient subsequently let me know her friend was referred to a genetic counselor and that she had tested positive for a BRCA mutation and was being seen by a gynecologist. The friend later contacted me to say thank you. Her pathology from the bilateral oophorectomies had shown a "precancerous" lesion on one ovary, and her gynecologist said that she had been destined for full-blown ovarian cancer if the surgery had not been done when it was.

♟ PROFILE IN PRACTICE

Jean Jenkins, PhD, RN, FAAN
National Institutes of Health, National Human Genome Research Institute, Bethesda, Maryland

Kathleen Calzone, MSN, RN, APNG, FAAN
National Institutes of Health, National Cancer Institute, Center for Cancer Research, Genetics Branch, Bethesda, Maryland

As cancer nurses, we (Jean Jenkins and Kathleen Calzone) began our journey together to integrate genetics and genomics into nursing practice and patient care in 1995, when a genetic counselor colleague suggested that we put together a workshop for nurses to explore the need for genetic education. At that time, genetic research was opening new doors to understanding the underlying genetics of an inherited susceptibility to breast cancer and influencing risk management, diagnosis, and treatment. We realized that these genetic discoveries would have a significant impact on oncology nursing practice and that nurses, including ourselves, were not prepared for this revolution in health care. We have since become "joined at the hip" and continue to work to move genetics and genomics into all nursing education and practice.

Our initial meeting was the Workshop on Genetics Education in Nursing, held at the National Institutes of Health in September 1995. Since then, we have collaborated to create the core competencies in cancer genetics for advanced practice nurses, initiate a nursing genetics and ethics study, and publish books and articles on these topics. One of our proudest accomplishments has been the publication of a series of peer-reviewed articles by genetics nurse specialists on genetics and genomics science and health care applications, showcasing important implications for nursing practice in the *Journal of Nursing Scholarship* over a 2-year period. This article series is now available as an educational resource for nurses (www.genome.gov/17515679) (Jenkins, 2007).

Another of our exciting endeavors was a 2-year initiative to establish essential competencies in genetics and genomics for all nurses. This culminated with an invitational consensus conference that brought together key nursing organizations at the American Nursing Association headquarters in September 2005 to finalize these competencies. This foundational meeting of 50 nursing organizations led to the consensus and publication of the *Essentials of Genetic and Genomic Nursing: Competencies, Curricula Guidelines, and Outcome Indicators* in 2005 and a second edition in 2008 (Consensus Panel on Genetic/Genomic Nursing Competencies, 2008), which defined the minimum genetics and genomics competencies needed by all registered nurses regardless of their educational preparation, clinical specialty, or role. To date, 49 nursing organizations have endorsed the *Essential Nursing Competencies,* many of which are developing their own genetic and genomic educational and outreach efforts.

The next steps in the competency initiative focused on making the *Essential Nursing Competencies* a living, useful document. In October 2006, we convened the group of endorsing organizations and some key stakeholders to develop a 5-year, multifaceted strategic implementation plan for the integration of the genetics and genomics competencies into nursing curricula, NCLEX, specialty certifications, continuing education, and accreditation, a process that involves collaboration among nursing and academic organizations and federal agencies both nationally and internationally.

A "toolkit" for academic faculty was developed, launched, and disseminated in February 2010 and can be accessed at www.g-2-c-2.com. As the toolkit is developed and disseminated, we are also working to establish an interdisciplinary consortium because achieving competency in genetics and genomics is an issue for all members of the health care community. In the next year we will be working with the American Academy of Nursing to hold meetings that will help to establish a national nursing research outcomes agenda for genetic and genomic nursing.

Our vision for all nurses is that (1) they become fluent in genetics and genomics so that they can communicate with their patients, families, and communities, and (2) they competently use genetic and genomic information to develop personalized plans to improve health care outcomes. Nurses are the keystone of the health care community and, as such, are fundamental to closing the gap between patients and the genetic and genomic discoveries that could optimize their health care.

INTRODUCTION: WHY GENETICS AND GENOMICS?

The human genome was completely mapped and sequenced in 2003. Discoveries from this human genome research are increasing our understanding of the role genes play in health and both rare and common diseases. A new era of health care—called *genomic health care*—is rapidly advancing. *Genomic Health Care* means that health care providers now have accessible new tools for tailoring health care to the individual by using a person's unique genomic information to design and prescribe the most effective treatment for each patient. These advances are ushering in new directions in the provision of health care and will have a significant impact on nurses and all other health care providers. Nurses in all practice settings will increasingly be expected to use genetic- and genomic-based approaches and technologies in their patient care. In recognition of the implications of genomic health care for nurses, the *Essentials of Genetic and Genomic Nursing: Competencies, Curricula Guideline, and Outcome Indicators* (Consensus Panel on Genetic/Genomic Nursing Competencies, 2008) was published. This chapter is founded on the *Essentials of Genetic and Genomic Nursing* and presents genetic and genomic discoveries and applications from yesterday to today, as well as for tomorrow. Applications of genetics and genomics to nursing and health care are addressed, including family history assessment, genetic screening and testing, pharmacogenetics and pharmacogenomics, and direct-to-consumer (DTC) genetic testing. Ethical and social issues related to genetics and genomics are also described. Genetics and genomics educational and clinical resources are provided to support the needs of all nurses wanting to learn more about and provide competent genomic health care, as noted in the *Essentials of Genetic and Genomic Nursing*:

Because essentially all diseases and conditions have a genetic or genomic component, options for care for all persons will increasingly include genetic and genomic information along the pathways of prevention, screening, diagnostics, prognostics, selection of treatment, and monitoring of treatment effectiveness. The clinical application of genetic and genomic knowledge has major implications for the entire nursing profession regardless of academic preparation, role, or practice setting. (Consensus Panel, 2008, p. 7)

Box 16-1 provides a listing of basic genetic terms and their definitions as a beginning step for nurses to become familiar with and knowledgeable about genetics and genomics.

Yesterday's Genetics

It was not until the late 1800s that scientists first began to discover the basic genetic structures—*chromosomes*—the threadlike structures inside of cells that contain genes. And it was not until the early 1900s that inherited diseases were linked to chromosomes. Scientific research and discoveries from the 1950s through the 1980s helped

scientists to develop genetic tests for genetic conditions such as Down syndrome, cystic fibrosis, and Duchenne muscular dystrophy. During those years, genetic testing was used to confirm a diagnosis of a genetic condition and to screen newborns for conditions such as phenylketonuria (PKU) so that early treatments and interventions could be administered (Genetics Home Reference, 2014a). Therefore nurses practicing in neonatal and pediatric settings were the first nurses to become informed about and involved with genetics in their practice with the advent of genetic testing for newborns and pediatric patients and their families. But were those nurses prepared with genetics knowledge so that they could provide competent and informed patient care? Not necessarily. The recognition that nurses did not have adequate knowledge of genetics to practice genetics health care was first documented in the nursing literature of 1979 (Cohen, 1979).

Today's Genetics and Genomics

Mapping and sequencing of the entire human genome was completed in 2003 after 15 years of research. Knowledge of the human genome has opened new doors to understanding the role of genes in health and disease. As an example, genetic discoveries have led to the development of an increasing number of genetic tests that can be used to identify a trait, diagnose a genetic disorder, and/or identify individuals who have a genetic predisposition to diseases, such as cancer or heart disease. Our understanding of genes and their roles in health and disease has expanded beyond genetics, which involves the study of individual genes and their impact on relatively rare, single-gene disorders. A new field of research called *genomics* involves the study of all of the genes in the human genome together, including their interactions with one another, their interactions with the environment, and the influence of other cultural and psychosocial factors (Consensus Panel, 2008; Guttmacher & Collins, 2002). In the pre-genome era, health care providers used a "one size fits all" approach to treating their patients. In the post-genome era, health care providers will increasingly use genomic information to tailor treatments to the individual patient and to personalize their care (National Human Genome Research Institute, 2014).

Genetics and genomics are therefore becoming an integral part of health care for patients from preconception to adulthood. Patients, families, and communities

BOX 16-1 Common Genetic and Genomic Terms

Allele—One of the variant forms of a gene at a particular location on a chromosome. Different alleles create variation in inherited characteristics such as hair color or blood type.

Chromosome—One of the threadlike "packages" of genes and other DNA that are located in the nucleus of a cell. Humans have 23 pairs of chromosomes, 46 in all: 44 autosomes and 2 sex chromosomes. Each parent contributes one chromosome to each pair, so children get half of their chromosomes from their mothers and half from their fathers.

Deoxyribonucleic acid (DNA)—The chemical inside the nucleus of a cell that carries genetic instructions for making living organisms.

Double helix—The structural arrangement of DNA, which looks something like an immensely long ladder twisted into a helix, or coil. The sides of the "ladder" are formed by a backbone of sugar and phosphate molecules, and the "rungs" consist of nucleotide bases joined weakly in the middle by hydrogen bonds.

Gene—The functional and physical unit of heredity passed from parent to offspring. Genes are pieces of DNA, and most genes contain the information for making a specific protein.

Genetic disorders—A disease caused in whole or in part by a "variation" (a different form) or "mutation" (alteration) of a gene.

Genetics—A term that refers to the study of genes and their role in inheritance; the way certain traits or conditions are passed down from one generation to another.

Genomics—A relatively new term that describes the study of all of a person's genes, including interactions of those genes with one another and with the person's environment.

Mendelian inheritance—The way in which genes and traits are passed from parents to children. Examples of Mendelian inheritance include autosomal dominant, autosomal recessive, and sex-linked genes.

Protein—A large complex molecule consisting of one or more chains of amino acids. Proteins perform a wide variety of activities in the cell.

Ribonucleic acid (RNA)—A chemical similar to a single strand of DNA. In RNA, the letter U, which stands for "uracil," is substituted for T in the genetic code. RNA delivers DNA's genetic message to the cytoplasm of a cell, where proteins are made.

Data from National Human Genome Research Institute (2012). *Genetics and Genomics for Patients and the Public*. Retrieved from www.genome.gov/19016903; and National Human Genome Research Institute (2013). *Talking Glossary of Genetic Terms*. Retrieved from www.genome.gov/glossary.

will increasingly expect all registered nurses and nurse specialists to be familiar with and use genetic and genomic information and technologies when providing care (Consensus Panel, 2008). Nurses at all levels and in all areas of practice will soon be taking an active role in risk assessment for genetic conditions and disorders, explaining genetic risk and genetic testing, and supporting informed health decisions and opportunities for early intervention (Skirton, Patch, & Williams, 2005).

ESSENTIALS OF GENETIC AND GENOMIC NURSING

In recognition of the need for all nurses to become proficient in incorporating genetics and genomics into their practice, nursing leaders from clinical, research, and academic settings came together to create "the minimum basis by which to prepare the nursing workforce to deliver competent genetic- and genomic-focused nursing care" (Consensus Panel, 2008, p. 1). The *Essentials of Genetic and Genomic Nursing* was developed based on several sources and resources, including (1) review of peer-reviewed published work that has

reported practice-based genetic and genomic competencies, guidelines, and recommendations; (2) input from nurses who were representatives to the National Coalition for Health Professional Education in Genetics (NCHPEG) in 2005; (3) public comment from the nursing community at large; and (4) statements during open comment periods from the nurses who attended a 2-day meeting of key stakeholders held in September 2005. The *Essentials of Genetic and Genomic Nursing* that were developed apply to the practice of all registered nurses regardless of their academic preparation, practice setting, role, or specialty. To date, more than 49 nursing organizations have endorsed the *Essentials of Genetic and Genomic Nursing* (Consensus Panel, 2008).

The *Essentials of Genetic and Genomic Nursing* is broken down into two categories: professional responsibilities and professional practice domain. The professional responsibilities are consistent with the nursing scope and standards of practice that were developed by the American Nurses Association (American Nurses Association, 2004). They include the incorporation of genetic and genomic technologies and information into registered nursing practice and the ability to tailor genetic and genomic information and services to clients based on their knowledge level, literacy, culture, religion, and preferred language. The professional practice domain includes the following: competencies in nursing assessment (applying and integrating genetic and genomic knowledge); identification of clients who could benefit from genetic and genomic information and services as well as reliable genetic and genomic resources; referral activities; and provision of education, care, and support, such as using genetic- and genomic-based interventions and information to improve client outcomes (Consensus Panel, 2008).

The *Essentials of Genetic and Genomic Nursing* document includes strategies to implement the competencies into nursing practice. These strategies include participating in the NCLEX test development process and working with the American Hospital Association and other regulatory agencies to incorporate genetics and genomics practice content. Another strategy is to have all certification exams include test items that measure the knowledge of genetic and genomic information specific to the specialty for which nurses are being certified. Practicing nurses are encouraged to pursue genetic and genomic continuing education. Accreditation programs are encouraged to evaluate whether the curriculum they are creating is designed to meet the essential nursing core genetic and genomic competencies. Nursing faculty members are given ideas and solutions regarding how they can incorporate genetics and genomics as a central science into their curricula. Resources to support the *Essentials of Genetic and Genomic Nursing* are also provided (Consensus Panel, 2008). Box 16-2 provides examples of currently available genetics and genomics educational resources for practicing nurses and nurse educators.

APPLYING GENETICS AND GENOMICS IN NURSING PRACTICE

This section focuses on several examples of how nurses are applying genetics and genomics in their practice. Two important clinical tools are now available to health care providers to personalize screening, prevention, diagnosis, and treatment of individuals and their families. These two tools are family history and genetic testing. Based on the *Essentials of Genetic and Genomic Nursing*, nurses will be involved with family history collection and pedigree construction and in offering and explaining genetic testing. Nurses will also refer individuals and families for genetic services and consultation.

Family History

Knowing the role of family history in common and rare genetic conditions and disorders is an important first step in genetic and genomic risk assessment and early intervention. It is now known that individuals who have a family history of chronic diseases such as heart disease, diabetes, and cancer in close relatives are more likely to have a higher risk of developing these diseases. Having a first-degree relative with any one of these diseases has been shown to increase a person's risk for developing the disease, with the risk increasing even more when there are more affected relatives or if the disease was diagnosed at an early age (National Human Genome Research Institute, 2012). All health care providers, including nurses, have a responsibility to collect family history information and could take advantage of this information to provide specific clinical prevention and management interventions for those diseases that run in the patient's family (National Human Genome Research Institute, 2012).

In recognition of the importance of family history in health and disease, the U.S. Surgeon General, in cooperation with the U.S. Department of Health and Human Services and other government agencies, began a national public health campaign in 2004 called the *U.S. Surgeon General's Family History Initiative*. The *Initiative* encourages all American families to learn more about their family history and offers a computerized tool to help families create a portrait of their family health (U.S. Department of Health and Human Services, 2014). Nurses need to be able to gather a minimum of three generations of family health history information so as to help families learn about their family health history. Nurses can offer individuals and families information about the *U.S. Surgeon General's Family History Initiative* to begin this process.

In accordance with the *Essentials of Genetic and Genomic Nursing*, nurses also need to be prepared to construct a pedigree from the collected family history information using the standardized symbols and terminology (Consensus Panel, 2008). Figure 16-1 provides an example of a pedigree and standardized symbols. During the process of family history collection and pedigree construction, nurses need to be alert for clients who present with family histories with multiple generations affected with a particular disorder (e.g., autosomal dominant inheritance), those with multiple siblings who have a genetic disorder (e.g., autosomal recessive inheritance), and those affected with a disease or condition at an early age (e.g., multiple generations with early-onset breast or ovarian cancer). When a client is identified as having a family history of a possible inherited genetic disorder, the nurse discusses the family history with the health care team and lets the client know that he or she may have a risk factor for a specific disease. The nurse and health care team can then facilitate referrals for specialized genetic and genomic services (Consensus Panel, 2008).

Genetic Testing: What It Is and How It Is Used in Clinical Practice

One of the most significant applications of genomics to health care that has expanded rapidly since the mapping of the human genome is genetic testing. Genetic testing involves the use of a laboratory test to find genetic variations that are associated with a disease. Genetic testing results are used to confirm or rule out a genetic disorder or to determine the chance of a person to pass a mutation on to his or her children. Genetic testing can be done prenatally or after birth. Genetic screening involves the testing of a population for a particular genetic disease to identify a subgroup of individuals that may have the disease or the potential to pass the disease on to their children (National Human Genome Research Institute, 2013).

Genetic testing is now available for more than 1600 genetic disorders ranging from single-gene disorders, such as cystic fibrosis, to complex disorders, such as diabetes, cancer, and heart disease (GeneTests, 2015). A number of different types of genetic tests are used in health care today.

Carrier testing is a type of genetic testing that can tell individuals if they "carry" a genetic variation that can cause a disease. Carriers of the genetic variation do not usually show any signs of the disorder because they carry one normal version of the gene. However, carriers can pass on the genetic variation to their children, who may develop the disorder or become carriers themselves. Thus testing may be offered or sought when couples are considering pregnancy or during early pregnancy. Carrier testing is offered to couples who are from particular ethnic or racial backgrounds and who have an increased risk for being carriers of an autosomal recessive gene for disorders. Examples include African-American couples who have an increased chance to carry a gene for sickle cell anemia and couples of Ashkenazi Jewish ancestry who have an increased chance for being carriers of a gene for Tay-Sachs disease (Genetics Home Reference, 2014b).

Diagnostic testing identifies a genetic variation that is either causing a person to have a genetic condition or disease now or may cause a condition in the

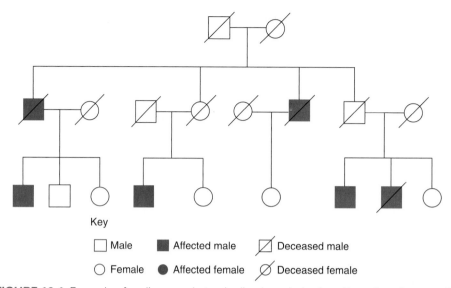

Key

☐ Male   ■ Affected male   ◻̸ Deceased male

◯ Female   ● Affected female   ◯̸ Deceased female

FIGURE 16-1 Example of pedigree and standardized symbols. A pedigree is a diagram of a family history that shows family members' relationships to each other and how a particular disease or trait is being passed on (inherited) in that family. For more information about how to construct a family history pedigree, go to the National Human Genome Research Institute, Your Family History, www.genome.gov/Pages/Education/Modules/YourFamilyHealth History.pdf. (From National Human Genome Research Institute. *Talking Glossary of Genetic Terms*. Retrieved from www.genome.gov/Pages/10002096.)

future. Results of diagnostic genetic testing can help with treatment decisions and management of the disorder. *Newborn screening* is used to test infants in the first few days of life to determine whether they have a genetic disorder that will cause problems with health and development. *Prenatal genetic testing* is offered during pregnancy to help identify fetuses that have certain diseases. *Preimplantation diagnostic genetic testing* is carried out in conjunction with in vitro fertilization to determine whether embryos for implantation carry genes that could cause disease (Genetics Home Reference, 2014a).

Research genetic testing helps scientists to learn more about how genes contribute to health and disease. Genetic and genomic research also helps with the development of gene-based treatments. The research genetic test results may not directly help the research participant; however, results may benefit others in the future by helping researchers expand their understanding of human genes and their roles in health and disease (National Human Genome Research Institute, 2012).

Nurses will be increasingly involved in the genetic testing process and will need to become knowledgeable

about the different types of genetic tests so that they can provide competent genetic- and genomic-based care. This knowledge will serve as the foundation to providing patients and families with interpretation of selective genetic and genomic information such as genetic testing results.

Referral for Genetic Counseling and Support Services

Nurses will benefit from knowing where to access specialized genetic and genomic services so that they are able to facilitate a genetics referral for clients who may have a genetic risk factor, abnormal genetic test result, or questions about a genetic or genomic condition or disorder. Genetics specialists are health care professionals who have specialized degrees and experience in medical genetics and counseling. Genetics professionals include medical geneticists, genetic counselors, and genetics nurses.

Genetic professionals work as members of health care teams to provide information and support to individuals and families who have genetic disorders or may be at risk for inherited conditions. Genetic professionals conduct the following activities during a genetic consultation:

- Assess the risk of a genetic disorder by evaluating and researching a family's history and evaluating medical records
- Consider the medical, social, and ethical decisions surrounding genetic testing
- Provide support and information to help a person make a decision about genetic testing
- Help to interpret the results of genetic tests and medical data
- Provide counseling and refer individuals and families to support services as needed
- Act as patient advocates
- Discuss and explain the possible treatments or preventive measures
- Review and discuss reproductive options (National Human Genome Research Institute, 2013)

A number of online resources provide comprehensive listings of genetics services that nurses can use to locate genetics professionals and services in their practice area. These include GeneTests (2015), which has a searchable genetics clinic directory, and the University of Kansas (2012), which offers a listing of genetics centers, clinics, and departments.

TOMORROW'S GENETICS AND GENOMICS: PERSONALIZED MEDICINE

Genetic and genomic research is revealing more every day about the role of genetics in how each person's body metabolizes and responds to certain medicines. This section describes new directions in use of genetic testing results for selection of treatments that are leading to more individualized health care, called *personalized medicine*. Pharmacogenetics and pharmacogenomics are defined and described. A new wave in personal genetic testing, called *direct-to-consumer (DTC) genetic testing*, is also discussed.

Pharmacogenetics and Pharmacogenomics

There are now two new fields of research and applications of genetics and genomics for medical treatment of disease—pharmacogenetics and pharmacogenomics. *Pharmacogenetics* is the field of research that looks at the difference in each individual's response to medications based on genetic variation. This field investigates how an individual's genetic information affects the way in which drugs are transported and metabolized in the person's body as a result of specific drug receptors. The goal of pharmacogenetics is to create an individualized drug treatment program that involves the best choice and dose of drugs for a particular patient. One example of the application of pharmacogenetics involves the drug warfarin, a blood thinner. Genetic testing can now be done for certain genes, called *CYP2C9* and *VKORC1*, that affect how warfarin is metabolized; this testing can guide the specific dosage and management to help prevent adverse side effects (Lea, Feero, & Jenkins, 2008).

Pharmacogenomics is the field of research that looks for genetic variations associated with drug discovery and development. Pharmacogenomic research is leading to the creation of new drugs that can be tailor-made for each specific patient and adapted to that person's particular genetic makeup. A person's diet, lifestyle, age, state of health, and environment can all affect that person's response to medicines. Now and in the future, in addition to considering these factors, an understanding of an individual's genetic makeup will increasingly help with the creation and prescription of personalized drugs that are most effective—and have fewer side effects—for a specific person (National Human Genome Research Institute, 2013). As an example, a test is now being used to determine whether a medicine called *trastuzumab* (Herceptin) will be effective in the treatment of breast cancer. The test determines whether a woman who has metastatic breast cancer also tests positive for human epidermal growth factor receptor 2 (HER2). Women who have a positive test result and have HER2-positive breast cancer have been found to have a more serious and aggressive form of the disease, with a greater chance of recurrence, poorer prognosis, and lower chance of survival, when compared with those women who have HER2-negative breast cancer. Herceptin, which is designed to target and block the function of HER2 protein overexpression, is now given to those women who test positive for HER2 (National Cancer Institute, 2013).

DIRECT-TO-CONSUMER GENETIC TESTING

Genomic research has also opened the door for a new approach to accessing genetic testing that allows people to order, via the Internet, genetic testing by sending a sample of their saliva or tissue to a laboratory that will perform the test. A growing number of for-profit companies offer this type of genetic testing, known as DTC genetic testing, to assess genetic status. The company analyzes the individual's gene-sequence data, interprets it for the risk information it reveals, and develops a report. The report is then sent directly to the consumer. Often a health care provider is not involved in this process. This means that individuals who have DTC genetic testing may bring the results to their health care providers, including nurses, to ask for their help in interpreting the complex genetic test results for common diseases. Most health care providers have insufficient knowledge, training, or clear guidelines on how to interpret and use these genetic test results (Hunter, Khoury, & Drazen, 2008).

Another concern about DTC is the accuracy of the test results. This concern led the Senate Special Committee on Aging to hold a hearing based on a year-long Government Accountability Office (GAO) investigation of the validity of the results of DTC testing. The GAO's investigation involved sending samples to a number of different DTC companies. The GAO determined that results and information that consumers received was often misleading and provided inconsistent predictions of diseases (National Human Genome Research Institute, 2012).

Other concerns raised by DTC genetic testing include the possibility that individuals may misinterpret the genetic information that is given directly to them or the possibility that they may order genetic tests that are inappropriate. Several organizations, including the National Human Genome Research Institute (NHGRI) and the National Institutes of Health, have developed resources to educate the general public and health care professionals about genetic testing (National Human Genome Research Institute, 2014).

Nursing practice will increasingly include these new directions in health care. Nurses will need to expand their knowledge and skills in tailoring genetic and genomic information and testing to their patients. Having knowledge of both the benefits and limitations of emerging genetic tests will enable nurses to assist their patients to be informed health care decision makers (Lea et al., 2008). Box 16-3 provides a listing of clinical genetics resources that nurses and their patients can use to learn more about genetic testing.

ETHICAL ISSUES IN GENETICS AND GENOMICS

The nursing profession has long recognized the importance of ethics as an integral component of professional nursing practice. In recognition of the importance of an ethical foundation in nursing practice, the American Nurses Association created the *Code of Ethics for Nurses*. The Code of Ethics "makes explicit the primary goals, values and obligations of the profession" (American Nurses Association, 2001, p. 5). Genetics and genomics raise a number of ethical issues of concern for nurses. These include informed decision making and consent; privacy and confidentiality of genetic and genomic information; social, cultural, and religious issues in genomic research; and concerns about insurance and employment discrimination based on a person's genetic and genomic information. This section provides information about social, cultural, and religious issues in genomic research, misuse of genetic and genomic information, and discrimination based on genetic information. The Code of Ethics for Nurses provides a foundation and guide for nurses when confronting these ethical issues in genetics and genomics. Readers are directed to Chapter 12 for an overview of ethical issues for nurses, including more information on informed decision making and consent, as well as privacy and confidentiality of medical information.

Social, Cultural, and Religious Issues in Genomic Research

Human genome research raises some difficult questions related to scientific, biomedical, and legal issues. Some of the most difficult questions, however, are related to social, cultural, or religious implications of new genetic knowledge and technology. Emerging knowledge about the history of our evolution and the small variations within an individual's genomes has the potential to affect concepts of race, ethnicity, and even gender. To address the challenges associated with the relationships among genomics, race, and ethnicity, researchers have now moved into the areas of social science and psychology to learn about genetic effects on behavior, as well as explore new dimensions of religious or philosophical concepts about identity, potentially redefining what it means to be human (Bonham, Warshauer-Baker, & Collins, 2005).

BOX 16-3 Genetics and Genomics Clinical Resources

Centers for Disease Control and Prevention (CDC)—Offers online resources for credible health information. One of their online resources is a "Diseases & Conditions A-Z Index" that includes genetic disorders: www.cdc.gov/DiseasesConditions

Genetic Alliance—Provides individuals and organizations with dynamic resources that emphasize expanded access to quality, vetted information, including information about specific diseases, support groups for specific diseases, family history, and other resources: www.geneticalliance.org

Genetics and Genomics for Patients and the Public—Created by the National Human Genome Research Institute; provides detailed information about genetic disorders, background on genetic and genomic science, the new science of pharmacogenomics, tools to create your own family health history, and a list of online health resources: www.genome.gov/19016903

Genetics and Rare Diseases Information Center (GARD)—Established by the National Human Genome Research Institute (NHGR) and the Office of Rare Diseases (ORD) to help members of the general public, including patients and their families, health professionals, and biomedical researchers find useful information about genetic and rare diseases. GARD has a website (http://rarediseases.info.nih.gov/GARD) and also provides immediate, virtually round-the-clock access to experienced information specialists who can furnish current and accurate information (in both English and Spanish) about genetic and rare diseases: www.genome.gov/10000409

Genetics Home Reference—Provides consumer-friendly information about the effects of genetic variations on human health: http://ghr.nlm.nih.gov

Genes in Life—Genes in Life is a website where people can learn about all the ways genetics is a part of their life. This site provides information about how genetics affects individuals and their families, why they should talk to their health care providers about genetics, how to get involved in genetics research, and much more. http://www.genesinlife.org/

GeneTests—Features expert-authored, peer-reviewed, current disease descriptions that apply genetic testing to the diagnosis, management, and genetic counseling of patients and families with specific inherited conditions. GeneTests also provides a directory of genetic clinics in the United States: www.genetests.org

National Institutes of Mental Health (NIMH)—Looking at My Genes: What Can They Tell Me? Frequently Asked Questions About Genome Scans and Genetic Testing: www.nimh.nih.gov/health/publications/looking-at-my-genes-what-can-they-tell-me.shtml

National Society of Genetic Counselors (NSGC)—The NSGC has a resource link to assist individuals and health professionals in locating genetic counseling services. Genetic counselors can be searched by state, city, counselor's name, institution, or areas of practice or specialization: www.nsgc.org/resourcelink.cfm

Office of Rare Diseases Research (ORDR)—Coordinates research and information on rare diseases at the NIH and for the rare diseases community. The ORDR website provides information for patients and their families with rare diseases and about NIH- and ORDR-sponsored biomedical research and scientific conferences: http://rarediseases.info.nih.gov

Personalized Medicine—Provides up-to-date information about a new era in health care, personalized medicine, which is creating new methods for earlier diagnoses and individualized interventions: www.ageofpersonalizedmedicine.org

U.S. Surgeon General's Family History Initiative, Family History Tool—This web-based tool helps users organize family history information and then print it out for presentation to the family doctor. In addition, the tool helps users save their family history information to their own computer and even share family history information with other family members: https://familyhistory.hhs.gov

---

In recognition of the potential for misuse of genetic and genomic information, the NHGRI created the Ethical, Legal and Social Implications (ELSI) program in 1990 as an important component of the Human Genome Project. Insights gained through the ELSI research help to inform development of regulations and legislation to safeguard against misuse of genetic information. ELSI–funded activities have included multiple research and education projects, books, articles, newsletters, websites, and television and radio programs, as well as conferences and other activities that focus on translating ELSI research into clinical and public health practices (NHGRI, 2012).

Nurses need to become familiar with ELSI research and be able to identify these social, cultural, and religious issues related to genetic and genomic information and technologies so that they can provide guidance and understanding to their patients, families, and communities (Consensus Panel, 2008).

Discrimination Based on Genetic and Genomic Information

Until recently, many individuals and families were worried about the possibility of insurance and employment discrimination based on their genetic test results and information. These concerns have led many people who could benefit from genetic testing to decide not to have the testing at all, or to pay for genetic testing on their own outside of their insurance company so that they would not be denied future health care coverage or employment (Genetics and Public Policy Center, 2009).

In May 2008, then-President George W. Bush signed the Genetic Information Nondiscrimination Act, called *GINA*. The GINA gives U.S. citizens protection from health insurance and employment discrimination based on their genetic information. The GINA is a major breakthrough for today's health care and has important implications for all health care providers, especially nurses. Nurses will need to become familiar with what protections GINA does and does not cover so that they can educate patients, families, and communities about this new federal protection law. The GINA prevents health insurers from denying coverage, adjusting premiums, or otherwise discriminating on the basis of a person's genetic information. Health insurers may not request that a person have a genetic test. Employers are prohibited from using genetic information to make decisions to hire, fire, compensate, or promote an individual. The law also significantly limits a health insurer's or employer's right to request, require, or purchase someone's genetic information. The new GINA legislation does not allow insurers and employers to use research participants' genetic information against them (Genetics and Public Policy Center, 2008).

The GINA also has important limitations that nurses should understand. The law does not prevent health care providers from recommending genetic tests to their patients. The GINA does not mandate coverage for any particular test or treatment, and it does not prohibit medical underwriting based on current health status. The GINA does not cover life, disability, and long-term care insurance, nor does it apply to members of the military (Hudson, Holohan, & Collins, 2008).

SUMMARY

Genetic and genomic research that has evolved since the human genome was mapped and sequenced is ushering in a new era of health care, genomic health care. Genomic health care involves the use of new knowledge and tools to tailor health care at the individual level by using a person's unique genetic and genomic information to guide care. This means that health care will be more personalized and will include the use of more effective gene-based screening, diagnostic, and treatment measures. Nurses in all practice settings will increasingly be called upon to use genetic- and genomic-based approaches and technologies in their patient care. Nursing leaders created the *Essentials of Genetic and Genomic Nursing: Competencies, Curriculum Guidelines, and Outcome Indicators* (Consensus Panel, 2008) in recognition of the implications of genomic health care for nurses. Having genetic and genomic knowledge and competency will enable nurses to provide the most effective and meaningful patient care.

SALIENT POINTS

- Genetic and genomic research has ushered in a new era of health care, called *genomic health care.*
- Genomic health care involves the use of new knowledge and tools to tailor health care to the individual by using a person's unique genetic and genomic information to guide care.
- Health care is becoming more personalized and includes the use of more gene-based screening, diagnostic, and treatment measures.
- All registered nurses in all areas of practice increasingly will be expected to use genetic- and genomic-based approaches and technologies in the care of patients, families, and communities.

- Nursing leaders created the *Essentials of Genetic and Genomic Nursing: Competencies, Curricula Guidelines, and Outcome Indicators* as a necessary foundation to prepare all nurses to provide genetic- and genomic-based nursing care.
- Two important tools that nurses will use to personalize screening, prevention, diagnosis, and treatment of individuals and families are family history and genetic tests.
- Based on the *Essentials of Genetic and Genomic Nursing*, nurses will be involved in conducting family history collection and pedigree construction, as well as in offering and explaining genetic testing.

- Nurses will participate in the referral of individuals and families to genetics specialty services, where they can get more detailed genetic and genomic evaluation, diagnosis, and information.
- Nurses need to become knowledgeable about the ethical issues in genomic research and concerns about

insurance and employment discrimination based on a person's genetic and genomic information.
- Nurses should become familiar with the scope and limitations of the Genetic Information Nondiscrimination Act (GINA) so that they can educate patients, families, and communities about the details of this new nondiscrimination legislation.

CRITICAL REFLECTION EXERCISES

1. As a nurse working in a family health clinic, you see a 40-year-old woman for a routine visit. During the visit, you update her family history. She informs you that she is concerned because her sister was just diagnosed with breast cancer at the age of 42. Since her sister's diagnosis, she has learned that one of her aunts (her father's sister) died of breast cancer at the age of 45. Also, that aunt's daughter, now 38, has a history of breast cancer. Her father's mother died at an early age from cancer as well. She tells you that her father's family has never wanted to talk about the family history of breast cancer; until recently, it was kept a secret. The woman asks you, "What does this mean for me?" How would you answer her question? What resources would you make available to her?

2. At a cardiovascular clinic, two patients who are waiting to be seen begin a conversation about their history of having strokes. They talk about how they are being treated with the blood thinner warfarin. One of the patients is receiving a much lower dose of warfarin than the other patient. When this patient sees the nurse, he talks about his conversation with the other patient and asks the nurse why he is getting a lower dose: "Why don't I have the same higher dose as the other patient? If I have the lower dose, doesn't this increase my risk for having another stroke?" How would you answer this patient's question?

3. A young husband and wife come to the obstetric clinic where you work. They tell you that they are planning to have a baby. When taking their family history, you learn that both of them are of African-American ancestry and that the husband's brother has a history of sickle cell anemia. The wife tells you, "We want to know what our risk is of having a baby with sickle cell anemia and whether there are any tests that can be done to help us find out." How would you respond to the couple's concerns? What resources could you make available to them to help answer their question?

4. A 50-year-old male has just learned that he has a history of early-onset colorectal cancer in his family. One of his brothers and a maternal uncle developed colorectal cancer at an early age. His physician has suggested that he and his family consider having genetic testing to determine whether they carry the gene that increases the risk for early-onset colorectal cancer. After seeing the physician, the patient tells you that he does not think he or his family members will want to have the genetic testing because "We don't want our insurance companies to deny us coverage." How would you respond to this patient's concerns about the possibility of his insurance company discriminating against him based on genetic information?

REFERENCES

American Nurses Association. (2001). *Code of ethics for nurses with interpretive statements*. Silver Spring, MD: American Nurses Association.

American Nurses Association. (2004). *Nursing: Scope and standards of practice*. Washington, DC: American Nurses Association. Retrieved from http://nursesbooks.org.

Bonham, V. L., Warshauer-Baker, E., & Collins, F. S. (2005). Race and ethnicity in the genome era: The complexity of the constructs. *American Psychologist, 60*(1), 9–15.

Cohen, F. (1979). Genetic knowledge possessed by American nurses and students. *Journal of Advanced Nursing, 4*(5), 493–501.

Consensus Panel on Genetic/Genomic Nursing Competencies. (2008). *Essentials of genetic and genomic nursing: Competencies, curricula guidelines, and outcome indicators*. Silver Spring, MD: American Nurses Association.

Genetics and Public Policy Center. (2008). *The Genetic Information Nondiscrimination Act*. Retrieved from http://www.dnapolicy.org/policy.issue.php?action=detail&issuebrief_id=37.

Genetics and Public Policy Center. (2009). *Genetic privacy & discrimination*. Retrieved from http://www.dnapolicy.org/policy.privacy.php.

Genetics Home Reference. (2014a). *What are the types of genetic tests?* Retrieved from http://ghr.nlm.nih.gov/handbook/testing/uses.

Genetics Home Reference. (2014b). *What is genetic testing?*. Retrieved from http://ghr.nlm.nih.gov/handbook/testing/genetictesting.

GeneTests. (2015). Retrieved from www.genetests.org.

Guttmacher, A. E., & Collins, F. S. (2002). Genomic medicine—A primer. *New England Journal of Medicine, 347*, 1512–1521.

Hudson, K. L., Holohan, M. K., & Collins, F. S. (2008). Keeping pace with the times: the Genetic Information Nondiscrimination Act. *New England Journal of Medicine, 358*(25), 2261–2263.

Hunter, D. J., Khoury, M. J., & Drazen, J. M. (2008). Letting the genome out of the bottle—will we get our wish? *New England Journal of Medicine, 358*(2), 105–107.

Jenkins, J. (Ed.). (2007). Genetics in nursing and healthcare. *nurseAdvance Collection series*. Indianapolis, IN: Sigma Theta Tau International.

Lea, D. H., Feero, F., & Jenkins, J. F. (2008). Warfarin therapy and pharmacogenomics: A step toward personalized medicine. *American Nurse Today, 3*(5), 12–13.

National Cancer Institute. (2013). *Trastuzumab*. Retrieved from http://www.cancer.gov/cancertopics/druginfo/trastuzumab.

National Human Genome Research Institute. (2012). *Frequently asked questions about genetic research*. Retrieved from http://www.genome.gov/19516792.

National Human Genome Research Institute. (2012). *GAO concludes that DTC genetic tests mislead consumers*. Retrieved from http://www.genome.gov/19518344.

National Human Genome Research Institute. (2012). *Genetics and genomics for patients and the public*. Retrieved from http://www.genome.gov/19016903.

National Human Genome Research Institute. (2012). *Guidelines and tools to assess family history of common diseases: Value of family history*. Retrieved from http://www.genome.gov/27527602.

National Human Genome Research Institute. (2012). *Social, cultural and religious issues in genetic research*. Retrieved from http://www.genome.gov/10001848.

National Human Genome Research Institute. (2013). *Frequently asked questions about genetic counseling*. Retrieved from http://www.genome.gov/19016905.

National Human Genome Research Institute. (2013). *Talking glossary of genetic terms*. Retrieved from http://www.genome.gov/Glossary/.

National Human Genome Research Institute. (2014). *Frequently asked questions about genetic testing*. Retrieved from http://www.genome.gov/19516567.

National Human Genome Research Institute. (2014). *Genetics, genomics and patient management*. Retrieved from http://www.genome.gov/27527600.

Skirton, H., Patch, C., & Williams, J. (2005). *Applied genetics in healthcare: A handbook for specialist practitioners*. New York: Taylor & Francis.

University of Kansas Medical Center. (2012). *Genetic centers, clinics and departments*. Retrieved from http://www.kumc.edu/gec/prof/genecntr.html.

U.S. Department of Health and Human Services. (2014). *My family health portrait: A tool from the surgeon general*. Retrieved from https://familyhistory.hhs.gov.

Global Rural Nursing Practice

Marianne Baernholdt, PhD, MPH, RN, FAAN, Julie Schexnayder, DNP, MPH, ACNP-BC and Mary Catherine T. Winston, DNP, RN, ANP-BC

http://evolve.elsevier.com/Friberg/bridge/

OBJECTIVES

After completion of this chapter, the reader will be able to:

- Describe challenges defining global rural location.
- Discuss the social determinants of health for global rural populations.
- Identify major health issues impacting global rural areas.
- Discuss the scope of global rural nursing practice.

- Identify common professional practice issues for nurses working in global rural areas.
- Apply knowledge of factors that impact rural health to develop provision of health care to global rural populations.

PROFILE IN PRACTICE

NURSE-RUN CLINICS IN SOUTH AFRICA
Julie Schexnayder, DNP, MPH, ACNP-BC

What role do nurses have in responding to the global HIV/AIDS epidemic? In the United States HIV-related health care services are generally provided through specialty medical practices. Indeed, many general practitioners in the United States are uncomfortable managing the complicated medication regimens used in treating HIV. For those living in rural and remote areas, the nearest HIV-trained provider may be located hours away. In resource-poor countries, chronic physician shortages have increased reliance on other cadres of health care workers to provide access to even basic medical care. Yet, widespread delivery of HIV care by non-physician providers has lagged because of the complexity of managing HIV disease. This has tremendous and potentially deadly implications for remote communities that lack access to a medical provider.

In countries hardest hit by the HIV/AIDS epidemic, task-shifting of HIV care to nurses is one approach that has been implemented to increase access to life-saving medical care. For example, in South Africa, a national policy change in 2010 allowed nurses in primary health care clinics to prescribe HIV treatments for infected patients in accordance with national treatment guidelines.

As a nurse practitioner (NP) specializing in HIV care in the United States, I became increasingly interested in whether such programs increase rural and remote access to HIV care, and ultimately improve patient outcomes. During my Doctor of Nursing Practice program at the University of Virginia, I had the great fortune of working with a rural primary health clinic (PHC) in Limpopo, South Africa for 2 months to learn more about nurse-led models of HIV care. Here nurses serve as first-line providers of publicly funded primary care. In a community with high rates of unemployment and poverty, transportation costs prevent many from accessing hospital-based services. Historically, this is where HIV treatment was provided.

Unlike my practice in the United States, HIV care in rural Limpopo is no longer a specialty. On any given day a clinic nurse may consult on a full range of medical and nursing problems, including labor and delivery, treating common injuries and illnesses, and managing chronic conditions such as hypertension or HIV. Clinic nurses described themselves as "jacks-of-all-trades," but also felt challenged as "masters of nothing" because of the numerous programs with which they were expected to be familiar. Using national guidelines and protocols to guide her practice, a nurse with a bachelor's level of training operates largely autonomously. Medical providers supplement nursing services through monthly clinic visits. Challenging cases or persons requiring physician prescription for certain medications can be scheduled for consultation during these visits.

HIV services are provided as part of integrated primary care. In this sense, the goal is for HIV testing, treatment, and follow-up to occur as extensions of routine care. For example, a woman presenting for contraceptives would be counseled on HIV factors and be offered testing as part of her visit. For those enrolled in an HIV treatment program, follow-up visits would be expected to include routine primary care screenings as appropriate. This change in the organization and delivery of HIV care has introduced both rewards and challenges.

Several described their feelings of helplessness with the old model of care, unable to intervene with necessary treatment for those presenting with symptoms of AIDS. Because of this nurses argued that PHC-based HIV services are a necessary response to community needs—particularly in remote communities. Since the beginning of the clinics HIV treatment program in 2011, more than 100 patients have been started on treatment by clinic nurses, with most still in care. Larger studies conducted in PHC in South Africa, Uganda, and other sub-Saharan Africa countries suggest that nurse-led treatment programs are comparable to physician-led HIV care in terms of mortality and retention in care. So what role do nurses have in responding to the global HIV/AIDS epidemic? For many HIV-infected patients in sub-Saharan Africa, they are the most accessible providers of both HIV-related and general medical care.

PROFILE IN PRACTICE

A GLOBAL RURAL HEALTH PRACTICE IN VIRGINIA
Mary Catherine T. Winston, DNP, RN, ANP-BC

My interest in global rural nursing has been evolving over a 35-year nursing practice, shaped by changing regional demographics and health needs in the southern Shenandoah Valley where I live and practice. I came to rural Virginia as a young BSN with about 3 years of nursing experience in an urban setting. After relocating, I was thrilled to find employment as a staff RN on the med-surg unit at the 20-bed local community hospital. Even though better wages could be earned working at a large regional hospital about an hour's drive from my home, I wanted to serve the people in the community where I lived. However, I quickly found I was ill prepared for the role required of a rural nurse on a unit that would commonly have infants with croup, seniors with multiple medical problems, as well as a mix of ENT, orthopedic, GYN, and general surgical patients.

Culture shock gradually dissipated and grew toward rural cultural competence with perseverance, commitment to learning the local ways, and mentoring from the nursing professionals with whom I worked. These nurses were mostly diploma program, ADN graduates or LPNs and I am afraid my first few months there did nothing to sway local opinion in support of the American Nurses Association decision at the time to move toward mandating the BSN as entry to practice, although with time and continuing education I integrated well into the nursing team and became quite comfortable delivering care in a variety of settings in that small community hospital, including med-surg, obstetrics, ER, ICU, and home health.

During that time I also gained a deeper understanding of the barriers to health experienced by members of my rural community. I also learned of emerging strategies for rural health promotion, including the 1977 Rural Health Clinic Services Act. This legislation addressed inadequate rural access to medical care by increasing the use of NPs and physician assistants in rural regions. These varied and rich experiences provided the foundation for my decision to enhance my scope of practice by becoming a NP.

My subsequent 25+-year NP career has been primarily in the same locale, serving the same rural community, although the population has gradually become more ethnically diverse, with increasing percentages of Hispanic permanent residents and seasonal migrant workers. Similar diversification in rural demographics can be observed in many rural regions in the United States. In addition to Hispanics, clusters of immigrants and resettled refugees from varied ethnicities reside across rural America. Language and cultural differences in these groups compound the health access barriers common to rural dwellers around the world related to remoteness and limited numbers of health care workers. Thus it is imperative that nurses recognize that global rural health concepts are applicable in many locales, including small town and rural America. A global rural health nurse needs both a wide range of nursing skills and the ability to incorporate cultural competencies specific to the locals who have resided there for generations as well as the diverse newcomers.

INTRODUCTION

About half of the world's population resides in rural areas (World Health Organization [WHO], October 2009). Nurses are often their first point of health care and in some instances the only one. Recognizing that resource-poor areas are similar across the world, this chapter focuses on nursing practice in global rural areas. We define global rural nursing practice as practice in *both* local and international rural contexts. To practice in these areas, nurses need knowledge, skills, and attitudes that enable them to understand world cultures and events, analyze global systems, appreciate cultural differences, and apply this knowledge and appreciation to their practice (Riner, 2011).

Global rural nursing practice encompasses learning and employment opportunities in rural and international areas—experiences increasingly in demand among nurses in the United States. It is widely understood that when nurses and other health care providers travel to and practice in resource-poor areas, communities benefit from much needed access to care. What is seldom recognized is the mutual learning that occurs between richer and poorer areas (Crisp, 2010). Nurses from richer areas gain personal development and a better understanding of the communities they serve; nurses in poorer areas gain professional training, development of services, and networking opportunities. Nurses from both richer and poorer areas gain valuable research and learning opportunities. None of this is apparent, however, without an understanding of what constitutes global rural nursing practice.

DEFINITION OF RURAL

There are several definitions for rural or remoteness, all contingent on geographic location and sociocultural differences (Farmer, Clark, & Munoz, 2010). The United Nations states: "the characteristics that distinguish urban from rural areas, the distinction between the urban and the rural population is not yet amenable to a single definition that would be applicable to all countries or, for the most part, even to the countries within a region" (United Nations Statistics Division Demographic and Social Statistics, n.d.). In the United States there are more than 15 definitions of rural used in federal programs (Coburn et al., 2007). For example,

some definitions relate to county, others zip codes, and yet others use census track. No matter the definition, the number of rural dwellers varies greatly by state. For example, in the 2000 United States census definition, Maine, Mississippi, Vermont, and West Virginia had more than 50% of their residents in rural areas, and states like California and Nevada had less than 10% (U.S. Census Bureau, 2012). In other words, rural is that which is not urban.

GLOBAL RURAL NURSING PRACTICE

Some argue rural nursing practice is a specialty area requiring unique competencies. Rural nurses are "expert generalists" who need knowledge in many areas of nursing practice (Baernholdt, Jennings, Merwin, & Thornlow, 2010; Bushy, 2012; Hegney, McCarthy, Rogers-Clark, & Gorman, 2002; Sharff, 2013). Rural nursing practice requires skill and knowledge development across the life span, and adaptability to a variety of health care settings. A commitment to ongoing professional development is essential in rural areas, as nurses may not perform a task or procedure more than once a year, yet have to maintain proficiency in task performance. Further, rural nurses are expected to work with a high degree of independence and initiate treatments that are typically provided by other members of the health care team in urban settings. Additionally, rural nurses often are working with limited or delayed access to resources. Finally, practicing in global rural areas involve a high degree of community visibility, including a unique interconnectedness between nurses and their communities (Baernholdt et al., 2010; Bushy, 2012), described as "permeability between the rural workplace and the community setting" (Zibrik, MacLeod, & Zimmer, 2010). Experienced rural nurses use their knowledge of their patients outside of the health care system to better plan for their care within the health care system (Baernholdt et al., 2010).

SOCIAL DETERMINANTS OF HEALTH

More than in any other practice area, nurses practicing in global rural areas care for people across the life span and in all health care settings. Further, nurses have to consider the social determinants of health that are often responsible for health inequities between urban and rural populations. Social determinants of health are the conditions in which people are born, grow, live, work, and age. These circumstances are shaped by the distribution of money, power, and resources at global, national, and local levels (WHO, 2013). Globally, efforts to improve living conditions in the world's least resourced areas have been guided by the United Nations Millennium Development Goals that target both social determinants and health outcomes (Box 17-1).

Because practicing rural nurses are most successful if they consider the social determinants of health, we discuss how seven determinants of health (rural culture, physical environment, social support, economic factors, education, personal characteristics, and access to health care) impact rural health and shape global rural nursing practice (Figure 17-1).

Rural Culture

I know I've had difficulty not being from here. I've had difficulty communicating with some of my patients, but [as you] work closely with the nurses that are from here, you're able to learn what the best way is to go about educating the patients.
(Baernholdt et al., 2010, p. 1351)

Culture is a specific set of beliefs and attributes for a group, region, or nation (Hofstede, 2001). Culture determines how a group thinks, feels, and acts. The rural culture is important to individuals' health and how health care is delivered (Baernholdt et al., 2010; Leipert & George, 2008; Pierce, 2001). Although there are different local rural cultures, there is an understanding of a different, more generalized culture—the "rural culture" (Kayser, n.d.). The problems and disadvantages

that rural areas experience may contribute to the often strong sense of a unique rural culture and connectedness found among rural residents. Changes in migration patterns, however, may change the rural culture.

In both Europe and the United States the middle classes, including professionals or executives, are retiring and migrating to rural areas at an increasing rate (Cromartie & Nelson, 2009; Kayser, n.d.). American people close to retirement age and above often choose rural and small-town destinations when they migrate. If the aging baby boomers (those born from 1946 to 1964) follow past migration patterns, the rural and small-town population of 55 to 75 year olds will increase two thirds between 2000 and 2020 from 8.6 million to 14.2 million (Cromartie & Nelson, 2009). This in-migration cannot help but have an influence on the rural culture (Kayser, n.d.). The retirees often tend to make up the largest and most well-off social group in the rural area. Some of them have roots in the area, but most of them do not. What can happen is a considerable effect in terms of "watering down" of the collective rural culture. Too many newcomers can cause the established rural culture to change significantly; perhaps to the point where the connectedness between rural families and friends is lost.

The values and beliefs in a rural culture not only influence how rural people define health, but also from whom they seek advice, treatment, and care. Nurses in rural areas have to be viewed as part of the community

---

BOX 17-1 The Eight Millennium Development Goals

1. Eradicate extreme poverty and hunger.
2. Achieve universal primary education.
3. Promote gender equality and empower women.
4. Reduce child mortality.
5. Improve maternal health.
6. Combat HIV/AIDS, malaria, and other diseases.
7. Ensure environmental sustainability.
8. Global partnership for development.

Data from United Nations. (2015). We can end poverty: millenium development goals and beyond 2015. Retrieved from http://www.un.org/millenniumgoals/

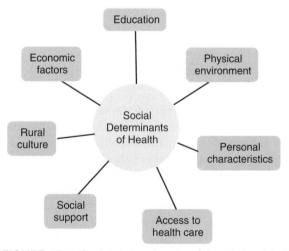

FIGURE 17-1 Social determinants of health in global rural communities.

to be able to practice in the area (Baernholdt et al., 2010; Bushy, 2012). On the one hand, knowledge of the rural culture is a basic requirement for nurses to effectively improve health in global rural areas; on the other hand, community connectedness, in which nurses and patients know one another outside the health care setting, can create boundary-related ethical conflicts (Nelson, Pomerantz, Howard, & Bushy, 2007). Delivering care consistent with local customs and beliefs yet understanding how to set limits to avoid ethical conflicts is essential for successful nurse practice in a rural area (Baernholdt et al., 2010).

Physical Environment

You go out here and get back in these mountains and just look at the scenery. … Makes you wonder why people want to leave and everything like this. You know it's God's creation and our mountains are ours—and we love them.
  (Coyne, Demian-Popescu, & Friend, 2006, p. 3)

A person's health is determined largely by the physical environment in which he or she lives, learns, and works. A natural physical environment with clean water and air, fertile soil, and thriving green spaces, and a built physical environment with healthy workplaces, good roads, safe housing, and communities are all factors promoting good health (WHO, 2013). Conversely, poor housing, inadequate sanitation, substandard roads and transportation systems, and weak community infrastructure negatively influence psychological and physical health (Centers for Disease Control [CDC], 2013). Globally the rural physical environment is different than the urban one. For those providing health care, there are unique challenges and opportunities in the rural setting.

The term *rural* brings to mind landmasses between urban areas or islands separated from urban areas by oceans. Varied landscapes are visualized, including isolated, quaint small towns, sparsely populated farmland, mountains, forests, and open ranges where successive generations have engaged in farming, ranching, mining, or logging. Quiet rural areas with abundant natural beauty, clean air, and closeness to nature are seen as the antithesis to crowded, noisy, polluted cities. Contact with nature and green spaces positively affects mental health (Bowler, Buyung-Ali, Knight, & Pullin, 2010).

Furthermore, people living in quiet rural areas perceive their quality of life to be better than their counterparts in noisy urban and rural areas (Shepherd, Welch, Dirks, & McBride, 2013). These health-promoting features are unfortunately offset by the numerous negative health outcomes that disproportionately affect rural populations.

Many rural regions in Europe, Australia, New Zealand, Canada, and the United States have higher rates of injuries related to occupational hazards (National Rural Health Association [NRHA], 2007; Smith, Humphreys, & Wilson, 2008). Rural industries (e.g., fishing, forestry, agriculture, mining) are the most dangerous occupations in the world and are associated with higher frequencies of fatal accidents compared with other industries (Smith et al., 2008). In the United States rural residents disproportionately die from unintentional injuries sustained in accidents (motor vehicle, occupational, and others) and gunshot wounds compared with urban dwellers (NRHA, 2007). These health risks are compounded by the isolated and remote rural physical environment. For example, longer emergency response times in isolated communities may be one of the factors contributing to higher rural accident-related death rates.

The effect of the rural physical environment as a single determinant of health is unclear (Smith et al., 2008). What is known is that rural populations in general have poorer health than their urban counterparts. Rural adults in the United States describe their health as fair or poor more frequently than urban adults (NRHA, 2007). Similarly, rates for chronic medical conditions such as hypertension, vascular disease, diabetes, and some cancers are higher in many rural regions compared with urban areas (NRHA, 2007; Smith et al., 2008). Finally, rates for behavioral health conditions are higher in rural areas in North America, Europe, Australia, and New Zealand (Smith et al., 2008). In the United States rural/urban behavioral health disparities include higher rural suicide rates among children and men, and higher rates of alcohol abuse and tobacco use among rural youth (NRHA, 2007). However, when socioeconomic variables such as age, gender, income, education, and ethnicity are controlled, many rural/urban health differentials are mitigated, suggesting a complex multifactorial and interrelated association among health, the rural environment, and other determinants of health (Smith et al., 2008).

Social Support

When a disease is so rare and there are no folks in your town, and few in your state who are going through what you are going through, you need a support group that encompasses people from all over the world. Getting to know people through the disorder has been an amazing experience and has created incredibly wonderful friendships and ties.

(Fox, 2011, p. 11)

Social support is *support* from families, friends, and communities. Greater social support is linked to better health (WHO, 2013). Social isolation is an independent risk factor for mortality (Pantell, Rehkopf, Jutte, Syme, Balmes, & Adler, 2013). Conversely, social support is associated with lower rates of depression (Mechakra-Tahiri, Zunzunegui, Preville, & Dube, 2009). In rural areas social isolation has been linked to higher mortality rates in Botswana (Clausen, Wilson, Molebatsi, & Holmboe-Ottesen, 2007), poorer cardiovascular health in Ecuador (Del Brutto, Tettamanti, Del Brutto, Zambrano, & Montalvan, 2013), and depression in Japanese elderly and U.S. elderly women (Buys, Roberto, Miller, & Blieszner, 2009; Kimura et al., 2012). Social support or social connectedness is a vital aspect of rural living for individuals and nurses (Bushy, 2012). It is often the sense of belonging to a community that draws people to rural areas (Baernholdt, 2012). Not surprisingly, data from Canada and the United States indicate rural individuals participate in community groups at a higher level than their urban counterparts (Keating, Swindle, & Fletcher, 2011; Stern, Adams, & Boase, 2011). Yet others have reported that compared with older adults in urban areas, rural elders have less social support (Baernholdt, Hinton, Yan, Rose, & Mattos, 2012; Cleary & Howell, 2006).

For nurses and other health care providers, rural practice settings can present a challenging social dichotomy and professional isolation. The dense social networks present in small, rural communities may result in dual relationships between nurses and their patients. Although some rural health care providers express satisfaction with having close community ties to their patients, such relationships also can introduce challenges to confidentiality (Brooks, Eley, Pratt, & Zink, 2012; Kenny, Endacott, Botti, & Watts, 2007). Despite opportunities for rich community involvement, limited access to other providers, peer support, and clinical mentorship factor prominently in rural nurse's negative descriptions of professional isolation (Williams, 2012).

For both rural dwellers and their nurses, the Internet offers an alternative approach to creating and maintaining social support across geographically isolated areas (Stern et al., 2011). In the United States 26% of Internet users read or watched someone else's experience regarding health or medical issues in the previous year and 16% went online to find others with similar health concerns as themselves (Fox & Duggan, 2013). For rural nurses who lack access to traditional resources and support, online forums and social media can provide opportunities to share ideas and practice challenges with colleagues (Barry & Hardiker, 2012). However, compared with urban dwellers, rural adults are less likely to report Internet use (Zickuhr, 2013) and countries with higher percentages of rural populations have less access to Internet services (The World Bank, 2013b).

Economic Factors

Take the death of this small boy this morning, for example. The boy died of measles. We all know he could have been cured at the hospital. But the parents had no money and so the boy died a slow and painful death, not of measles, but out of poverty.

(Narayan, Patel, Schafft, Rademacher, & Koch-Schulte, 2000, p. 36)

Economic factors include income, employment, and occupation (WHO, 2013). Higher incomes are associated with improved health, and conversely poverty contributes significantly to ill health. An absolute definition of poverty has been difficult to discern because of differing societal norms across the globe. However, there is agreement that poverty is a state that results in social and material deprivation (Halseth & Ryseth, 2010). Social deprivation includes lack of access to resources that could alleviate poverty and lack of power to make decisions that could enhance quality of life. Material deprivation encompasses hunger, insufficient housing, inadequate income, and lacking other goods that would be considered necessities within a given society (Halseth & Ryseth, 2010). Upper income countries have varying country-specific policies which delineate poverty thresholds. The World Bank (2013c) uses the following thresholds: percentage of a country's population living on less than $1.25/day as a measure of extreme poverty and less than $2/day as a measure of average poverty. In reality, the most evocative and meaningful definitions can be derived from statements made by those who live in poverty: "[Poverty] means the person is stuck. You cannot go anywhere or do anything to get out of the situation. You are not in a mood to rejoice. You can get rough with your children. You fear the future" (International Fund for Agricultural Development [IFAD], 2011, p. 54).

About 70% of the world's very poor populations reside in rural regions (IFAD, 2011). Rural poverty, although more prevalent in low income countries, also disproportionately affects rural populations in affluent countries. In 2012, the U.S. rural poverty rate was 17.7% compared with the urban poverty rate of 14.5% (Kusmin, 2013). Moreover, rural dwellers experience poverty differently than their urban counterparts (Halseth & Ryseth, 2010). Rural poverty is widely dispersed and might have pockets in marginalized areas with low agricultural or other economic potential and subsequently lacking in public or private investment (IFAD, 2011; Lichter & Parisi, 2008).

The path out of poverty is very complex; however, achievement of decent and full employment and diversification of income are targeted strategies for poverty eradication as put forth in the 2015 Millennium Development Goals (United Nations [UN], n.d.) (see Box 17-1). Dedication and commitment to work has been expressed as a core value by rural people in low income regions (Coyne et al., 2006; Freydberg, Strain, Tsuyuki, McAlister, & Clark, 2010) and middle income countries (IFAD, 2011). Diversification of income sources is common in rural households worldwide because it is necessary to alleviate risks associated with relying solely on crop production or livestock management. Income source diversity is seen across all income levels and higher household incomes are associated with higher rates of nonfarm employment (Brown & Weber, 2013; IFAD, 2011). In a sample of rural households in 15 Asian, Latin American, and sub-Saharan African countries, between 30% and 60% of those surveyed derived significant amounts of their annual incomes from nonfarm activities. Nonfarm rural occupations are highly variable and include trade, manufacturing, construction, agricultural-related businesses, and service industries (IFAD, 2011).

In the United States rural employment is also diversified. The stereotypical vision of rural family life in which the mother runs the household while the father manages the farm is no longer the norm, with merely 6.5% of the U.S. rural work force employed on the farm (Johnson, 2006). Moreover, in farming households, 91% had one or more family members working off the farm for pay. Off-farm employment for farm operators most commonly was in construction followed by various agricultural-related businesses, mining, and manufacturing, whereas employment for women was most commonly in health care or education (Brown & Weber, 2013).

Education

… if I had been to school, I could have had a good job in town. Of course I would still come to the village because there are so many fruits and other things to eat here. But it would be my decision. I would not be forced to stay here. I could be in a nice office, writing down things for other people to do. But you see, I am illiterate and I got married too early. That is precisely the problem of being illiterate. You have no way of knowing what the possibilities are out there. I can't know. All I know is farming.

(IFAD, 2011, p. 63)

Low education levels are linked with poor health, more stress, and lower self-confidence (WHO, 2013). In both low and high income countries, those with greater levels of education are more likely to be healthier and live longer (Cutler & Lleras-Muney, 2006). What differs is how level of education is measured. In low income countries ensuring access to primary education remains a struggle. In high income countries measures of educational level focus on completion of secondary and tertiary education programs. For both low and high income countries rurality matters when assessing educational opportunity: rural children are nearly twice as likely to be out of school as urban children (UN, 2013). With the inconsistencies between and across countries in levels of education as a result of lack of access to higher level education programs globally, literacy statistics provide a common measure of educational attainment.

Globally, 773.5 million adults lack basic reading and writing skills (UN Educational, Scientific, and Cultural

Organization, 2013). This disparity persists despite significant gains in primary school enrollment following inclusion of universal primary education as a 2015 Millennium Development Goal. Adult literacy rates range from less than 40% in Chad and Mali to greater than 99% among high income countries (The World Bank, 2013a). In the United States 14% of adults are unable to perform simple and everyday literacy activities (Kutner, Greenburg, Jin, & Paulsen, 2006). Health literacy is discussed in Chapter 13.

The relationships between education and health are at least partly explained by health literacy or the ability to use literacy skills in the processing of health-related information. The concept of health literacy is complex and has been defined in numerous ways. Among the most common is "the degree to which individuals have the capacity to obtain, process, and understand basic health information and services needed to make appropriate health decisions" (Institute of Medicine [IOM], 2004, p. 2). Health literacy is influenced by individual factors such as language and reading skills, as well as characteristics of health care systems (D. W. Baker, 2006; IOM, 2004). The ability of health care providers, including nurses, to provide easily understood health information is critical to improving health literacy across settings. Indeed, an objective of the United States Healthy People 2020 is to increase health literacy by improving provision of easy to understand health information at the provider level (U.S. Department of Health and Human Services, 2013).

Lower health literacy is associated with poorer health, poorer adherence to prescribed medical treatments, and higher rates of hospital admission (Kanj & Mitic, 2009). Rural areas have lower health literacy levels compared with urban areas. Results from a national health literacy survey in Taiwan revealed that 30% of adults had inadequate or marginal health literacy. Those with lower levels of health literacy tended to be older with lower household income, and live in rural areas (Lee, Tsai, & Ku, 2010). The disparity is also present in the United States, where 7.7% of rural adults have proficient health literacy skills (Zahnd, Scaife, & Francis, 2009), compared with 12% of the overall adult U.S. population (Kutner et al., 2006). More than 39% of rural adults had basic or below basic health literacy skills compared to 35% in urban areas (Zahnd et al., 2009). The overall burden of low health literacy in rural U.S. populations is notable and results in a disproportionate number of rural adults who are unable to understand and use health-related information to make appropriate decisions about their health care.

Personal Characteristics

Most people's biggest fear as you get older ... you start to think well you know I don't want to be cared for, I don't want to be unable to look after myself.

(Terrill & Gullifer, 2010, p. 713)

Personal characteristics influencing health include age, race/ethnicity, and gender (WHO, 2013). The makeup of global rural populations is somewhat different than urban populations. Differences are seen in all three personal characteristics.

Age. In both rural and urban areas the growth of the population 60 years and older is outpacing total population growth in almost all of the world regions (United Nations Population Fund and HelpAge International, 2012). Population aging in rural areas is happening more rapidly (Cai, Giles, O'Keefe, & Wang, 2012). By international standards, a society is aging when more than 10% of the population is 60 years and older. Major factors in population aging include declining fertility rates, increasing life expectancy, and population migration (Berry & Kirschner, 2013; Glascow & Brown, 2012). In 2005, the proportion of the Chinese population 60 years and older was 13.7% in rural areas compared with 12.1% in urban areas (Cai et al., 2012). The difference is explained by outward migration of younger adults. Indeed 82.1% of migration from rural to urban China occurred in adults less than 40 years of age (National Bureau of Statistics of China, 2008). Similar trends are seen in the United States, where 17.2% of rural residents are 65 years and older compared with 12.8% of urban residents (Werner, 2011). Young adults leave rural areas in search of work, whereas adults aged 55 years and older are less likely to migrate to metropolitan areas, but are increasingly migrating to rural communities for retirement (Berry & Kirschner, 2013).

The increased population aging has implications for the prevalence of chronic disease in rural communities. Overwhelmingly the burden of disease in older persons is from noncommunicable diseases. Ischemic heart disease, stroke, and chronic lung disease serve as the greatest causes of mortality worldwide although hearing and visual impairments, dementia, and osteoarthritis contribute the largest burden of disability (United Nations Population Fund and HelpAge International, 2012). Globally population aging is an important demographic trend affecting rural areas disproportionally.

Race/Ethnicity. There is great variation in racial/ethnic distributions in rural areas within and across countries. Low income countries, particularly in Africa, tend to have more ethnic diversity including in rural areas. Most notable is Uganda, which is ranked as the world's most ethnically diverse country (Alesina, Easterly, Devleeschauwer, & Wacziarg, 2003), with more than three-quarters of its population living in rural areas (Baker, 2001). In contrast, in high income countries minorities tend to be underrepresented in rural areas when compared with other urban areas. In the United States approximately 78% of the population in rural areas is white and non-Hispanic, compared with 64% of the population in the nation as a whole (Housing Assistance Council, 2012). However, rural America is becoming more diverse. From 2000 to 2010, more than half of all rural population growth was in Hispanic populations followed by African-American populations increasing by 2.9% and the Native American population by 7.5% (Housing Assistance Council, 2012). Dramatic growth was also observed in other rural minority populations, including, Asian, Native Hawaiian/Pacific Islanders, and persons of two or more races; however, in total these other rural minorities comprised less than 3% of the total rural population.

Gender. Rural areas have higher rates of women; especially in rural communities with high rates of older adults, reflecting the greater life expectancies for women (Inter-Agency Task Force on Rural Women, 2012). The experiences of women living in rural areas differ from their urban counterparts. Globally, rural women spend more time than urban women and men on reproductive and household work, including time spent obtaining water and fuel, caring for children and the sick, and processing food (Inter-Agency Task Force on Rural Women, 2012). Despite their active role in the household, women often lack decision-making authority over household concerns. In a recent survey in 37 low income countries with large rural populations, no more than 50% of women reported participating in decisions on large household purchases (UN Statistics Division Demographic and Social Statistics, n.d.). Further in many rural areas poor infrastructure

and culturally accepted gender roles limit women's participation in employment opportunities (Inter-Agency Task Force on Rural Women, 2012). With higher rates of unemployment women are disproportionately affected by poverty. Additionally, women in rural areas are adversely affected by health care access issues, including limited OB/GYN services (Bennett, Lopes, Spencer & van Hecke, 2013). Finally, intimate partner violence (IPV) has a set of different problems in rural areas. Although rural women experience IPV at similar rates as urban women (Alexander & Castillo, 2004; Breiding, Ziembroski, & Black, 2009), rural IPV may be more easily concealed (Burholdt & Dobbs, 2012). In rural Southwest Ontario, women attributed this to the dense social relationships common in rural communities. Rural health providers and police may have familial or other relationships with abusers and their families, presenting challenges to confidentiality in the reporting of abuse (Leipert & George, 2008). In addition, fewer resources exist in rural areas for preventing IPV (Breiding et al., 2009).

ACCESS TO HEALTH CARE

Not long ago we had an OB with a baby, small for gestational age, and at the same time we got two ambulances 5 minutes apart, and they were both cardiac with chest pain. While that was happening there was surgery going on, and there was somebody in the unit. I don't know if God is watching you or what, but for the most part, things seem to come out ok in the end.

(Sharff, 2013, p. 253)

Access to health care includes having access to services and the quality of those services, both of which contribute to a person's health status (CDC, 2013). Access to health care is a prominent concern in rural regions around the world in both low and high income countries as remote regions similarly have limited communications, transport options, and medical resources (Strasser, 2003). Indeed, access to quality health care was the top concern of rural residents participating in the U.S. Rural Healthy People 2020 survey (Bolin & Bellamy, 2011). Compared with urban areas health care providers, specialized services, and facilities are in shorter supply in rural areas (IOM, 2005). Whereas nearly half of the world population lives in rural areas, only 38% of the world's nurses and less than 25% of doctors work in rural areas (WHO, 2009). The uneven distribution is similar in the United States. Although 19% of the U.S. population resides in rural areas, only 10% of the nation's physician and 18% of nurse practitioner practices in rural areas (American Association of Nurse Practitioners, 2013; NRHA, 2007). Mental health providers are absent in 20% of rural counties compared with 5% of metropolitan counties.

Across all states there are fewer physicians for the rural population compared with the urban. For example, 40% of Missouri's population lives in rural areas, but only 25% of the state's physicians practice there; in Minnesota 13% of population live in rural areas with 5% physicians practicing there; and in Kentucky 43% population is rural with 28% of physicians practicing there (Center for Workforce Studies Association of American Medical Colleges, 2012). The number of nurses are also lower in rural areas. In the United States the proportion of registered nurses (RNs) who live in rural areas grew from 14.9% to 18% from 1980 to 2004, but the number of nurses who reside and work in a rural area decreased (86.1% versus 62.9%) (Skillman, Palazzo, Hart, & Butterfield, 2007). With more nurses living in a rural area but commuting to work in an urban area, rural areas have fewer nurses and vacancies that are hard to fill.

Recruitment and retention strategies have to be tailored to a specific country's circumstances because nurses' preferences for different human resource policy interventions vary between countries. In Kenya and South Africa, better educational opportunities or rural allowances would be most effective in increasing nurses in rural areas, whereas in Thailand better health insurance coverage would have the greatest impact (Blaauw et al., 2010). Given that nurse residency programs reduce turnover (Bratt, Baernholdt, & Pruszynski, 2012; Krugman et al., 2006; Romyn, Linton, Giblin, & et al., 2009), several U.S. rural nurse residency programs are in place (Bratt et al., 2012; Keahey, 2008). A challenging retention strategy is providing continuing education for rural nurses. Rural nurses have voiced how not being able to access continuing education readily is a major drawback to practicing in rural areas (Baernholdt et al., 2010; Bushy, 2012). The challenges globally include distance to educational offerings and lack of technology to access online learning opportunities (Francis & Mills, 2011; IOM, 2005).

Specialized services and facilities are sparse in rural areas, but providing more services without community input may not be beneficial. In rural Australia health care services were more likely to be provided because of available funding for that service rather than because of community needs (Allan, Ball, & Alston, 2007). Additionally community preferences may be different, so rural patients bypass their local community hospital in favor of urban hospitals (Escarce & Kapur, 2009). In Central America availability of services and proficient health care providers made small rural hospitals preferable to rural residents in Honduras, whereas rural residents from Costa Rica and Panama traveled significant distances to urban hospitals where they felt they would get better care (Leon, 2003). For some rural areas improving access to services may be better by partnering with urban hospitals and using telehealth technologies for diagnosing and managing patients (Arora et al., 2011).

IMPLICATIONS FOR NURSING PRACTICE

Nurses desiring positions in global rural practices must understand the expert generalist role required for health care delivery in these settings. Preparation for the role necessitates broad-based education and clinical experience that might be best achieved in rural nurse residency programs in which essential knowledge and skills can be attained within the local cultural context. Rural connectedness is an important aspect of rural living. To connect and integrate with the rural community a nurse will likely face challenges related to confidentiality, trust, and various roles associated with being a community member, neighbor, and health care professional.

The rural nurse will be highly visible in his or her community and thus will be well positioned for leadership in rural health advocacy initiatives targeted at removing negative determinants of health. Although local circumstances dictate the rural nurse's activities, Healthy People 2020's four foundational health measures (general health status, health-related quality of life and well-being, determinants of health, and disparities) provide an excellent start to examine the rural community's needs (U.S. Department of Health and Human Services, 2013). Activities can range from initiatives focused on individual patients, to those focused on local communities, to those focused on global rural health policy. At the individual level, nurses must recognize that the remote and isolated physical environment affects physical and mental health as well as professional development. Nurses must advocate for and be adept at accessing Internet-based patient and professional development resources, including telehealth service, information for clinical decision support, and continuing education. Further, to be most effective rural nurses must accurately identify patients with inadequate health literacy using validated health literacy assessment tools, and not rely on "gut feeling" to identify those who need help (Macabasco-O'Connell & Fry-Bowers, 2011). Only with accurate determination of an individual's health literacy can the rural nurse tailor health education to help a patient achieve more effective self-management.

At the community level rural nurses need to engage with other professionals and lay community members to perform community needs assessments to plan interventions beneficial to their specific community. Memberships in rural nursing and other organizations are helpful for networking and forming coalitions to address both local and global rural health issues.

Several global rural issues will need attention. There are greater concentrations of older people in rural areas and thus increased demand for care for chronic medical conditions. Older individuals experience unique challenges related to accessing health care, including dependence on caretakers. With nursing leadership strategies to develop improved outreach or home-based health services in one vital solution to meet the rural elderly's health needs.

Another global rural health problem the nurse practicing in rural areas need to address is poverty, which disproportionately affects rural populations. The nurse must ensure that poor people are full partners in planning and implementation of anti-poverty measures so that they are not simply recipients of aid or nursing care, but are empowered to make decisions and act on these to improve their situations (International Council of Nurses [ICN], 2009). The nurse needs to lobby for policies that create jobs, assure fair wages, and improve education because these strategies have been proved to relieve poverty (United Nations, 2013). Nurses should also advocate for and design local educational programs aimed at preparing workers to address local needs.

SUMMARY

Practicing in global rural areas is a unique experience sought by many U.S. nurses (Winston, 2014). Whether for short-term or more permanent assignments, nurses have to prepare to practice in a rural area just as they would for any other specialty position. Information that will prepare nurses for global rural practice is not in one place. Nurses need to access a multitude of resources, including reading reports, books, and article describing ideas, models, and lessons addressing local delivery

challenges in rural areas (Farmer et al., 2010). In addition to the multiple clinical and cultural competencies needed for delivery of quality global rural health care, nurses need a deep understanding and appreciation for the complex inter-related social determinants of health applied to rural settings. Nonetheless, although rural areas may differ from country to country and even within a country, lessons learned in one country can be useful information for rural nurses in other countries.

SALIENT POINTS

- We define global rural nursing practice as practice in both local and international rural contexts.
- A global rural nurse is an expert generalist with a broad knowledge base and skill sets that can be applied within rural contexts.
- Definitions of "rural" vary across the globe.
- The social determinants of health are the conditions in which people are born, grow, live, work and age. In this chapter we have considered rural culture, physical environment, social support, economic factors,

- education, personal characteristics and access to healthcare as social determinants of rural health.
- Rural culture is a separate entity comprised of a set of beliefs and attributes differing from those generally held in urban settings.
- The effect of the rural physical environment as a single determinant of health is unclear, but statistically, rural populations have poorer health than urban dwellers.
- Lack of social support or social isolation is associated with poor health throughout the world. However,

social connectedness is an important characteristic of rural communities that nurses practicing in rural regions need to embrace.

- Approximately 70% of the world's poor live in rural areas. The economic factor of poverty influences health in a cyclical pattern, each state causing worsening of the other resulting in an unabated downward spiral.
- Education and health literacy levels are lower in rural areas and associated with poor health.
- The personal characteristics such as age, race/ethnicity, and gender affect health. Globally, rural populations are disproportionately older and female. Rural ethnic and racial distributions vary greatly worldwide.
- Limited communications, transport options, and medical resources are common barriers to health care access in rural regions worldwide.
- Professional isolation is an important barrier to recruitment, retention, and competency of rural nurses.

CRITICAL REFLECTION EXERCISES

1. Discuss factors that influence a rural nurse's success in improving health in her/his community.
2. In what ways can the strengths of rural communities offset factors causing poorer health outcomes?
3. For nurses in rural and remote settings, discuss advantages and disadvantages of online resources for clinical support and continuing education.
4. You have decided to participate in a humanitarian medical mission in a medically underserved region in rural El Salvador. You have all the necessary information concerning personal health and safety. What are some of the challenges you might encounter in providing health care in that setting? Discuss how you might prepare for clinical practice in that region.

WEBSITE RESOURCES

AHRQ—Health Literacy Universal Precautions Toolkit, AHRQ—Health Literacy Universal Precautions Toolkit. http://www.ahrq.gov/professionals/quality-patient-safety/quality-resources/tools/literacy-toolkit/index.html#sthash.WAwYYpTq.dpuf

Carsey Institute. http://carseyinstitute.unh.edu/policy/rural-america

CMS Toolkit for Making Written Material Clear and Effective. http://www.cms.gov/Outreach-and-Education/Outreach/WrittenMaterialsToolkit/index.html?redirect=/WrittenMaterialsToolkit/

Global Health Council. http://www.globalhealth.org/

Global Health Delivery Online. www.ghdonline.org/

Healthy People 2020. http://www.healthypeople.gov/2020/about/default.aspx

International Council of Nurses. http://www.icn.ch/

Migrant Clinicians Network. http://www.migrantclinician.org/

National Association of Rural Health Clinics. http://narhc.org/

National Rural Health Association. http://www.ruralhealthweb.org

Office of Rural Health Policy. http://www.hrsa.gov/ruralhealth/

Partners in Health. http://www.pih.org/

Rural Assistance Center. http://www.raconline.org/topics/rural-health-clinics/

Rural Health Research Institute. http://www.gatewayresearch.ca/

Rural Nurse Organization. http://www.rno.org/

Things you can do to fight poverty. http://billmoyers.com/2013/05/12/twelve-things-you-can-do-to-fight-poverty-now/

United States Department of Agriculture. http://www.usda.gov/wps/portal/usda/usdahome

United States Department of Health and Human Services. http://www.globalhealth.gov/

University of Virginia Rural and Global Health Care Center. http://www.nursing.virginia.edu/global/about_rural_global/

World Health Organization. http://www.who.int/hrh/retention/guidelines/en/

REFERENCES

Alesina, A. F., Devleeschauwer, A., Easterly, W., Kurlat, S., & Wacziarg, R. (2003). Fractionalization. *Journal of Economic Growth, 8*(2), 155–194. Retrieved from http://link.springer.com/article/10.1023%2FA%3A1024471506938#page-1.

Allan, J., Ball, P., & Alston, M. (2007). Developing sustainable models of rural health care: A community development approach. *Rural and Remote Health, 7*(4), 818. Retrieved from http://www.rrh.org.au/articles/subviewnew.asp?ArticleID=818.

Alexander, J., & Castillo, G. (2004). Injury and violence prevention in rural areas: A literature review. In L. D. Gamm, L. L. Hutchison, B. J. Dabney, & A. M. Dorsey (Eds.), *Rural Healthy People 2010: A companion document to Healthy People 2010* (pp. 89–106). Retrieved from http://www.srph.tamhsc.edu/centers/rhp2010/Volume_3/rhp2010v3_ILR_Injvio.pdf.

American Association of Nurse Practitioners. (November 2013). *NP fact sheet.* Retrieved from http://www.aanp.org/all-about-nps/np-fact-sheet.

Arora, S., Kalishman, S., Dion, D., Som, D., Thornton, K., Bankhurst, A., & Yutzu, S. (2011). Partnering urban academic medical centers and rural primary care clinicians to provide complex chronic disease care. *Health Affairs, 30*(6), 1176–1184. Retrieved from http://dx.doi.org/10.1377/hlthaff.2011.0278.

Baernholdt, M. (2012). Rural health. In J. J. Fitzpatrick, & M. W. Kazer (Eds.), *Encyclopedia of nursing research* (3rd ed.). New York: Springer.

Baernholdt, M., Hinton, I., Yan, G., Rose, K., & Mattos, M. (2012). Factors associated with quality of life in older adults in the United States. *Quality of Life Research, 21*(3), 527. Retrieved from http://dx.doi.org/10.1007/s11136-011-9954-z.

Baernholdt, M., Jennings, B. M., Merwin, E., & Thornlow, D. (2010). What does quality care mean to nurses in rural hospitals? *Journal of Advanced Nursing, 66*(6), 1346–1355. Retrieved from http://dx.doi.org/10.1111/j.1365-2648.2010.05290.x.

Baker, D. W. (2006). The meaning and the measure of health literacy. *Journal of General Internal Medicine, 21*(8), 878–883. Retrieved from http://dx.doi.org/10.1111/j.1525-1497.2006.00540.x.

Baker, W. G. (2001). *Uganda: The marginalization of minorities.* Retrieved from the Minority Rights Group International http://www.minorityrights.org/1042/reports/uganda-the-marginalization-of-minorities.html.

Barry, J., & Hardiker, N. (2012). Advancing nursing practice through social media: A global perspective. *The Online Journal of Issues in Nursing, 17.* (3). Retrieved from http://dx.doi.org/10.3912/OJIN.Vol17No03Man05.

Bennet, K., Lopes, J. E. Jr., Spencer, K., & van Heck, S. (January 2013). *Rural Women's Health.* [policy brief] Retrieved from National Rural Health Association website: http://www.ruralhealthweb.org/download.cfm?downloadfile=F5A503E1-3048-651A-FE066957562D3AC7&typename=dmFile&fieldname=filename.

Berry, E. H., & Kirschner, A. (2013). Demography of rural aging. In N. Glascow, & E. H. Berry (Eds.). *Rural aging in 21st century America: Understanding population trends and processes: vol. 7.* (pp. 17–36). Dordrecht: Springer. Retrieved from http://dx.doi.org/10.1007/978-94-007-5567-3.

Blaauw, D., Erasmus, E., Pagaiya, N., Tangcharoensathein, V., Mullei, K., Mudhune, S., & Lagarde, M. (2010). Policy interventions that attract nurses to rural areas: A multicountry discrete choice experiment. *Bulletin of the World Health Organization, 88*(5), 350–356. Retrieved from http://dx.doi.org/10.2471/BLT.09.072918. 10.2471/BLT.09.072918.

Bolin, J., & Bellamy, G. (2011). *Rural healthy people 2020.* Retrieved from http://www.srph.tamhsc.edu/centers/srhrc/rural-healthy-people-2020.html.

Bowler, D., Buyung-Ali, L., Knight, T. & Pullin, A. S. (2010). The importance of nature for health: Is there a specific benefit of contact with green space? CEE review 08–003 (SR40). Retrieved November 15, 2013, from www.environmentalevidence.org/SR40.html

Bratt, M. M., Baernholdt, M., & Pruszynski, J. (2012). Are rural and urban newly licensed nurses different? A longitudinal study of a nurse residency programme. *Journal of Nursing Management.* Retrieved from http://dx.doi.org/10.1111/j.1365-2834.2012.01483.x. Advance online publication.

Breiding, M. J., Ziembroski, J. S., & Black, M. C. (2009). Prevalence of rural intimate partner violence in 16 US states, 2005. *Journal of Rural Health, 25*(3), 240–245. Retrieved from http://dx.doi.org/10.1111/j.1748-0361.2009.00225.x.

Brooks, K. D., Eley, D. S., Pratt, R., & Zink, T. (2012). Management of professional boundaries in rural practice. *Academic Medicine, 87*(8), 1091–1095. Retrieved from http://dx.doi.org/10.1097/ACM.0b013e31825ccbc8.

Brown, J., & Weber, J. (2013). *The off farm occupations of U.S. farm operators and their spouses.* Retrieved October 17, 2013, from http://www.ers.usda.gov/publications/eib-economic-information-bulletin/eib117.aspx#.UoZOSeLjWdw.

Burholdt, V., & Dobbs, C. (2012). Research on rural ageing: Where have we got to go and where we are going in Europe? *Journal of Rural Studies* (28), 432–446. Retrieved from http://dx.doi.org/10.1016/j.jrurstud.2012.01.009.

Bushy, A. (2012). The rural context and nursing practice. In D. Molinari, & A. Bushy (Eds.), *The rural nurse. Transition to practice* (pp. 3–22). New York: Springer.

Buys, L., Roberto, K. A., Miller, E., & Blieszner, R. (2009). Prevalence and predictors of depressive symptoms among rural older Australians and Americans. *International Journal of Geriatric Psychiatry, 24*(11), 1226–1236. Retrieved from http://dx.doi.org/10.1111/j.1440-1584.2007.00948.x.

Cai, F., Giles, J., O'Keefe, P., & Wang, D. (2012). *The elderly and old age support in rural China: Challenges and prospects* (No. 67522). Washington, DC: The World Bank. Retrieved from http://dx.doi.org/10.1596/978-0-8213-8685-9.

Center for Workforce Studies Association of American Medical Colleges. (2012). *Recent studies and reports on physician shortages in the US*. Washington, DC: Association of American Medical Colleges.

Centers for Disease Control. (2013). *Social determinants of health*. Retrieved from http://www.cdc.gov/socialdeterminants/FAQ.html.

Clausen, T., Wilson, A. O., Molebatsi, R. M., & Holmboe-Ottesen, G. (2007). Diminished mental- and physical function and lack of social support are associated with shorter survival in community dwelling older persons of Botswana. *BMC Public Health, 7* (144). Retrieved from http://dx.doi.org/10.1186/1471-2458-7-144.

Cleary, K. K., & Howell, D. M. (2006). Using the SF-36 to determine perceived health-related quality of life in rural Idaho seniors. *Journal of Allied Health, 35*(3), 156–161. Retrieved from http://www.ingentaconnect.com/content/asahp/jah;jsessionid=4tnnsik8i5hrg.alexandra.

Coburn, A. F., MacKinney, A. C., McBride, T. D., Mueller, K. J., Slifkin, R. T., & Wakefield, M. K. (March 2007). *Choosing rural definitions: Implications for health policy* (Issue brief No. 2). Columbia, MO: Rural Policy Research Institute.

Coyne, C. A., Demian-Popescu, C., & Friend, D. (2006). Social and cultural factors influencing health in southern West Virginia: A qualitative study. *Preventing Chronic Disease, 3*(4), A124.

Crisp, N. (2010). *Turning the world upside down: The search for global health in the 21st century*. Boca Raton, FL: CRC Press.

Cromartie, J., & Nelson, P. (2009). *Baby boom migration and its impact on rural America*. (Economic Research Service Report No. 79). Retrieved from United States Department of Agriculture Economic Research Service http://www.ers.usda.gov/publications/err-economic-research-report/err79.aspx#.UpvtNaWzjbw.

Cutler, D. M., & Lleras-Muney, A. (2006). *Education and health: Evaluating theories and evidence* (Working Paper No. 12352). Retrieved from the National Bureau of Economic Research http://www.nber.org/papers/w12352.

Del Brutto, O. H., Tettamanti, D., Del Brutto, V. J., Zambrano, M., & Montalvan, M. (2013). Living alone and cardiovascular health status in residents of a rural village of coastal Ecuador (the Atahualpa Project). *Environmental Health & Preventive Medicine, 18*(5), 422–425. Retrieved from http://dx.doi.org/10.1007/s12199-013-0344-8.

Escarce, J. J., & Kapur, K. (2009). Do patients bypass rural hospitals? Determinants of inpatient hospital choice in rural California. *Journal of Health Care for the Poor and Underserved, 20*, 625–644. Retrieved from http://dx.doi.org/10.1353/hpu.0.0178.

Farmer, J., Clark, A., & Munoz, S. (2010). Is a global rural and remote health research agenda desirable or is context supreme? *The Australian Journal of Rural Health, 18*, 96–101. Retrieved from http://dx.doi.org/10.1111/j.1440-1584.2010.01140.x.

Fox, S. (2011). *Peer-to-peer healthcare: Many people—especially those living with chronic or rare diseases—use online connections to supplement professional medical advice*. Washington, DC: Pew Research Center's Internet & American Life Project.

Fox, S., & Duggan, M. (2013). *Health online 2013*. Washington, DC: Pew Research Center's Internet & American Life Project.

Francis, K. L., & Mills, J. E. (2011). Sustaining and growing the rural nursing and midwifery workforce: Understanding the issues and isolating directions for the future. *Collegian, 18*(2), 55–60. Retrieved from http://dx.doi.org/10.1016/j.colegn.2010.08.003.

Freydberg, N., Strain, L., Tsuyuki, R. T., McAlister, F. A., & Clark, A. M. (2010). "If he gives in, he will be gone…": The influence of work and place on experiences, reactions and self-care of heart failure in rural Canada. *Social Science & Medicine* (1982), *70*(7), 1077–1083. Retrieved from http://dx.doi.org/10.1016/j.socscimed.2009.11.026 10.1016/j.socscimed.2009.11.026.

Glascow, N., & Brown, D. L. (2012). Rural ageing in the United States: Trends and contexts. *Journal of Rural Studies* (28), 422–431. Retrieved from http://dx.doi.org/10.1016/j.jrurstud.2012.01.002.

Halseth, G., & Ryseth, L. (2010). *A primer for understanding issues around rural poverty*. Prince George, British Columbia, Canada: University of Northern British Columbia, The Community Development Institute.

Hegney, D., McCarthy, A., Rogers-Clark, C., & Gorman, D. (2002). Retaining rural and remote area nurses. The Queensland, Australia experience. *The Journal of Nursing Administration, 32*(3), 128–135.

Hofstede, G. (2001). *Culture's consequences* (2nd ed.). Thousand Oaks, CA: Sage.

Housing Assistance Council. (2012). *Rural research notes: Race and ethnicity in rural America* (Electronic). Washington, DC: Housing Assistance Council.

Institute of Medicine. (2004). *Health literacy: A prescription to end confusion*. Washington, DC: The National Academies Press.

Institute of Medicine. (2005). *Quality through collaboration. The future of rural health*. Washington, DC: The National Academies Press.

Inter-Agency Task Force on Rural Women. (2012). *Facts & figures: Rural women and the millennium development goals*. Retrieved from http://www.un.org/womenwatch/feature/ruralwomen/facts-figures.html.

International Council of Nurses. (2009). *ICN on poverty and health: Breaking the link. Nursing Matters*. Retrieved from http:// www.icn.ch/images/stories/documents/publications/fact_sheets/10d_FS-Poverty_Health.pdf

International Fund for Agricultural Development. (2011). *Rural poverty report*. Retrieved from http://www.ifad.org/rpr2011.

Johnson, K. M. (2006). *Demographic trends in rural and small town America* (No. Paper 5). Durham, NH: The Carsey Institute at the Scholars' Repository.

Kanj, M., & Mitic, W. (2009). *Health literacy and health promotion*. Geneva: World Health Organization.

Kayser, B. (n.d.). Culture and rural development: Culture, and important tool in rural development. Retrieved from http://ec.europa.eu/agriculture/rur/leader2/rural-en/biblio/culture/art03.htm

Keahey, S. (2008). Against the odds: Orienting and retaining rural nurses. *Journal for Nurses in Professional Development, 24*(2). Retrieved from http://journals.lww.com/jnsonline/Fulltext/2008/03000/Against_the_Odds__Orienting_and_Retaining_Rural.15.aspx.

Keating, N., Swindle, J., & Fletcher, S. (2011). Aging in rural Canada: A retrospective and review. *Canadian Journal on Aging, 30*(3), 323–338. Retrieved from http://dx.doi.org/10.1017/S0714980811000250.

Kenny, A., Endacott, R., Botti, M., & Watts, R. (2007). Emotional toil: Psychosocial care in rural settings for patients with cancer. *Journal of Advanced Nursing, 60*(6), 663–672. Retrieved from http://dx.doi.org/10.1111/j.1365-2648.2007.04453.x.

Kimura, Y., Wada, T., Okumiya, K., Ishimoto, Y., Fukutomi, E., Kasahara, Y., & Matsubayashi, K. (2012). Eating alone among community-dwelling Japanese elderly: Association with depression and food diversity. *Journal of Nutrition, Health & Aging, 16*(8), 728–731. Retrieved from http://dx.doi.org/10.1007/s12603-012-0067-3.

Krugman, M., Bretschneider, J., Horn, P. B., Krsek, C. A., Moutafis, R. A., & Smith, M. O. (2006). The national post-baccalaureate graduate nurse residency program: A model for excellence in transition to practice. *Journal for Nurses in Professional Development, 22*(4). Retrieved from http://journals.lww.com/jnsonline/Fulltext/2006/07000/The_National_Post_Baccalaureate_Gradua_te_Nurse.8.aspx.

Kusmin, L. (2013). *Rural poverty at a glance.* Retrieved from http://www.ers.usda.gov/publications/eb-economicbrief/eb24.aspx#.UoaK8OLjWdw.

Kutner, M., Greenburg, E., Jin, Y., & Paulsen, C. (2006). *The health literacy of America's adults: Results from the 2003 national assessment of adult literacy* (No. NCES 2006-483). Washington, DC: U.S. Department of Education.

Lee, S. D. I.T.T., Tsai, Y., & Ku, K. N. (2010). Health literacy, health status, and healthcare utilization of Taiwanese adults: Results from a national survey. *BMC Public Health, 10*, 614. Retrieved from http://dx.doi.org/10.1186/1471-2458-10-614.

Leipert, B. D., & George, J. A. (2008). Determinants of rural women's health: A qualitative study in southwest Ontario. *Journal of Rural Health, 24*(2), 210–218. Retrieved from http://dx.doi.org/10.1111/j.1748-0361.2008.00160.

Leon, M. (2003). Perceptions of health care quality in Central America. *International Journal in Health Care, 15*(1), 67–71.

Lichter, D. T., & Parisi, D. (2008, Fall). *Concentrated poverty and the geography of exclusion.* Durham, NH: Carsey Institute. Retrieved from http://carseyinstitute.unh.edu/publications/PB-Lichter-Parisi.pdf

Macabasco-O'Connell, A., & Fry-Bowers, E. (2011). Knowledge and perceptions of health literacy among nursing professionals. *Journal of Health Communication, 16*, 295–307. Retrieved from http://dx.doi.org/10.1080/10810730.2011.604389.

Mechakra-Tahiri, S., Zunzunegui, M. V., Preville, M., & Dube, M. (2009). Social relationships and depression among people 65 years and over living in rural and urban areas of Quebec. *International Journal of Geriatric Psychiatry, 24*(11), 1226–1236. Retrieved from http://dx.doi.org.proxy.its.virginia.edu/10.1002/gps.2250.

Narayan, D., Patel, R., Schafft, K., Rademacher, A., & Koch-Schulte, S. (2000). The definitions of poverty. In Authors (Ed.), *Can anyone hear us? Voices from 47 countries.* New York: Oxford University Press.

National Bureau of Statistics of China. (2008). *Communique on major data of the second national agricultural census of China* (No. 5). Retrieved from http://www.stats.gov.cn/english/newsandcomingevents/t20080303_402465584.htm.

National Rural Health Association. (2007). *What's different about rural health care?*. Retrieved from http://www.ruralhealthweb.org/go/left/about-rural-health.

Nelson, W., Pomerantz, A., Howard, K., & Bushy, A. (2007). A proposed rural healthcare ethics agenda. *Journal of Medical Ethics, 33*(3), 136–139. Retrieved from http://dx.doi.org/10.1136/jme.2006.015966.

Pantell, M., Rehkopf, D., Jutte, D., Syme, S. L., Balmes, J., & Adler, N. (2013). Social isolation: A predictor of mortality comparable to traditional clinical risk factors. *American Journal of Public Health, 103*(11), 2056–2062. Retrieved from http://dx.doi.org/10.2105/AJPH.2013.301261.

Pierce, C. (2001). The impact of culture on rural women's descriptions of health. *Journal of Multicultural Nursing & Health, 7*(1), 50–56.

Riner, M. E. (2011). Globally engaged nursing education: An academic program framework. *Nursing Outlook, 59*(6), 308–317. Retrieved from http://dx.doi.org/10.1016/j.outlook.2011.04.005.

Romyn, D., Linton, N., Giblin, C., et al. (2009). Successful transition of the new graduate nurse. *International Journal of Nursing Education Scholarship, 6.* (1). Retrieved from http://dx.doi.org/10.2202/1548-923X.1802.

Sharff, J. E. (2013). The distinctive nature and scope of rural nursing practice: Philosophical bases. In C. A. Winters (Ed.), *Rural nursing. concepts, theory, and practice* (4th ed.) (pp. 241–258). New York: Springer.

Shepherd, D., Welch, D., Dirks, K. N., & McBride, D. (2013). Do quiet areas afford greater health-related quality of life than noisy areas? *International Journal of Environmental Research and Public Health, 10*(4), 1284–1303. Retrieved from http://dx.doi.org/10.3390/ijerph10041284.

Skillman, S. M., Palazzo, L., Hart, L. G., & Butterfield, P. (2007). *Changes in the rural registered nurse workforce from 1980 to 2004* (Final Report No. 115). Seattle, WA: WWAMI Rural Health Research Center, University of Washington.

Smith, K. B., Humphreys, J. S., & Wilson, M. G. A. (2008). Addressing the health disadvantage of rural populations: How does epidemiological evidence inform rural health policies and research? *The Australian Journal of Rural Health, 16*(2), 56–66. Retrieved from http://dx.doi.org/10.1111/j.1440-1584.2008.00953.x.

Stern, M. J., Adams, A. E., & Boase, J. (2011). Rural community participation, social networks, and broadband use: Examples from localized and national survey data. *Agricultural and Resource Economics Review, 40*(2), 158–171. Retrieved from http://ageconsearch.umn.edu/bitstream/117769/2/ARER%2040-2%20pp%20158-171%20Stern%20Adams%20Boase.pdf.

Strasser, R. (2003). Rural health around the world: Challenges and solutions. *Family Practice, 20*(4), 457–463.

Terrill, L., & Gullifer, J. (2010). Growing older: A qualitative inquiry into the textured narratives of older, rural women. *Journal of Health Psychology, 15*(5), 707–715. Retrieved from http://dx.doi.org/10.1177/1359105310368180.

The World Bank. (2013a). *Data: Education*. Retrieved from http://data.worldbank.org/topic/education.

The World Bank. (2013b). *Data: Infrastructure*. Retrieved from http://data.worldbank.org/topic/infrastructure.

The World Bank. (2013c). *Poverty overview*. Retrieved from http://www.worldbank.org/en/topic/poverty/overview.

United Nations. (n.d.). *United Nations millennium development goals*. Retrieved from http://www.un.org/millenniumgoals/poverty.shtml

United Nations. (2013). *Millennium development goals report 2013*. New York: Author.

United Nations Educational, Scientific, and Cultural Organization. (2013). *Adult and youth literacy: UIS fact sheet* (No. 26). UNESCO Institute for Statistics. Retrieved from http://www.uis.unesco.org/literacy/Documents/fs26-2013-literacy-en.pdf.

United Nations Population Fund and HelpAge International. (2012). *Ageing in the twenty-first century*. New York: Author.

United Nations Statistics Division Demographic and Social Statistics. (n.d.). Population density and urbanization. Retrieved from http://unstats.un.org/unsd/demographic/sconcerns/densurb/densurbmethods.htm

U.S. Census Bureau. (2012). *U.S. Census Bureau, statistical abstract of the United States: 2012*. Retrieved from http://www.census.gov/compendia/statab/2012/tables/12s0029.pdf.

U.S. Department of Health and Human Services. (2013). *Healthy people 2020: Health communication and health information technology*. Retrieved from http://www.healthypeople.gov/2020/topicsobjectives2020/objectiveslist.aspx?topicId=18.

Werner, C. A. (2011). *The older population: 2010* (2010 Census Briefs No. C2010BR-09). Washington, DC: U.S. Census Bureau.

Williams, M. A. (2012). Rural professional isolation: An integrative review. *Journal of Rural Nursing and Health Care, 12*(2).

Winston, M. (2014). *Addressing challenges to providing health care in a short term medical mission: diabetes outcomes in migrant farm workers* (Doctor of Nursing Practice Capstone). Charlottesville, VA: University of Virginia.

World Health Organization. (October 2009). *Monitoring the geographical distribution of the health workforce in rural and underserved areas* (Spotlight on Health Workforce Statistics No. 8). Geneva: Author.

World Health Organization. (2013). *Social determinants of health*. Retrieved from http://www.who.int/social_determinants/sdh_definition/en/index.html.

Zahnd, W. E., Scaife, S. L., & Francis, M. L. (2009). Health literacy skills in rural and urban populations. *American Journal of Health Behavior, 33*(5), 550–557. Retrieved from http://dx.doi.org/10.5993/AJHB.33.5.8.

Zibrik, K. J., MacLeod, M. L., & Zimmer, L. V. (2010). Professionalism in rural acute-care nursing. *The Canadian Journal of Nursing Research, 42*(1), 20–36.

Zickuhr, K. (2013). *Who's not online and why*. Washington, DC: Pew Research Center.

CHAPTER 18

Violence Against Women: An Epidemic and a Health Issue

Camille Burnett, PhD, MPA, APHN-BC, DSW and Kathryn Laughon, PhD, RN, FAAN

ⓔ http://evolve.elsevier.com/Friberg/bridge/

OBJECTIVES

At the completion of this chapter, the reader will be able to:

- Understand the global issue of violence against women and girls.
- Identify the health consequences of violence against women.
- Describe the various forms of violence against women.
- Describe the terms *intimate partner violence* and *intimate partners*.
- Discuss the health consequences of intimate partner violence.
- Identify opportunities to assess intimate partner violence in health care settings.
- Describe assessment tools and techniques to screen patients for intimate partner violence.
- Describe the steps to take after a positive screen for intimate partner violence.
- Identify strategies, approaches, and supports to address violence against women.

PROFILE IN PRACTICE

Natalie McClain, RN, PhD, CPNP
Northeastern University School of Nursing, Boston, Massachusetts

Various forms of violence, including intimate partner and sexual violence, are experienced by men, women, and children around the world each day. After experiencing sexual violence or intimate partner violence, survivors may seek health care either for documentation of the assault or for treatment of injuries. Sexual assault nurse examiners (SANEs) are specially trained forensic nurses who provide health evaluations, treatment, and evidence collection to victims of sexual and intimate partner violence.

My first experience working as a SANE was in a clinic in which children, adolescents, and young adults who were victims of sexual abuse were referred for forensic services, including medical examinations, treatment, and evidence collection. My role at the clinic included conducting examinations to document any injuries, treating health needs, collecting evidence, and providing expert testimony in both civil and criminal cases. Later, I worked as a SANE in an emergency department in a university teaching hospital, providing forensic services for adults

and children who had experienced either sexual violence or intimate partner violence. In both of these settings I found that combining concepts essential to nursing—compassion and caring—with the need for detailed evidence collection and forensic documentation resulted in a more positive experience for survivors.

I find working with survivors of violence in their hour of need to be personally rewarding. Looking into the eyes of rape survivors, holding their hands, letting them know they are in a safe place, and listening to their words are the reasons I became a nurse. I wanted to care for others when they needed help. Sexual assault nurse examiners help make an uncomfortable and often embarrassing examination more kind and humane while obtaining evidence crucial to prosecuting the crime. Perhaps there is no other time in a person's life when he or she needs another person more than after surviving a violent attack.

In addition to the professional responsibilities of caring for survivors of sexual and physical violence, SANEs are also active in shaping the evolving practice.

Much is still unknown about the best practices for evidence collection and physical assessment of injuries after sexual and physical assault. As a member of a SANE team and a nurse researcher, I have had opportunities to be active in research that will affect future practice and public policy for survivors of violence. As experts in the field, SANEs are essential to the growing science and debate over public policy that affects survivors of trauma.

The number of forensic nurses specializing in sexual and physical violence continues to grow. Nurses have successfully identified a wonderful way of expanding the nursing role to provide highly skilled and compassionate forensic care to survivors of trauma. As the specialty continues to grow, nurses may find themselves presented with an opportunity to work in forensic nursing. I encourage nurses to pursue interests in working with survivors of violence. Although I found working with victims and survivors of sexual assault to be emotionally challenging, I believe working as a SANE allowed me to provide forensic services with the compassionate care at the heart of nursing.

INTRODUCTION

Violence against women is a global epidemic affecting 35% of women worldwide (WHO, 2013, http://apps.who.int/iris/bitstream/10665/85239/1/9789241564625_eng.pdf). It is a major international public health concern adversely affecting the lives of women and negatively impacting their health outcomes and quality of life. Sadly, in the most severe of cases, violence against women leads to death. Violence against women is defined by the United Nations as "any act of gender-based violence that results in, or is likely to result in, physical, sexual or mental harm or suffering to women, including threats of such acts, coercion or arbitrary deprivation of liberty, whether occurring in public or in private life" (WHO, 2013). There are many forms of violence against women that include acts of sexual violence (rape, sexual assault, trafficking, genital mutilation) and sexual coercion, physical violence (hitting, slapping, kicking, punching), psychological violence (belittling, name calling, isolation), economic, and femicide (the killing of a woman). Globally 70% of women will experience violence in their lifetime (UN, 2011). Exposure to violence creates numerous costs and consequences to women, families, and communities. In the United States it is estimated that one in four women experience physical violence by an intimate partner in her lifetime (Black, 2011; Tjaden & Thoennes, 2000). However, due to the under-reported nature of this crime the rates are suspected to be even higher. It has been reported that one third of women killed in the United States are murdered by an intimate partner (UN, 2011).

Intimate partner violence (IPV) is the most common form of violence against women, which has also been called by many terms such as partner or spousal abuse; woman abuse; domestic violence; or termed spousal assault, wife abuse, and wife battering (Hart & Jamieson, 2002). Intimate partners are "current and former husbands and wives, same-sex partners, boyfriends, and girlfriends" (Saltzman, Fanslow, McMahon, & Shelley, 1999, p. 12). The U.S. Department of Justice Office on Violence Against Women (2013) defines domestic violence as "a pattern of abusive behavior that is used by an intimate partner to gain or maintain power and control over the other intimate partner" (http://www.ovw.usdoj.gov/domviolence.htm). Intimate partner violence or domestic violence can be physical, sexual, emotional, economic, or psychological actions or threats of actions that influence another person. This includes any behaviors that intimidate, manipulate, humiliate, isolate, frighten, terrorize, coerce, threaten, blame, hurt, injure, or wound someone (United States Government Department of Justice, 2013).

Violence against women creates many health consequences that often extend beyond the obvious dangers of injuries and death related to the assault. This chapter explores the various forms of violence against women and its health consequences and identifies current strategies and trends of importance to health care professionals in addressing violence against women.

BACKGROUND ON VIOLENCE AGAINST WOMEN

Understanding violence against women requires insight into the gendered nature of violence against women. Women are disproportionately victims of intimate partner violence and are at an increased risk of intimate partner violence than their male counterparts (Ansara & Hinton, 2011; Tjaden & Thoennes, 2000). This reflects its rootedness in male dominance and unequal power relations between men and women (UN, 2006), and also societal gender attitudes that include various manifestations of power and control. The rates of physical abuse of women by intimate partners in the United States during their lifetimes ranges from 25% to 33%, according to two large nationally representative studies (Plichta, 1997; Tjaden & Thoennes, 2000). Between 3% and 12% of women have been physically assaulted in the past year and more than 7% of women are sexually assaulted by an intimate partner in their lifetimes (Tjaden & Thoennes, 2000). Most reported IPV is perpetrated by men against women; approximately 85% of the victims of serious IPV are women (Rennison & Welchens, 2000). Although women can abuse men, the pattern of repeated violence in a context of coercive, controlling behaviors is most commonly directed against women. Abuse can also occur within same-sex couples, although little research has specifically focused on violence in same-sex couples (Renzetti, 1998). One of the few population-based studies of IPV that included same-sex couples suggests that the prevalence of IPV in male homosexual couples was similar to that of heterosexual couples and was slightly lower for female homosexual couples (Tjaden & Thoennes, 2000).

Violence against women creates many costs and the magnitude of its impact is enormous. The National Center for Injury Prevention and Control (2003) of the Centers for Disease Control and Prevention report estimates the annual cost of IPV using 1995 data sources to be $5.8 billion based on 5.3 million IPV victimizations per year. Of the $5.8 billion in costs, $4.1 billion are directly related to mental and medical health care expenditures and the remaining costs are associated with lost productivity and lifetime earnings of the victim (National Center for Injury Prevention and Control, 2003). Although enormous, these costs do not account for criminal justice, social services, or other specific medical costs and hence do not reflect the full extent of the costs associated with IPV. What is known is even though the associated financial costs are quite high, personal costs are even higher and affect many domains of a woman's overall health and well-being.

HEALTH EFFECT OF VIOLENCE AGAINST WOMEN

Violence against women contributes to poorer physical and mental health, and diminished quality of life among female survivors that continues well beyond the abuse (Banyard, 2008; Campbell, 2002; Devries et al., 2011; Gilliam, Bybee, & Sullivan, 2003; Goodkind, Gilliam, Bybee, & Sullivan, 2003; Montero et al., 2011; Rodriguez, 2008). Women exposed to IPV are more likely to experience specific health problems (Campbell, 2002; Campbell & Soeken, 1999; Kendall-Tackett, Marshall, & Ness, 2003; McNutt, Carlson, Persaud, & Postmas, 2002; Wilson, Silberberg, Brown, & Yaggy, 2007) that include chronic pain, gastrointestinal symptoms/irritations, headaches, depression, diminished self-esteem (Campbell, 2002; Campbell & Soeken, 1999; Forte, Cohen, DuMont, Hyman, & Romans, 2005; Hill, Schroeder, Bradley, Kaplan, & Angel, 2009; Wilson et al., 2007) and more likely to engage in unhealthy behaviors such as substance overuse (Eby, 2004; Hathaway, Mucci, Silverman, Brooks, Mathews, & Pavlos, 2000; Tomasulo & McNamara, 2007). It is clear that IPV has serious health consequences. The most obvious physical consequence is injury. In 2011, 42% of assaults result in injury, and roughly 20% of women seek health care services related to the assault (Catalano, 2013). Other physical health problems include increased rates of upper respiratory problems, urinary tract infections, pelvic pain, painful intercourse, increased rates of sexually transmitted infections, and irritable bowel syndrome.

The cause of these health problems is not fully understood. Some indications suggest the chronic stress of living with IPV may adversely alter immune function (Woods, 2005). Forced sex may result in cervical and pelvic injuries that could partially explain chronic pelvic pain. Abusive partners also may refuse to use condoms or have multiple sexual partners, thus placing their female partners at greater risk for sexually transmitted infections (El-Bassel et al., 2001; Neighbors, O'Leary, & Labouvie, 1999; Wingood & DiClemente, 1997). The World Health Organization (WHO) also reports that both IPV and sexual violence can lead to other negative health outcomes, such as unintended pregnancies, induced abortions, gynecological problems, and increased sexually transmitted infections (WHO, 2013).

Sadly, women's experiences with violence do not disappear during pregnancy and as a result experiencing IPV during pregnancy is associated with a number of poor pregnancy outcomes, including increased likelihood of miscarriage, stillbirth (WHO, 2013) lower-birth-weight babies, more preterm labor, increased rates of smoking, and fetal trauma (Campbell et al., 2003; Silverman, Decker, Reed, & Raj, 2006). Given the breadth and scope of all of these issues, it is not surprising these women have a higher use of services (Coker, Reeder, Fadden, & Smith, 2004; Duterte, et al., 2008; Ulrich et al., 2003) and frequently access (Campbell, 2002; Ford-Gilboe et al., 2009) and use health services (Coker, Reeder, Fadden, & Smith, 2004; Macy, Nurius, Kernic, & Holt, 2005; Tomasulo & McNamara, 2007; Ulrich et al., 2003). However, the most severe outcome is death, which globally accounts for 38% of murders of women (WHO, 2013).

Femicide

Death is the most severe outcome of IPV. Femicide (or the homicide of a woman) is the seventh leading cause of premature death for women overall in the United States among African-American women aged 15 to 34 years (CDC, 2005). As many as one half of murdered women are killed by a current or former intimate partner (Langford, Isaac, & Kabat, 1998) and pregnant women appear to have two to three times the risk for femicide compared with nonpregnant women (Krulewitch, Pierre-Louis, de Leon-Gomez, Guy, & Green, 2001; Krulewitch, Roberts, & Thompson, 2003; McFarlane, Campbell, Sharps, & Watson, 2002). Although intimate partner homicides have declined since the 1970s, the decline has mostly occurred among male victims, with the rate holding nearly steady for women (Campbell, Glass, Sharps, Laughon, & Bloom, 2007). Among those women, as many as 70% of IPV murder victims were previously battered by their partner (Campbell et al., 2007). Nearly half of these murder victims used the health care system—and thus might have had access to help, had someone asked the women about violence before their deaths (Sharps et al., 2001; Wadman & Muelleman, 1999).

An 11-city case-control study of risk factors for intimate partner femicide found that specific risk factors are associated with victims of completed and attempted femicide, as compared with women who had been abused by an intimate partner but had not experienced lethal or near-lethal violence (Campbell et al., 2003). Also, victims of femicide or attempted femicide were more likely to have a partner who was unemployed but not looking for work, have a partner who had access to a gun, have been threatened with a weapon, have a child who was not the biological child of the perpetrator

in the home, and be estranged or separated from the perpetrator.

Mental Health Consequences

Intimate partner violence has been consistently associated with depression and posttraumatic stress disorder (PTSD) in the literature (Goodman, Smyth, Borges, & Singer, 2009; Hill et al., 2009; Mechanic, Weaver, & Resick, 2008; Rodriguez et al., 2008). In one large population-based study, women experiencing abuse were three times more likely than nonabused women to have experienced depression in the prior month and more than twice as likely to have been anxious (Hathaway et al., 2000). Women who are depressed may be more likely to enter into and stay in abusive relationships, but there is evidence that in some cases the depression did not occur until after the abuse. A relationship between the severity of the abuse and the severity of the depression also has been publicized (Campbell & Soeken, 1999; Silva, McFarlane, Soeken, Parker, & Reel, 1997).

Posttraumatic stress disorder and its related symptoms are associated with experiencing IPV (Campbell, 2002). One study of residents of a shelter for battered women found that increasing levels of dangerousness are associated with increased numbers of PTSD symptoms (Sato-DiLorenzo & Sharps, 2007). Symptoms of PTSD included re-experiencing the trauma through memories of the event that will not go away (intrusive thoughts) or recurring dreams; avoidance behaviors such as a general numbing of emotions or avoiding places, sights, smells, or sounds that might trigger memories of the event; increased arousal and difficulty falling asleep; exaggerated startle responses; and irritability and other persistent, unpleasant feelings. A formal diagnosis of PTSD requires exposure to a traumatic event that places a person in fear of bodily harm or death. Many battered women are exposed to psychological trauma that does not meet the requirements of the formal diagnosis; however, several studies illustrate that these women have similar symptom profiles to women experiencing severe physical and sexual trauma (Kaysen, Resick, & Wise, 2003). Furthermore, the diagnosis of PTSD requires the clinician to screen for exposure to a traumatic event. In addition to experiencing higher stress levels (Eby, 2004) and PTSD, women also experience sleep difficulties, eating disorders, emotional distress, and suicide attempts (WHO, 2013). Many studies propose an association between violence against women and postpartum depression (Garabedian, Lain, Hansen, Garcia, Williams, & Crofford, 2011). All of these facts lead a nurse to understand the importance of listening to women's details of their lives.

IMPACT OF INTIMATE PARTNER VIOLENCE OR DOMESTIC VIOLENCE ON CHILDREN

Intimate partner violence or domestic violence is an adverse childhood event that often causes direct and/or indirect harm to children. Children witness, hear, and see abusive incidents that can harm them psychologically and emotionally. According to Graham-Bermann and Seng (2005), children exposed to violence display child traumatic symptoms and have more health problems such as headaches, gastrointestinal concerns, and asthma. Older children exposed to IPV have more behavioral problems, more difficulty in school, more social problems, and poorer health than do children who are not exposed (Dube, Felitti, Dong, Giles, & Anda, 2003; Kernic et al., 2002; McFarlane, Groff, O'Brien, & Watson, 2003). Babies born to mothers who experience IPV during pregnancy are more likely to have low birth weight than their peers whose mothers did not experience IPV (El-Kady, Gilbert, Xing, & Smith, 2005; Silverman et al., 2006; Yost, Bloom, McIntire, & Leveno, 2005). Regardless of age, children can be inadvertently injured as bystanders and others are injured by unknowingly placing themselves in harm's way if they try to intervene. Intimate partner violence in the home is also associated with a significant increase in child abuse (Campbell & Lewandowski, 1997). With violence in the home, children can become displaced should they accompany their abused parent in seeking refuge at a shelter or be removed from the home without a parent for their own protection. Additionally, perhaps as many as 2500 children each year experience the death of one parent by the other (Laughon, Steeves, Parker, Sawin, & Knopp, 2008). Although minimal research can be found to explain the specific effects of this event, the children generally lose both parents in one sudden event: One is dead and the other in prison for many years or also dead (in the case of murder-suicides). Even though this portrays a grim reality, at least one research study presented evidence that assessment

and interventions for the mother dramatically improve outcomes for her children (McFarlane et al., 2003).

RISK FACTORS FOR INTIMATE PARTNER VIOLENCE AND SEXUAL VIOLENCE

The World Health Organization (WHO; 2013) outlines various risk factors for being a perpetrator and victim of IPV and sexual violence:

- Risk factors for being a perpetrator include low education, exposure to child maltreatment or witnessing violence in the family, harmful use of alcohol, attitudes accepting of violence and gender inequality.
- Risk factors for being a victim of intimate partner and sexual violence include low education, witnessing violence between parents, exposure to abuse during childhood, and attitudes accepting violence and gender inequality.

Situations of conflict, post conflict, and displacement may exacerbate existing violence and present new forms of violence against women (WHO, 2013). Research by Simister (2010) investigating violence against women, suggests a strong link between higher levels of education associated with less violence. Although the study focus was on female genital mutilation there appears to be support for the applicability to other forms of violence. Additionally, there is some evidence of effectiveness of school-based programs targeting violence prevention in youth relationships (dating violence) in higher-income settings. In low-income settings microfinance initiatives that accompany gender equality training, community-based initiatives to address gender inequality and communication and relationship skills are promising (WHO, 2013).

OPPORTUNITIES IN THE HEALTH CARE SYSTEM

Role of the Nurse

Most of the challenges women exposed to violence face have serious health consequences and diminish the social determinants of health of this already very vulnerable population. Nurses are highly visible at many points of access across the system of care. They are ideally situated to help and support abused women through screening and brief counseling for IPV, referrals, system navigation, providing resources, and connecting them across the system. As such, nurses witness the impact of violence in the lives of women and children. From this purview, nurses can advocate to inform, influence, and shape health policy directions that: (1) raise awareness of the conditions that create barriers to optimizing the health of these women; (2) inform how best to support abused women; (3) identify opportunities within the system to improve the health of women exposed to violence; and (4) inform intervention work with abused women. All of these actions contribute to protecting women and improving women's quality of life and well-being. Nurses can engage in political action at multiple levels through letter writing; collectively lending their voices to issue related to violence against women through professional associations, boards, and commissions; holding political office; or engaging at various strategic points along the political process (i.e., meeting with government officials, forming grassroots coalitions working with political parties to bring relevant issues to the forefront).

Nurses are also important critical players in health research and education. As researchers, nurses conduct studies that generate knowledge of benefit to women and children exposed to violence for those working to eliminate violence against women and who support these families such as cross-sectoral service providers, law enforcement, and government. Nursing research in this field also inform broader system functioning such as interagency coordination of services. They can also address various levels of policies pertaining to violence against women and policies across sectors that impact the lives of involved women such as housing, income support policies, and so on. Nursing research identifies knowledge gaps, challenges, barriers, intervention strategies related to abused women and highlights areas for further research. Nurses have knowledge and expertise of the needs of abused women and children that sheds light on clinical practice, policy, decision making, and closing system gaps related to violence against women. Drawing on nurses' historical social justice lens, nurses bring an approach that gives primacy to women's multiple social locations and recognizes women's multiple experiences. This fosters the valuing women's experiences of abuse and helps to minimize re-victimization.

On March 23, 2010 the Patient Protection and Affordable Care Act (also referred to as Obama Care or the ACA) was signed into law (https://www.healthcare.gov/where-can-i-read-the-affordable-care-act/). With this law came sweeping health reforms, particularly in the area of preventive health services for women, which now must be covered copay-free by health plans. Screening and brief counseling for domestic and interpersonal violence are listed among the 22 required preventive health services for women (https://www.healthcare.gov/what-are-my-preventive-care-benefits/#part=2). This is an important milestone for all women because few women report being assessed for IPV at their health care visits (Glass, Dearwater, & Campbell, 2001). More than 40% of women who were murdered by an intimate partner used the health care system for an injury or mental health issue in the year before their deaths (Sharps et al., 2001). Therefore assessing women as they come in contact with the health care system is an ideal opportunity to offer care. Assessment does work; women who screen positive for IPV are nine times more likely to experience physical violence in the year before their deaths than women who do not have a positive screen (Koziol-McLain, Coates, & Lowenstein, 2001). Screening creates a window of opportunity for nurses to explore violence in the lives of women who they encounter at multiple system access points. In doing so, nurses can begin a conversation that offers support, referral, and a more comprehensive insight into the overall health status, including the factors affecting the health of each woman. Findings from both quasi-experimental and experimental studies have demonstrated that a nurse-delivered intervention significantly increases women's safety-promoting behaviors and reduces the severity and frequency of IPV experienced by women (McFarlane et al., 2004; Parker, McFarlane, Silva, Soeken, & Reel, 1999).

ASSESSMENT FOR INTIMATE PARTNER VIOLENCE

Nurses and other health care professionals should assess all women, not just women with identifiable risk factors. *Futures Without Violence* offers several patient provider resources and a toolkit for screening as well as brief counseling (http://www.futureswithoutviolence.org/section/our_work/health/_toolkit/_provider_tools) and the CDC has compiled a comprehensive document of validated screening tools for assessing IPV (http://www.cdc.gov/ncipc/pubres/images/ipvandsvscreening.pdf).

Several evidence-based tools are available for screening patients; some have been more widely used than others. The Abuse Assessment Screen (AAS) has been used in a variety of clinical settings. It includes a question about abuse during pregnancy that can be omitted if the woman is not pregnant. It also includes a body map for documenting areas of injury. The tool is reliable and valid with white, African-American, and Hispanic women (Soeken, McFarlane, Parker, & Lominack, 1998). It was recently updated to include strangulation behaviors, so the newest version of the instrument should be used (Laughon, Renker, Glass, & Parker, 2008). The Woman's Experience with Battering (WEB) scale is a longer, 10-item instrument. This tool screens for coercive behavior and psychological abuse, as well as for physical and sexual abuse (Smith, Earp, & DeVellis, 1995).

All these instruments can be self-administered or read to patients. Some researchers suggest that face-to-face screening increases disclosure. However, evidence also indicates this varies by ethnicity (Torres et al., 2000). Ideally women would have the opportunity to complete both a written screening and a face-to-face screening by a health care provider. Regardless of how the screening is conducted, the woman should be ensured privacy while answering the questions. No one should accompany the client when the questions are asked, including children older than 3 years of age. This is also an ideal time to ask questions about other sensitive topics such as history of pregnancies, abortions, and miscarriages; sexually transmitted infections; and mental health diagnoses and treatments.

Some women may not disclose abuse but nevertheless have signs that suggest it is possible to the nurse. A client may present with injuries not consistent with the explanation of how they occurred. Multiple injuries in various stages of healing, especially when they appear on the head, trunk, or genitals, can also indicate abuse. In such cases the nurse can gently confront the inconsistency, making statements such as, "In my experience, this kind of injury doesn't usually happen from what you've described."

Other clients present with less clear-cut signs and symptoms of injury. A pattern of somatic symptoms of unknown origin (e.g., chronic pelvic and other pain, neurological symptoms, gastrointestinal symptoms, frequent sexually transmitted diseases), a pattern of difficulty in keeping appointments, increased anxiety when the partner is present, or a partner's refusal to allow the client private time with the provider can all

indicate IPV. In the past providers could document that IPV was not disclosed, note "injuries consistent with abuse" or "IPV suspected," and provide the client with written information on abuse "to share with a friend." However, with required IPV screening and brief counseling through the ACA, nurses must screen all women regardless of signs and symptoms for abuse. In all cases the nurse should inform the client that she is available if needed in the future. If possible, a follow-up visit should be scheduled.

Although providers are often concerned that women will be offended by routine IPV screening, research indicates that both abused and nonabused women support routine screening in health care settings (Glass et al., 2001; Renker & Tonkin, 2006). A variety of studies highlighted that abused women supported screening and believed such screening would make obtaining help easier for women when needed (Gielen et al., 2000; Rodriguez, McLoughlin, Nah, & Campbell, 2001; Sachs, Koziol-McLain, Glass, Webster, & Campbell, 2002).

AFTER A POSITIVE SCREEN

When clients disclose abuse, the nurse's first response should be to listen empathetically and nonjudgmentally. The woman may never have previously disclosed abuse or may not have been believed in the past. Statements such as "I believe you" and "The abuse is not your fault" are helpful and supportive. Women often believe they have no choices or that their only choice is to leave the abuser. Women can contact the police and press charges, contact police and obtain a restraining order, engage in safety planning around staying or leaving at a future date, contact a shelter or a hotline, attend support groups related to IPV/domestic violence, try to get her partner into a program for abusers, or any combination of these activities. The woman should hear that she does have options and people will help her. Findings should be documented; the records can be used in court for criminal and civil proceedings.

Assess the client's immediate safety by asking, "Are you safe to go home right now?" If the woman answers no, assist her in developing a plan. The plan should include how she will exit the office and building, who will assist her in leaving safely (e.g., security officers, police officers), and where she will go (e.g., to a friend's house, women's shelter). Available resources (e.g., police and security phone numbers, shelter hotline, social work, depending on the setting) should be identified by office staff before they are needed. The nurse should also ask whether the client has a safe place from which to make the calls, and if not, provide her with a phone in the health care facility from which she can make private phone calls. Know the local shelter hotline number and the state hotline number and provide these to the client. The woman can be moved to another room within the setting and assisted with calling an abuse hotline while practitioners see other clients, if needed. Remember that having access to a phone where the abuser cannot hear her call or track the calls she makes and where she has some privacy can be enormously empowering for a woman in a battering relationship. Also note that although some areas do not have local hotlines, state hotline numbers are available in all areas. The national hotline, which will refer women to the appropriate local programs and provide direct assistance, is 800-799-SAFE (7233).

If the woman feels safe to leave at that time, she can be assisted in identifying her current level of safety and developing an appropriate safety plan. This can be done in several ways, depending on the setting. At a minimum, the nurse should let the client know she has options to help her stay safer while in an abusive relationship, encourage her to think about her safety and that of her children, and provide her with the appropriate hotline numbers and other local resources so she can discuss safety planning. If the nurse is in a setting where more elaborate safety planning can be done, information is provided in the following.

Finally, offer information on local resources to the client. Most programs have informational cards small enough to be slipped into a shoe.

Ideally, in addition to the minimum interventions discussed in the preceding, the nurse should obtain a thorough history of the abuse; perform a physical examination focusing on the injuries; document thoroughly; and make referrals to social service, criminal justice, mental health, and specialty medical services as needed. A critical pathway for IPV has been developed and can serve as a guide for assessment and interdisciplinary referrals (Dienemann, Campbell, Wiederhorn, Laughon, & Jordan, 2003). Consensus guidelines for assessing and intervening for IPV have been developed, including forms and assessment tools, and can be accessed online (http://endabuse.org /programs/healthcare).

ADDRESSING VIOLENCE AGAINST WOMEN

Globally, violence against women is being addressed through a multitude of international declarations, conventions, state policies, and community level intervention such as the Convention on the Elimination of All Forms of Discrimination Against Women; the United Nations Development Fund for Women, the Beijing Platform for Action and the UN Declaration on the Elimination of Violence Against Women. (Commission on the Status of Women; Office of the United Nations High Commissioner for Human Rights; United Nations, General Assembly Declaration 48/104; United Nations Development Fund, 2009). Frequent calls to intensify efforts and reaffirm commitment to eliminate violence against women have ensued (United Nations Security Council, Resolution 1325; United Nations Security Council, Resolution 1820; UN Secretary-General's database on violence against women).

The WHO (2013) has proposed ways to address the priority of ending violence against women that include:
- Strengthening research and research capacity to assess interventions to address partner violence
- Developing technical guidance for evidence-based intimate partner and sexual violence prevention and for strengthening the health sector responses to such violence
- Disseminating information and supporting national efforts to advance women's rights and the prevention of and response to violence against women
- Collaborating with international agencies and organizations to reduce/eliminate violence globally.

Nationally the U.S. Department of Justice created the Office on Violence Against Women through the passage of the Violence Against Women Act (VAWA) in 1994 to implement VAWA and fund programs and special initiatives to respond to violence by administering both financial and technical assistance to communities; and supporting the creation of programs, policies, and practices aimed at ending violence against women (United States Government Department of Justice, 2013). The VAWA was reauthorized in 2000, 2005 and again in 2013 demonstrating the priority to end violence against women by influencing how societal and criminal justice views violence against women. With the added support of routine IPV screening and brief counseling in the Affordable Care Act, addressing the issue of violence against women is increasingly more visible in the United States.

Women have sought formal and informal support to alleviate the effects and challenges of abuse. Such supports provide a protective mechanism for women (Bybee & Sullivan, 2005; Sullivan & Bybee, 1999) and enhances a woman's health, well-being (Ford-Gilboe et al., 2009; Harris, Stickney, Grasley, Hutchinson, Greaves, & Boyd, 2001; Morales-Campos, Casillas, & McCurdy, 2009). Many agencies such as abused women's shelters, sexual assault agencies, domestic violence services, social services, and community partners (victim advocates, police officers, prosecutors, judges, probation and corrections officials, health care professionals) Inter-professionals work in tandem to respond to violence in the lives of women. With all of these services and cross-sector interaction, a coordinated community response to violence is important and critical to fully address the needs of abused women and their children.

SUMMARY

Violence against women is a serious health problem. Women who live with violence experience a range of poor physical and mental health problems and are at risk for femicide. Children living in the home are also at direct and indirect risk. Nurses have an essential role to play in assessing women for violence and providing competent, empathic, and thorough interventions.

Nursing interventions, which have been demonstrated to be effective, are an essential part of making the health care system an empowerment zone for "battered women and their children to find safety, to find respite, and affirmations for their strengths" (Campbell, Rose, Kub, & Nedd, 1998, p. 744).

SALIENT POINTS

- Violence against women is pervasive worldwide and occurs in many forms that includes but is not limited to various types of physical, sexual, emotional, and psychological abuse.
- Intimate partner violence is the most common form of violence against women and includes current and former husbands and wives, same-sex partners, boyfriends, and girlfriends. Intimate partner violence is either physical or sexual violence, both physical and sexual violence, or threats of either.
- A wide range of health consequences are associated with IPV, including injuries, death, headaches, fainting, chronic pain syndromes, upper respiratory problems, sexually transmitted infections, urinary tract infections, and pelvic pain.
- Sexual assault nurse examiners (SANEs) are specially trained forensic nurses who provide health evaluations, treatment, and evidence collection to victims of sexual and intimate partner violence.
- The prevalence of depression in abused women is two to four times higher than the rate of depression in the general population.
- Posttraumatic stress disorder is present in 64% of battered women. Posttraumatic stress disorder symptoms include intrusive thoughts, avoidance behaviors, exaggerated startle responses, and insomnia.
- Death from IPV is the seventh most common cause of premature death for women overall in the United States and the second leading cause of death in African-American women aged 15 to 34 years.
- Intimate partner violence screening and brief counseling for women is required in accordance with the Affordable Care Act and can be done using various screening tools.
- Nurses can facilitate disclosure of abuse through therapeutic interactions with the client, provision of a safe environment, use of valid screening tools, and referral to available resources.
- In the event of a disclosure of IPV, the nurse should listen empathetically, offer options available to the client, document all findings, perform a safety assessment, and assist the client in developing a safety plan.
- The role of the nurse in addressing violence against women is multidimensional and includes policy, advocacy research, and education at multiple levels.

CRITICAL REFLECTION EXERCISES

1. Explore the *Futures Without Violence* (http://www.futureswithoutviolence.org/section/our_work/health/_toolkit/_provbider_tools)and/or the Center for Disease Control and Prevention (CDC) (http://www.cdc.gov/ncipc/pub-res/images/ipvandsv screening.pdf) websites. Select two validated screening tools. Compare and contrast the usefulness of the two tools for adoption in your practice setting. Present your findings in a class discussion.

2. Consider the degree to which your nursing practice incorporates assessments for risk of intimate partner violence or sexual violence. Given the prevalence and impact associated with violence against women and children, what opportunities exist for you to enhance your professional practice and nursing assessment skills? Identify two opportunities to enhance your practice and discuss with your peers.

REFERENCES

Ansara, D., & Hinton, M. (2011). Psychosocial consequences of intimate partner violence for women and men in Canada. *Journal of Interpersonal Violence, 26*, 1628–1645.

Banyard, V. (2008). Consequences of teen dating violence: Understanding intervening variables in ecological context. *Violence Against Women, 14*(9), 998–1013.

Black, M. C. (2011). Intimate partner violence and adverse health consequences: Implications for clinicians. *American Journal of Lifestyle Medicine, 5*(5), 428–439.

Bybee, D., & Sullivan, C. (2005). Predicting re-victimization of battered women 3 years after exiting a shelter program. *American Journal of Community Psychology, 36*(1/2), 85–96.

Campbell, J., & Lewandowski, L. (1997). Mental and physical health effects of intimate partner violence on women and children. *Psychiatric Clinics of North America, 20*, 353–374.

Campbell, J., Webster, D., Koziol-McLain, J., Block, C., Campbell, D., Curry, M. A., et al. (2003). Risk factors for femicide in abusive relationships: Results from a multisite case control study. *American Journal of Public Health, 93*(7), 1089–1097.

Campbell, J. C. (2002). Violence against women and health consequences. *The Lancet, 359*, 1331–1336.

Campbell, J. C., Glass, N., Sharps, P. W., Laughon, K., & Bloom, T. (2007). Mortality related to intimate partner violence: A review of research and implications for the advocacy, criminal justice and health care systems. *Trauma, Violence, & Abuse, 8*(3), 246–269.

Campbell, J. C., Rose, L., Kub, J., & Nedd, D. (1998). Voices of strength and resistance: A contextual and longitudinal analysis of women's responses to battering. *Journal of Interpersonal Violence, 13*, 743–762.

Campbell, J., & Soeken, K. (1999). Women responses to battering over time: An analysis of change. *Journal of Interpersonal Violence, 14*, 21–40.

Catalano, S. (2013). *Intimate Partner Violence: Attributes of Victimization, 1993–2011*. Washington, DC: U.S. Department of Justice Office of Justice Programs, Bureau of Justice Statistics.

Centers for Disease Control and Prevention. (2003). Retrieved from http://www.cdc.gov/violenceprevention/pdf/ipvbook-a.pdf

Centers for Disease Control and Prevention. (2003). *Costs of intimate partner violence against women in the United States*. Retrieved from http://www.cdc.gov/violenceprevention/pdf/ipvbook-a.pdf.

Centers for Disease Control and Prevention. (2005). *Web-based injury statistics query and reporting system (WISQARS)*. Retrieved from http://www.cdc.gov/ncipc/wisqars.

Centers for Disease Control and Prevention. (2013). *Intimate partner violence consequences*. Retrieved from http://www.cdc.gov/violenceprevention/intimatepartnerviolence/consequences.html.

Coker, A., Reeder, C., Fadden, M., & Smith, P. (2004). Physical partner violence and medicaid utilization and expenditures. *Public Health Reports, 119*, 557–567.

Devries, K., Watts, C., Yoshihama, M., Sachraiber, L., Deyessa, N., Heise, L., & WHO Multi-Country Study Team (2011). Violence against women is strongly associated with suicide attempts: Evidence from the WHO multi-country study on women's health and domestic violence against women. *Social Science Medicine, 73*(1), 79–86.

Dienemann, J., Campbell, J., Wiederhorn, N., Laughon, K., & Jordan, E. (2003). A critical pathway for intimate partner violence across the continuum of care. *Journal of Obstetric, Gynecologic, and Neonatal Nursing, 32*, 594–603.

Dube, S. R., Felitti, V. J., Dong, M., Giles, W. H., & Anda, R. F. (2003). The impact of adverse childhood experiences on health problems: Evidence from four birth cohorts dating back to 1900. *Preventive Medicine, 37*, 268–277.

Duterte, E., Bonomi, A., Kernic, M., Schiff, M., Thompson, R., & Rivara, F. (2008). Correlates of medical and legal help seeking among women reporting intimate partner violence. *Journal of Women's Health, 17*(1), 85–95.

Eby, K. (2004). Exploring the stressors of low income women with abusive partners: Understanding their needs and developing effective community responses. *Journal of Family Violence*, 19(4), 221–232.

El-Bassel, N., Fontdevila, J., Gilbert, L., Voisin, D., Richman, B. L., & Pitchell, P. (2001). HIV risks of men in methadone maintenance treatment programs who abuse their intimate partners: A forgotten issue. *Journal of Substance Abuse*, 13, 29–43.

El-Kady, D., Gilbert, W. M., Xing, G., & Smith, L. H. (2005). Maternal and neonatal outcomes of assaults during pregnancy. *Obstetrics & Gynecology*, 105, 357–363.

Ford-Gilboe, M., Wuest, J., Varcoe, C., Davies, L., Merritt-Gray, M., Campbell, J., & Wilk, P. (2009). Modeling the effects of intimate partner violence and access to resources on women's health in the early years after leaving an abusive partner. *Social Science and Medicine*, 68, 1021–1029.

Forte, T., Cohen, M., DuMont, J., Hyman, I., & Romans, S. (2005). Psychological and physical sequelae of intimate partner violence among women with limitations in their activities of daily living. *Archives of Women's Health*, 8(4), 248–256.

Garabedian, M., Lain, K., Hansen, W., Garcia, L., Williams, C., & Crofford, L. (2011). Violence against women and postpartum depression. *Journal of Womens Health*, 20(3), 447–453.

Gielen, A. C., O'Campo, P. J., Campbell, J. C., Schollenberger, J., Woods, A. B., Jones, A. S., et al. (2000). Women's opinions about domestic violence screening and mandatory reporting. *American Journal of Preventative Medicine*, 19(4), 279–285.

Gilliam, T., Bybee, D., & Sullivan, C. (2003). The impact of family and friends' reaction on the well-being of women with abusive partners. *Violence Against Women*, 9, 347–373.

Glass, N., Dearwater, S., & Campbell, J. (2001). Intimate partner violence screening and intervention: Data from eleven Pennsylvania and California community hospital emergency departments. *Journal of Emergency Nursing*, 27(2), 141–149.

Goodkind, J., Gilliam, T., Bybee, D., & Sullivan, C. (2003). The impact of family and friends' reactions on the well-being of women with abusive partners. *Violence Against Women*, 9, 347–373.

Goodman, L., Smyth, K., Borges, A., & Singer, R. (2009). When crises collide: How intimate partner violence and poverty intersect to shape women's mental health and coping? *Trauma, Violence, Abuse*, 10(4), 306–329.

Graham-Bermann, S., & Seng, J. (2005). Violence exposure and traumatic stress symptoms as additional predictors of health problems in high-risk children. *Journal of Pediatrics*, 146(30), 349–354.

Harris, R., Stickney, J., Grasley, C., Hutchinson, G., Greaves, L., & Boyd, T. (2001). Searching for help and information: Abused women speak out. *Library & Information Science Research*, 23, 123–141.

Hart, L., & Jamieson, W. (2002). *The National Clearinghouse report on family violence: intimate partner abuse against women*. Retrieved from http://www.phac-aspc.gc.ca/ncfv-cnivf/pdfs/women%20abuse%20-%20e.pdf.

Hathaway, J., Mucci, L., Silverman, J., Brooks, D., Mathews, R., & Pavlos, C. (2000). Health status and health care use of Massachusetts women reporting partner abuse. *American Journal of Preventive Medicine*, 19(4), 302–307.

Hill, T., Schroeder, R., Bradley, C., Kaplan, L., & Angel, R. (2009). The long-term health consequences of relationship violence in adulthood: an examination of low-income women from Boston, Chicago, and San Antonio. *American Journal of Public Health*, 99(9), 1645–1650.

Kaysen, D., Resick, P. A., & Wise, D. (2003). Living in danger: The impact of chronic traumatization and the traumatic context on posttraumatic stress disorder. *Trauma, Violence, Abuse*, 4, 247–264.

Kendall-Tackett, K., Marshall, R., & Ness, K. (2003). Chronic pain syndromes and violence against women. *Women & Therapy*, 1, 45–56.

Kernic, M. A., Holt, V. L., Wolf, M. E., McKnight, B., Huebner, C. E., & Rivara, F. P. (2002). Academic and school health issues among children exposed to maternal intimate partner abuse. *Archives of Pediatric and Adolescent Medicine*, 156, 549–555.

Koziol-McLain, J., Coates, C. J., & Lowenstein, S. R. (2001). Predictive validity of a screen for partner violence against women. *American Journal of Preventive Medicine*, 21, 93–100.

Krulewitch, C. J., Pierre-Louis, M. L., de Leon-Gomez, R., Guy, R., & Green, R. (2001). Hidden from view: Violent deaths among pregnant women in the District of Columbia, 1988–1996. *Journal of Midwifery and Women's Health*, 46, 4–10.

Krulewitch, C. J., Roberts, D. W., & Thompson, L. S. (2003). Adolescent pregnancy and homicide: Findings for the Maryland Office of the Chief Medical Examiner, 1994–1998. *Child Maltreatment*, 8, 122–128.

Langford, L., Isaac, N., & Kabat, S. (1998). Homicides related to intimate partner violence in Massachusetts: Examining case ascertainment and validity of the SHR. *Homicide Studies*, 2, 353–377.

Laughon, K., Renker, P., Glass, N., & Parker, B. (2008). Revision of the Abuse Assessment Screen to address non-lethal strangulation. *Journal of Obstetric, Gynecologic, & Neonatal Nursing*, 37(4), 502–507.

Laughon, K., Steeves, R., Parker, B., Sawin, E., & Knopp, A. (2008). Forgiveness, and other themes, in women whose fathers killed their mothers. *Advances in Nursing Science* PMID: 18497591.

Macy, R., Nurius, P., Kernic, M., & Holt, V. (2005). Battered women's profiles associated with service help-seeking efforts: Illuminating opportunities for intervention. *Social Work Research*, 29(3), 137–150.

McFarlane, J., Campbell, J. C., Sharps, P., & Watson, K. (2002). Abuse during pregnancy and femicide: Urgent implications for women's health. *Obstetrics & Gynecology*, 100, 27–36.

McFarlane, J. M., Groff, J. Y., O'Brien, J. A., & Watson, K. (2003). Behaviors of children who are exposed and not exposed to intimate partner violence: An analysis of 330 black, white, and Hispanic children. *Pediatrics, 112*(3), E202–E207.

McFarlane, J., Malecha, A., Gist, J., Watson, K., Batten, E., Hall, I., et al. (2004). Increasing the safety-promoting behaviors of abused women. *American Journal of Nursing, 104,* 40–50.

McNutt, L., Carlson, B., Persaud, M., & Postmus, J. (2002). Cumulative abuse experiences, physical health and health behaviours. *Annals of Epidemiology, 12*(2), 123.

Mechanic, M., Weaver, T., & Resick, P. (2008). Mental health consequences of intimate partner abuse—A multidimensional assessment of four different forms of abuse. *Violence Against Women, 14*(6), 634–654.

Montero, I., Escriba, V., Ruiz-Perez, I., Vives-Cases, C., Martin-Baena, D., Talavera, M., & Plazaola, J. (2011). Interpersonal violence and women's psychological well-being. *Journal of Womens Health, 20*(2), 295–301.

Morales-Campos, D., Casillas, M., & McCurdy, S. (2009). From isolation to connection: Understanding a support group for Hispanic women living with gender-based violence in Houston, Texas. *Journal of Immigrant and Minority Health, 11*(91), 57–65.

National Center for Injury Prevention and Control. (2003). *Costs of intimate partner violence against women in the United States.* Atlanta: Centers for Disease Control and Prevention. Retrieved from http://www.cdc.gov/violenceprevention/pdf/ipvbook-a.pdf.

Neighbors, C. J., O'Leary, A., & Labouvie, E. (1999). Domestically violent and nonviolent male inmates' responses to their partners' requests for condom use: Testing a social-information processing model. *Health Psychology, 18,* 427–431.

Parker, B., McFarlane, J., Silva, C., Soeken, K., & Reel, S. (1999). Testing an intervention to prevent further abuse to pregnant women. *Research in Nursing and Health, 22,* 59–66.

Plichta, S. (1997). Violence, health and the use of health services. In M. Falik, & K. Collins (Eds.), *Women's health: The Commonwealth Fund survey* (pp. 237–272). Baltimore, MD: Johns Hopkins University Press.

Renker, P. R., & Tonkin, P. (2006). Women's views of prenatal violence screening: Acceptability and confidentiality issues. *Obstetrics & Gynecology, 107*(2), 348–354.

Rennison, C., & Welchens, S. (2000). *Intimate partner violence.* Washington, DC: (Rep. No. Publication NCJ 183781). U.S. Department of Justice.

Renzetti, C. M. (1998). Violence and abuse in lesbian relationships: Theoretical and empirical issues. In R. K. Bergen (Ed.), *Issues in intimate violence* (pp. 117–127). Thousand Oaks, CA: Sage.

Rodriguez, M., Heilemann, M., Fielder, E., Ang, A., Nevarez, F., & Manigone, C. (2008). Intimate partner violence, depression, and PTSD among pregnant Latina women. *Annals of Family Medicine, 6*(1), 44–52.

Rodriguez, M. A., McLoughlin, E., Nah, G., & Campbell, J. C. (2001). Mandatory reporting of domestic violence injuries to the police: What do emergency department patients think? *Journal of the American Medical Association, 286,* 580–583.

Sachs, C. J., Koziol-McLain, J., Glass, N., Webster, D., & Campbell, J. (2002). A population-based survey assessing support for mandatory domestic violence reporting by health care personnel. *Women & Health, 35*(2–3), 121–133.

Saltzman, L. E., Fanslow, J. L., McMahon, P. M., & Shelley, G. A. (1999). *Intimate partner violence surveillance: Uniform definitions and recommended data elements.* Atlanta: Centers for Disease Control and Prevention.

Sato-DiLorenzo, A., & Sharps, P. W. (2007). Dangerous intimate partner relationships and women's mental health and health behaviors. *Issues in Mental Health Nursing, 28*(8), 837–848.

Sharps, P. W., Koziol-McLain, J., Campbell, J., McFarlane, J., Sachs, C., & Xu, X. (2001). Health care providers' missed opportunities for preventing femicide. *Preventive Medicine, 33,* 373–380.

Sharps, P. W., Laughon, K., & Giangrande, S. K. (2007). Intimate partner violence and the childbearing year: Maternal and infant health consequences. *Trauma, Violence, & Abuse, 8*(2), 105–116.

Silva, C., McFarlane, J., Soeken, K., Parker, B., & Reel, S. (1997). Symptoms of post-traumatic stress disorder in abused women in a primary care setting. *Journal of Women's Health, 6,* 543–552.

Silverman, J. G., Decker, M. R., Reed, E., & Raj, A. (2006). Intimate partner violence around the time of pregnancy and breastfeeding behavior among U.S. women. *Journal of Women's Health, 15,* 934–940.

Simister, J. (2010). Domestic violence and female genital mutilation in Kenya: Effects of ethnicity and education. *Journal of Family Violence, 25,* 247–257.

Smith, P. H., Earp, J. A., & DeVellis, R. (1995). Development and validation of the Women's Experience with Battering (WEB) scale. *Women's Health, 1,* 273–288.

Soeken, K., McFarlane, J., Parker, B., & Lominack, M. C. (1998). The Abuse Assessment Screen: A clinical instrument to measure frequency, severity, and perpetrator of abuse against women. In J. C. Campbell (Ed.), *Empowering survivors of abuse: Healthcare for battered women and their children* (pp. 195–203). Thousand Oaks, CA: Sage.

Sullivan, C., & Bybee, D. (1999). Reducing violence using community based advocacy for women with abusive partners. *Journal of Consulting and Clinical Psychology, 67*(1), 43–53.

Tjaden, P., & Thoennes, N. (2000). *Full report of the prevalence, incidence, and consequences of violence against women* (Rep. No. NCJ 183781). Washington, DC: U.S. Department of Justice, Office of Justice Programs.

Tomasulo, G., & McNamara, J. (2007). The relationship of abuse to women's health status and health habits. *Journal of Family Violence, 22,* 231–235.

Torres, S., Campbell, J., Campbell, D. W., Ryan, J., King, C., Price, P., et al. (2000). Abuse during and before pregnancy: Prevalence and cultural correlates. *Violence & Victims, 15*(3), 303–321.

Ulrich, C., Cain, K., Sugg, N., Rivara, F., Rubanowice, D., & Thompson, R. (2003). Medical care utilization patterns in women with diagnosed domestic violence. *American Journal of Preventative Medicine, 24*(1), 9–15.

United Nations, (2006). *Unite to end violence against women: United Nations Secretary General's campaign.* Fact Sheet. Retrieved from http://www.un.org/women/ endviolence/docs/vaw.pdf.

United Nations, (2009). *Commission on the status of women overview.* Retrieved from www.un.org/womenwatch/daw/csw/.

United Nations, (2010). *UN high commissioners for human rights concept note.* Retrieved from http://www2.ohchr.org /engish/issues/women/docs/ConceptN ote_VAWworkshop.pdf.

United Nations, (2011). *Unite to end violence against women: United Nations Secretary General's campaign.* Fact Sheet. Retrieved from http://endviolence.un.org/pdf/pressmaterials/unite_the_situation_en.pdf.

United Nations Development Fund. (2009). *30 years United Nations convention on the elimination of all forms of discrimination against women.* Retrieved from http://www.unifem.org/cedaw30/about_cedaw/.

United Nations General Assembly. (1994). *Declaration on the elimination of violence against women, General Assembly Resolution, 48/104 of 20 December 1993.* Retrieved from http://www.unhchr.ca/huridocda/huridoca.nsf/(Symbol)/A.RES.48.104.En.

United Nations Security Council. (2000). *Security Council 4213 Meeting. Resolution 1325.* Retrieved from http://www.un.org/ga/search/view_doc.asp?symbol=s/ res/1325(2000).

United Nations Security Council. (2008). *Security Council Meeting 5916. Resolution 1820.* Retrieved from http://www.un.org/ga/search/view_doc.asp?symbol+s/res/1820(2008).

United Nations Secretary General. (2009). *The UN secretary-general's database on violence against women.* Retrieved from http://webapps01.un.org/vawdatabase/about.action.

United States Government. (2013). *Healthcare.gov.* Retrieved from https://www.healthcare.gov/where-can-i-read-the-affordable-care-act/.

United States Government Department of Justice. (2013). *Department of Justice Office on Violence Against Women.* Retrieved from http://www.ovw.usdoj.gov/docs/about-ovw-factsheet.pdf.

Wadman, M. C., & Muelleman, R. L. (1999). Domestic violence homicides: ED use before victimization. *American Journal of Emergency Medicine, 17*(7), 689–691.

World Health Organization. (2013). *Violence Against women: Intimate partner and sexual violence against women.* Fact sheet number 239. Retrieved from http://www.who.int/mediacentre/factsheets/fs239/en/index.html.

Wilson, K., Silberberg, M., Brown, A., & Yaggy, S. (2007). Health needs and barriers to healthcare of women who have experienced intimate partner violence. *Journal of Women's Health, 16,* 1485–1498.

Wingood, G. M., & DiClemente, R. J. (1997). Effects of having a physically abusive partner on the condom: Use and sexual negotiation rates of young adult African American women. *American Journal of Public Health, 2,* 53–60.

World Health Organization. (2013). *Violence against women intimate partner and sexual violence against women.* Fact sheet N239. Retrieved from http://www.who.int/mediacentre/factsheets/fs239/en/.

World Health Organization Report. (2013). *Global and regional estimates of violence against women.* Retrieved from http://apps.who.int/iris/bitstream/10665/85239/1/9789241564625_eng.pdf.

Woods, S. J. (2005). Intimate partner violence and post-traumatic stress disorder symptoms in women: What we know and need to know. *Journal of Interpersonal Violence, 20,* 394–402.

Yost, N. P., Bloom, S. L., McIntire, D. D., & Leveno, K. J. (2005). A prospective observational study of domestic violence during pregnancy. *Obstetrics & Gynecology, 106,* 61–65.

19 CHAPTER

Telehealth

Audrey E. Snyder, PhD, RN, ACNP- BC, CEN, CCRN, FAANP, FAEN

ⓔ http://evolve.elsevier.com/Friberg/bridge/

OBJECTIVES

At the completion of this chapter, the reader will be able to:

- Define telemedicine and telehealth.
- Describe the components of telehealth technology.
- Discuss the implications of telehealth for nursing practice.
- Articulate the advantages and challenges of telehealth technology.
- Identify health policy concerns for telehealth.
- Evaluate local telehealth capabilities.

👤 PROFILE IN PRACTICE

Karie Wilson, MSN, CWOCN, AG-ACNP-BC
Wound, Ostomy, Continence Nurse, Clinician IV, University of Virginia Health System, Charlottesville, Virginia

I am a certified wound, ostomy, and continence nurse at a university hospital, and an adult-gerontology acute care nurse practitioner. My passion lies in providing education and support to patients with new ostomies and their families. I have witnessed first-hand how our ostomy patient population often falls through the cracks in terms of education and support. The soon-to-be ostomy patient is typically met the morning of surgery by an ostomy specialist for preoperative stoma site marking. The patient is next visited on postoperative day #1 and subsequent days for postoperative stoma site teaching. Many days of this postoperative course often fail to deliver teachable moments because of an alteration in sensorium, pain, and nausea. The patient is then discharged from the hospital to the home setting often ill prepared to care for his or her new stoma independently.

Some patients call when they struggle at home and can be assisted via the telephone; some patients simply do not call but try to manage on their own; other patients call but need more assistance than the phone can allow. These experiences are frustrating not only for the patient and family, but also for the ostomy provider. These experiences coupled with my continuing education encouraged me to brainstorm for a better way. This led me down the path to telemedicine as a viable option to connect ostomates with ostomy specialists. After all, telemedicine has been an effective option for many disciplines and has been found to decrease health care cost, improve access to care, and increase patient satisfaction.

The experience of establishing a telemedicine ostomy clinic has been both rewarding and challenging. The rewarding aspect is providing specialty care to remote areas while saving the patient driving time and cost. The challenging part has been that there is a paucity of research data on telemedicine use with ostomy patients and thus it has been difficult to find remote health care clinics willing to partner with me and be the hands-on piece for the clinic visit. So far, two clinics have agreed and three others are considering. The next steps include providing ostomy education to the staff of the remote sites, advertising this new and exciting service to the public and other health care providers, and expanding to sites all over Virginia. I am hopeful that with advertising and expansion, the patients will come! My goal is to show a reduction in peristomal skin complications and improvement in patient satisfaction and quality of life by providing specialized ostomy support preoperatively, postoperatively, and after discharge. The next step is the use of telemedicine to follow and assess patients with wounds, which is well documented in the literature.

Currently the telemedicine ostomy clinic connects UVA wound, ostomy NPs with ostomates in Wise and Bland, Virginia. The staff in the clinics are instrumental in preparing the patient for the visit. We are able to adjust the camera remotely from Charlottesville, Virginia, to evaluate the stoma. We have had several successes in which we were able to identify and correct peristomal skin problems owing to either incorrect pouching methods or the use of the wrong appliance. We are also connecting via telemedicine with a clinic in Liberia (for wounds, but with the potential for ostomies). We are in the process of expanding to other satellite clinics, prisons, and dialysis centers.

PROFILE IN PRACTICE

Teresa Gardner, DNP, FNP-BC, RN, FAANP

Executive Director, The Health Wagon, Wise and Clintwood, Virginia

I am a family nurse practitioner in a small free clinic in the heart of central Appalachia, where the economic tumultuous coal mining industry is the lifeblood of the region. I have worked in this health clinic for 20 years and have seen firsthand the desperation for health care resources and the daily struggle to ration health care to a population that is vulnerable and largely without hope for adequate access. Addressing the paramount prevalence of health disparities are incapacitating at times to providers here, and social equity is often far too illusory to this general population. This population has been entrenched in chronic poverty and plagued with social problems that have contributed to this certain vulnerability. It is a daily battle in the clinic to address patients who present to the clinics as "train wrecks" with multiple co-morbid conditions that are often life threatening. They have simply foregone care for too long or were not aware of the services of the clinic. We have to sort through the myriad illnesses and address those that are most critical, hoping in the not-too-distant future to get the patient back on the overly crowded schedule within the coming weeks to address further crucially important issues.

Sometimes for the provider and patients, desperately needed resources are as elusive as the air that is lacking and killed the "canary in the coal mine" many years ago. I have worked for all my years at this clinic to forge partnerships, alliances, and resources to repudiate the severe dearth of health inequalities that permeate the region. Our telemedicine partnership with the University of Virginia Health Systems has been one of the most successful resources that we have been able to provide for our patients. Patients are able to access specialty health care all without leaving their community. Those patients with no insurance are covered under a grant from Anthem BCBS of Virginia, which helps to alleviate the barrier of cost. The transportation obstacle is also removed in that patients are saved a 12-hour round-trip drive. Far too often, our patients do not have reliable transportation and the gas is too costly for patients who are just getting by day to day. I fondly recall our very first telemedicine encounter. We had told the patient that her visit would be over TV. She showed up all dressed up in makeup and a new hairstyle because she thought she would be on actual TV. This was the first of many wonderful telemedicine encounters over the past 10 years. Clinical consults that have been provided to our patients include cardiology, nephrology, endocrinology, psychiatry, pediatric cardiology, radiology, dermatology, gastroenterology, and gynecology, to name a few. All of these patients would not have had access to specialty care without the wonderful advancement of telemedicine. This year we have added other clinics via videoconferencing, such as a colposcopy clinic, an ostomy clinic, and a wound care clinic, availing resources to a population in desperate need of quality health care. Telemedicine provides a new way to get that access delivered.

INTRODUCTION

Telehealth provides the opportunity for health care providers to meet the challenges facing health care delivery. It is often considered an alternative method of health care delivery. It is not a specialty in and of itself but has the potential to facilitate care provided by various specialties. It has been marketed as a tool for providing care in rural areas, for underserved populations, and when patients may have transportation difficulties, yet there are urban settings in which it may be beneficial. Nurses can use telehealth technologies to assess patients, make clinical decisions, and support or intervene with patients.

The American Telemedicine Association defines *telemedicine* as "the use of medical information exchanged from one site to another via electronic communications to improve a patient's clinical health status." *Telehealth* often has a broader definition of remote health care and may not involve clinical services (ATA, 2012).

This definition has evolved as health care specialties, and not just medicine, use telemedicine. The term *telehealth* is used for the remainder of this chapter.

Telehealth technology has evolved over the last three decades. In the acute care high-technology environment, monitors transmit physiological parameters directly into medical records. Many pumps are electronic and can be programmed to adjust based on imputed patient data. Electronic medical records for retrieval of patient data are a standard today. Although information technology improves patient care and reduces health care cost, Simpson (2005) found that nursing has been slow to adopt information technology for nursing purposes. Since that time a gap is found in the literature that specifically addresses its use for nursing care–specific activities, including electronic record capture of nursing-sensitive quality indicators and cost.

Videoconferencing has been used for distance learning in education, especially for rural or underserved areas. Virtual classrooms have existed for the last two decades. Nursing curriculums may now employ virtual clinical practicums as well, like the innovative program developed in Pennsylvania for a rural area (Grady, 2011). Nurses have adopted electronic health records and videoconferencing as avenues for education, and now they need to adopt technology such as telehealth for evaluation of patients. This chapter provides an overview of telehealth technology and case examples of its use in the health care arena.

MODES OF TELEHEALTH

There are four modes of telehealth technology transmission. The first and oldest is the use of voice only via telephone; for example, to perform telephone triage or management of disease in specific populations, such as people with diabetes who are followed in an endocrinology clinic in which telephone triage protocols help manage care (Vinson, McCallum, Thornlow, & Champagne, 2011). The second is *store and forward* of video images, in which data are collected and then sent to a specialist. Historically radiology has used store and forward methods of evaluation, such as the picture archiving and communications systems (PACS) and teleradiology. An example of this is the forwarding of radiographs from a rural hospital to a radiologist at a distant tertiary center for reading. The third mode is data exchanged via computer; for example, the transmission of physiological data from a home unit to a hospital electronic medical record. The fourth mode is interactive live videoconferencing, in which there is virtual contact with the patient to assess, manage, treat, or educate and counsel patients. Telehealth can be done with low or high bandwidth, although images and data transfer require higher bandwidth. Regardless of the level of technology, practitioners in three evaluation studies were satisfied with the encounters (Winters & Winters, 2007).

TELEHEALTH CENTERS

Because of the rapid explosion of demand and use of telehealth technology, *Telehealth Resource Centers* (TRCs) were developed. Telehealth Resource Centers are funded by the U.S. Department of Health and Human Services Administration (HRSA) Office for the Advancement of Telehealth, which is division of the Office of Rural Health Policy. There are 12 regional TRCs in the United States and two telehealth technology assessment centers. Telehealth Resource Centers exist to improve the understanding of telehealth and how it can be used to improve access to and quality of care in rural and other medically underserved areas, and to help develop telehealth programs that match the needs of a practice or community. For example, the Mid-Atlantic Telehealth Resource Center (MATRC) was established in September 2011 and covers the states of Delaware, Kentucky, Maryland, North Carolina, Virginia, Washington, DC, and West Virginia. Their website has many resources for nurses and other health care providers and systems (www.MATRC.org) (What is a telehealth resource center?, 2012).

EQUIPMENT

To operate, telehealth technology requires a *computer platform*, *network protocol,* and *network*. The computing platform is the hardware and software framework that together allow the software to run. A network protocol is a set of digital rules for exchange of data between computers. A network can be a local area network (LAN) for a small geographical area, for example, in a hospital building or a wide area network (WAN) that encompasses a larger geographical area and also includes leased telecommunication lines.

ADVANTAGES OF TELEHEALTH TECHNOLOGY

Telehealth reaches patients in their home or home community. Encounters via telehealth technology can empower patients to participate actively in their care from home and promotes independence. Maintaining a level of independence translates into improved health status and quality of life for older adult patients experiencing chronic health problems. Increased patient satisfaction also may be an outcome of telehealth. In the managed care environment telehealth can increase patient contacts without the expense of a hands-on visit. Access to a specialist who may not be readily available in a rural community is an advantage. Medical errors were decreased for seriously ill or injured pediatric patients in rural underserved hospitals when telemedicine was used to consult pediatric critical care colleagues at a larger academic medical center (Dharmar, 2013). A Cochrane Review evaluating telemedicine versus face-to-face patient care identified no detrimental effects for telemedicine interventions (Currell, Urquhart, Wainwright, & Lewis, 2010).

Multiple demonstration studies have documented cost savings. Telehealth can save travel time for patients, care providers, and specialists, and reduce out-of-pocket expenses (Loh et al., 2013). One academic institution that has developed 125 telehealth sites in the Commonwealth of Virginia documented 38,000 encounters since inception of the telemedicine program with 8.7 million miles saved for patients (Cattell-Gordon, 2014). A longitudinal analysis of Medicare data for a demonstration clinic for patients with congestive heart failure (CHF), chronic obstructive pulmonary disease (COPD), or diabetes using a telehealth system for care management demonstrated a 15% decrease in mortality and an 18% reduction in inpatient admissions (Baker et al., 2013). The program strongly correlated with fewer admissions for COPD and decreased mortality for those with CHF (Baker et al., 2013).

USE OF TELEHEALTH

Televisits can be used to assess, monitor, support, coach, and provide medical care. More than one of these intervention types may occur in the same visit. Chronic care management through remote monitoring has grown rapidly. It allows nurses to monitor and assess for complications early. It lends itself to patients with heart disease, diabetes, asthma, psychiatric illness, and wounds. Home monitoring programs are using equipment for physiological measurements. Assessments may include heart rate, blood pressure, pulse oximetry, weight, spirometry, glucose level, electrocardiogram tracing, and temperature (Kleinpell, 2007). Stethoscopes, cameras, otoscopes, ophthalmoscopes, and videophones can be used for assessment. Video with magnifying capability can assess wounds and monitor healing. Nurses also can use the camera to view labels on medication bottles. Electronic medication dispensing devices that are controlled remotely can increase medication regimen adherence. Home telehealth should be integrated with hospital electronic medical records so the nurses and other care providers can access patient medical information to help make care decisions. Telehealth allows clinicians to safely manage high caseloads by obtaining physiological data (Chetney, 2008).

Monitoring at home has evolved to prevent readmissions and potential Medicare penalties. At hospital discharge nurses identify at-risk patients and coordinate patient transitions to home with activation of daily provider monitoring and clinical coordination using clinical review software and reporting, while documenting outcomes of readmission, population health, costs, and satisfaction. One home health agency documented cost savings for both hospitals and home care by decreasing emergency department visits and readmissions for cardiac patients by 72% (Chetney, 2008). Use of telehealth in schools for patients with asthma reduced days of school missed by 61%, emergency department visits by 70%, and hospital admissions by 86% for middle school age children. Remote monitoring can improve self-efficacy and disease management with patient support (Suter, Suter, & Johnston, 2011).

Experienced ICU nurses and physicians can use electronic intensive care units (e-ICU) to help monitor and treat intensive care patients, at a remote location. They assess the patient by video and have access to the patient's medical records and electronic monitoring results. This monitoring prevents untoward outcomes, such as reintubation or unplanned extubation, and improves patient outcomes by recognizing changes in patient trends (Williams et al., 2012). In a review of one health system's use of eICU, 594 nursing interventions were identified; 80% of these were independent nursing interventions, the remaining involved a physician or pharmacist collaboration, and 26% were rescue or prevention interventions (Williams et al., 2012).

Another innovative use of telehealth is the Telestroke programs that assist in the evaluation of individuals experiencing symptoms of a cerebrovascular accident living in rural areas. Upon arrival to the emergency department with symptoms of a potential ischemic cerebrovascular accident, the cerebrovascular accident specialist can examine a patient, obtain medical history, and review computed tomography studies remotely. Patients can receive tissue plasminogen activator (tPA) before transfer to a tertiary medical center if warranted. In non-rural areas robots using telehealth technology also may be used to allow the on-call neurologist to see the patient faster instead of coming in from home. This allows the patient to receive tPA faster (Martin, 2013). Physicians can make clinical decisions based upon data rather than using the telephone alone. Both of these telestroke interventions allow the patient to be treated faster, enhancing outcomes for cerebrovascular accident patients.

With the national shortage of health care providers in the area of psychiatry, telepsychiatry has blossomed. Even in urban areas, smaller hospitals may not have a specialist on call to evaluate for suicidal or homicidal risk. Instead of risking transport of the patient to a hospital with a mental health specialist, the assessment can be made through videoconferencing.

Cameras support store and forward capabilities or direct videoconferencing. With teleophthalmology, rural clinic staff can be taught to use a retinal camera to complete the yearly diabetic retinopathy screening. The images can be forwarded to a distant ophthalmologist, who reads the images and provides consultation back to the clinic. During videoconferencing an enterostomal nurse can observe new ostomies. In the past if the patient called the specialty clinic with a concern, the patient may have been instructed to travel to the specialty clinic, which may have been a long distance away and incurred cost for the patient. Now when there is a concern the patient can go to a nearby clinic and connect remotely through videoconferencing with a specialist, who can use the camera to zoom in on the ostomy and evaluate the concern.

Keeping patients close to home is a goal of many evolving telehealth programs. Telehealth allows high-risk obstetrical patients to have their appointments with a high-risk obstetrician via telehealth at a clinic closer to home until they near their delivery date. The Virginia Department of Corrections is using telehealth sites in the prisons to decrease the cost and risks associated with transport of prisoners to distant sites for health care appointments. For patients who have an abnormal pap smear, the next step is a colposcopy procedure in which a camera or colposcope is used to examine the vagina and cervix and biopsy any areas of concern. A pilot program using nurse practitioners to perform the procedure with supervision by a gynecologist oncologist at a distant center via videocolposcopy has shown 100% patient satisfaction (Snyder, 2013). Videocolposcopy is an intervention to help overcome the shortage of providers and expand the role of the nurse in rural southwest Virginia.

In third world countries there is often limited access to specialists for both natives and visitors. With worldwide travel today, visitors to remote locations may experience medical or trauma concerns in which a specialist consultation could impact outcomes. The Swinfen Charitable Trust is one organization that assists the poor, sick, and disabled in developing countries by establishing telemedicine links between medical practitioners in the developing world and expert medical and surgical specialists.

As telehealth evolves there will be expansion to other environments of care. The use of telehealth in nursing homes to evaluate acute complaints may help prevent transfer to the emergency department and early recognition of a change in patient condition may prevent readmission. A pilot project using a mobile platform for evaluation of patients in the prehospital arena for cerebrovascular accident symptoms may allow ischemic cerebrovascular accident patients to receive tPA faster (Swensen, 2014). With an aging population, and with cerebrovascular accident currently being the third leading cause of death, the use of this technology may impact morbidity and mortality from cerebrovascular accident.

TELE-EDUCATION

Videoconferencing is an effective means of both patient and nursing education. Diabetes education can be transmitted by one educator to multiple sites at one time and provide a vehicle for group support to manage this chronic illness. The education session can promote health in this population. Physicians working in remote areas can benefit from continuing medical education when paired with an academic institution. Surgical grand rounds are teleconferenced monthly to Rwanda from the University of Virginia. Surgeons in both countries present patients (Cattell-Gordon, 2013).

Nurses also can receive training via telehealth. A program for preoperative and oncology assessment in rural communities in Canada provided the education intervention to teach the nurses to conduct the assessments normally performed by physician during a 1-day education session via videoconferencing. A survey identified learning needs before the education sessions. Post survey the nurses reported it provided the opportunity to talk to nurses doing similar jobs and gave them time to brainstorm (Sevean et al., 2008). Telehealth is a valid method for providing continuing education to nurses in rural area.

CHALLENGES

Challenges to the use of telehealth include the quality of technology, cost, confidentiality and security, physical distancing from patients, licensure across state lines, and lack of reimbursement. There is a lack of broadband networks in many rural areas, which limits access to telehealth. The initial cost to establish a telemedicine network is high, usually requiring capital investment. Confidentiality of patient data is paramount. There is the potential for hackers, and security systems are evolving to prevent access to patient data.

Telehealth technology can create a physical distance between the nurse and the patient and a perception of distance for the patient. This theme may be a bias of nurses and other health care providers (Schlachta-Fairchild, Varghese, Deickman & Castelli, 2010). Undergraduate students demonstrated more consistent eye contact in a study of simulated practitioner–patient interactions with televisits. In the study students turned their backs to the patient only during the face-to-face interviews (Winters & Winters, 2007). Nurses have demonstrated therapeutic interactions and caring through their actions to promote health and healing (Nagel, Pomerleau, & Penner, 2013). The role of the nurse in telemedicine is evolving. Advanced practice nurses are developing ways to be with the patient

before, during, and after their virtual visits by reading about their patients before the visit, transmitting information to the patient in advance, listening and communicating, using verbal and nonverbal messaging, and following up with phone calls or monitoring of physiological parameters using telehealth (Schlachta-Fairchild, Varghese, Deickman & Castelli, 2010).

Practicing across state lines is a concern because the practitioner must be licensed in the state in which he or she practices. Nurses may have a compact state agreement that allows them to be in one state but practice by telemedicine in another state. This model has not been adopted for medicine. A physician is required to be licensed in both the state in which he or she practices and the state in which the patient is receiving care.

There exists a lack of reimbursement for remote patient monitoring. Medicare reimbursement is limited to the type of services provided, geographical location, type of institution delivering the services, and type of health provider. There is a need for federal telehealth legislation and reimbursement by Medicare and other payers to improve access to care by remote monitoring (Prinz, Cramer, & Englund, 2008; Suter, Suter, & Johnston, 2011).

NURSES' ROLE

The role of the nurse in telehealth is evolving. Education and training are important to any telehealth program. Nurses need to learn how to use and troubleshoot the technology and should know their resources. Undergraduate and graduate education should include telehealth technology and simulation experiences to facilitate the transition to practice and comfort with the technology. Telehealth has great potential to expand the roles of advanced practice nurses. The availability of training for simulation is associated with greater use according to a survey of nurse faculty (Nguyen, Zierler, & Nguyen, 2011). To prepare nurse practitioners for the current health care environment, clinical experiences incorporating telehealth applications must be integrated into the curriculum (Hawkins, 2012).

Practicing nurses also need education on telehealth applications. In the use of telehealth for cerebrovascular accident assessment, 1-hour training was sufficient and provided competency in the equipment (Winters & Winters, 2007). Training needs to meet the needs of the practitioner and simulation can help assess if the provider is competent in using the technology.

A literature review by While and Dewsbury (2011) identified nurses as participants in the delivery of health care interventions by telehealth, but noted little detail related to the specific activities, roles, frequency, or dosage of the nursing interventions performed. This is an area for growth of outcomes evaluation and evidence-based research in telehealth.

There are many successful models for telehealth, such as the Arizona Telemedicine Program that was established in 1997 to enhance care delivery for underserved populations (Krupinski et al., 2011). Education and training have been documented as strategic to the success of any telehealth program. Nurses using telehealth should evaluate patient satisfaction, care transition, and care coordination, and report the outcomes of their work.

SUMMARY

Telehealth is revolutionizing health care delivery. The greatest use is in management of chronic health problems through remote assessment or monitoring, education, and support in keeping patients at home or their own communities. Telehealth empowers patients to self-manage their disease and improves quality of life. Nurses need to become familiar with the technology, equipment, and understand the language used. Nursing students in undergraduate and graduate programs should be educated in the use of telehealth as an avenue of patient care. As more patients are cared for in their home environment, telehealth can improve patient outcomes.

SALIENT POINTS

- Telemedicine is medical information exchanged from one site to another via electronic communications to improve a patient's clinical health status.
- Telehealth may not involve clinical services.
- Nurses use telehealth to provide comprehensive care to patients.
- Nurses can use telehealth technologies to assess patients, make clinical decisions, and support or intervene with patients.
- Telehealth Resource Centers exist to improve the understanding of telehealth and how it can be used to improve access to and quality of care in rural and other medically underserved areas, and to help develop telehealth programs that match the needs of a practice or community.
- Encounters via telehealth technology can empower patients to participate actively in their care from home, promoting independence.

- Telehealth can save travel time for patients, care providers, and specialists, and reduce out-of-pocket expenses.
- eICUs can prevent untoward outcomes, such as re-intubation or unplanned extubation, and improve patient outcomes by recognizing changes in patient trends.
- Telestroke programs provide more rapid evaluation of cerebrovascular accident patients and allow tPA to be administered sooner.
- Telehealth is a valid method for providing continuing education to nurses in rural areas.
- Challenges to telehealth include the quality of technology, cost, confidentiality and security, physical distancing from patients, licensure across state lines, and lack of reimbursement.
- Nurses need to integrate telehealth technologies into their nursing practice.
- Undergraduate and graduate nursing curriculums should incorporate telehealth.

CRITICAL REFLECTION EXERCISES

1. Identify a telemedicine center in your area. What resources are available through this center? What types of specialty services are available for patient consultation?
2. Conduct a literature review to see if there are outcomes data for use of telehealth with a specific patient population or patient disease. Focus on your specialty area. How could the use of telehealth impact your practice?
3. Consider how you could make a patient feel your presence when using telehealth to provide support.

REFERENCES

American Telemedicine Association. (2012). *What is telemedicine?* Retrieved from http://www.american telemed.org/learn/what-is-telemedicine#.UuW9dk0o7cs.

American Telemedicine Association. (2013). *Telemedicine and telehealth services.* Retrieved from http://www.americantelemed.org/docs/default-source/policy/medicare-payment-of-telemedicine-and-telehealth-services.pdf?sfvrsn=14.

Baker, L. C., Macaulay, D. S., Sorg, R. A., Diener, M. D., Johnson, S. J., & Birnbaum, H. G. (2013). Effects of care management and telehealth: A longitudinal analysis using Medicare data. *Journal of the American Geriatrics Society, 61*(9), 1560–1567. Retrieved from http://dx.doi.org/10.1111/jgs.12407.

Cattell-Gordon, D. (October 26, 2013). Personal communication.

Cattell-Gordon, D. (January 27, 2014). Personal communication.

Chetney, R. (2008). Using telehealth to avoid urgent care and hospitalization. *Home Health Care Management & Practice, 20*(2), 154–160.

Currell, R., Urquhart, C., Wainwright, P., & Lewis, R. (2010). Telemedicine versus face to face patient care: Effects on professional practice and health care outcomes. *Cochrane Database System Review, 2*(2).

Dharmar, M., Kuppermann, N., Romano, P. S., Yang, N. H., Nesbitt, T. S., Phan, J., et al. (2013). Impact of critical care telemedicine consultations on children in rural emergency departments. *Critical Care Medicine, 132*(6), 1090–1097.

Grady, J. L. (2011). The virtual clinical practicum: An innovative telehealth model for clinical nursing education. *Nursing Education Perspectives, 32*(3), 189–194. Retrieved from http://dx.doi.org/10.5480/1536-5026-32.3.189.

Hawkins, S. (2012). Telehealth nurse practitioner student clinical experiences: An essential educational component for today's health care setting. *Nurse Education Today, 32*(8), 842–845. Retrieved from http://dx.doi.org/10.1016/j.nedt.2012.03.008.

Kleinpell, R., & Avitall, B. (2007). Integrating telehealth as a strategy for patient management after discharge for cardiac surgery: Results of a pilot study. *Journal of Cardiovascular Nursing, 22*, 38–42.

Krupinski, E., Patterson, T., Norman, C., Roth, Y., Elnasser, Z., Abdeen, Z., … Freedman, M. (2011). Successful models for telehealth. *Otolaryngologic Clinics of North America, 44*(6), 1275–1288.

Loh, P. K., Sabesan, S. S., Allen, D. D., Caldwell, P. P., Mozer, R. R., Komesaroff, P. A., … Withnall, D. D. (2013). Practical aspects of telehealth: Financial considerations. *Internal Medicine Journal, 43*(7), 829–834. Retrieved from http://dx.doi.org/10.1111/imj.12193.

Martin, S. (May 23, 2013). Robots roam hospital halls, and patients love it. *USA Today*, p.1B.

Nagel, D. A., Pomerleau, S. G., & Penner, J. L. (2013). Knowing, caring, and telehealth technology: "Going the distance" in nursing practice. *Journal of Holistic Nursing, 31*(2), 104–112. Retrieved from http://dx.doi.org/10.1177/0898010112465357.

Nguyen, D. N., Zierler, B., & Nguyen, H. Q. (2011). A survey of nursing faculty needs for training in use of new technologies for education and practice. *Journal of Nursing Education, 50*(4), 181–189. Retrieved from http://dx.doi.org/10.3928/01484834-20101130-06.

Prinz, L., Cramer, M., & Englund, A. (2008). Telehealth: A policy analysis for quality, impact on patient outcomes, and political feasibility. *Nursing Outlook, 56*(4), 152–158.

Schlachta-Fairchild, L., Varghese, S., Deickman, A., & Castelli, D. (2010). Telehealth and telenursing are live: APN policy and practice implications. *Journal for Nurse Practitioners, 6*(2), 98–106. Retrieved from http://dx.doi.org/10.1016/j.nurpa.2009.12.019.

Sevean, P., Dampier, S., Spadoni, M., Strickland, S., & Pilatzke, S. (2008). Bridging the distance: Educating nurses for telehealth practice. *Journal of Continuing Education in Nursing, 39*(9), 413–418. Retrieved from http://dx.doi.org/10.3928/00220124-20080901-10.

Simpson, R. (2005). Nursing informatics. From tele-ed to telehealth: The need for IT ubiquity in nursing. *Nursing Administration Quarterly, 29*(4), 344–348.

Snyder, A., Merwin, E., Mahone, I., & Hinton, I. (2013). Preventing cervical cancer in rural impoverished women. Unpublished data.

Suter, P., Suter, W., & Johnston, D. (2011). Theory-based telehealth and patient empowerment. *Population Health Management, 14*(2), 87–92. Retrieved from http://dx.doi.org/10.1089/pop.2010.0013.

Swensen, E. (January 6, 2014). Using tablets, telemedicine to speed stroke treatment. *UV Today*. Retrieved from http://news.virginia.edu/content/using-tablets-telemedicine-speed-stroke-treatment.

Vinson, M. H., McCallum, R., Thornlow, D. K., & Champagne, M. T. (2011). Design, implementation, and evaluation of population-specific telehealth nursing services. *Nursing Economic$, 29*(5), 265–277.

What is a telehealth resource center (TRC)? (Summer 2012). *Virginia Rural Health News, 13*, 7.

While, A., & Dewsbury, G. (2011). Nursing and information and communication technology (ICT): A discussion of trends and future directions. *International Journal of Nursing Studies, 48*(10), 1302–1310. Retrieved from http://dx.doi.org/10.1016/j.ijnurstu.2011.02.020.

Williams, L. M., Hubbard, K. E., Daye, O., & Barden, C. (2012). Telenursing in the intensive care unit: Transforming nursing practice. *Critical Care Nurse, 32*(6), 62–69.

Winters, J., & Winters, J. (2007). Videoconferencing and telehealth technologies can provide a reliable approach to remote assessment and teaching without compromising quality. *Journal of Cardiovascular Nursing, 22*(1), 51–57.

Patient Safety

Vicki S. Good, MSN, RN, CENP, CPPS and Kimberly R. Cash, RN, MSN, CNML

e http://evolve.elsevier.com/Friberg/bridge/

OBJECTIVES

At the completion of this chapter, the reader will be able to:

- Describe the RN's central role in patient safety.
- Illustrate the regulatory requirements specific to patient safety.
- Characterize a "just culture."
- Explain the role of a healthy work environment and culture on patient safety.
- Demonstrate the utilization of key tools to enhance patient safety.

PROFILE IN PRACTICE

Sonya A. Flanders, MSN, RN, ACNS-BS, CCRN

Clinical Nurse Specialist for Internal Medicine Services, Baylor University Medical Center, Dallas, Texas

As a nurse with over 25 years of clinical and leadership experience in critical care, administration, cardiovascular services, care coordination, patient safety, and internal medicine, I have seen many examples of the dedication exhibited by professional nurses in providing safe patient care. I have also come to recognize the necessity to mitigate threats to patient safety inherent to the complex environments in which nurses, physicians, and other health care team members work.

Although the concept of patient safety has always been embedded in my clinical and leadership work, patient safety became my primary area of focus a few years ago. Because ineffective communication is a known threat to patient safety, my earliest formal patient safety work was to help design a standardized educational presentation and tools for nurses to learn and apply the Situation-Background-Assessment-Recommendation (SBAR) standardized communication method. SBAR communication guides nurses to articulate a patient situation or problem to a physician or other health care professional in a clear, concise, and assertive way. Developing SBAR education and tools (such as pocket cards and posters placed near telephones) that all nurses in the organization could use was a step aimed at fostering consistent and effective interdisciplinary communication. Not only does SBAR help nurses convey information more effectively, but it also provides a framework for the receiver to get the information necessary to act on a patient problem. The recommendation step in SBAR encourages nurses to state what they think the patient may need to address a problem, a step some nurses may omit without this structured communication method. Examples of recommendations include requesting a new medication order, suggesting transfer to a higher level of care, or asking a physician to assess the patient. A recent survey of a sample of physicians within our organization indicated many providers prefer receiving patient information in SBAR format.

Building on the SBAR work, next steps were to collaborate with other patient safety nurses, physicians, and team members to train our peers and interdisciplinary colleagues about the value of teamwork and the ways in which effective teamwork and communication contribute to building a culture of patient safety. Together we developed a training program that included general concepts about patient safety, human factors, characteristics of high reliability organizations, and SBAR. Over time, new content has been added to include other patient safety practices and concepts. During the training, a variety of examples are used to convey this very critical message: Patient safety is everyone's responsibility. Regardless of education level, job title, or position within the organization, everyone has the right to speak up about patient safety concerns and is supported when doing so. A culture that supports excellent teamwork and communication gives patients and care-givers alike an added layer of protection because there are more eyes and ears working synergistically to identify and eliminate patient safety risks. Nurses are in an ideal position to contribute to this positive patient safety culture because we are often at the hub of patient care and interdisciplinary communication.

Another patient safety activity I worked on involved implementing a multihospital program focused on The Joint Commission's National Patient Safety Goals (NPSGs). The goals of the program have been to enhance overall awareness of the NPSGs, ensure a shared understanding of what the expectations are for each goal, clarify how each goal applies in clinical practice, measure performance, and act on opportunities to improve patient safety processes. A complementary part of the NPSGs program has been to enhance patient, family, and visitor awareness of the NPSGs by placing posters and cards explaining the goals in public areas of the hospitals. This is one way to encourage patients and families to ask questions and speak up about patient safety concerns—as we know, involving them is another valuable patient safety strategy.

My career path has continued to evolve, and I now practice as a clinical nurse specialist in a large acute-care hospital, but patient safety is still very much a part of my work. As nurses and steadfast patient advocates, almost everything we do involves a component of providing safe care. From performing appropriate infection prevention measures, to correctly identifying every patient before administering every medication, to participating in a "time out" before a surgical or invasive procedure, nurses are on the front lines of patient safety. As the science of patient safety matures, I think nurses in all practice environments have an opportunity to take an active role in patient safety activities and programs. Nurses have the ability and responsibility to continually assess and identify actual and potential threats to patient safety, develop plans and processes to eliminate or minimize risks, evaluate effectiveness of patient safety activities, and act as role models and entrepreneurs in the area of patient safety. Together with our colleagues, patients, and families, we must be leaders in achieving the goal of providing patients the safest possible care.

INTRODUCTION

Fourteen years have passed since the Institute of Medicine (IOM) published *To Err Is Human: Building a Safer Health System,* a report that is considered a milestone in the history of patient safety (Ilan & Fowler, 2005; Wachter, 2010). The report estimated that as many as 98,000 hospitalized patients die each year from errors in hospital care (IOM, 2000). It also illustrated that although human beings are not perfect and will continue to make errors, the responsibility lies with health care systems to identify processes leading to errors and design improvements to decrease errors, with the ultimate goal of mitigating and eliminating health care errors. Because professional nurses have the greatest amount of interaction with patients throughout the hospital stay, they are in a key position to identify and implement process improvements to enhance patient safety. Professional nurses have the ability to intercept medical errors as much as 90% of the time owing to the frequency of interaction nurses have with patients (Lin & Liang, 2007; Tregunno, Jeffs, & McGillis Hall, 2009).

Americans continue to advocate for a safer health care delivery system, and practitioners continue to struggle with the provision of a safe health care delivery system. Some progress has been made toward a safer health care system, but challenges remain (Gluck, 2012). This chapter focuses on the central role of the nurse on regulatory requirements for patient safety, establishing and sustaining a culture of patient safety, and defining key processes to enhance patient safety.

REGULATORY OVERVIEW

The Joint Commission

As the *To Err Is Human* report was being released by the IOM, The Joint Commission began its journey toward developing standards to ensure a safer health care system. In 1999, The Joint Commission's mission statement (Box 20-1) was revised to explicitly reference patient safety as a key initiative (The Joint Commission, 2009a, 2009b; The Joint Commission Online, 2009).

The Joint Commission continued pursuing patient safety by introducing the National Patient Safety Goals (NPSGs) in 2002. The purpose of the NPSGs is to promote patient safety improvements based on

BOX 20-1   The Joint Commission Mission Statements

Mission Statement 1999

To continuously improve the safety and quality of care provided to the public through the provision of health care accreditation and related services that support performance improvement in health care organizations.

Mission Statement 2009

To continuously improve health care for the public, in collaboration with other stakeholders, by evaluating health care organizations and inspiring them to excel in providing safe and effective care of the highest quality and value.

From The Joint Commission. (2009). The Joint Commission mission statement. Retrieved October 21, 2013, from http://www.jointcommission.org/assets/1/18/Mission_Statement_8_09.pdf. © The Joint Commission, 2010. Reprinted with permission.

TABLE 20-1   Department of Health and Human Services Resources for Patient Safety

RESOURCE	WEBSITE
Agency for Healthcare Research and Quality (AHRQ)	www.ahrq.gov
Agency for Toxic Substances and Disease Registry (ATSDR)	www.atsdr.cdc.gov
Centers for Disease Control and Prevention (CDC)	www.cdc.gov
Centers for Medicare and Medicaid Services (CMS)	www.cms.hhs.gov
Food and Drug Administration (FDA)	www.fda.gov
Health Resources Services Administration (HRSA)	www.hrsa.gov
National Institutes of Health (NIH)	www.nih.gov
Quality & Safety Education for Nurses	http://qsen.org
Substance Abuse and Mental Health Services Administration (SAMHSA)	www.samhsa.gov

recommendations made from sentinel event alerts, the Patient Safety Advisory Group, and review of current patient safety literature. The NPSGs address the complex health care environment by providing specific requirements for a variety of settings, including ambulatory, behavioral health care, critical access hospitals, home care, hospital, laboratory, long-term care, and office-based surgery centers.

In 2002 the initial hospital goals consisted of six goals focused on the accuracy of patient identification; effectiveness of communication among caregivers; medication safety; elimination of wrong-site, wrong-patient, wrong-procedure surgery; safety of infusion pumps; and effectiveness of clinical alarm systems. Each year the goals are analyzed based on current trends in patient safety, and recommendations are made for goals to be retained, be revised, or moved to The Joint Commission standards (The Joint Commission, 2006). Accredited health care organizations are required to demonstrate ongoing NPSGs compliance using specific requirements established by The Joint Commission. The NPSGs' requirements are more prescriptive than The Joint Commission standards, but they do allow facilities flexibility in process implementation to meet the requirements (The Joint Commission, 2006).

In addition to NPSGs requirements, The Joint Commission demonstrates its commitment to patient safety by providing guidance to health care delivery systems

in a variety of efforts. These efforts include sentinel event policy, sentinel event alerts, patient safety advisory groups, universal protocol, office of quality monitoring, patient safety research, patient safety education, and the Speak Up Initiative. Although The Joint Commission takes a multidisciplinary view of patient care, the professional nurse plays the central role in implementing many of the safety programs as the primary coordinator of patient care. Health care organizations rely on the professional nurse as a team leader to design process improvement with colleagues (e.g., pharmacy, respiratory therapy) to continuously meet NPSGs requirements. Information on The Joint Commission's patient safety initiatives can be found at www.jointcommission.org/topics/patient_safety.aspx.

U.S. Department of Health and Human Services

The U.S. Department of Health and Human Services (DHHS) is charged with protecting the health of all Americans and providing services for those who cannot provide for themselves. As a part of this responsibility, the DHHS has initiated several programs with the specific goal of improving patient safety. Table 20-1 outlines agencies within DHHS that play key roles in defining and regulating patient safety initiatives. These

DHHS agencies work with the health care team to coordinate and collaborate on initiatives to improve the health and safety of Americans. The Agency for Healthcare Research and Quality (AHRQ) serves as the lead organization for quality of care and patient safety research (both the provision of research and the synthesis of published research evidence). One of the goals of AHRQ is to promote the use of evidence-based practice in routine health care. Therefore AHRQ partners with key regulatory agencies such as the Centers for Medicare and Medicaid (CMS), The Joint Commission, and other partners such as the National Quality Forum to move evidence-based practice into health care (Couig, 2005; Taylor et al., 2009).

The professional nurse is the primary advocate for the patient and is responsible for ensuring that all regulatory requirements are met during patient care activities. The professional nurse can identify key patient care process improvements to meet and exceed regulatory requirements. When key processes are not carried out as intended, the professional nurse has been described as the clinician on the "sharp end" of patient care or the clinician closest to the patient care delivery—thus often the last line of defense to potentially mitigate or avoid medical errors (Hughes, 2008).

Patient Safety and Quality Improvement Act of 2005

Learning from health care errors is a foundational principle to mitigate and prevent future occurrences of errors. A key way of learning from errors is for practitioners and organizations to share information with others. Unfortunately, providers remain cautious about sharing information regarding errors and the lessons learned from those errors. This caution arises out of fear of litigation, potential professional sanctions, and potential damage to professional reputations (Catalano, 2008). Recognizing the importance of designing systems to mitigate errors, the Patient Safety and Quality Improvement Act of 2005 was signed into law on July 29, 2005. The primary purpose of the act was to amend Title IX of the Public Health Service Act, encouraging a culture of safety by facilitating the sharing of information through patient safety organizations (PSOs) that are administered through AHRQ. These PSOs create a secure environment within the organization titled a *Patient Safety Evaluation System*,

in which the organization can share, aggregate, and analyze information, thus improving patient care by identifying trends and patterns amenable to risk prevention and reduction, and program improvement. The Patient Safety and Quality Improvement Act of 2005 is divided into three distinct divisions. First, all PSOs must be certified and meet patient safety criteria in order to influence the learning from numerous patient safety events. Second, PSOs must maintain strict confidentiality of patient safety work products. *Patient Safety Work Product* is any information the organization collects and designates for the purpose of reporting to a PSO; information may include but not be limited to data, reports, written and verbal statements, and event investigation analysis. Patient safety work products are protected from any proceedings and legal actions against providers and health care facilities. Finally, PSOs report to the Secretary of Health and Human Services, who is then responsible to report to Congress all successful strategies that have reduced medical errors, thus increasing patient safety across the United States (AHRQ, 2010, Catalano, 2008).

The Patient Protection and Affordable Care Act of 2010 (ACA) incentivizes hospital participation in a PSO. The ACA required states to create health insurance exchanges by January 1, 2014. The goal of the exchanges is to expand coverage for uninsured individuals, reduce costs, and target prevention (Gable, 2011). Beginning on January 1, 2015, the ACA requires hospitals with 50 beds or more to participate in a PSO in order to contract with a qualified health insurance plan that is part of a health insurance marketplace. The health care organization must also establish a patient safety evaluation system and begin reporting safety events to the PSO to meet the full requirements of the ACA. The ultimate goal of requiring participation in a PSO is to improve the safety, affordability, and quality of patient care by allowing health care providers to learn from aggregated information on medical errors.

PATIENT SAFETY CULTURE

Many industries have demonstrated success in reducing and preventing errors, not by changing processes but by changing the culture to maintain vigilance for detection of potential errors, analysis of actual errors when they occur, and addressing those errors. In organizations with a high focus on patient safety culture, the administrative team demonstrates an unyielding commitment to a safety culture by ensuring that appropriate organizational resources are dedicated to patient safety, including training, human resource policies, budget, and personnel (Fagan, 2012; Feng, Bobay, & Weiss, 2008; IOM, 2000). The nurses in these organizations demonstrate a sense of personal responsibility and shared ownership for promoting a work environment supportive of patient safety (Armstrong, Laschinger, & Wong, 2009; Hughes, Chang, & Mark, 2009). Applying principles from industry partners such as aviation and nuclear power, health care has identified many key concepts fundamental to ensuring a culture of patient safety. Concepts central to the role of the professional nurse that will be explored in this chapter include establishing a just culture, building and sustaining a healthy work environment, and facilitating teamwork among colleagues (Leonard, Graham, & Taggart, 2004).

Just Culture

Human factors science, simply stated, is the science of determining how human beings interact with the environment (e.g., devices, policies and procedures, work space). Human factors research has assisted health care practitioners to shift focus when medical errors occur, from the individual person to the system or processes that led to the error. Despite several years working on human factors in health care, health care organizations continue to lack progress toward an error-free care delivery system. Many argue that this is a result of the fact that most organizations have not devoted adequate resources and attention to analyzing organizational and system processes but have continued to focus on the individual (Henriksen, Dayton, Keyes, Carayon, & Hughes, 2008; Kaissi, 2006; Marx, 2009). Focusing on the individual creates a culture of blame in which practitioners become more reluctant to report errors and failures of the system. To overcome the culture of blame and to increase organizational learning from health care errors, *just culture* philosophies are increasing across health care. Just culture philosophy encourages open and active reporting of errors and learning from mistakes, while holding practitioners and organizations accountable as indicated (Gorzeman, 2008; IOM, 2000).

There are two primary types of failures or errors within the health care literature. First is an *active failure,* which is an unsafe act committed by a clinician who is in direct contact with the patient—"the sharp end." The second type is a *latent failure,* which is a system problem that is not within the direct control of the clinician—for instance, poor system design, organizational structure, and policies and procedures, often referred to as the "blunt end" (Henriksen et al., 2008). Latent failures lead to organizational accidents or medical errors more often than do active failures. Latent failures in health care may include poor design, communication, planning and training, policies and procedures, and situational awareness (van Beuzekom, Boer, Akerboom, & Hudson, 2012)

The fundamental challenge for health care organizations, and nurses in particular, is to move prevention of medical errors from a system focusing on active failures or the individual to a system approach focusing on latent failures or the organization. Organizations such as commercial air travel and nuclear power have achieved inspiring safety records and are therefore referred to as *high reliability organizations* (HROs). An HRO is an organization that recommends systems to produce consistent results and to quickly detect deviations and/or potential errors within the system before the error reaches the patient (Hughes, 2008). A defining factor for an HRO is mindfulness, keeping all practitioners acutely aware of all processes that could potentially go wrong and ways to quickly identify and recover from errors when they occur.

There are five mindful processes that comprise the core of an HRO. As a key member of the health care team, the professional nurse has a key role in all five processes. First, the nurse must have a constant preoccupation with failure. Nurses must confidently share their inner voice of concern with the rest of the health care team. Often, prior to a patient becoming extremely unstable, a nurse has reported "a feeling" that something is not right with the patient. Unfortunately, many nurses do not confidently act on these concerns (Henriksen et al., 2008; Weick & Sutcliffe, 2001). Second, nurses must be reluctant to simplify interpretations and not accept conventional explanations that are obvious. The professional nurse who has strong collaborative relationships is in a position to facilitate the health care team's performance of thorough investigations when errors occur. Third, nurses must maintain situational awareness during all clinical exchanges. *Situational awareness,* a term commonly used in the airline industry, means that the entire team demonstrates an understanding of all team members' roles and responsibilities and of the progress the team is making toward the ultimate outcome. Nurses have a full understanding of the complex roles outside of their own role; therefore they serve as "clinical glue," helping the team maintain situational awareness. Fourth, nurses must be committed to resilience. *Resilience* is the ability to quickly recover when an error does occur, thus mitigating any adverse consequences of the error. Nurses continuously demonstrate their commitment to resilience in numerous ways—for example, maintaining supplies and equipment in key locations and maintaining continual competency in using such devices for the safety of their patients. Fifth, nurses in HROs show deference to expertise, allowing decisions to be made by those clinicians with the expertise, resources, and ability to assist the patient. High reliability organizations that demonstrate deference to expertise have less rigid hierarchical structure and team members are treated with mutual respect. Typically, nurses can cite several examples of how misplaced deference is granted to physicians; on the other hand, it is not uncommon for nurses to automatically assume that those with "less experience" are unable to make decisions for patients (Cohen, 2013; Henriksen et al., 2008; Weick & Sutcliffe, 2001).

High reliability organizations place emphasis on strategies to develop a just culture in which practitioners are encouraged to report errors and concerns free from blame, humiliation, and retaliation. Recently, critics have raised the concern that a blame-free culture is risky and could lead to unsafe clinical practice. However, the purpose of a just culture is to balance the need to learn from mistakes with the need to hold practitioners accountable (Marx, 2001). In a just culture, nurses are protected from disciplinary action both within the facility and within regulatory agencies when reporting injuries, errors, and near misses in which they are personally involved (Gorzeman, 2008). Such protection should not be granted in three important exceptions. These exceptions are criminal behavior (e.g., a nurse who treats a patient while under the influence of drugs or alcohol), active malfeasance (e.g., a nurse who actively or purposely violates safety protocols), and an injury or incident that has not been reported in a timely manner (IOM, 2004a).

Healthy Work Environment

Fundamental to any patient safety culture is the work environment in which the nurse practices. Nursing literature supports the fact that unhealthy work environments lead to decreased quality outcomes of patient care and decreased nursing satisfaction, which can result in challenges to recruitment and retention of staff nurses (Aiken, Clarke, Sloane, Lake, & Cheney, 2008; Browne, 2009). Ironically, although patients come to health care facilities seeking an environment in which to heal, that very environment can often be toxic to the extent that patient safety is in jeopardy. Recognizing these concerns, after the release of the IOM's *To Err Is Human* report, the American Association of Critical-Care Nurses (AACN) began landmark work exploring the work environment of nursing staff. As a result of the exploration, the AACN Healthy Work Environment Standards were introduced (AACN, 2005; Browne, 2009).

The AACN Healthy Work Environment Standards are divided into six areas (Table 20-2): skilled communication, true collaboration, effective decision making, appropriate staffing, meaningful recognition, and authentic leadership. The standards provide a framework for nurses to establish and sustain a healthy work environment. They are not all-inclusive and other factors such as regulatory requirements, unique clinical needs, and patient outcomes must be considered. The standards are interdependent; for example, in order for the environment to provide meaningful recognition, nurses must possess both skilled communication and authentic leadership (Good, 2009).

KEY PROCESSES

Once a healthy work environment and culture are established, nurses must engage key processes that are fundamental to patient safety. Depending on the maturity of the clinical practice environment, processes can range from basic to advanced concepts. For example, an immature environment/culture may need to focus first on basic teamwork and basic communication processes, whereas a mature environment

TABLE 20-2 AACN Standards for Establishing and Sustaining Healthy Work Environments

Skilled communication	Nurses must be as proficient in communication skills as they are in clinical skills.
True collaboration	Nurses must be relentless in pursuing and fostering collaboration.
Effective decision making	Nurses must be valued and committed parties in making policy, directing and evaluating clinical care, and leading organizational operations.
Appropriate staffing	Staffing must ensure an effective match between patient needs and nurse competencies.
Meaningful recognition	Nurses must be recognized and must recognize others for the value each brings to the work of the organization.
Authentic leadership	Nurse leaders must fully embrace the imperative of a healthy work environment, authentically live it, and engage others in the achievement.

From American Association of Critical-Care Nurses. (2005). AACN standards for establishing and sustaining healthy work environments: A journey to excellence. Retrieved from http://www.aacn.org/wd/hwe/docs/hwestandards.pdf

may choose to focus on more advanced communication processes. An example of a more advanced concept is "Stop the Line," a communication process that has been adopted from the Toyota Production System into health care. In this process, all staff members are empowered to draw attention to any potential error. At Toyota, at the time a potential error is identified, any employee has the authority to stop the production line; in the case of health care, all staff members have the authority to stop the procedure until clarification is sought and corrective action is taken if applicable. "Stop the Line" means more than merely stopping a procedure. The goal of this process is to establish a culture in which it is every team member's responsibility to speak up in order to identify and mitigate errors effectively (Leonard et al., 2004; Liker & Meier, 2006; O'Grady, Parmentier, & Woltmann, 2012). Although this chapter only focuses on the processes of teamwork, communication, and clinical tools to support these processes, numerous processes exist and

continue to be developed to enhance patient safety (Gluck, 2012). Many of these tools can be found on the websites identified in Table 20-1, especially those of the AHRQ, CMS, and TJC.

Teamwork

The complexity and diversity of the health care team continue to transform at a rapid rate. Previously the health care team consisted of the physician and the nurse; now a health care team may consist of the physician, nurse, pharmacists, therapists, dietitian, social workers, care coordinators, and others. Often there is an automatic belief that when a group of individuals is referred to as a *team,* they will function as a team (i.e., communicating, collaborating) but this simply is not reality. The majority of traditional health care educational programs (nursing and medical alike) do not teach teamwork or collaboration in the basic curriculum or in postgraduate residencies and/or internships. Patient safety experts have demonstrated that patient safety increases when teamwork and collaboration skills are taught and empowered; when teamwork and collaboration are not present, medical errors will result (Leonard et al., 2004). Nursing leadership must take an active role in promoting a collaborative work environment in which the nurse feels comfortable participating as an equal partner on the health care team (Clark, 2009; Hughes, 2008; Leonard et al., 2004). When nurses accept this responsibility, the patient will benefit from the teamwork and collaboration.

One of the more successful models for teamwork training was developed by the AHRQ in partnership with the Department of Defense. Team Strategies and Tools to Enhance Performance and Patient Safety (TeamSTEPPS) is an evidence-based curriculum that integrates teamwork principles and skills in the entire health care team. TeamSTEPPS involves a three-phase approach to creating and sustaining a culture of safety. In Phase I the institution conducts a pretraining assessment to determine readiness for the training. During Phase 2 the institution trains members of the health care team to become the onsite trainers for the curriculum. Phase 3 consists of the implementation and sustainment of the teamwork training across the institution. Teamwork training should begin initially in high-risk departments such as obstetrics, intensive care, or the operating room, and then progress to other departments until the entire organization has been trained. The initial departments should become leaders and role models to other areas and serve as change agents, promoting and sustaining the teamwork model of care delivery. The TeamSTEPPS curriculum is a flexible system that allows customization of materials to the institution or departmental needs. The curriculum consists of presentations, pocket guides, video vignettes, workshop materials, and a variety of case studies, all available on DVD/CD-ROM.

Beyond TeamSTEPPS, other teamwork training programs exist, each offering advantages and disadvantages to individual programs. For any teamwork training program, the primary element of success is the full support of nursing leadership, physician leadership, administration, and other informal change agents within the facility. Without this network of support, teamwork training will not be successful (Clark, 2009; Leonard et al., 2004).

Communication

One of the primary trainable teamwork skills is communication, a foundational element to a healthy work environment and patient safety. Failures in communication continue to be the leading cause of preventable patient injuries and death according to TJC (2014). Common communication mistakes in health care include providing patient care with incomplete or missing information; poor patient handoffs among nurses, physicians, and other clinical staff; failing to share known information; and making assumptions regarding patient outcomes and safety (Leonard et al., 2004). Communication is as critical to patient safety as having trained, competent staff; unfortunately, many clinicians, including nurses, struggle with this skill. The reasons for the challenges nurses experience with communication are numerous; one problem is inadequate education for staff nurses on how to communicate with other health care professionals. Despite efforts to remove hierarchical communication patterns, power struggles and hierarchy continue to exist, while the ever-changing health care environment becomes increasingly complex.

On a basic level, *communication* can be defined as the exchange of information from one individual to another; this exchange can be verbal or nonverbal. Nurses and physicians are educated to communicate in very different styles. Physicians are taught and expected to communicate in brief, succinct, problem-oriented styles. On the other hand, nurses are taught to communicate in narrative styles, describing an event or condition rather than using a focused approach. This has led to frustrations and miscommunications among nurses and physicians, putting the patient at risk for receiving suboptimal care (Flicek, 2012; IOM, 2004b; Leonard et al., 2004; Nadzam, 2009; Scalise, 2006; Shojania, Fletcher, & Saint, 2006).

Enhancing communication among the health care team requires a systematic approach, beginning with establishing a culture that emphasizes open communication and proceeding with intentional training on communication strategies. As part of The Joint Commission's National Patient Safety Goals, health care organizations are required to establish consistent processes and strategies to improve the effectiveness of communication. Each organization can choose to meet minimum requirements or elect to maximize communication opportunities to provide optimal patient safety.

Because of the variability in practitioner training, cultural issues, hierarchical concerns, and the critical nature of health care, utilization of structured communication techniques becomes essential to enhance the consistency of communication. *Structured communication techniques* offer the benefit of the entire team having a shared model through which to communicate, thus helping to reduce incidents of miscommunication. Table 20-3 outlines proven structured communication techniques to enhance communication among the health care team. In each of these techniques the professional nurse plays an essential role in the dialogue as both a facilitator and participator (IOM, 2004b; Leonard et al., 2004; Meginniss, Damian, & Falvo, 2012; Nadzam, 2009; Simpson, James, & Knox, 2006). Communication is addressed in Chapter 8.

TABLE 20-3   **Structured Communication Strategies**

STRATEGY	KEY FEATURES	TECHNIQUES	USES
Briefings	Briefings are structured interactions in which the team shares the goals of the procedure or shift to ensure all members have the current information regarding the patient's care.	When utilizing a briefing, always be concise in message delivery, involve the entire team, use first names, and make eye contact facing the individual(s) communicating.	This tool can be used in a variety of circumstances, including procedural areas, ambulatory care to develop a plan for the day's activities, as situations change, and during handoffs. A "time-out" is one example of a briefing.
SBAR	SBAR represents a particular type of briefing by defining the specific information that is to be communicated during each patient interaction.	*Situation*—What is going on with the patient? *Background*—What is the clinical background? *Assessment*—What are the current patient assessment data? *Recommendation*—What should be done or what is needed?	This technique is especially helpful during nurse-to-physician interactions by assisting to bridge any potential communication style gaps. Other uses include handoffs of patient information during critical times (i.e., after a rapid response call or code), interdisciplinary communication, and handoffs post procedures.
Debriefing	Debriefings are constructive conversations held after an event or procedure in which the team can analyze activities to enhance organizational learning.	During the debriefing, utilize the following questions to guide the discussion: What went well? What should be done differently next time? Were there any system issues that impeded the success of the event, such as equipment, incomplete data, policies, and/or procedures? What did the team learn from the event? Who will accept the responsibility for following up on any system problems or other issues that need follow-up?	Debriefing conversations should be positive in nature, while maintaining specific focus to ensure that lessons learned can be identified.

Data from Institute of Medicine, 2004a; Leonard, Graham, & Taggard, 2004; Meginniss, Damian, & Falvo, (2012); Nadzam, 2009; and Simpson, James, & Knox, 2006.

SUMMARY

Patients enter the hospital or other health care organizations at a time of great vulnerability. These patients expect safe, high-quality care from the health care team, whether the ultimate goal is being healed or being provided a dignified end-of-life experience. As a key member of the health care team, the professional nurse has the most interaction with a patient during the course of treatment. The nurse's ability to assess, identify problems, and plan, implement, and evaluate the care rendered to a patient has been shown to be directly linked to the outcomes the patient achieves. This places the professional nurse in a central role to keep patients safe.

In order for any health care worker to successfully keep patients safe, a culture of safety must exist in the organization. If an organization maintains a culture of safety, that organization is constantly examining existing and new processes to enhance patient safety through prevention, mitigation, and process improvement. The organization does this not because of regulatory requirements, but because of a desire to achieve the safest environment possible for patients. The professional nurse is the essential advocate for the patient, continually examining all processes for improvement, identifying potential and actual errors to mitigate potential harm to the patient, and maintaining a just culture that offers the opportunity to learn from *any* event.

SALIENT POINTS

- The Joint Commission (TJC) introduced National Patient Safety Goals (NPSGs) in 2002 to promote patient safety, addressing the complex health care environment by defining key safety requirements for all accredited organizations.
- The Agency for Healthcare Research and Quality (AHRQ) serves as the lead organization within the Department of Health and Human Services for research on quality of care and patient safety.
- Patient safety organizations (PSOs) were created by the "Patient Safety and Quality Improvement Act of 2005" to provide a secure environment to share information surrounding adverse events to facilitate a safer health care environment.

- Just culture philosophy and practice encourages open and active reporting of errors and learning from mistakes, while holding practitioners and organizations accountable.
- Healthy work environment standards are fundamental to a patient safety culture. Standards include skilled communication, true collaboration, effective decision making, appropriate staffing, meaningful recognition, and authentic leadership.
- Teamwork skills must be taught just as any other clinical skill.
- Common communication mistakes in health care include incomplete or missing information, poor patient handoffs among clinicians, and making assumptions regarding patients.

CRITICAL REFLECTION EXERCISES

1. Reflect on a recent adverse event or near miss in which you were involved and identify all active and latent failures that were involved in the case. Define strategies to mitigate failures in the future.
2. Identify an element of the Healthy Work Environment. Which standard is the most challenging for the unit to embrace? What interventions would

be recommended to facilitate adoption of the standard?
3. According to the literature, what are the key fundamental elements of a high function team? Define the key members of the health care team. Assess the greatest need(s) of the team to enhance its effectiveness. What interventions would be recommended to close the gap?

REFERENCES

Agency for Healthcare Research and Quality. (n.d.) TeamSTEPPS National Implementation. [Online]. Retrieved October 21, 2013, from http://www.pso.ahrq.gov/regulations/guidance.htm.

Agency for Healthcare Research and Quality. (2010). Department of health and human services guidance regarding patient safety organizations' reporting obligations and the patient safety and quality improvement act of 2005. Retrieved October 20, 2013, from http://www.pso.ahrq.gov/regulations/guidance.htm.

Aiken, L. H., Clarke, S. P., Sloane, D. M., Lake, E. T., & Cheney, T. (2008). Effects of hospital care environment on patient mortality and nurse outcomes. *Journal of Nursing Administration*, 38(5), 223–229.

American Association of Critical-Care Nurses. (2005). AACN standards for establishing and sustaining healthy work environments: A journey to excellence. *American Journal of Critical Care*, 14(3), 187–197

Armstrong, K., Laschinger, H., & Wong, C. (2009). Workplace empowerment and magnet hospital characteristics as predictors of patient safety climate. *Journal of Nursing Care Quality*, 24(1), 55–62.

Browne, J. A. (2009). Healthy workplaces and ethical environments: A staff nurse's perspective. *Critical Care Nursing Quarterly*, 32(3), 253–261.

Catalano, K. (2008). Proposed regulations for enforcement of the patient safety and quality improvement act of 2005. *Plastic Surgical Nursing*, 28(2), 96–98.

Clark, P. R. (2009). Teamwork: Building healthier workplaces and providing safer patient care. *Critical Care Nursing Quarterly*, 32(3), 221–231.

Cohen, N. L. (2013). Using the ABCs of situational awareness for patient safety. *Nursing*, 64–65.

Couig, M. P. (2005). Patient safety: A priority in the US Department of Health and Human Services. *Nursing Administration Quarterly, 29*(1), 88–96.

Fagan, M. J. (2012). Techniques to improve patient safety in hospitals: What nurse administrators need to know. *The Journal of Nursing Administration, 42*(9), 426–430.

Feng, X., Bobay, K., & Weiss, M. (2008). Patient safety culture in nursing: A dimensional concept analysis. *Journal of Advanced Nursing, 63*(3), 310–319.

Flicek, C. L. (2012). Communication: A dynamic between nurses and physicians. *Medsurg Nursing, 21*(6), 385–387.

Gable, L. (2011). The Patient Protection and Affordable Care Act, public health, and the elusive target of human rights. *Journal of Law, Medicine, and Ethics, 39*(3), 340–354.

Gluck, P. A. (2012). Patient Safety: Some progress and many challenges. *Obstetrics & Gynecology, 120*(5), 1149–1159.

Good, V. S. (2009). The critical care environment. In K. Carlson (Ed.), *Advanced critical care nursing.* St Louis: Saunders.

Gorzeman, J. (2008). Balancing just culture with regulatory standards. *Nursing Administration Quarterly, 32*(4), 308–311.

Henriksen, K., Dayton, E., Keyes, M. A., Carayon, P., & Hughes, R. (2008). Understanding adverse events: A human factors framework. In R. G. Hughes (Ed.), *Patient safety and quality: An evidence-based handbook for nurses* (Vol. 1). (AHRQ Publication NO. 08-0043). Rockville, MD: Agency for Healthcare Research and Quality.

Hughes, L. C., Chang, Y., & Mark, B. A. (2009). Quality and strength of patient safety climate on medical-surgical units. *Health Care Management Review, 34*(1), 19–28.

Hughes, R. G. (2008). Nurses at the 'Sharp End' of patient care. In R. G. Hughes (Ed.), *Patient safety and quality: An evidence-based handbook for nurses* (Vol. 1, pp. 1-7-1–35). (AHRQ Publication No. 08-0043). Rockville, MD: Agency for Healthcare Research and Quality.

Ilan, R., & Fowler, R. (2005). Brief history of patient safety culture and science. *Journal of Critical Care, 20*(1), 2–5.

Institute of Medicine. (2000). *To err is human: Building a safer health system.* Washington, DC: National Academy Press.

Institute of Medicine. (2004a). *Keeping patients safe: Transforming the work environment of nurses.* Washington, DC: National Academy Press.

Institute of Medicine. (2004b). *Patient safety: Achieving a new standard for care.* Washington, DC: National Academy Press.

The Joint Commission. (2006). Introduction to National Patient Safety Goals. [Online]. Retrieved December 8, 2009, from http://www.jointcommission.org/PatientSafety/NationalPatientSafetyGoals/npsg_intro.htm.

The Joint Commission. (2009a). A journey through the history of the Joint Commission. [online]. Retrived December 8, 2009, from http://www.jointcommission.org/AboutUs/joint_commission_history.htm.

The Joint Commission. (2009b). Facts about patient safety. [online]. Retrived December 8, 2009, from http://www.jointcommission.org/General Public/PatientSafety.

The Joint Commission on Accreditation of Healthcare Organizations. (2005). *Sentinel event statistics.* Oak Brook, IL: Author.

The Joint Commission on Accreditation of Healthcare Organizations. (2014). *Summary data of sentinel events reviewed by the joint commission.* Retrieved November 28, 2014, from http://www.jointcommission.org/assets/1/18/2004_to_2014_2Q_SE_Stats_-_Summary.pdf.

The Joint Commission Online. (2009). The Joint Commission updates its mission, creates vision statement. Retrieved December 8, 2009, from http://www.jointcommission.org/NR/rdonlyres/2F04C126-906D-4155-B16F-1F1A6570C387/0/jconlineAug1209.pdf.

Kaissi, A. (2006). An organizational approach to understanding patient safety and medical errors. *Health Care Manager, 25*(4), 292–305.

Leonard, M., Graham, S., & Taggart, B. (2004). The human factor: Effective teamwork and communication in patient strategy. In M. Leonard, et al. (Ed.), *Achieving safe and reliable healthcare: Strategies and solutions.* Chicago: Healthcare Administration Press.

Liker, J. K., & Meier, D. (2006). *The Toyota way fieldbook: A practical guide for implementing Toyota's 4Ps.* New York: McGraw-Hill.

Lin, L., & Liang, B. A. (2007). Addressing the nursing work environment to promote patient safety. *Nursing Forum, 42*(1), 20–30.

Marx, D. (2001). *Patient safety and the "Just Culture": A Primer for health care executives.* Funded by a grant from the National Heart, Lung, and Blood Institute, National Institutes of Health (Grant RO1 HL 53772, Harold S. Kaplan, M.D., Principle Investigator). New York: Trustees of Columbia University.

Marx, D. (2009). *Whack a mole: The price we pay for expecting perfection.* Plano, TX: By Your Side Studios.

Meginniss, A., Damian, F., & Falvo, F. (2012). Time out for patient safety. *Journal of Emergency Nursing, 38*(1), 51–53.

Nadzam, D. M. (2009). Nurses' role in communication and patient safety. *Journal of Nursing Care Quality, 24*(3), 184–188.

O'Grady, D., Parmentier, D., & Woltmann, J. (2012). The journey to zero. *The Journal of Continuing Education in Nursing, 43*(5), 199–200.

Scalise, D., & Clinical communication and patient safety (2006). *Hospitals & Health Networks, 80*(8), 49–54.

Shojania, K. G., Fletcher, K. E., & Saint, S. (2006). Graduate medical education and patient safety: A busy—and occasionally hazardous—intersection. *Annals of Internal Medicine, 145*(8), 592–598.

Simpson, K. R., James, D. C., & Knox, G. E. (2006). Nurse-physician communication during labor and birth: Implications for patient safety. *Journal of Obstetric, Gynecologic, & Neonatal Nursing, 35*(4), 547–556.

Taylor, S. L., Ridgley, M. S., Greenberg, M. D., Sorbero, M. E. S., Teleki, S. S., Damberg, C. L., & Farley, D. O. (2009). Experiences of agency for healthcare research and quality-funded projects that implemented practices for safer patient care. *Health Services Research, 44*(2), 665–683.

Tregunno, D., Jeffs, L., & McGillis Hall, L. (2009). On the ball: Leadership for patient safety and learning in critical care. *Journal of Nursing Administration, 39*(7/8), 334–339.

Van Beuzekom, M., Boer, F., Akerboom, S., & Hudson, P. (2012). Patient safety in the operating room: An intervention study on latent risk factors. *BMC Surgery, 12*(10), 1–11.

Wachter, R. M. (2010). Patient safety at ten: Unmistakable progress, troubling gaps. *Health Affairs, 29*(1), 165–173.

Weick, K., & Sutcliffe, K. (2001). *Managing the unexpected: Assuring high performance in an age of complexity.* San Francisco: Jossey-Bass.

INDEX

A

AACN. *see* American Association of Colleges of Nursing (AACN).
Abstract, definition of, 248
Abuse Assessment Screen (AAS), 326–327
Academic Search Complete, 243
Accessibility, of nursing programs, 32
Accountable Care Organizations (ACOs), 149–150
Accreditation, of nursing education programs, 31
Accreditation Commission for Education in Nursing (ACEN), 31
Acquired immunodeficiency syndrome (AIDS), 219
ACRL. *see* Association of College and Research Libraries (ACRL).
Active failure, 346
Active learning, 189
Active listening, 163–164
    focus of, 163–164
    selective attention and habituation in, 163–164
    silence and, 164
    therapeutic responses and, 164–165
Acute care nurse practitioner (ACNP) programs, 16
Acute care nurse specialist, 14–15, 15f
Adaptation, 75
Adaptation model, Roy's, 75
    assumptions about the individual, 75
    concepts of, 75
        adaptive level, 75
        adaptive modes, 75
        adaptive system, 75
    environment and, 75
    health and illness, 75
    nursing and, 75
    overview of, 75
    theoretical perspectives, comparison of, 82t
Adaptive level, determination of, 75
    contextual stimuli, 75
    focal stimulus, 75
    residual stimuli, 75
Adaptive model, 272
Adaptive modes, 75
    interdependence, 75
    physiological, 75
    role function, 75
    self-concept, 75
Adaptive system, control processes of, 75
    cognator subsystem, 75
    regulator subsystem, 75
Adjourning phase, of groups, 169
Adjudicatory power, 210
Administrative law, 208
    in nursing, 208–211
ADN. *see* Associate degree in nursing (ADN).
Adolescent
    smoking in, 278–279
    tobacco advertisements for, 101
Advanced practice nurses (APNs), 25, 56

Advanced practice nursing
    in clinical settings, 14–17
    critical elements in, 56f
Advanced practice registered nurses (APRNs), laws governing, 209
Advanced specialists, advanced practice nurses as, 56
Advocacy
    economic concepts for, 133–136
    nursing role in, 54
Advocate, nurse as, 54–55
Affective learning objective, 199
African American, HIV in, 261
African-American nurses, 11–12
Africans, respecting authority, 198
Age, health and, 312–313
Agency for Healthcare Research and Quality (AHRQ), 102, 344–345
Allan, Janet, 102
Allele, 295b
Allostasis, 284
Allostatic load, 284
America, diversification of, 262–263
American Association of Colleges of Nursing (AACN), 10–11, 183
    clinical nurse leader and, 16–17, 55
American Association of Critical Care Nurses (AACCN), 15, 103
    Healthy Work Environment Standards, 347, 348t
American Civil War, 7–8
American Dental Association, expert testimony by, 104
American Medical Association (AMA), 9
    expert testimony by, 104
American Nurses Association (ANA), 228, 234–235
    African-American nurse membership in, 12
    code of ethics for, 300
    expert testimony by, 104
    health policy and, 89
    nursing process and, 179
American Nurses Credentialing Center (ANCC), 103
American Public Health Association (APHA), expert testimony by, 104
American Red Cross
    disaster nursing through, 218–219
    volunteer nurses' aides program and, 11
American Telemedicine Association, 335–336
Americans with Disabilities Act (ADA), 211
America's Health Insurance Plans, 55
ANA. *see* American Nurses Association (ANA).
Analysis/nursing diagnoses, nursing process and, 180–181
Analyticity, 175
Anger
    management of, 280–281
    suppression of, 280
    wellness and, 280
APN. *see* Advanced practice nurses (APNs).
Applied ethics, 224–225
Apprenticeship, in professional nursing education, 42
Apprenticeship model of nursing, 4
Appropriation bill, 96
Arizona Telemedicine Program, 340
Army Nurse Corps, 8

Page numbers followed by "b", "f" and "t" indicate boxes, figures and tables respectively.